The Lupus Encyclopedia

A Johns Hopkins Press Health Book

Donald E. Thomas, Jr.,
MD, FACP, FACR

The Lupus

ENCYCLOPEDIA

*A Comprehensive
Guide for Patients
and Health Care
Providers*

SECOND EDITION

 JOHNS HOPKINS UNIVERSITY PRESS   BALTIMORE

Note to the Reader. This book is not meant to be a substitute for medical care of people with lupus, and treatment should not be based solely on its contents. Instead, treatment must be developed in a dialogue between the individual and their physician. This book has been written to help with that dialogue. The author, contributing chapter editors, and publisher are not responsible for any adverse consequences resulting from the use of information in this book.

Drug dosage. The author, contributing chapter editors, and publisher have made reasonable efforts to determine that selection and dosage of drugs discussed in this text conform to the practices of the general medical community. The medications described do not necessarily have specific approval by the US Food and Drug Administration for use in the diseases and dosages for which they are recommended. In view of ongoing research, changes in governmental regulations, and the constant flow of information relating to drug therapy and drug reactions, the reader is urged to check the package insert of each drug for any change in indications and dosage and for warnings and precautions. This is particularly important when the recommended agent is a new and/or infrequently used drug.

Disclaimers. The opinions and assertions expressed herein are those of the author and contributing chapter editors and do not necessarily reflect the official policy or position of the Uniformed Services University, the Department of Defense, the National Institutes of Health, or the United States Government. This research was supported in part by the Intramural Research Program of the National Institute of Arthritis and Musculoskeletal and Skin Diseases of the National Institutes of Health.

Dr. Donald E. Thomas, Jr., is on the Speaker's Bureaus for AstraZeneca (manufacturer of Saphnelo, chapter 34), Aurinia Pharmaceuticals (manufacturer of Lupkynis, chapter 34), GlaxoSmithKline (manufacturer of Benlysta, chapter 34), and Exagen, Inc. (AVISE and CB-CAPS lab testing).

© 2023 Johns Hopkins University Press
All rights reserved. Published 2023
Printed in the United States of America on acid-free paper
9 8 7 6 5 4 3 2 1

Johns Hopkins University Press
2715 North Charles Street
Baltimore, Maryland 21218
www.press.jhu.edu

Library of Congress Cataloging-in-Publication Data

Names: Thomas, Donald E., Jr., 1961– author.
Title: The lupus encyclopedia : a comprehensive guide for patients and health care providers /
    Donald E. Thomas, Jr., MD, FACP, FACR.
Description: Second edition. | Baltimore : Johns Hopkins University Press, 2023. |
    Series: A Johns Hopkins Press health book | Includes bibliographical references and index.
Identifiers: LCCN 2022046173 | ISBN 9781421446837 (hardcover) | ISBN 9781421446844 (paperback) |
    ISBN 9781421446851 (ebook)
Subjects: LCSH: Systemic lupus erythematosus—Encyclopedias.
Classification: LCC RC924.5.L85 T46 2023 | DDC 616.7/72—dc23/eng/20221114
LC record available at https://lccn.loc.gov/2022046173

A catalog record for this book is available from the British Library.

Figures 1.1, 10.1, 11.1, 12.1, 12.2, 13.1, 14.3, 15.1, 16.1, 17.1, 21.1, 24.1, 24.2, 26.1, 28.1, 28.2, 28.3, 30.1, 30.5, 33.1, 33.2, 33.3, 33.4, 37.1, 37.2, and 38.1 are by Jacqueline Schaffer.

Special discounts are available for bulk purchases of this book. For more information, please contact Special Sales at specialsales@jh.edu.

CONTENTS

Health Insurance for Lupus Patients: Affordable Health Care is online at lupusen
cyclopedia.com/health-insurance-for-lupus-patients-affordable-health-care.

Can You Work with Lupus? Lupus patients and the ADA are online at lupusencyclo
pedia.com/can-you-work-with-lupus-lupus-patients-and-the-ada.

Patient Resources are at lupusencyclopedia.com/patient-resources
    Here you will find information about and links to financial help for medications,
patient advocacy groups, lupus blogs and forums, lupus educational websites, and
other useful books about lupus and related topics.

References are at lupusencyclopedia.com/references.
    Here you will find all the medical journal articles, books, and research used to
compile *The Lupus Encyclopedia*.

Jemima Albayda, MD Assistant Professor, Division of Rheumatology, Johns Hopkins University School of Medicine; Director, Rheumatology Fellowship Program; Director, Musculoskeletal Ultrasound and Injection Clinic, Baltimore, Maryland: Chapter 7.

Divya Angra, MD Dermatology Chief Resident at Howard University Hospital in Washington, DC: Chapter 8.

Alan N. Baer, MD Professor of Medicine, Johns Hopkins University School of Medicine; Director, Jerome L. Greene Sjögren's Center, Baltimore, Maryland: Chapter 14.

Sasha Bernatsky, MD, PhD James McGill Professor and Senior Scientist, Centre for Health Outcomes Research and Division of Clinical Epidemiology at the Research Institute, McGill University Health Centre, Montreal, Quebec, Canada; member of the Systemic Lupus International Collaborating Clinics: Chapter 23.

George Bertsias, MD, PhD Associate Professor in Rheumatology-Clinical Immunology, Rheumatology Clinic, University Hospital of Heraklion, University of Crete Medical School: Chapter 32.

Ian N. Bruce, MD, FRCP Professor Rheumatology, Arthritis Research UK Centre for Epidemiology, The Kellgren Centre for Rheumatology, University of Manchester; National Institute for Health Research Senior Investigator at the Centre for Epidemiology Versus Arthritis, Centre for Musculoskeletal Research, Division of Musculoskeletal and Dermatological Sciences, Manchester, UK; and past Chair of the Systemic Lupus International Collaborating Clinics: Chapter 1.

Jill P. Buyon, MD Sir Deryck and Lady Va Maughan Professor of Medicine, New York University Grossman School of Medicine, Director of Rheumatology, Director of the NYU Lupus Center, New York; Director of The US National Research Registry for Neonatal Lupus: Chapter 41.

Yashaar Chaichian, MD Clinical Assistant Professor, Director, Stanford Lupus Clinic, Division of Immunology & Rheumatology, Department of Medicine, Stanford University School of Medicine, Stanford, California: Chapter 30.

Maria Chou, MD Arthritis and Pain Associates of Prince George's County, Greenbelt, Maryland: Chapter 6.

Sharon Christie, Esq Social Security Disability Lawyer, Disability Associates, Towson, Maryland: Chapter on Working and Dealing with Disability (online).

Angelique N. Collamer, MD, FACP, Col, USAF, MC Clinical Professor of Medicine, Uniformed Services University; Chief Medical Officer, RAF Lakenheath, United Kingdom: Chapter 36.

Ashté Collins, MD, FASN Associate Professor of Medicine, Division of Kidney Diseases and Hypertension, Department of Medicine, George Washington School of Medicine and Health Sciences, Washington, DC: Chapter 4.

Caitlin O. Cruz, MD, FACP Assistant Professor of Medicine, Uniformed Services University, Bethesda, Maryland; Naval Medical Center Portsmouth, Department of Rheumatology; Portsmouth, Virginia: Chapter 17.

Mark M. Cruz, MD, FACP Assistant Professor of Medicine, Uniformed Services University, Bethesda, Maryland; Naval Medical Center Portsmouth, Department of Endocrinology, Portsmouth, Virginia: Chapter 26.

Dana DiRenzo, MD, MHS Instructor of Medicine, Johns Hopkins University School of Medicine; Johns Hopkins Jerome L. Greene Sjögren's Center, Johns Hopkins Arthritis Center, Johns Hopkins Division of Rheumatology, Baltimore, Maryland: Chapter 39.

Jess D. Edison, MD Associate Professor of Medicine, Department of Medicine, Uniformed Services University of the Health Sciences; Division Director, Rheumatology, Bethesda, Maryland: Chapter 31.

Titilola Falasinnu, PhD Assistant Professor, Stanford School of Medicine, Stanford, California: Chapter 19.

Andrea Fava, MD Assistant Professor of Medicine, Lupus Center, Division of Rheumatology, Johns Hopkins University School of Medicine, Baltimore, Maryland: Chapter 33.

Cheri Frey, MD Assistant Professor, Program Director, Department of Dermatology, Howard University College of Medicine, Washington, DC: Chapter 8.

Neda F. Gould, PhD Associate Professor, Department of Psychiatry and Behavioral Sciences; Director, Mindfulness Program, Johns Hopkins University School of Medicine, Baltimore, Maryland: Chapter 39

Nishant Gupta, MD, MS Director, Interstitial and Rare Lung Disease Program, Division of Pulmonary, Critical Care and Sleep Medicine, University of Cincinnati, Cincinnati, Ohio: Chapter 10.

Sarthak Gupta, MD Associate Research Physician, Lupus Clinical Trials Unit, National Institute of Arthritis and Musculoskeletal and Skin Diseases, National Institutes of Health, Bethesda, Maryland: Chapters 40 and 43.

Sarfaraz Hasni, MD, MSc Director Lupus Clinical Research, National Institute of Arthritis and Musculoskeletal and Skin Diseases, National Institutes of Health, Bethesda, MD: Chapter 37.

David Hunt, MB, BChir, PhD Wellcome Trust Senior Clinical Fellow, Neuroinflammation Group Leader, United Kingdom Dementia Research Institute at University of Edinburgh, Edinburgh, UK; Head of Neuroinflammatory Medicine, NHS Lothian, UK: Chapter 13.

Mariana J. Kaplan, MD Chief, Systemic Autoimmunity Branch; Acting Director, Lupus Clinical Trials Unit, National Institute of Arthritis and Musculoskeletal and Skin Diseases, National Institutes of Health, Bethesda, Maryland: Chapter 21.

Alfred Kim, MD, PhD Associate Professor of Medicine, Founder and Co-Director, Washington University Lupus Clinic, Washington University School of Medicine, St. Louis, Missouri: Chapter 5.

Deborah Lyu Kim, DO, FACR Arthritis and Pain Associates of Prince George's County, Clinton, Maryland: Chapter 42.

Rukmini Konatalapalli, MD Arthritis and Pain Associates of Prince George's County, Greenbelt, Maryland: Chapter 27.

Fotios Koumpouras, MD Associate Professor of Medicine, Rheumatology Training Program Director, Director Yale Lupus Program, Yale School of Medicine, New Haven, Connecticut: Chapter 12.

Vasileios C. Kyttaris, MD Assistant Professor of Medicine, Harvard Medical School, Director, Rheumatology Training Program, Beth Israel Deaconess Medical Center, Boston, Massachusetts: Chapter 38.

Jerik Leung, MPH Department of Behavioral, Social, and Health Education Sciences, Rollins School of Public Health, Emory University, Atlanta, Georgia: Chapter 5.

Hector A. Medina, MD Assistant Professor of Medicine, Uniformed Services University of the Health Sciences, Bethesda, Maryland; Chief, Rheumatology, Landstuhl Regional Medical Center, Landstuhl, Germany: Chapter 25.

Timothy Niewold, MD Vice Chair of Medicine for Research; Director, Barbara Volcker Center for Women and Rheumatic Diseases, Hospital for Special Surgery, New York, New York: Chapter 34.

Julie Nusbaum, MD Assistant Professor of Medicine, New York University (NYU) Long Island School of Medicine, Department of Medicine, Division of Rheumatology, Mineola, New York: Chapter 18.

Ginette A. Okoye, MD, FAAD Professor & Chair, Department of Dermatology, Howard University College of Medicine, Washington, DC: Chapter 8.

Sarah L. Patterson, MD Assistant Professor, UCSF Department of Medicine, Division of Rheumatology; Affiliated Faculty, UCSF Osher Center for Integrative Medicine: Chapter 38.

Ziv Paz, MD Chief, Department of Rheumatology, Chief Innovation Officer, Galilee Medical Center, Galilee, Israel: Chapter 30.

Darryn Potosky, MD, AGAF Clinical Assistant Professor of Medicine, University of Maryland School of Medicine, Baltimore, Maryland; Capital Digestive Care, Columbia, Maryland: Chapter 15.

Rachel C. Robbins, MD, FACP, MAJ, USA, MC Assistant Professor of Medicine, Uniformed Services University; Program Director, Rheumatology Fellowship, Walter Reed National Military Medical Center, Bethesda, Maryland: Chapter 11.

Neha S. Shah, MD Assistant Professor of Medicine—Immunology & Rheumatology, Program Director, Adult Rheumatology Fellowship, Stanford University School of Medicine, Stanford, California: Chapter 39.

Matthew A. Sherman, MD Division of Rheumatology, Children's National Hospital, Washington, DC: Chapter 20.

Yevgeniy Sheyn, MD, MPH, FACR Arthritis and Pain Associates of Prince George's County, Greenbelt, Maryland: Chapter 24.

Julia F. Simard, ScD Associate Professor, Department of Epidemiology & Population Health, Division of Immunology and Rheumatology Stanford School of Medicine, Stanford, California: Chapter 19.

Jonathan Solomon, MD Adjunct-Assistant Professor, Cornea, Cataract, and Refractive Surgery, Department of Ophthalmology and Visual Sciences, University of Maryland School of Medicine; Director of Research, Bowie Vision Institute, Bowie Health

Campus, Bowie, Maryland; Refractive/Cataract Director, Solomon Eye Physicians & Surgeons, Greenbelt, Maryland: Chapter 16.

Rodger Stitt, MD Lebanon VA Medical Center, Lebanon, Pennsylvania: Chapter 28.

George Stojan, MD Assistant Professor of Medicine, Johns Hopkins University School of Medicine, Baltimore, Maryland (all contributions were completed while employed at Johns Hopkins and is currently employed at UCB S.A. Belgium as Global SLE Medical Affairs Director): Chapter 29.

Sangeeta Sule, MD, PhD Chief, Division of Rheumatology, Children's National Hospital, Washington, DC: Chapter 20.

Barbara Taylor, CPPM, CRHC Office Administrator, Arthritis and Pain Associates of Prince George's County, Greenbelt, Maryland: Chapter on Health Insurance (online)

George C. Tsokos, MD Professor of Medicine, Harvard Medical School; Chief, Division of Rheumatology and Clinical Immunology, Beth Israel Deaconess Medical Center, Boston, Massachusetts: Chapters 3 and 22.

Ian Ward, MD, FACP, FACR Assistant Professor of Medicine, Department of Medicine, Uniformed Service University, Bethesda, MD; Chief, Rheumatology Service, Department of Medicine, Dwight D Eisenhower Army Medical Center: Chapter 35.

Emma Weeding, MD Rheumatology Fellow, Division of Rheumatology, Johns Hopkins University School of Medicine, Baltimore, Maryland: Chapter 9.

Arthur Weinstein, MD, FACP, FRCP, MACR Clinical Professor of Medicine (Rheumatology), Loma Linda University, Clinical Professor Emeritus of Medicine (Rheumatology), Georgetown University: Chapter 2.

Sean A. Whelton, MD, FACP, FACR Associate Professor of Medicine, Division of Rheumatology, Allergy, and Immunology; Internal Medicine Residency Program Director and Vice-Chair for Medical Education in the Department of Medicine, Internal Medicine Residency Program, Georgetown University, Medstar Georgetown University Medical Center, Washington, DC: Chapter 4.

* Color version available at lupusencyclopedia.com/book-photos.

I am honored to have been asked to write the foreword for the tour de force that is the second edition of Dr. Thomas's encyclopedia on lupus, one of the most challenging diseases. I have been humbled by the disease itself for many years. Lupus is enigmatic: it is difficult to understand where it comes from and where it might strike next. I have learned many things over my years of diagnosing and taking care of people with lupus and performing clinical research on this complex disease. The first is always to keep an open mind. While many of the myriad systemic manifestations of lupus are diagnoses of exclusion, meaning that many other entities have to be ruled out, I have learned never to say reflexively that a certain symptom or manifestation just could not be caused by lupus. The list of common and uncommon clinical and laboratory manifestations of lupus and related conditions is ever-expanding. The human immune system and the development of autoimmunity are incredibly complicated. With ongoing intense research into the immune system and the exposures and events related to the development of lupus, increasing complexity in these biologic systems and pathways is being unearthed. The immunologic system of checks and balances is intricate. Its dissection has led to new targeted biologic medications for lupus even within the last year. I hope that there will be more soon.

Like Dr. Thomas and many of us in lupus-focused rheumatology, I clearly recall my first encounter with lupus. As a second-year medical student, I had never heard of lupus before being assigned to the complex case of a young woman with many strange systemic manifestations. Not only was her case an excellent teaching vehicle because all of the human bodily systems were involved, which my fellow students and I attempted to divide and conquer in our learning, but I found it both intellectually and existentially challenging. The young woman was about the same age that I was at that time. I was puzzled at the idea that the immune system could turn on itself and recognize its own proteins, leading to autoantibodies, immune complexes, and a panoply of organ system involvement such as the young woman in the case presented. To this day, my work is motivated by trying to figure out who is at risk for developing this autoimmune disease and identifying potentially modifiable factors and pathways that can turn off the autoimmunity before it causes irreversible organ and tissue damage.

Lupus presents a challenge for primary care physicians, other health care providers, people affected, and their loved ones to understand as well. This encyclopedia is incredibly accessible, and I have learned a huge amount from reading it. Dr. Thomas has done a tremendous job of cataloging and explaining this complicated disease. He first discusses the most recent science about how we think it develops and then tackles lupus-related laboratory results, which are evolving, but also confusing. His explanations and key points to remember make these often- impenetrable lab tests much more understandable. He then explains the breadth of the disease in a system-by-system approach, starting with the constitutional symptoms that are often the most vague and difficult to quantify and treat. He takes on each organ system, which is how we approach treatment of this heterogeneous disease, with a comprehensive discussion of the state-of-the-art treatment and monitoring.

The presentation and clinical course of lupus are extremely varied. Some patients present with an explosion of symptoms of systemic inflammation involving multiple organ systems and a "full house" of autoantibodies. Others have nonspecific symptoms mimicking other conditions, such as other autoimmune diseases, infections, cancer, or fibromyalgia, for years prior to receiving the correct diagnosis. We know that these delays in lupus diagnoses contribute to poor outcomes. Despite the enormous heterogeneity of lupus at the onset and across its clinical course, there are important patterns that have been recognized over the years and that help guide treatment choices and prognostic decisions. Dr. Thomas does an excellent job of describing these patterns, including, for example, how a patient with new-onset lupus nephritis may present compared with someone with skin rashes of discoid lupus, a patient with the manifestations of antiphospholipid antibody syndrome, or someone who suffers primarily from arthritis and body pain. Earlier recognition of these patterns of abnormal laboratories, symptoms, and organ involvement will contribute to earlier diagnosis and more appropriate management, screening, and therapy. This, in turn, can only improve outcomes for people with lupus. Dr. Thomas's contribution to improving these outcomes is enormous.

It is also proven that people with lupus have better outcomes when managed by multidisciplinary teams with excellent communication between team members and between patients and health care providers. Understanding the disease and how the medications prescribed for it may affect the immune system, as well as their possible side effects, including the risk of cancer and infections, are essential for all medical specialists and for informed patients who want to take an active part in decisions about their care. Dr. Thomas's encyclopedia will advance the care of patients across the spectrum of lupus in all these ways.

KAREN COSTENBADER, MD, MPH
Chair, Medical-Scientific Advisory Council, Lupus Foundation of America
Professor, Rheumatology, Harvard University Medical School
Director, Brigham and Women's Hospital

How to Use This Book

While many people want to know only the basics and straightforward treatment instructions regarding an illness, others want to know all the medical facts, including the meaning of any abnormal lab results. I wrote this book with both groups in mind. Most of the information is presented in an easy-to-understand format using nonmedical terms. Where any complex medical terms are required, they are accompanied by explanations. Lupus patients may wish to look up their doctors' medical terminology in the index and read about it in the referred text to better understand what is going on.

The book is divided into five parts:

Part I explains what lupus is, what causes it, what other immune disorders are associated with it, which laboratory tests diagnose the disease, and which ones are used to follow lupus disease activity.

Part II details how the immune system attacks different body parts in systemic lupus erythematosus (SLE) patients. It is divided into chapters based on organ systems.

Part III is devoted to other lupus complications that may occur for reasons other than immune system activity. Examples of such complications are osteoporosis and fibromyalgia.

Part IV discusses lupus treatments.

Part V covers other practical matters, such as talking to your doctor, how women may have a successful pregnancy, preparing for surgery, and traveling. The final chapter in this part of the book gives you my Lupus Secrets checklist.

In addition, chapters on insurance, disability, and patient resources as well as the book's references can be found in the online version of *The Lupus Encyclopedia* at:

lupusencyclopedia.com/health-insurance-for-lupus-patients-affordable-health
-care

lupusencyclopedia.com/can-you-work-with-lupus-lupus-patients-and-the-ada

lupusencyclopedia.com/patient-resources

lupusencyclopedia.com/references

If you have lupus, there are several things you can do to help manage your illness. I recommend that the reader perform the following steps in order. This will increase your chances of learning the most useful, important information first.

Step 1: Include the Lupus Secrets into your lifestyle. Copy the Lupus Secrets in chapter 44 and read over the checklist regularly. Work on practicing all these measures as a matter of routine. Once an activity on the list becomes a natural and constant part of your life, you can put a checkmark next to it. Your goal is to make all the activities regular habits. At first, do these things even if you do not understand their importance. As you read this book, their purposes will become clear. If you would like to have a reason or explanation more quickly, each recommendation in the checklist tells you which sections of the book discuss that particular Lupus Secret.

If I had to pick the three most important things to do first, they would be to make sure that you (1) take hydroxychloroquine (or chloroquine), (2) practice ultraviolet light protection perfectly, and (3) take vitamin D (if your level is lower than 40 ng/mL). Read about each of these (look them up in the index) to understand their importance. Also, get into the habit of never missing any doses of medications. This is one of the best habits you can get into right away. If your doctor has not prescribed an antimalarial (hydroxychloroquine or chloroquine) and vitamin D (if your level is low), ask them if it is possible to do so. This is the standard of medical care worldwide.

Step 2: Get a copy of your records, notes, lab tests, x-rays, and other results. Learn exactly how your doctors diagnosed your lupus and how you are doing. Keep these records yourself, just in case you need them for future reference or if you need to give them to other doctors. You may have to pay a fee to have them copied, but if you ask for a copy of the previous visit's note, lab results, and any other test results at each appointment, there is rarely a charge. Use the index of this book to look up every term, lab test, word, or diagnosis in your notes. It will direct you to the parts of the book that discuss subjects specific to your lupus. We have tried to be as complete as possible, so most problems from lupus are included. If anything in your records is not listed, discuss it with your doctor. Look at your lab results. Look up each abnormal result in the index. Chapter 4 is dedicated to laboratory tests. Make sure to read the section on collecting a urine specimen accurately. This is one of the most important tests we need, and doing it properly makes a big difference in accuracy. This exhaustive chapter is primarily a reference tool to help you understand what lab results may mean—and what they do *not* mean.

Step 3: Read the chapters listed below. These chapters give essential information that makes it easier to understand what lupus is and why it is important to do many things that your doctor recommends. They are listed in the order I consider most helpful and practical.

Chapter 43 takes some of the mystery out of effectively dealing with your doctor. Knowing how to navigate your doctor's office and communicating effectively with your doctor and their staff can go a long way in your doing well.

Chapter 40 discusses important symptoms you may encounter and how to deal with them.

Chapters 21 and 22 are devoted to the most common causes of death in persons with SLE. Learn the measures you should take to decrease your risk of developing these problems and learn to live longer.

Chapter 23 is all about cancer. Some cancers are more common in SLE patients, and there are things you can do to prevent them.

Chapter 24 discusses osteoporosis, which occurs commonly with SLE and is a silent killer. It contains practical prevention advice and how to treat it if it occurs.

Chapters 26 and 31 should be read by people taking steroids. These chapters give detailed information about steroids and practical advice on preventing side effects.

Chapter 29 talks about general lupus treatment principles. It discusses how to evaluate the potential for drug side effects and gives information on taking and managing medications properly.

Chapter 30 covers the antimalarial drugs that all SLE patients should be taking (as long as they can). It also covers the important eye tests that should be done regularly.

Chapter 38 explains that treating lupus is not just about taking pills. It also includes lifestyle changes such as protecting yourself from ultraviolet light, eating a diet that lowers inflammation, exercising, getting enough sleep, and learning to reduce stress.

Chapter 39 reports on new research that points toward practices such as mindfulness, breathing exercises, yoga, tai chi, and ingesting substances such as ginger and turmeric (curcumin) as possibly helping inflammatory disorders such as lupus. Learn what the science shows and how you can include these in your life. I also discuss medical marijuana and CBD.

Chapter 14 is for those with dry mouth, dry eyes, or dry skin, or those who have problems with vaginal dryness. Many people with lupus also have Sjögren's disease, which is covered in this chapter.

Chapter 20 is for you if you are a child or teenager with lupus or if you are the guardian of someone with pediatric SLE. It is new to this edition of the book.

Chapter 1 explains what lupus is and how doctors diagnose it. Having this information will make it easier for you to communicate with health professionals about exactly what type of lupus you have and what problems it causes you.

Chapter 3 discusses the causes of lupus. Some of these causes are controllable. In other words, you can actually make changes in your life to decrease the severity of lupus by knowing what things cause it or make it worse. I also discuss what your family members and children can do to lower their risk of developing SLE.

Chapter 4 should not be read from start to finish. Instead, read the first part of the chapter through the section on collecting a urine sample. Then refer to specific sections (using the index) regarding any abnormal lab test results you may get so that you can understand them.

Chapter 19 lists the factors that can cause some people with lupus to have more severe disease. While many of these things are uncontrollable (such as age and gender), many are within your control.

Step 4: Read in detail other chapters pertaining to your situation; skim other chapters that sound interesting. This book contains a lot of information about lupus and related health care concerns. Whenever a new problem occurs with your lupus or a new test becomes abnormal, use the index to learn more.

Step 5: Consult the Patient Resources at www.lupusencyclopedia.com/patient-resources/. Many resources are available to help people with SLE. These include patient support groups, financial assistance, and other books on lupus.

Step 6: Check my blog at www.lupusencyclopedia.com and follow me on Twitter @lu puscyclopedia to find out the latest lupus news. Medical knowledge and lupus treatments are constantly changing. A third edition with these additions hopefully will be published in the future. Until then, I will keep you updated on the website.

Step 7: If you have any comments or recommendations, please email me at lupusen cyclopedia@gmail.com and let me know what you would like to see in a future book edition. This book is for you, the reader. When I revise it in the future, I want it to be even better and ensure I do not omit anything important. If I have missed any topics or made any comments that you do not understand or do not think are correct or appropriate, I would like to know. I take all comments and recommendations seriously.

New to This Edition

I received many helpful suggestions from readers of the first edition. I have included as many as possible in this new edition.

It contains practical information for health care providers (non-lupologist doctors, physician assistants, nurse practitioners, and nurses) that will help them improve care for lupus patients.

Worldwide experts have contributed their specialized knowledge to this edition of *The Lupus Encyclopedia*. They scrutinized each chapter that I wrote to ensure the highest accuracy and that the latest medical information was included. This is a method usually reserved for the highest-quality medical textbooks. Lupus is such a complex disorder, however, that a patient education book (and non-lupologist health care provider management book) deserves the same approach. If you know these doctors or are a patient of one of them, please give them a sincere "thank you!" for donating their valuable time and expertise to this endeavor.

New topics and updates include:

- Rare SLE complications
- New SLE classification criteria (chapter 1)
- "Leaky gut" (the microbiome) and lupus (chapters 3 and 38)
- Updated pregnancy and breastfeeding guidelines (chapters 18 and 41)
- A prognosis chapter that addresses health care disparities (chapter 19)

- A pediatric lupus chapter (chapter 20)
- Some drugs should be stopped at specific times for vaccines to work best. Learn how. (chapter 22)
- COVID-19 (chapter 22)
- New Recommendations for hydroxychloroquine dosing, other drug levels, and proper eye screening (chapter 30)
- New FDA-approved drugs: voclosporin and anifrolumab (Lupkynis and Saphnelo, chapter 34)
- Expanded discussion of non-drug treatments and complementary medicine (chapters 38 and 39)
- Anti-inflammatory diet (chapter 38)
- Medical marijuana, CBD, and lupus (chapter 38 and online)

For Health Care Providers

You may find it strange that this book states it is for both patients and health care providers. However, I was approached by doctors, physician assistants, and nurse practitioners who told me how much the first edition helped them care for their lupus patients better by providing practical, easy-to-find information. Therefore, I have expanded on this type of information in this new edition.

One place to start is to read the last chapter: "The Lupus Secrets." I give this list of "dos and don'ts" to all my lupus patients. After reading this, you will sense how complex it is to care for SLE patients. Please consider making copies of this list and giving it to your patients.

Lupus is an incredibly complicated disease with many nuances in lab test meanings, disease manifestations, and management. This book clarifies many of these. Note that the index is purposefully comprehensive. There, you can look up almost any lab test, disease manifestation (even rare complication), and medication. For example, if one of your patients has a high amylase and lipase level, looking up both "amylase" and "lipase" in the index will direct you to text that will inform you that it is not uncommon for SLE patients to have elevated levels without having pancreatitis. This sort of information can help prevent misdiagnoses and unnecessary tests.

The chapters on the disease's manifestations (chapters 5 through 18) include the most appropriate testing and which medications may be best. The medication sections are designed to be concise and practical. For example, they discuss what to do with each drug in terms of dosing, surgery, pregnancy, and breast-feeding. However, these sections do not replace sources for reviewing important drug interactions and more complex issues.

Chapters 38 and 39 include important information about dietary and dental habits (including microbiome effects) that may help reduce SLE inflammation. They also include many "wellness" measures.

Of course, as we all know, medical information is constantly expanding and improving. All medical texts will have incorrect information as new research makes information obsolete. For example, soon after the first edition was published, hydroxychloroquine dosing recommendations changed. Therefore, please always double-check information in this book with the latest research. Never hesitate to ask your doctor.

Please be brief in your email, and please do not relate personal patient information. I cannot give any medical advice about anyone's medical problems. Only a doctor who has done a thorough evaluation can do this. However, I can give general advice.

Thank you, and I wish you the best in life and health.

I thank each contributing chapter editor. I appreciate that you donated your valuable time and expertise. This is a form of teamwork that we usually see in high-quality medical textbooks. I hope you realize how many lives you will help beyond your own patients. You kept me honest by ensuring I included information using the best medical evidence and minimizing my biases and personal opinions. For any future edition of this book, I hope you strongly consider continuing to participate, helping improve the lives of lupus patients worldwide.

I am thankful for Joe Rusko, my editor at Johns Hopkins University Press. He has had great ideas and suggestions. He has been open to my special requests. I appreciate his patience. It took a lot longer to hand in the manuscript (way past the deadline in my contract). When I felt bad for taking so long, he immediately made me feel comfortable and never made me feel rushed. I believe that this has resulted in a much stronger book.

I am blessed to have my animal companions who kept me company and cheerful during the writing of this second edition:

- Timmy (our talkative Timneh African grey parrot who makes me melt every time he says, "Donny, I love you")

- Musette (our lapdog Bichon Frise who is built for comfort)

- Clairvaux (our guard dog Coton de Tulear who thinks she is keeping our home safe from the Amazon delivery people and mail delivery personnel)

- Siroe (our regal Savannah cat who constantly demands more food as if he were starving).

PART I

Definitions, Causes, and Diagnosis of Autoimmune Diseases

What Is Lupus and How Is It Diagnosed?

Ian N. Bruce, MD, FRCP, *Contributing Editor*

Lupus, the Latin word for "wolf," was first used to refer to a disease in 959 CE by the Catholic bishop of Leodicum (today known as Liège, Belgium). He allegedly wrote in an affidavit: "Ego Eraclius . . . morbo, qui Lupus dicitur, graviter attritus, & fere ad mortem deductus . . ." This is translated as "I, Eraclius . . . being gravely affected and nearly taken to death by the disease called Lupus . . ."

A later text (approximately twelfth century) called the "Miraculi beati Martini," or "The Miracles of Saint Martin," states: "The bishop of Leodicum, Hildricus by name . . . troubled with a disease that is popularly called lupus . . . so severely was the strength of the illness raging, consuming, nibbling away at, devouring the man's flesh . . . the deeply rooted disease, though sometimes feeding on the outside, nevertheless was consuming his internal matter" (translation from Latin). This account speaks to two understandings of lupus—as a disease that causes skin damage ("devouring the man's flesh") and as a disease that attacks the internal organs ("consuming his internal matter"). These problems are strikingly similar to the disease we call systemic lupus erythematosus (SLE).

This chapter describes lupus and how it is diagnosed. It is important to realize that lupus is not a cancer, such as breast cancer or leukemia. Nor is it a contagious disease, like chickenpox or the flu. A person with lupus cannot spread it to another person.

The Immune System

Lupus is an autoimmune disease. "Auto-" comes from the Greek word for "self," and "immune" refers to the body's immune system, which protects the body from illnesses. An autoimmune disease is one in which the immune system does the opposite: it attacks the body. A look at how the immune system normally works will help you to understand autoimmune diseases such as lupus.

The immune system is the part of the body that usually protects us from, for example, infections, chemicals (such as medicines), allergens (such as animal skin dander or pollen), and even cancer cells. The immune system is composed largely of white blood cells, or WBCs (such as leukocytes; see chapter 9).

Lymph nodes are an important part of the immune system. Lymph nodes are small, ball-shaped structures linked by lymph vessels that are located in the neck, armpits, groin, and other areas. Leukocytes can travel to and from the blood along these lymph vessels to the lymph nodes.

3

The lymph nodes are a meeting place for immune cells to communicate with each other when the body encounters infections, allergens (substances we are allergic to), or anything else that stimulates the immune system. You may have noticed that your lymph nodes can swell when you have an infection (commonly referred to as "swollen glands"). Suppose you have strep throat (due to a bacterial infection in the tonsils, throat, and back of the mouth). Strep throat may cause the lymph nodes in the front of your neck to become swollen and tender. This occurs because the lymph nodes fill up with WBCs attacking the bacteria in the throat. The skin, intestines, and spleen (an organ located in the left upper part of the abdomen, under the ribcage) are other important immune system components.

The primary job of WBCs is to act as bodyguards. WBCs recognize something that does not belong by its chemical structure. They use molecules called antibodies against these invaders. Antibodies recognize chemical structures, known as antigens, on the invader. There are millions of unique antigens for which the immune system must develop millions of unique antibodies in response.

When WBCs encounter invading foreign antigens, they alert other WBCs by releasing chemical messages (cytokines) that other WBCs recognize and respond to in a particular way. Think of cytokines as a way that WBCs talk to each other. As foreign substances (pollen, bacteria, viruses, cancer cells, poison, and so on) invade the body, cytokines signal other WBCs to enter the affected area and defend the body.

WBCs can attack invaders in several ways. One is for the WBCs to swallow the invaders, or, in technical terms, to use phagocytosis (*phago-* means "eat" and *-cytosis* refers to cells). Once they swallow the invaders, WBCs use chemicals and enzymes to digest them.

Mild infections occur daily as we encounter germs and other foreign substances that could cause us harm. During these frequent mild infections, the immune system gets rid of the bad germs without our realizing it. This continuous protection is a good example of the immune system working well.

The immune system is complex. To simplify how one part of the immune system works, figure 1.1 shows how the immune system responds to poison ivy. Poison ivy is a good example because most people can easily visualize the skin inflammation and damage it causes.

There are four common consequences of inflammation: discomfort, redness, warmth, and swelling. Pain occurs due to tissue damage; redness, warmth, and swelling occur due to increased blood flow into the area.

In people sensitive to poison ivy, the immune system considers the oils of the poison ivy plant to be an invading and dangerous substance. In trying to protect the body, the immune system causes inflammation, which is temporary and involves only parts of the skin. The following is what happens step by step:

1. Poison ivy contacts the skin and encounters WBCs called antigen-presenting cells (APCs). The immune system is a large army of protectors with different jobs. The job description of APCs is to be the initial identifiers of "invaders" (such as poison ivy, viruses, fungus, bacteria, and even cancer cells) and to tell other members of the immune system to attack these invaders. (This first step is similar to what occurs in the person with lupus after sunlight or other sources of ultraviolet light damages the person's skin

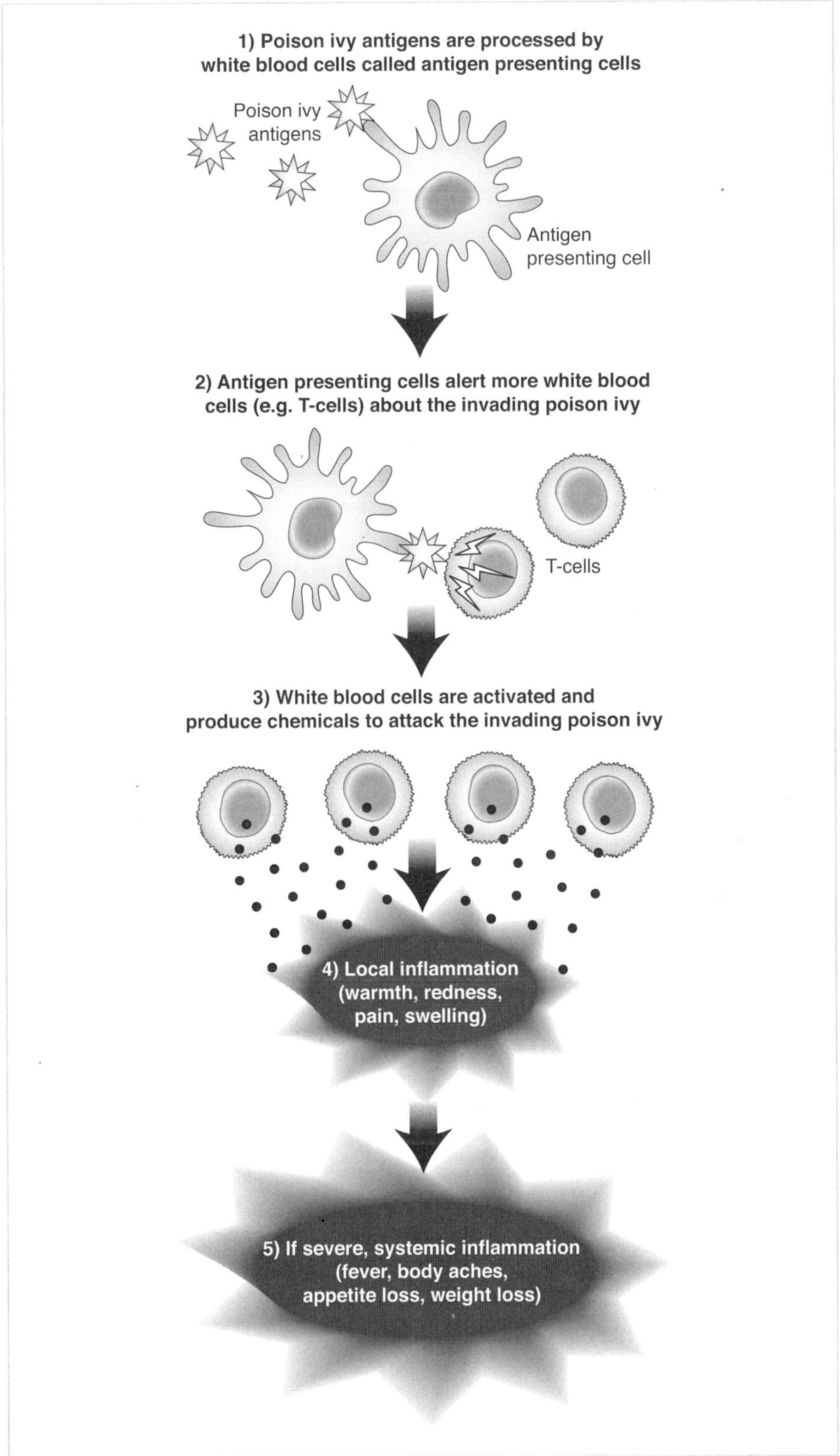

Figure 1.1 How the immune system causes inflammation

cells; see chapters 8 and 38). When poison ivy touches the skin, APCs identify the plant's oils as "bad."

2. APCs absorb parts of the invading poison ivy oil and break down the oil's chemical structures into tiny pieces called antigens. The APCs carry these foreign antigens through the lymph vessels to lymph nodes. They communicate with other WBCs called T lymphocytes (also called T cells) by showing these foreign antigens to them.

3. These T cells secrete cytokines to alert other WBCs to become more active.

4. The entire army of alerted members of the immune system travels to the area of skin exposed to poison ivy and attacks the invading substances. These WBCs release chemicals that cause the skin's blood vessels to swell. This allows more WBCs to come to the area and enter the affected skin. The swollen blood vessels and increased blood flow allow more WBCs to go to the site.

However, the swollen vessels also cause redness and warmth. Fluid can leak out of the blood vessels and cause swelling under the skin. Some of the fluid produces painful blisters. The WBCs release irritating chemicals in their attempts to protect us. The nerves and skin are affected, and the person suffers from red, warm, swollen, itchy skin with oozing blisters. Although the immune system is trying to protect us from poison ivy, the inflammation it causes makes us miserable.

After the poison ivy oil is removed from the skin by washing, the immune system reaction is not needed anymore. The WBCs realize that the foreign invader is gone, and the battle has been won. These WBCs then release other types of cytokines that tell invading WBCs to "calm down" and stop coming to the affected site. Instead of increasing inflammation the way that the initially released cytokines (inflammatory cytokines) did, these cytokines decrease inflammation (anti-inflammatory cytokines). The body can now go through the slow process of healing. If the injury is mild, the affected area recovers. If the injury is severe, permanent damage and scar tissue may be left.

5. If the poison ivy exposure is severe, intense inflammation caused by the immune system may affect the entire body, adding fever, body aches, loss of appetite, and weight loss to the picture. These complications of inflammation can also occur with systemic infections (such as those caused by viruses and bacteria), cancers, and diseases such as systemic lupus.

Immunodeficiency Disorders versus Autoimmune Disorders

Sometimes the immune system underperforms. For example, when the human immunodeficiency virus (HIV) infects someone, the virus destroys T cells. Without T cells, the person infected with HIV cannot properly fight off certain other infections and could die from AIDS (acquired immunodeficiency syndrome) if not treated. AIDS is an immunodeficiency disease. The immune system is deficient (or lacking) and stops protecting the person from foreign intruders and even cancer cells. Because of this, people with HIV get certain cancers more commonly than other people.

There are many different types and potential causes of immunodeficiency disorders. Chapter 3 will discuss how the genes and DNA we are born with can make it more likely for some people to have lupus. Some of these genes can cause the immune system to become abnormal, including causing immunodeficiency and autoimmunity. Because of this, many people with lupus (an autoimmune problem) are also at increased risk for developing infections due to an immunodeficiency problem (discussed in chapter 22).

Many normal chemical structures in the body can act as antigens and interact with the immune system's antibodies. During infancy, the immune system learns that the baby's own antigens are part of themselves and eventually comes to ignore these antigens and not attack them. We say the body "recognizes itself" and call this important immune system process "tolerance."

In people with autoimmune diseases, however, something goes wrong at some point. The immune system "forgets" that certain antigens in the body belong there; it loses tolerance for them. In a person who develops rheumatoid arthritis (another autoimmune disease), the immune system thinks that the joints' normal antigens are foreign invaders and begins to attack them. This ends up causing inflammation within the joints.

There are many different autoimmune diseases (chapter 2), and some attack a single (organ-specific) part of the body. Type 1 diabetes, sometimes called juvenile diabetes, is an example of an organ-specific autoimmune disease. In type 1 diabetes, the immune system does not recognize the pancreas cells that make insulin as being a normal part of the body. Therefore, the immune system attacks and destroys these cells. As a result, the pancreas cannot produce insulin, which is needed to keep glucose sugar levels normal. Thus, someone with type 1 diabetes must inject themselves with insulin every day for the rest of their life.

While some autoimmune diseases affect only one organ, others can affect multiple organs that make up a body system. An example of a body system is the musculoskeletal system, which includes bones, muscles, ligaments, tendons, and bursas. When an autoimmune disease affects multiple organs, it is called a systemic autoimmune disease. One of the most common systemic autoimmune diseases is rheumatoid arthritis, or RA (chapter 2). In addition to affecting the joints, the immune system in RA can attack the skin, causing lumps called rheumatoid nodules. It can also attack the lining of the lungs (pleurisy) or heart (pericarditis), causing fluid buildup and chest pain. Lung inflammation in RA can also result in scarring and shortness of breath. RA can even cause eye inflammation and lead to blindness if untreated.

Other common terms, used by some doctors, for "systemic autoimmune disease" include "connective tissue disease" and "collagen vascular disease." Some systemic autoimmune diseases are scleroderma (which causes thickening of the skin), Sjögren's disease (which causes dry mouth and dry eyes), polymyositis and dermatomyositis (which cause muscle weakness), and vasculitis (which causes blood vessel inflammation), as well as SLE. All systemic autoimmune disorders can cause joint pain (arthralgia) or joint inflammation (arthritis). That is why arthritis doctors (rheumatologists) became the experts in diagnosing and treating them.

Lupus

SLE is a classic example of a systemic autoimmune disease.

One of the features of SLE is that it stimulates the production of many different types of antibodies directed toward the body's own cells and tissues. B cells are a type of white blood cell of the immune system. They produce antibodies used in fighting off foreign invaders, such as bacteria and viruses. Normally, the body's immune system learns not to make antibodies against itself (tolerance, discussed earlier). However, in SLE, it begins to do just that. The immune system in SLE does not believe that some molecules (antigens) of the body's own cells belong there. It produces antibodies against these antigens. These antibodies that attack the person's body are called autoantibodies ("auto-" meaning self).

We can check for many of these autoantibodies by blood tests. The most common autoantibodies produced by SLE are directed toward molecules within the nucleus of cells. These are called antinuclear antibodies (ANAs). Almost all people with SLE are positive for antinuclear antibodies (chapter 4). If a doctor thinks that someone could have SLE, they order an ANA blood test.

SLE can produce many other types of autoantibodies. Some, such as anti-Smith and anti-ribosomal-P, are rarely seen in people who do not have lupus, while many others, such as anti-SSA, anti-RNP, and ANA, can be seen in any of the systemic autoimmune diseases. Chapter 4 discusses all these autoantibodies in detail.

SLE can potentially affect any organ system of the body. The areas of the body that lupus attacks are different from person to person, so people with SLE can present very different problems. For example, in many people with SLE, the immune system attacks the cells that line the joints or tendons, causing pain and sometimes swelling, warmth, and joint redness (the signs of inflammation). Most people with SLE have joint pain or arthritis at some point.

One might ask, *"If all of these systemic diseases can produce similar autoantibodies, affect multiple organ systems, and cause arthritis, how do you know it is SLE instead of one of the other diseases?"*

Each systemic autoimmune disease has characteristics that set it apart. For example, SLE can affect the kidneys in some people, causing glomerulonephritis, or "lupus nephritis" for short. SLE can also cause low blood counts, such as decreased platelets or a type of anemia (reduced red blood cells) called autoimmune hemolytic anemia. Such blood cell problems do not occur as commonly in other systemic autoimmune disorders. SLE also frequently affects the skin in distinctive ways. For example, some people with SLE develop a butterfly-shaped rash on the cheeks (the malar area) and the nose. The malar rash usually worsens with exposure to light; it is a sun-sensitive or photosensitive condition. SLE can also cause a red, scarring, oval-shaped rash called discoid lupus. A biopsy of these rashes can confirm a lupus diagnosis.

Blood tests can also help distinguish SLE from other systemic autoimmune diseases. Some blood tests are specific to lupus. They include anti-Smith, Crithidia anti-double-stranded DNA (anti-ds DNA), BC4d, and anti-ribosomal-P (see chapter 4). If any of these is positive, it can help diagnose SLE. For example, if someone appears to have a systemic autoimmune disease, is positive for antinuclear antibodies, has lupus-specific problems (discoid lupus, a low platelet count, autoimmune hemolytic anemia, or lupus nephritis), and is positive for anti-Smith or anti-ribosomal P, the chances of their having SLE are high.

Putting all the above together, we can come up with a layperson's definition of SLE: SLE is a systemic autoimmune disease in which the immune system treats various organs of the body as though they were foreign invaders and attacks them. It produces autoantibodies (especially ANAs) as a feature of the disease. Many problems set it apart from other systemic autoimmune diseases (for example, RA, scleroderma, and Sjögren's). These problems can include lupus nephritis, low platelet counts, autoimmune hemolytic anemia, discoid lupus, and butterfly (malar) rashes. Some blood tests, such as anti-Smith, anti-ribosomal-P, and BC4d, also distinguish it from other diseases.

SLE is one type of lupus, but there are four types of lupus: SLE, drug-induced lupus, cutaneous lupus, and neonatal lupus. Throughout the book, "SLE" refers specifically to patients who have systemic lupus and not necessarily the other three forms of lupus. "Lupus" includes patients with any form of lupus (systemic, cutaneous, neonatal, or drug-induced). The other three forms of lupus are discussed below.

Drug-Induced Lupus

Some medicines can cause the immune system to become overactive, which can, in turn, result in a form of lupus. This is called drug-induced lupus (DIL). Most people with DIL experience joint pain or arthritis. Other common problems include fever, muscle pain, acute cutaneous and subacute cutaneous lupus rashes (see chapter 8), and inflammation around the lining of the heart (pericarditis, chapter 11) or lungs (pleurisy, chapter 10).

There are some differences between SLE and DIL. The most important is that when the offending drug is stopped, the lupus gradually goes away. SLE, however, is a life-long condition, usually requiring medications that calm down the immune system for the person's entire life.

While DIL affects men and women equally, 90% of those with SLE are women. In addition, DIL affects more white than Black people. However, SLE is more common in people of color (such as Black, non-white Hispanic, American Indian, and Native Alaskan). And while the average age for DIL is about 60, for SLE it is 20 to 30.

DIL is also usually less severe than SLE. Several SLE problems are not commonly seen in DIL, including discoid lupus rash, low blood counts, lupus nephritis, and brain involvement.

Immune system lab tests can help tell the difference between DIL and SLE. For example, SLE can cause positive anti-Smith and anti-dsDNA antibodies and low C3 and C4 complement levels (chapter 4), yet these rarely occur in DIL.

Histone antibodies are a type of autoantibody. They occur in around 95% of people with DIL. However, many people with SLE also have histone antibodies, so being positive for histone antibody does not automatically mean that someone has DIL. Its utility for diagnosis is when anti-histone is negative, in which case DIL is less likely.

There are some exceptions to these abnormal lab test results. For example, a group of medications called TNF inhibitors (adalimumab, etanercept, infliximab, golimumab, and certolizumab) can cause DIL with anti-ds DNA, antichromatin, and anti-cardiolipin antibodies (all discussed in chapter 4).

Antineutrophil cytoplasmic antibodies (ANCA, chapter 4) can also be present with DIL due to minocycline, hydralazine, propylthiouracil, and methimazole.

DIL usually does not occur until a person takes a DIL-inducing medication for at least a month. When someone with DIL stops using that medicine, DIL resolves, although it can take weeks to months for it to completely go away.

Since the early 2000s, the drugs that have most commonly caused DIL include adalimumab (Humira), etanercept (Enbrel), infliximab (Remicade), procainamide, and hydralazine. The first three are used to treat rheumatoid arthritis and other systemic inflammatory diseases. Procainamide (a blood pressure medicine) causes DIL in approximately one out of three people who take it. Around one in ten people who take hydralazine (another blood pressure medicine) will develop DIL.

Over 100 medications can cause DIL. Drugs known to definitely cause DIL are listed in table 1.1. Others may do as well, so this list will probably continue to grow.

Although the drugs listed in table 1.1 may cause drug-induced lupus, most of them are safe for lupus patients to take. They rarely cause someone with lupus to develop worsening lupus disease activity (called flares, chapter 5). For example, suppose someone with SLE has high blood pressure. In that case, it is acceptable for the doctor to treat them with hydralazine, because it would be unusual for hydralazine to worsen SLE. Similarly for someone with SLE who has recurrent seizures: it would be appropriate for the doctor to prescribe an anti-epileptic medicine such as Dilantin (phenytoin), even though it can potentially cause drug-induced lupus.

An important exception are sulfonamide antibiotics such as trimethoprim-sulfamethoxazole (TMP-SMX, also known as Bactrim). People with SLE should generally not take TMP-SMX. Sulfonamide antibiotics (often shortened to sulfa antibiotics) have a high potential for causing lupus flares or other reactions in people with lupus (chapter 5).

Another exception is estrogen prescribed for menopause symptoms (such as hot flashes). Women who take estrogen for menopause are at increased risk for mild to moderate lupus flares if they already have SLE.

Cutaneous Lupus

Cutaneous lupus occurs when lupus causes skin inflammation ("cutaneous" is a medical term referring to the skin). Cutaneous lupus is discussed in detail in chapter 8.

Neonatal Lupus

"Neonatal" is the medical term for a newborn. Neonatal lupus may occur when the mother has certain antibodies in her blood, especially anti-SSA (also known as anti-Ro). Neonatal lupus is discussed in detail in chapters 18 and 41.

Table 1.1 Drugs That Can Cause Drug-Induced Lupus

adalimumab (Humira)	minocycline (Minocin)
chlorpromazine	nivolumab (Opdivo)
etanercept (Enbrel)	pembrolizumab (Keytruda)
hydralazine	penicillamine (Cuprimine)
infliximab (Remicade, Truxima)	procainamide
interferon-alfa (Intron A)	quinidine
ipilimumab (Yervoy)	terbinafine (Lamisil)
isoniazid	TNF inhibitors (tumor necrosis factor inhibitors)
methyldopa	

How Is SLE Diagnosed?

SLE is often difficult to diagnose for many reasons. At first, SLE may start very gradually, causing minor problems the person doesn't notice. It may be impossible to pinpoint exactly when the disease began. There may not be any definitive blood test abnormalities to help identify the problem as SLE. New problems may then develop slowly over time, producing one problem at a time.

For example, SLE may first cause some fatigue and achiness for a few weeks. Or it may cause mildly low blood cell counts that do not make the person feel ill. A few months later, it may cause the fingers to turn pale when the cold winter weather arrives (Raynaud's phenomenon, chapter 11). If these episodes are mild, the individual affected may feel this is just a nuisance and brush them off.

That person may feel well for a year or so and then develop painful joints. During this stage, the person may realize that something is wrong and see a doctor. Recognizing that the pattern of fatigue, Raynaud's phenomenon, and joint pains can potentially be seen in systemic autoimmune diseases such as SLE, as well as other disorders such as fibromyalgia and some infections, the doctor will usually order tests, including an antinuclear antibody (ANA) test. If only the ANA comes back positive, and all other tests are normal, it may be impossible for a doctor to determine whether the symptoms are due to SLE or something else. The doctor may diagnose this condition as an undifferentiated connective tissue disease (chapter 2). Later, if problems occur that are typical for SLE (such as discoid lupus, low platelet counts, or positive anti-Smith antibody), the doctor would be more confident in diagnosing the problem as SLE instead of one of the other systemic autoimmune diseases.

SLE can affect virtually any body part. The doctor must consider all diseases that can do the same things. For example, some infections such as parvovirus, hepatitis C, and Lyme disease can cause arthritis, fatigue, rash, and many other blood abnormalities just as SLE can. These infections can also cause a positive ANA, which further adds to the difficulty in telling the difference between these infections and lupus.

Other disorders, such as fibromyalgia, chronic fatigue syndrome (CFS), anxiety disorder, and depression, may cause fatigue, joint pain, and muscle pain, just as SLE does. If someone has any of these conditions and is also positive for ANA (which is commonly positive in healthy people; see chapter 4), it may be difficult to distinguish the problem (fibromyalgia or CFS, for example) from SLE.

The same is true of many autoimmune diseases, such as multiple sclerosis, rheumatoid arthritis, and autoimmune thyroid disease, which can also show a positive ANA. Other conditions that can cause problems like those seen in lupus include cancer, liver diseases, lung diseases, kidney diseases, and more.

A person may need to see several specialists to assess different problems. The first step in the evaluation process is for the doctor to talk to the patient to determine what has been happening (taking a history, chapter 43) and perform a physical examination. The doctor will ask the person whether they have had any unusual symptoms. Symptoms are what the individual has been feeling or noticing, and they alert the doctor to consider a range of possible causes. For example, if a person with specific symptoms works in a daycare center, those symptoms could be the result of a parvovirus infection, rather than SLE, which has similar symptoms.

If SLE is suspected, the doctor will look for a variety of clues during the physical examination. The doctor will look at the skin for lupus rashes, examine the mouth and nose for ulcers, listen to the lungs for possible inflammation or fluid and the heart for abnormal sounds or murmurs, study the joints looking for inflammation, and so on.

After the history and physical examination, if lupus continues to be a possibility, additional tests, especially blood and urine tests, are needed. The most important first test is the ANA, because virtually everyone with SLE is ANA positive before diagnosis (see chapter 4 for exceptions). If the test is negative, SLE is highly unlikely. If the ANA test is positive, it does not stop there, especially since 15% to 20% of healthy people are also positive for ANA. As noted above, non-lupus illnesses can cause a positive ANA. These include not only diseases that cause systemic inflammation, but also autoimmune disorders that are not systemic, such as thyroid disease and multiple sclerosis. The doctor will need to think about ordering additional tests to exclude other possibilities.

These tests will include a complete blood count, which can detect a low WBC count, a low platelet count, or autoimmune hemolytic anemia, all of which can occur in SLE. Other tests can also find liver or kidney inflammation, as well as a number of other issues. If any of these is abnormal, the doctor considers other diseases that can look like SLE. For example, if liver function tests are high, the person could have other liver problems, such as viral hepatitis C infection, hepatitis B, or autoimmune hepatitis. Like SLE, these diseases can also cause joint pain, rashes, and a positive ANA.

The doctor will also order other immune system blood tests. Some are specific for SLE, meaning that when these tests are positive, it is more likely that SLE is causing the test result, rather than something else. These tests include Crithidia anti-double-stranded DNA, anti-Smith, anti-ribosomal-P antibodies, and BC4d. However, even these specific tests are not 100% accurate. A doctor cannot diagnose systemic lupus based on one immunologic test result.

Doctors may also need to order other kinds of tests. A chest x-ray can look for fluid around the lungs, which can occur in lupus pleuritis (chapter 10). It can also check for inflammation or scarring of the lungs from SLE, or find diseases that mimic SLE. For example, lymph-gland swelling shown on the x-ray could indicate sarcoidosis, which, like SLE, can also cause rashes, arthritis, low blood counts, fatigue, and a positive ANA. Other tests include an ECG (short for electrocardiogram), which can look for evidence of inflammation around the heart due to SLE, and an echocardiogram (an ultrasound of the heart), which can check if fluid is around the heart from SLE.

Doctors sometimes need to order a biopsy, which is a minor surgical procedure in which the doctor numbs up a body part and removes a small piece of tissue that will be examined under a microscope. This examination can detect characteristics of specific diseases and thus help make a correct diagnosis. For example, a skin biopsy of lupus looks different from skin affected by sarcoidosis.

Making a diagnosis of SLE involves putting all these pieces of the puzzle together. The doctor combines the history, physical examination, blood and urine tests, and other medical test results. They will then consider other diseases that can cause each problem and eliminate those that do not make sense or are unlikely. The doctor determines that the affected person has SLE if nothing else fits.

SLE Criteria

Due to the difficulty in making a diagnosis of SLE, in 1982, the American College of Rheumatology (ACR) came up with a set of classification criteria. These aimed to ensure that only people with SLE (and not diseases mimicking SLE) enrolled in lupus research. These criteria were revised in 1997 with the addition of antiphospholipid antibodies (see chapter 4). The ACR is a professional medical organization made up of doctors, scientists, and other health professionals worldwide. It is a leader in calling for research and education for all forms of musculoskeletal disorders (diseases that affect the muscles, bones, joints, ligaments, and tendons), including systemic autoimmune diseases like lupus.

There are now three different sets of classification criteria for SLE. They are described below.

1997 ACR Classification Criteria

The 1997 revision of the 1982 ACR classification criteria requires 4 out of the following 11 criteria:

1. Malar rash (chapter 8)

2. Discoid rash (chapter 8)

3. Photosensitive rash (chapter 8).

4. Oral ulcers (chapter 8)

5. Arthritis (chapter 7)

6. Serositis (chapters 10, 11, and 15)

7. Renal disorder (chapter 12).

8. Neurologic disorder—specifically seizures and psychosis (chapter 13)

9. Hematologic disorder—specifically low platelets, low white blood cells, low lymphocytes, and autoimmune hemolytic anemia (chapter 9)

10. Immunologic disorder—specifically anti-dsDNA, anti-Smith, or antiphospholipid antibodies (anti-cardiolipin, anti-beta-2 glycoprotein I, or lupus anticoagulant; chapter 4)

11. ANA

2012 SLICC Classification Criteria

The Systemic Lupus International Collaborating Clinics (SLICC) was formed to combine information from many experts and patients worldwide to improve lupus research. In 2012, the SLICC group developed classification criteria for SLE. As with the ACR classification criteria, these were also designed to ensure better SLE research.

Someone meets the 2012 SLICC criteria for SLE by two possible means. The first is if they have lupus nephritis (proven by a kidney biopsy) and a positive ANA or anti-dsDNA blood test. Otherwise, doctors look at two sets of criteria, clinical criteria and immunologic criteria. A person must have at least four total criteria: one criterion from each of these two sections as well as two more from either section to classify as having SLE.

The SLICC clinical criteria include the following:

1. Acute or subacute cutaneous lupus (chapter 8).

2. Chronic cutaneous lupus erythematosus (chapter 8)

3. Oral and nasal ulcers (chapter 8)

4. Non-scarring alopecia (chapter 8)

5. Synovitis (or inflammatory arthritis) in at least two joints (chapter 7).

6. Serositis, which occurs as pericarditis (chapter 11), pleuritis (chapter 10), and peritonitis (chapter 15).

7. Renal or kidney disorder (chapter 12).

8. Neurological disorders—specifically, seizures, psychosis, mononeuritis multiplex, myelitis, peripheral neuropathy, cranial neuropathy, and acute confusion (chapter 13).

9. Autoimmune hemolytic anemia (chapter 9).

10. Leukopenia or lymphopenia (chapter 9)

11. Thrombocytopenia (chapter 9)

The SLICC immunologic criteria are as follows:

1. ANA (chapter 4)

2. Anti-ds DNA (chapter 4)

3. Anti-Smith (chapter 4)

4. Antiphospholipid antibodies (chapter 4)

5. Low C3, C4, or CH50 complements (chapter 4)

6. Direct Coombs' antibody (chapter 4)

2019 EULAR-ACR Classification Criteria

In 2019, the European League Against Rheumatism (EULAR) and the ACR developed newer criteria, which are outlined in table 1.2. There are 21 criteria, and each is assigned different points. Someone is said to have SLE for a research study if they have 10 points or higher.

For example, having a fever would contribute a score of only 2, while having biopsy-proven lupus nephritis gets 8–10 points. Assigning different scores to different problems makes a lot of sense. Some problems (such as fever, arthritis, thinning of the hair, and mouth sores) commonly occur in people with disorders other than lupus, so they are assigned fewer points to decrease the risk of making an incorrect diagnosis of SLE. Other lupus problems (such as lupus nephritis and discoid lupus) occur only in people with lupus, so these contribute a much higher number of points to the final score.

Research studies suggest that these criteria may be superior to the previous ACR and SLICC criteria. This newer set seems to have higher accuracy in identifying people with SLE. One downside is that it is more complex, making it more difficult for doctors to use.

Table I.2 2019 ACR-EULAR SLE Classification Criteria

All patients must have a positive ANA of 1:80 or higher. Need 10 points or higher to be classified as having SLE. Only include the problem with the highest score in each group (for example, if someone has both low platelets and low white blood cell counts, the person would receive 4 points for hematologic problems).

	Points
CLINICAL PROBLEMS	
Constitutional	
Fever	2
Hematologic	
Low white blood cell count	3
Low platelet count	4
Autoimmune hemolytic anemia	4
Neurologic	
Delirium, severe mental confusion	2
Psychosis, hallucinations	3
Seizures	5
Skin (mucocutaneous)	
Nonscarring alopecia, hair loss	2
Oral ulcers, mouth sores	2
Subacute cutaneous or discoid lupus	4
Acute cutaneous lupus	6
Serositis	
Pleural or pericardial effusion, fluid around lungs or heart	5
Acute pericarditis, inflammation around the heart	6
Joint (musculoskeletal)	
Joint involvement	6
Kidney (renal)	
Protein in urine > 500 mg/24 hours	4
WHO Class II or V lupus nephritis	8
WHO Class III or IV lupus nephritis	10
IMMUNOLOGIC LABS	
Antiphospholipid antibodies	
Lupus anticoagulant, anticardiolipin or β2 glycoprotein I antibodies	2
Complements	
Low C3 OR low C4	3
Low C3 AND low C4	4
Lupus-specific antibodies	
Anti-ds DNA OR anti-Smith antibody	6

Classification Criteria versus Diagnostic Criteria

Notice in the preceding paragraphs that the term "classification criteria" is used rather than "diagnostic criteria." This is because diagnostic criteria identify almost all individuals with a disorder. With a complex disease such ase SLE, this is impossible to do at this time. Instead, classification criteria supply a worldwide tool to ensure doctors enter similar groups of SLE patients into research studies. Even so, classification criteria can fail to identify many people with SLE.

Suppose someone has discoid lupus, a very high positive ANA test, repeatedly positive lupus anticoagulant, joint aches (without actual arthritis), recurrent fevers (in the absence of infection), and fatigue. Even though they have only three ACR and SLICC classification criteria (discoid lupus, ANA, and lupus anticoagulant) and only 8 points using the EULAR/ACR criteria, they most likely have SLE. This is because they show evidence of immune system problems seen in SLE (lupus anticoagulant and ANA), a highly specific lupus problem (discoid lupus), and common SLE symptoms (joint pains, fevers, and fatigue). This illustrates how someone can have SLE yet not meet classification criteria.

A 2017 study from New York looked at all the SLE patients at the Hospital for Special Surgery and Weill Cornell Medical College. They showed that if they had used only the 1997 ACR criteria, they would have missed the diagnosis in half of their SLE patients. In other words, many of them had fewer than four ACR criteria.

A rule of thumb for the three types of classification criteria discussed above is that any given criterion should be counted only if there is no more likely alternative.

Take, for example, low WBC (leucopenia) and neutrophil counts (neutropenia). These low counts can be normal for some individuals with African ancestry (due to genetics). But they can also be low due to lupus. It can be impossible to distinguish between the two except when the blood counts improve when their lupus is under good control and decrease when their lupus worsens. Or consider someone of African heritage who has neutropenia, a low positive ANA, recurrent aphthous ulcers in the mouth, and hair loss. In this case, it could be a mistake to automatically say that that person has SLE even though there are four criteria present. The low WBC count could be normal for that person, given their ancestry; healthy people are frequently positive for ANA; aphthous ulcers are common; and the hair loss could be genetic or from other causes. In other words, the criteria used to diagnose SLE can have causes other than SLE (table 1.3).

A person can also satisfy SLE criteria yet have a different non-lupus disease. Someone with rheumatoid arthritis (RA) could have inflammatory arthritis, pleurisy due to their RA, a low WBC count (which can happen with RA), and a positive ANA (which occurs in 30% of RA). If the SLICC or the 1997 ACR classification criteria were incorrectly used as diagnostic criteria, this person could be incorrectly diagnosed with SLE since they meet four criteria in each set. The doctor would probably need to order additional tests or follow the person over time before determining if they have SLE or RA. Sometimes it may be impossible, even for the best rheumatologists, to do so definitively.

Nevertheless, it is the case that the more criteria a person meets, the more likely it is to be SLE. Consider someone with increased protein in the urine, inflammatory arthritis, seizures, thrombocytopenia (low platelet cell count), photosensitive rash, pleurisy,

Table I.3 Non-Lupus Causes of Some SLE Classification Criteria

Criterion	Common Non-Lupus Causes
ANA	Inflammation, infections, drugs, age
Fever	Infections, drugs, cancer
Leucopenia, neutropenia	Drugs, infection, genetics
Lymphopenia	Age, drugs, infection
Delirium	Drugs, infection
Psychosis	Drugs, schizophrenia, brain tumor
Seizures	Drugs, stroke, genetics, glucose or sodium problems, brain tumor
Hair loss	Genetics, stress, damage from hairstyles and chemicals, iron deficiency, thyroid problems, aging, central centrifugal cicatricial alopecia (CCCA; chapter 8)
Oral ulcers	Aphthous ulcers, drugs, infection, other rheumatic diseases (Crohn's, Behçet's)
Malar rash	Seborrheic dermatitis, rosacea, sun-sensitivity due to fair skin
Sun sensitivity	Fair skin, drugs, polymorphic light eruption
Arthritis	There are over 100 other causes of arthritis and joint pains
Proteinuria	Numerous other kidney diseases

painless ulcers on the roof of the mouth, and ANA-positive results (eight ACR and SLICC criteria). SLE would likely be the correct diagnosis. That is, it would be unlikely that something else would be causing all these problems—but then that is not impossible.

Why Does Diagnosing Lupus Take Such a Long Time?

Studies performed by the lupus patient advocacy group LUPUS UK in the United Kingdom and another by the Lupus Foundation of America (LFA) separately showed that it took six years (on average) after symptoms began before SLE was diagnosed in their members. These studies also showed that doctors made at least one other diagnosis in 45% of SLE patients before the correct diagnosis of SLE. In addition, the LFA study showed that patients saw an average of four doctors before a proper diagnosis. These problems highlight the need for better and more accurate diagnostic tests.

In a further illustration of how difficult it is to diagnose SLE, the Lupus Clinical Unit at the University of Florida did a study assessing the accuracy of an SLE diagnosis in patients referred to them. The lupus experts examined the patients again and followed them over time. They found that about half the patients ended up not having SLE at all. More than 25% did not even have an autoimmune disease, and 15% were inappropriately

LUPUS IN FOCUS

It took an average of four years to diagnose SLE in a German clinic

A 2021 study from Düsseldorf, Germany, showed that it took an average of 4 years from the onset of symptoms to diagnose SLE in 585 patients.

In addition, this German study noted that those patients who took longer to get a correct diagnosis ended up with more organ damage, worse disease, worse fatigue, and worse quality of life. This finding points to the importance of early diagnosis.

treated with steroids (some at very high doses). Too many people are incorrectly diagnosed with lupus. They are then treated inappropriately with medications with potentially significant side effects.

In that University of Florida study, while 25% of those referrals from other rheumatologists were incorrect, the referring rheumatologists were four times more likely to correctly diagnose SLE than other types of doctors. Rheumatologists are the doctors who most commonly diagnose and treat people with lupus. They typically do a three-year internal medicine or pediatric residency. They then spend two to three years in a rheumatology fellowship learning about diagnosing and managing musculoskeletal disorders, including SLE. Even after all that training, they continue to learn the subtleties and potential pitfalls of diagnosing SLE by caring for many patients over many years. Experienced rheumatologists realize that diagnosing SLE is much more complex than just using the classification research criteria presented above. Understanding these criteria can make it easier to begin to understand diagnosing SLE.

How Common Is Lupus?

In 2002, the Centers for Disease Control and Prevention (CDC) showed that there was a 70% higher death rate in female SLE patients aged 45 to 64 (compared to healthy women) and that 36% of all lupus deaths occurred between the ages of 15 and 45. These facts prompted the CDC and the Lupus Foundation of America to set up a system of five large lupus registries to identify how often SLE occurs and how different ethnic groups are affected. These registries included the Georgia Lupus Registry and the Michigan Lupus Epidemiology and Surveillance Program. To have an adequate number of Hispanic and Asian patients, the CDC established the Manhattan Lupus Surveillance Program (in New York) and the California Lupus Surveillance Project. To include Native Americans and Native Alaskans, the CDC used data from the Indian Health Service (IHS) from Alaska, Phoenix, Arizona, and Oklahoma.

However, some experts think these results underestimate how many people have lupus for several reasons. First, most SLE diagnoses were determined using the ACR classification criteria. As discussed earlier in this chapter, these criteria identify a certain population of lupus patients who can participate in research. However, it misses a significant number of patients with SLE.

Second, some registries relied on hospital, laboratory, and clinic reports. A significant number of these locations did not report any SLE diagnoses. Not having any cases of SLE from numerous sites would be unusual.

Third, most of the registries did not include data from primary care doctors. Patients with mild lupus are often treated by primary care providers such as family practice doctors and general internists and never see a rheumatologist.

Fourth, inaccuracies are inevitable when trying to read handwritten notes, which can be illegible. Also, this data was collected using historical information. The problem with performing a study using historical data (called a retrospective study) is that many data that could be useful in diagnosing SLE are missing. Another problem with retrospective data is that the assignment of ethnicity and race can be inaccurate due to relying on chart-assigned results rather than insisting upon self-assigned designations (asking the patients directly).

Last, most patients with chronic cutaneous lupus erythematosus (CCLE, like discoid lupus) do not have systemic lupus. These registries did not include patients with CCLE but without SLE. Therefore, the number of people with lupus is likely more than twice these numbers.

When assessing these results, the estimate of 92 out of every 100,000 people in the Georgia registry is most likely one of the more accurate results. This estimate used ACR criteria and included diagnoses of lupus made by rheumatologists (even if they did not meet criteria) and patients with lupus nephritis who may not achieve ACR criteria.

The CDC registries estimate that there are 200,000 to 300,000 Americans with SLE. If you double this to account for those with CCLE without other organ involvement, you realize that we have at least 400,000 to 600,000 Americans with lupus.

An Important Recommendation about Your Medical Records

As you now know, diagnosing SLE can be difficult. When a rheumatologist evaluates someone diagnosed with SLE by a previous doctor, they usually want to confirm that the diagnosis is correct. About 20% of people with SLE under good control with medication can have a negative ANA, making it virtually impossible for the new doctor to confirm SLE. A negative ANA may cause the new rheumatologist to be skeptical about the SLE diagnosis.

People with SLE should protect themselves by keeping a copy of their records. Patients may see new doctors for any number of reasons—a doctor retires or moves away, a patient moves, the patient's insurance changes and forces them to switch rheumatologists, or the patient wishes to obtain a second opinion.

You should keep copies of the initial notes, laboratory test results, biopsy results, x-rays, and consultation notes that helped your first doctor make the SLE diagnosis. Store these records permanently at home. You can give copies to any new doctors you see in the future. Some people do not keep their medical records because they think they are easy to get. This is not true. Doctors must store paper records only for a certain period (typically seven years). It can be expensive to store large amounts of paper records. Many offices will have older charts destroyed to make room for newer documents.

Electronic health records (EHRs) take up less space, but they have their own vulnerabilities. For example, medical practices can be subject to ransomware attacks that cause them to lose all their patients' electronic records (notes, labs, x-rays, biopsy results). EHR systems can also be incompatible. For instance, if a rheumatology practice or hospital system acquired an established rheumatology practice that used a different EHR than they use, the patient data from the acquired rheumatologist's EHR would usually have to be entered by hand into the other ERH. After the new practice saw the acquired rheumatologist's patients for a while (such as a year), the acquired rheumatologist's EHR would likely be abandoned since it would be expensive to continue using it. This could result in the loss of numerous patient visit notes and test results.

An easy method for collecting your information is to ask the receptionist at each visit for a copy of the previous office visit's note, lab results, and x-ray results. Note that it is your legal right to get copies of your health records and results. This way, you can get them in small amounts without paying a fee. If you wait and ask for all your documents at once, most medical practices will charge a payment due to the work involved.

I (Don Thomas, MD) have had several patients who developed severe SLE flares when they moved or had to see other rheumatologists due to insurance coverage. All three had negative ANAs due to their SLE being well controlled on medications. Their new rheumatologists did not believe their SLE diagnoses and stopped their medications. One ended up with a severe stroke from SLE-associated thrombotic thrombocytopenic purpura (chapter 9), one developed lung inflammation from SLE, and the other had a severe SLE flare that resulted in severe oxygen-requiring pulmonary hypertension (chapter 10).

We cannot overemphasize the importance of keeping all records starting at the beginning of your diagnosis.

KEY POINTS TO REMEMBER

1. SLE is a systemic autoimmune disease. It is due to a person's overactive immune system attacking multiple areas of the body.

2. SLE is not contagious (you cannot catch it from someone else), nor is it cancer.

3. Almost everyone with SLE is positive for antinuclear antibody (ANA). However, ANA is also positive in other autoimmune diseases, infections, cancers, and some inflammatory diseases. Also, around 15%–20% of healthy people are positive for ANA.

4. There are four main types of lupus: SLE, drug-induced lupus, cutaneous lupus, and neonatal lupus.

5. The key first step in making a diagnosis of lupus is to consider the possibility. So, if you think you may have lupus, mention this to your doctor, and they can have it in their mind as they evaluate you.

6. SLE is a great imitator, mimicking many other diseases. Therefore, the doctor must consider many other diagnoses when evaluating a person who may have lupus.

7. SLE can sometimes come on gradually over time, making it difficult to diagnose. A correct diagnosis can take months or even years and require more than one doctor to make.

8. Doctors use the 1997 revision of the ACR Classification Criteria, the 2012 SLICC Classification Criteria, and the newer 2019 EULAR-ACR Classification Criteria to classify someone as having SLE for the purposes of research. The more criteria someone has, the greater the chances of having SLE. However, some people can have SLE even though they have only two or three criteria.

9. Keep copies of the laboratory test results, biopsies, and initial doctors' notes that led to your diagnosis of SLE in a safe, permanent place so that any new doctors you see can review the work done by your previous doctors.

Autoimmune Diseases

Arthur Weinstein, MD, FACP, FRCP, MACR, *Contributing Editor*

Systemic autoimmune diseases were defined in chapter 1. They are disorders in which the person's immune system attacks more than one organ of the body. Each well-defined systemic autoimmune disease (table 2.1) can cause similar symptoms and blood test abnormalities, including a positive antinuclear antibody (ANA) test. Each also has unique features. One person can have more than one systemic autoimmune disease (such as SLE and rheumatoid arthritis). Also, a person may develop characteristics of a connective tissue disease—for example, the person may have inflammatory arthritis and a positive ANA test—yet not fall neatly into one diagnosis (such as SLE). Rheumatologists often diagnose these people as having an undifferentiated connective tissue disease.

Different doctors may use different terms for these diseases, which can create confusion. Although "systemic autoimmune disease" is the term used in this book, other rheumatologists may use the phrases "collagen vascular disease" (CVD) or "connective tissue disease" (CTD). We prefer "systemic autoimmune disease" because some diseases that are not autoimmune in nature can also be called CVDs or CTDs.

All systemic autoimmune diseases involve the immune system attacking multiple organs and systems of the body. It is not out of the ordinary for these diseases to occur in members of the same family. For example, someone with SLE can have a maternal aunt with Sjögren's disease and a mother with rheumatoid arthritis. This shows that hereditary factors are important. However, it is not clear why one person would develop one condition, and another person in the family would develop a different one.

Undifferentiated Connective Tissue Disease (UCTD)

Undifferentiated connective tissue disease (UCTD) is a diagnosis used when someone has problems that can be caused by an autoimmune disease (such as those in table 2.2) along with evidence of autoimmunity on their blood work (such as ANA, anti-RNP, anti-SSA, or RF; see chapter 4). At the same time, though, the person does not have anything specific that helps pinpoint an exact diagnosis (such as discoid lupus rash for SLE or skin thickening for scleroderma) or does not meet classification criteria for a well-defined systemic autoimmune disease (as listed in table 2.1).

The term "undifferentiated" implies that in the future the patient's illness could become a well-defined (or differentiated) systemic autoimmune disease (or connective tissue disease) such as lupus or scleroderma. However, some patients stay undifferentiated.

Table 2.1 Systemic Autoimmune Diseases

Systemic lupus erythematosus

Sjögren's disease

Rheumatoid arthritis

Relapsing polychondritis

Systemic sclerosis (scleroderma)

Polymyositis and dermatomyositis (inflammatory myositis)

Vasculitis

Mixed connective tissue disease

Note: Systemic autoimmune diseases are also sometimes called collagen vascular diseases or connective tissue diseases.

Since many of the problems seen in UCTD are seen in SLE, the condition is sometimes called "lupus-like disease" or "incomplete lupus." However, only about 20%–30% of UCTD patients develop SLE over the years. So, I prefer UCTD over lupus-like disease and incomplete lupus.

UCTD is a common diagnosis, accounting for 10% to 35% of all referrals to major medical center rheumatologists. Sometimes a systemic autoimmune disease will start slowly and cause nonspecific problems (table 2.2) and laboratory test results (such as a positive ANA, anti-SSA, anti-RNP, and RF) that can occur in most systemic autoimmune diseases. These labs show autoantibodies produced by the immune system, but they are not specific for any autoimmune disease. Therefore, someone with arthritis and a positive ANA and rheumatoid factor (RF) cannot confidently be diagnosed with rheumatoid arthritis or SLE until other specific features appear. If problems listed in table 2.2 occur without something more specific going on, an exact diagnosis may not be possible, and the label "UCTD" would apply.

Or suppose someone begins to have problems with their fingers turning white and blue with exposure to cold (Raynaud's phenomenon), develops joint pain without definite inflammatory arthritis, anemia of inflammation (chapter 9), and has a positive ANA and anti-SSA. This person could have any of the disorders listed in table 2.1. Recall from chapter 1 that someone with SLE could first have nonspecific problems (such as joint pains and Raynaud's) and then over time develop more specific problems (such as discoid lupus or positive anti-Smith antibody) that help clinch the diagnosis. All systemic autoimmune diseases can begin gradually in this way. During the early stage of the disease, when it is clear that the person has a systemic autoimmune disease, but the problems are nonspecific, we use the term "UCTD." Think of UCTD as being the early stages of SLE in this example.

Or let's say that the person above who starts off with a UCTD with joint pains, Raynaud's, ANA, and anti-SSA then develops swollen salivary glands, dry mouth, and dry eyes. In this example, the person had Sjögren's disease (described later in this chapter) the entire time. We called it a UCTD in the early stages because the symptoms that indicate Sjögren's had not yet appeared.

Table 2.2 Problems Seen in Most Systemic Autoimmune Diseases

Arthralgia (joint pain)

Arthritis (joint inflammation)

Myalgia (muscle pain)

Myositis (muscle inflammation)

Fatigue

Raynaud's phenomenon (chapter 11)

Eye problems: scleritis, episcleritis, conjunctivitis, uveitis (chapter 16)

Lung problems: pleuritis, interstitial lung disease (chapter 10)

Pericarditis (chapter 11)

Nephritis (kidney inflammation)

Peripheral neuropathy (nerve inflammation or damage)

Reddish-colored or bruised-appearing rashes

Blood count problems: anemia of inflammation and leukopenia (chapter 9)

Positive ANA, anti-RNP, anti-SSA, and RF (chapter 4)

Many other conditions, such as infections, can mimic a systemic autoimmune disorder. One such infection is parvovirus, which can cause arthritis, anemia, rash, and a positive ANA and RF. Parvovirus can be diagnosed using blood tests (IgM parvovirus test), as can some other infections. However, blood tests are often not available to detect many viral infections. Since most viral infections resolve within four to six weeks, doctors may choose to wait and see if the problems go away on their own before considering a diagnosis of a UCTD.

What eventually happens in people who have UCTD? There are several possibilities. One is that the condition could go away on its own. One study showed that about one-third of people diagnosed with UCTD ended up having no persistent disease at all after following them for over ten years. We assume that these were due to a disorder, such as an infection, that the body got rid of.

However, about one out of every three diagnosed with UCTD will ultimately evolve into one of the well-defined systemic autoimmune diseases (table 2.1), especially SLE, scleroderma, Sjögren's disease, and rheumatoid arthritis.

The other possibility is that UCTD may never worsen or evolve into anything definitive. In this case, the diagnosis would remain UCTD. Having the term "undifferentiated" as part of a diagnosis can be frustrating. However, it should be reassuring that the long-term outlook is usually significantly better with UCTD than full-blown SLE or one of the other diseases. Persistent UCTD cases can be considered milder forms of a systemic autoimmune disease.

A diagnosis of UCTD does not mean that it cannot be treated adequately. This is because the milder symptoms caused by the different systemic autoimmune diseases are usually treated the same, no matter which one is causing that issue. For example, blood pressure medicines are useful in treating Raynaud's phenomenon (they dilate and open the arteries to the fingers and toes, increasing the blood flow). Similarly,

Pregnancy and UCTD

UCTD patients have a slightly increased risk of pregnancy complications, as do women with SLE. We recommend that pregnant UCTD patients read and abide by the suggestions in chapters 18 and 41 to increase the chances of a successful pregnancy.

Pregnant UCTD patients also have a higher chance of developing a well-defined systemic autoimmune disease (such as SLE). One study showed that 20% of pregnant UCTD patients developed either SLE or systemic sclerosis over 8 years, while only 5% of nonpregnant UCTD patients did. This development was more common in pregnant patients with a history of low blood counts or low C4 levels.

anti-inflammatory drugs and medicines that calm the immune system (such as hydroxychloroquine and methotrexate) may be useful for inflammatory arthritis, eye inflammation, or pleurisy.

The Chances of UCTD Evolving to SLE

As discussed in chapter 3, systemic autoimmune disorders such as SLE develop in people born with genes that predispose them to these diseases. However, something in the person's environment is usually needed to trigger increased immune system activity to the point of producing clinical symptoms. Increased immune system activity can occur for many years before the person feels bad or develops any disease symptoms even though autoantibodies are being produced during this period. Autoantibodies such as ANA and anti-SSA can be detected in blood tests for years before the disease becomes clear.

One of the most helpful studies to show this came from the US military, where blood samples from recruits are stored for many years. Researchers examined old blood samples of military personnel who developed SLE later. The study showed that 88% of the military personnel who eventually developed SLE had autoantibodies up to nine years before their SLE was diagnosed. The earliest autoantibodies commonly produced included ANA, antiphospholipid, and anti-SSA antibodies (chapter 4). These particular antibodies can be present in any systemic autoimmune disease. Eventually, more specific SLE autoantibodies, such as anti-dsDNA antibodies, appeared in many patients.

This period when the person has no symptoms but has autoantibodies detected in blood tests can be called the preclinical period. One way to visualize how lupus develops over time is illustrated in figure 2.1. It is important to realize that not everyone with detectable autoantibodies will develop clinical SLE.

The earliest part of the preclinical period (when the least specific antibodies are produced) is called the time of benign autoimmunity. "Benign" is a medical term meaning "not doing anything bad." The military study showed that the antibodies that prove SLE (anti-Smith and anti-dsDNA) tend to appear later, closer to the time of diagnosis.

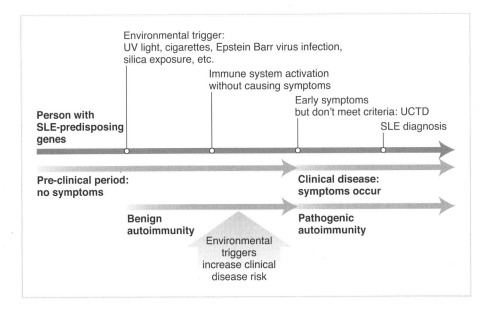

Figure 2.1 How lupus develops over time

Other studies (such as from the Oklahoma Medical Research Facility and one from Sweden) showed that in addition to autoantibodies, other immune system proteins (cytokines such as interferon, chapters 33 and 34) become more abundant during this preclinical time. After the immune system becomes more active, the person can develop symptoms. These initial symptoms may be mild or nonspecific, such as joint pains, fatigue, or Raynaud's. Later, more specific lupus problems may occur, such as kidney inflammation (lupus nephritis), butterfly rash, discoid lupus (chapter 8), and specific autoantibodies.

The emergence of SLE as the causative disease can occur very soon after an environmental exposure (trigger) in some people. One example is when someone gets sick with new-onset SLE after getting a bad sunburn at the beach and is admitted to the hospital with new-onset kidney inflammation (lupus nephritis) and a butterfly rash.

For others, it may take up to ten years or more to develop SLE, as occurred in some of members of the military. In these situations, the causative environmental triggers may not be identifiable. For example, all of us are continuously exposed to ultraviolet (UV) light from the sun and indoor light bulbs. UV light is a well-known trigger. People who have a longer period of milder and nonspecific symptoms (before a diagnosis of SLE can be made) tend to have milder SLE (with less severe major-organ involvement) than those who have an abrupt onset. However, there are certainly exceptions.

Some autoantibodies may cause particular problems. For example, anti-SSA can increase the risk of sun sensitivity and the lupus skin rash called subacute cutaneous lupus erythematosus (SCLE) or the annular erythema rash of Sjögren's disease (chapter 14). Suppose this person also develops another problem more indicative of SLE, such as discoid lupus, a butterfly rash, or a low platelet count. In that case, this person can accurately be diagnosed as having SLE earlier on. However, if this person developed dry

LUPUS IN FOCUS

Effects of antimalarials on military recruits with lupus

Military personnel deployed to areas with malaria sometimes took chloroquine (related to hydroxychloroquine) to prevent malaria. Those who took chloroquine developed fewer autoantibodies and developed lupus later than those who did not take an antimalarial.

mouth and dry eyes, then Sjögren's is the most likely diagnosis. Antimalarial medications, such as hydroxychloroquine (HCQ), may delay SLE evolution from preclinical to clinical.

Studies show that about 10% to 20% of people with UCTD develop SLE within five years. Over a long period, 20% to 35% of UCTD patients evolve into some form of a well-defined systemic autoimmune disease, including SLE.

Clinical researchers have tried to find out which patients with UCTD have the highest risk of developing SLE. Some risk factors are listed in table 2.3. However, it is essential to point out that someone with UCTD can still have these factors and combinations of features yet never develop SLE.

Many rheumatologists treat UCTD with HCQ (chapter 30). Studies show that HCQ can prevent severe SLE in some people with UCTD. People with UCTD who later develop SLE while taking HCQ tend to have a milder illness with fewer autoantibodies than patients not taking HCQ.

Overlap Syndromes

Occasionally more than one systemic autoimmune disease may occur in the same person. "Overlap syndrome" is the term for this occurrence. Having Sjögren's disease and another disorder is one of the most common combinations. About one-third of people with SLE will have an added systemic autoimmune disease (an overlap syndrome). A study from the Hospital for Special Surgery in New York showed that 38% of their SLE patients had an overlap syndrome. One out of 20 of their SLE patients even had two or more other autoimmune diseases. Of their rheumatoid arthritis patients, 8% also had SLE. Likewise, 8% of their Sjögren's patients also had SLE. The same study also showed that diagnoses could change repeatedly over time. These changing diagnoses and overlaps with other autoimmune diseases can confuse patients and their doctors. However, one of the known characteristics of systemic autoimmune diseases is that they can evolve over time.

Overlap syndrome patients tended to be older, which probably is an indication of the additive nature of these diseases over time. Having an overlap syndrome also complicates treatment. For instance, some rheumatoid arthritis (RA) drugs are avoided in SLE, so an overlap of these two diseases requires selecting effective and safe treatments for both.

Having three or more autoimmune disorders is called polyautoimmunity or multiple autoimmune syndrome. A large 2019 Spanish study of 3,679 SLE patients showed that 14% of them had polyautoimmunity. The other most common other autoimmune

Table 2.3 Factors That Increase the Risk of UCTD Progressing to SLE

- Having a family member with lupus (especially parent, sibling, or child)
- African ancestry
- Exposure to known triggers (smoking, low vitamin D levels, sun exposure, etc.)
- Young age (especially teenagers and young adults)
- Fevers unrelated to infections or other causes
- Sun sensitivity
- Malar (butterfly) rash
- Discoid lupus
- Mouth ulcers
- Hair loss
- Inflammatory arthritis
- Pleurisy
- Autoimmune hemolytic anemia or low white blood cell count
- Proteinuria (excessive protein in the urine)
- Organ damage
- Hypergammaglobulinemia (high IgG blood levels)
- High ANA (especially if ≥ 1:1080)
- ≥ 2 autoantibodies (in addition to ANA)
- ANA positive plus direct Coombs', anti-C1q, anti-dsDNA, anti-Smith, or antiphospholipid antibodies (cardiolipin antibody, beta-2 glycoprotein I antibody, false-positive syphilis test, or lupus anticoagulant)
- Low C3 or C4 complements
- High cell-bound complement activation products (CB-CAPS) such as EC4d and BC4d
- Have 3 of the 1987 ACR classification criteria (chapter 1)

disorders were (in decreasing frequency) Sjögren's disease (chapter 14), antiphospholipid syndrome (chapter 9), and autoimmune thyroid disease (chapter 17). Having anti-SSA, anti-SSB, or anti-RNP antibodies increased the risk of polyautoimmunity. Those SLE patients taking antimalarials such as hydroxychloroquine were half as likely to develop polyautoimmunity.

Sjögren's Disease

Sjögren's (pronounced SHŌ-grĭnz) disease is one of the most common systemic autoimmune diseases. In Sjögren's, the immune system primarily attacks the glands that secrete fluids (exocrine glands). It most commonly affects the lacrimal glands (which secrete tears), causing dry eyes, and salivary glands (which secrete saliva), causing dry mouth. However, it can affect other exocrine glands, causing dryness of the skin, ears, nose, and other areas.

Note that in the first edition of this book, we used the term "Sjögren's syndrome." In this book we refer to it as "Sjögren's disease," rather than "syndrome," or just "Sjögren's" (see chapter 14).

Rheumatoid Arthritis

Rheumatoid arthritis (RA) is the most well-known systemic autoimmune disease, affecting about 1% of the US population. As with SLE and Sjögren's, it affects more women than men; two to three women have RA for every man who has it. RA is a systemic autoimmune disease, a surprise to many people who think of it as "just arthritis."

RA can affect many body organs, including the eyes, lungs, heart, skin, liver, and kidneys. Its primary target is the tissue lining the joints and tendons (the synovium). RA causes this synovial lining to become inflamed (a condition called synovitis). The inflamed synovium attacks and destroys the cartilage (the cushioning of the joints) and the nearby bones, leading to bone erosions. This can cause crippling deformities that can be devastating. Fortunately, there are many effective therapies for RA. Most RA patients can go into remission or low disease activity if proper treatment is given quickly.

RA and SLE can cause inflammatory arthritis and similar abnormal lab tests (ANA and RF). Therefore, it can be difficult to tell if someone has SLE or RA early on. One clue is the presence of bone erosions at the joints on x-rays, in magnetic resonance imaging (MRI), or during an ultrasound examination. These erosions are more typical of RA and are less common in lupus arthritis. Also, a blood test called cyclic citrullinated peptide (CCP) antibody (chapter 4) is much more common in RA. RA and SLE can occasionally occur in the same person. Rheumatologists sometimes call this overlap syndrome rhupus.

Scleroderma (Systemic Sclerosis)

Scleroderma, or systemic sclerosis, is a systemic autoimmune disorder that affects the body's tissues, especially the skin. *Sclero-* comes from the Greek word for "hard," and *-derma* means "skin." This disease essentially causes the skin to thicken, especially on the hands, fingers, and face.

It also causes similar problems in other areas of the body, especially the blood vessels. Almost everyone with scleroderma will have Raynaud's phenomenon. Sometimes, the scleroderma can affect the intestinal tract muscles, causing persistent heartburn, constipation, and inefficient absorption of nutrients. Scarring of the lungs (interstitial fibrosis or interstitial lung disease), pulmonary hypertension (increased blood pressure in the lung blood vessels), and kidney disease can also occur.

Around 8% of scleroderma patients also have SLE overlap syndrome. A 2018 study at the University of Toronto, Canada, showed that their scleroderma-SLE overlap patients tended to be younger and was more common in Asian patients. They were also more likely to have the type of scleroderma called limited systemic sclerosis rather than the type known as diffuse systemic sclerosis. In other words, patients with lupus who also had scleroderma tend to have the less severe form of scleroderma.

Polymyositis and Dermatomyositis

People with SLE can develop inflammatory myositis (muscle inflammation), which causes muscle achiness and muscle weakness. However, myositis can also occur alone

LUPUS IN FOCUS

Scleroderma-SLE overlap and pulmonary hypertension

The Toronto Scleroderma Project demonstrated that half of scleroderma-SLE overlap patients have a potentially dangerous complication called pulmonary hypertension (chapter 10). If caught early, it is treatable. All SLE patients with scleroderma overlap need to have an annual echocardiogram (usually done by a cardiologist) plus annual pulmonary function tests (usually done by a pulmonologist) to catch this at an early stage if it occurs.

as a systemic autoimmune disease called polymyositis. Individuals with myositis develop weakness in the muscles of the upper arms, neck, and upper legs. This causes difficulty raising the arms (as in brushing your hair) and standing up from a chair without using your hands to push yourself up. Most people with polymyositis have no pain, but occasionally there can be muscle discomfort.

Dermatomyositis (DM) occurs when someone with polymyositis also gets skin (*dermato*-) inflammation, causing red-, purple-, or pink-colored rashes. A DM rash can also appear on the face and look like a lupus rash. Around 1 out of 20 people with SLE will also have an overlap syndrome with inflammatory myositis.

Doctors diagnose these diseases by finding muscle weakness on physical examination and discovering elevated muscle enzymes on blood tests (e.g., CPK, aldolase, LDH, AST, and ALT levels; see chapter 4). An EMG (electromyogram) test can check for abnormal electrical activity of the muscles. Muscle MRI and muscle biopsies are also useful for diagnosis. It is essential to diagnose and treat this disease quickly. If left untreated, the muscle weakness can progress to difficulty with breathing and swallowing. Persistent untreated myositis can lead to permanent weakness due to muscle scarring.

Adults with DM have an increased risk of cancer (children with DM do not). The reason for this is unknown. The cancer may occur before the doctor makes the DM diagnosis or at any time afterward and can happen in any part of the body. Therefore, the physician of a patient with DM will take a thorough history and perform a complete a physical examination followed by cancer screening tests.

Vasculitis

"Vasculitis" means "blood vessel inflammation." The problems it causes depend on which parts of the body are affected. When blood vessels become inflamed from vasculitis, blood flow to that part of the body is reduced, causing tissue damage because of lower oxygen and nutrient supply. The blood vessels can also leak blood and fluids, causing swelling and bruising of the affected area, especially the skin.

Leukocytoclastic vasculitis (LCV) is one of the most common types. LCV occurs when the skin's small blood vessels are affected with inflammation and capillary damage. This results in small red or purple areas (like raised blood spots) on the skin, especially the lower legs. A common cause of this type of vasculitis is an immune reaction to certain medications.

Henoch-Schönlein purpura is one type of leukocytoclastic vasculitis. It is found primarily in children. In addition to the skin, it can also affect the intestinal tract (causing bloody stools and abdominal pain) and kidneys (causing blood and protein in the urine).

Other areas commonly affected by vasculitis include the lungs, nerves, eyes, and kidneys. Some vasculitides (plural for vasculitis) can be positive for an autoantibody called ANCA (anti-neutrophil cytoplasmic antibody; chapter 4). Polyangiitis with granulomatosis, formerly called Wegener's granulomatosis, which can affect the kidneys, lungs, and sinuses, and microscopic polyangiitis, which often involves the lungs and kidneys, are examples of ANCA-associated vasculitides.

Giant cell arteritis (also called temporal arteritis) occurs in people over 50 and often much older. It affects the arteries of the head and neck and usually causes headaches. If it affects the main artery going to the eye, it can cause permanent blindness. It is diagnosed with a temporal artery biopsy, just underneath the skin at the temple (hence the name temporal arteritis). Treatment with steroids and tocilizumab (Actemra) alleviates headaches and prevents vision loss. Giant cell arteritis can also be associated with a very painful disease of the muscles and joints called polymyalgia rheumatica (PMR). PMR responds amazingly well to steroids. PMR, without giant cell arteritis, can also occur on its own.

These are a few of the types of vasculitis. Describing the others in more detail are beyond the scope of this book. All systemic autoimmune diseases, including SLE, can cause vasculitis.

Mixed Connective Tissue Disease

Mixed connective tissue disease (MCTD) is another systemic autoimmune disease. It has features of different systemic autoimmune diseases occurring in the same person. These individuals also have a positive ANA and high RNP antibody level but without having other autoantibodies that are suggestive of another autoimmune disease (see chapter 4). For example, they cannot have anti-Smith or anti-dsDNA (as seen in SLE), anti-Scl-70 (as seen in scleroderma), or anti-Jo-1 (as seen in polymyositis), just to name a few. High RNP antibody levels occur in everyone with MCTD.

Most MCTD patients have Raynaud's phenomenon. The other most common problems include inflammatory arthritis, muscle pain and weakness, and swollen fingers.

LUPUS IN FOCUS

Leukocytoclastic vasculitis

"Leukocytoclastic" comes from the Greek *leukocyte* (meaning white blood cell), and *-clast* (meaning broken). "Leukocytoclastic" refers to how a piece of involved skin biopsy looks under the microscope. Neutrophils (a type of leukocyte or white blood cell) are present around inflamed blood vessels (vasculitis). Many of these neutrophils have undergone leukocytoclasia—that is, they have died (appear "crushed") and released their cellular contents.

Over time, MCTD sometimes evolves into more of an SLE-like disease in some people. In other individuals, it will act more like scleroderma. Doctors should follow MCTD patients closely to look for pulmonary hypertension (see chapter 10).

Merely being positive for RNP antibody does not mean that someone has MCTD. About 30% to 40% of people with SLE are anti-RNP positive. Those positive for anti-RNP have an increased chance of having the same problems as people with MCTD, including Raynaud's and pulmonary hypertension.

MCTD is often confused with UCTD (undifferentiated connective tissue disease, discussed above). However, people with UCTD usually have a better long-term health outcome than those with MCTD. In some people with UCTD, their symptoms disappear over time or remain mild and not worsen. By contrast, those with MCTD have a long-lasting disease and may require treatment all their lives.

MCTD is often incorrectly used when "overlap syndrome" is the proper term. If someone satisfies classification criteria for more than one systemic autoimmune disease, "overlap syndrome" is usually correct. This is especially true if autoantibodies are present typical of other conditions (such as anti-dsDNA, anti-Smith, anti-ribosomal-P, anti-Jo1, ANCA, and anti-SSA).

To Make Things Even More Confusing . . .

SLE can be so variable that it seems like different diseases in different patients. For example, does the person and SLE with recurrent blood clots and nephritis have the same condition as someone with pleurisy and a butterfly rash or as someone with a sun-sensitive rash, arthritis, and dry mouth? Most experts think of SLE as an umbrella term that includes many different diseases. Our diagnostic tests (such as blood work) are just not advanced enough to tell those diseases apart at this point in time.

Organ system involvement and laboratory test results can even change over time. These fluctuations in problems and labs can cause disagreements over the diagnosis, such as whether the person actually has SLE, Sjögren's, RA, MCTD, or UCTD.

Even so, it is important to try to fit a person into one disease category or another. Specific problems are more common in some diseases than in others and may require different treatments and different tests over time. For example, doctors must evaluate people with SLE regularly to ensure they do not develop lupus nephritis. MCTD and scleroderma patients need close monitoring to ensure they do not develop pulmonary hypertension. Sjögren's needs to be evaluated for persistently swollen lymph glands, since large, firm lymph nodes that do not get better can potentially be due to lymphoma (a cancer of the lymph glands).

Treatment is often based on the organ system involved and not necessarily on the specific diagnosis. For example, treatment for inflammatory arthritis includes NSAIDs, hydroxychloroquine, methotrexate, mycophenolate, azathioprine, and steroids, no matter if that person has RA, SLE, UCTD, scleroderma, Sjögren's, or MCTD.

Due to these difficulties with diagnosis, it is never wrong to get a second opinion from another rheumatologist. Most rheumatologists feel more than happy to have patients see another rheumatologist for a second opinion. If you decide to get a second opinion, make sure that you get copies of all labs, test results, and doctors' notes to show to the new doctor. Having all this information will simplify the second opinion process and improve the accuracy of this second evaluation. It could be quite expensive to have all the tests needlessly repeated. If you happen to get a negative reaction from a doctor because you want a second opinion, you may be better off changing doctors anyway.

Organ-Specific Autoimmune Diseases

Suppose the immune system attacks one type of cell in one organ of the body. In that case, it is labeled an organ-specific autoimmune disease. These diseases do not generally attack other organs. This is contrary to systemic autoimmune diseases, which may attack multiple organs.

Around 25% of people with an autoimmune disease (both organ-specific and systemic) also develop another autoimmune disease. Some of these diseases have a higher chance of occurring alongside other autoimmune disorders, while others do not. For example, vitiligo (causes light-colored skin) and Addison's disease (causes adrenal insufficiency) commonly occur with other autoimmune diseases. Autoimmune thyroid disease commonly occurs along with systemic autoimmune diseases. Other organ-specific autoimmune disorders (such as type I diabetes) usually occur alone.

Many of these diseases appear to be associated with similar genes seen in systemic autoimmune diseases. In contrast, others may have unique genetic associations and environmental triggers.

Many organ-specific autoimmune diseases have been reported in people with lupus. Four organ-specific autoimmune diseases occur so often with SLE that they are included in the SLE classification criteria (chapter 1): autoimmune hemolytic anemia, autoimmune neutropenia, immune thrombocytopenic purpura, and autoimmune pericarditis.

KEY POINTS TO REMEMBER

1. In systemic autoimmune diseases the immune system can attack more than one organ. SLE is one of these diseases.

2. Other terms used for systemic autoimmune disease include collagen vascular disease and connective tissue disease.

3. These diseases can cause similar clinical problems (including Raynaud's phenomenon, interstitial lung disease, inflammatory arthritis, inflammation of the eyes, and rashes).

4. All these diseases can cause similar blood test abnormalities. These include positive ANA, anti-RNP, anti-SSA, RF, and anemia of chronic disease (table 2.2). These blood tests are nonspecific in diagnosing any particular systemic autoimmune disease. Some blood tests are more specific for one condition, such as anti-ds DNA and anti-Smith antibodies for lupus and anti-centromere and anti-Scl-70 antibodies for scleroderma.

5. When someone has evidence of a systemic autoimmune disease but has problems commonly found in all of these diseases, and this person does not fulfill classification criteria for any particular disorder, doctors may label that person as having an undifferentiated connective tissue disease (UCTD).

6. UCTD may evolve into one of the definite systemic autoimmune diseases (such as SLE or RA), or it may remain undifferentiated. It can even go away.

7. Approximately 20% of people with UCTD eventually develop SLE; taking hydroxy-chloroquine may decrease this chance.

8. People with SLE can also have any other systemic autoimmune disease (called overlap syndrome).

9. Mixed connective tissue disease (MCTD) and undifferentiated connective tissue disease (UCTD) are not the same disorders. Even doctors commonly misuse these terms.

10. Consider getting a second opinion from another rheumatologist if you are at all uncomfortable with your diagnosis. Please supply copies of all your earlier results to the doctor doing the second opinion.

11. Organ-specific autoimmune diseases affect only one organ; many occur more commonly in people who have lupus.

What Causes Lupus?

George C. Tsokos, MD, *Contributing Editor*

While we do not know all the causes of lupus, our understanding does take into account many factors, including genetics, the environment, epigenetics, aspects of immune system regulation, and sex hormones. For lupus to develop, you must be born with genes that increase the risk of developing lupus. We will call these "lupus-related genes" in this chapter. Yet, being born with those genes does not mean you'll develop lupus. Most people born with the genes never do. It's the combination of factors that makes the difference: the more there are, the higher the chances of developing lupus (figure 3.1). For example, if you are a male born with just one lupus-causing gene from one parent, have never smoked cigarettes, and have not had excessive sun exposure, you have a lower chance of developing lupus. However, if you are a female who has inherited multiple lupus genes from your father and mother, smoked cigarettes, had a stressful life, and suntanned regularly, you have a much higher chance of developing SLE.

Genetic Predisposition

Genes are a set of biological instructions for much of what makes us who we are as individuals. Genes from our mothers and fathers decide if we are born with blue eyes or a big nose. Collections of genes are strung together in a twisted string (or strand) called DNA. DNA exists inside the nucleus (package found toward the middle of cells) and mitochondria of most cells in our body. Mitochondria are structures in cells that produce energy. They contain small amounts of DNA that are handed down from the mother's side of the family. However, the vast majority of DNA is located in the nuclei (plural of nucleus). The DNA contains the genetic code that tells each cell what substances to produce and how the cell should function.

Lupus tends to be more common in some ethnic and racial groups. According to the Lupus Foundation of America, lupus occurs in 1 out of 700 Caucasian American women between 15 and 64 years old, while it appears in 1 out of 250 to 350 African American women of the same age. Other countries have similar findings about racial differences. Certain ethnic groups, such as those of African, Indigenous (such as Native American and Aboriginal Australians), and non-white Hispanic descent, have a higher number of people affected by lupus than others. The best explanation for this is the genes passed down from each generation.

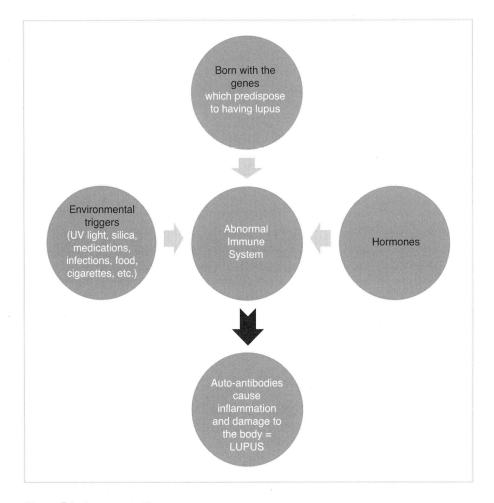

Figure 3.1 The causes of lupus

The importance of genetics is also evident in twins. Identical twins are born with the same genes. When an identical twin has SLE, there is a 25% chance that the other twin will also develop SLE. If lupus genes were the only cause, then 100% of identical twins with these genes would develop lupus. So, other factors must also play a role.

In fraternal (nonidentical) twins, the chance of both twins developing lupus is only 5%. Fraternal twins do not have the same genes. Their genetic differences are like those of siblings born at different times to the same mother and father. Even so, their chances of developing SLE are higher than for people who do not have a sibling with SLE. But then if someone has a sibling (who is not an identical twin) with SLE, that person is 30 times more likely to develop SLE than someone who does not have a sibling with SLE.

When someone is born with lupus-related genes, we say that that person has a "genetic predisposition" for developing lupus, but the genes do not guarantee it. The lupus-causing genes someone is born with contribute around 25% of the probability of getting lupus. The other 75% is due to other factors discussed in this chapter.

Some SLE patients have identifiable immune system abnormalities that play an important role in developing lupus. One immune system abnormality involves complements (also called complement proteins). Complements are proteins that help the body's white blood cells fight off foreign invaders, like bacteria. They are abbreviated C, followed by a number, which represents the order of discovery (C1 was discovered before C2).

Someone can be born with a deficiency in some of these complements (especially C1q, C4, and C2), in which case they have a high chance of developing SLE.

C1q, C2, and C4 are crucial for safely ridding the body of dying cells. When cells become old, they don't function as well, so they retire and die (a process called apoptosis, mentioned in chapters 9 and 34). These older cells are full of useful proteins and other components that can be used as building blocks for new cells. Therefore, the body is very efficient at recycling the contents of these older cells. C1q, C2, and C4 help the immune system recognize that these cells and their inner contents are part of the body and not foreign invaders. The body then knows it can safely recycle their contents.

However, if there is not enough C1q, C2, or C4, these old, dying cells and their inner contents look like foreign invaders to the immune system. White blood cells (specifically B cells, chapter 33 and 34) produce antibodies directed toward the cell contents, instructing the immune system to attack other cells in the body with similar contents. These antibodies that attack the body itself are called autoantibodies (*auto-* means "self"). The production of multiple types of autoantibodies is a hallmark of SLE. Therefore, people with complete genetic deficiencies in either of these complements can have SLE or an autoimmune disease that looks like SLE.

C1q, C2, and C4 are also important for the ability of the immune system to identify and destroy bacteria. When harmful bacteria are present, complements bind to the bacteria, alerting the immune system to get rid of them. Therefore, frequent bacterial infections are often the most dangerous part of C1q, C2, and C4 deficiencies.

People with a complete genetic lack of these complements are rare. Since only one gene abnormality is involved, their lupus is called a monogenic (one gene) disease. Monogenic SLE is rare, occurring in only 10% of SLE patients younger than ten. The vast majority of SLE patients have multiple lupus-related genes (polygenic SLE).

So far, doctors have found more than 180 lupus-related genes. Variants of these genes increase the chances of developing lupus. Some of these genes are very common, occurring in up to 30% of people who do not have SLE. The more lupus-related genes that someone inherits, the higher the likelihood of SLE. Also, some genes are much more likely to cause lupus than others. Together, the number of lupus-related genes someone has plus the likelihood of their playing a role in that person's developing lupus yield what is known as someone's "genetic risk." People with a high genetic risk tend to be younger, have more severe disease with more organ damage, and test positive for more autoantibodies than people with low genetic risk.

Some lupus-related genes increase the risk for other autoimmune diseases such as Sjögren's, scleroderma, vitiligo, Hashimoto's thyroiditis, and rheumatoid arthritis. For example, genes called STAT4 and PTPN22 have been linked to lupus, rheumatoid arthritis, and diabetes type I. (Genes are often named after the enzymes or chemical reactions they are associated with. Initials are used instead of the complete names, such as **S**ignal **T**ransducer and **A**ctivator of **T**ranscription in the case of STAT, to simplify the discussion.) It is common for people with lupus to have other family members with other autoimmune diseases. These shared genes help explain this.

Testing for lupus-related genes can reliably be done only in research settings. We are unable to test for these genes in the clinic.

Why Do More Women Have Lupus than Men?

Around 90% of people with lupus are women. Possible factors include the presence of genes that cause lupus occurring on the X-chromosome (the female sex chromosome), the effects of hormones on the immune system, and a phenomenon called microchimerism.

The X-Chromosome Dose Effect

Each human body cell normally has 46 chromosomes existing as 23 pairs. One chromosome of each pair comes from the mother, and one comes from the father. One of these chromosome pairs is composed of sex chromosomes. There are two types of sex chromosomes, Y and X. A female usually has just two X-chromosomes (one from her mother and one from her father); a male usually has an X-chromosome and a Y-chromosome paired together (the X came from his mother, and the Y came from his father). With rare exceptions, being XX or XY decides whether a person is born as a female (XX) or male (XY).

Some of the genes that have been linked to lupus, including IRAK1, TLR7, and MECP2, have been found on the X-chromosome. Because women have two X-chromosomes and men usually have only one, women are twice as likely to inherit these lupus-related genes. Normally, one of the X-chromosomes in women becomes inactive. Yet, some lupus-related genes on the x-chromosome do not become inactive (x-chromosome gene inactivation escape). If a woman has these genes, they remain active and increase her risk for having SLE.

Sometimes the sex chromosomes do not transfer perfectly from one generation to the next. One out of every 1,000 women is born with three X-chromosomes (XXX) instead of just two. Having this extra X-chromosome markedly increases the risk of developing SLE.

Another example is the genetic disorder called Klinefelter syndrome (KS). KS occurs when a baby with XY sex chromosomes receives one or more extra X-chromosomes and is born as a baby identified as a boy. Most boys with KS are XXY (instead of the usual XY). However, other variations may also occur, such as receiving three X-chromosomes and one Y-chromosome. KS occurs in 1 out of 600 boys born. Boys with KS tend to be taller, have little body hair, broad hips, narrow shoulders, and smaller testicles, and are usually infertile. Men with KS are 15 times more likely to develop SLE. This increased risk is partially related to inheriting more lupus genes on the extra X-chromosome.

Hormone Influences

There is quite a bit of evidence pointing to the effects of sex hormones on the immune system. It is most common for SLE to develop in adolescent girls and women of reproductive age (and therefore have high female sex-related hormones). The number of women who develop SLE during childbearing years far outweighs the number of men who develop SLE in this same age range. By contrast, in children (before the onset of

The X-chromosome dose effect

The more X-chromosomes a person is born with (the X-chromosome dose), the more likely that person is to develop lupus. A genetic inheritance called trisomy X, in which a woman is born with three X-chromosomes, occurs in 1 out of every 1,000–2,000 women. This occurrence increases their risk of getting either SLE or Sjögren's disease (1 out of every 400 women with SLE or Sjögren's has three X-chromosomes rather than two X-chromosomes).

puberty) and older adults (after menopause), the difference between the numbers of females and males who develop lupus is not as dramatic. The influence of sex hormones seems to be the most likely explanation.

It is not unusual for SLE to flare during menstruation. Lupus can become more active during the hormonal changes of pregnancy or soon after delivery in approximately 25% of women. Women who begin menstruation earlier than average have an increased risk of developing SLE. Women who take high-estrogen birth control pills and postmenopausal women who take estrogen also have an increased chance of developing SLE. There have even been reports of lupus developing in women on high estrogen-producing fertility treatments.

Some studies have shown abnormal sex hormone levels in both women and men who have SLE. SLE patients with higher levels of the female hormone prolactin (a hormone important for breast milk production) tend to have increased lupus disease activity. Women with active SLE tend to have lower levels of male sex hormones (androgens). Some men with SLE have lower testosterone (a male sex hormone) and higher estrogen levels (female hormones).

The female hormones estrogen and prolactin cause increased inflammation and stimulate various portions of the immune system in humans. The male hormone dehydroepiandrosterone (DHEA) may decrease lupus disease activity, and some doctors use it to treat lupus.

It should not be surprising, then, that sex hormones have important immune system interactions. We often learn a lot about humans with SLE by studying breeds of research mice that are prone to getting SLE. SLE-prone mice exposed to female hormones, such as estrogen, have an increased chance of developing SLE. Exposure to the male hormone testosterone decreases this chance.

Although it is not clear exactly how hormones increase the risk of developing lupus, in 2014 scientists at Ohio State University showed that estrogen could activate genes important in producing proteins for toll-like receptors (TLRs). TLRs are proteins on white blood cell surfaces that are important for the immune system working properly. If they function abnormally (or become overactive), they can cause increased immune system activity. The interaction of estrogen and TLRs may be an important link to lupus. One of the most important medications used to treat lupus (hydroxychloroquine) works by preventing TLRs from working properly. Therefore, TLR activity in the immune system is important in lupus, and estrogens may increase TLR production and result in increased lupus immune system activity.

Microchimerism

In Greek mythology, the chimera is a female monster whose body parts are made up of a lion, a goat, and a snake. Science has borrowed the word "chimera" to mean an animal composed of cells from two separate animals. The state of being a chimera is called chimerism.

Chimerism can occur in humans. The placenta is the organ that acts as a barrier to keep unwanted materials from the mother from entering the fetus (and vice versa). This barrier is not perfect. Some of the cells of the unborn baby may accidentally pass into the mother's blood. The opposite can also occur. Some of the mother's cells may pass into the baby.

Normally, the immune system would identify the baby's cells as not being part of the mother (labeled as "foreign" cells). The immune system would then attack and dispose of these foreign cells (from the baby) to protect the mother from this "invasion." However, in some people, the immune system cannot get rid of the baby's cells, and they persist. The result is microchimerism ("micro-" meaning tiny). Some child cells continue in the mother's body (or vice versa) on a microscopic level.

A 2006 study found that the kidneys of women affected by lupus nephritis (kidney inflammation) had male chimeric cells twice as often as kidneys not involved with lupus nephritis. Women without SLE in the study had no male chimeric cells. How this abnormal presence of male cells in the kidney contributes to disease is unknown.

Environmental Triggers

Most people born with lupus-related genes never get lupus. As with most autoimmune diseases, doctors believe that something in the environment must interact with the immune system in these genetically predisposed individuals for the disease to occur. Environmental factors refer to anything outside of the body's cells. These can be external environmental factors (such as cigarette smoke, pollution, or sunlight) or internal environmental factors (such as hormones, bacteria in the gut, or low vitamin D levels).

The environmental factors needed to interact with these lupus genes are called triggers (figure 2.1). Lupus appears to have many possible triggers. Experts do not know whether triggers instantly cause lupus or whether it takes repetitive trigger exposures over time. For example, it is not unusual for SLE to develop after a lot of sun exposure during a beach vacation. Others can pinpoint their first lupus symptoms as developing after they had mononucleosis (Epstein Barr virus). The question then arises as to whether it was this one instance of sun exposure or this one bout with mono that triggered their lupus, or whether sun exposure or mono caused a tipping point in a person who had already been exposed to multiple triggers (such as UV light, low vitamin D levels, and cigarette smoke).

Most of the rest of this chapter discusses potential environmental triggers (other than hormonal triggers discussed earlier) of lupus. But first, it would be helpful to discuss epigenetics.

Epigenetics

Before diving into the many potential environmental triggers of lupus, it is important to understand a concept called epigenetics. It is thought that many of these triggers may cause lupus by causing epigenetic changes.

Earlier in this chapter, we talked about how genes can lead to someone developing lupus. The collection of genes and DNA in our cells is called the "genome." The term "genetics" refers to the study of these genes.

While DNA molecules supply the instructions for how our bodies are to be made and perform, they do not work in isolation. Other molecules and structures surround the DNA (genome) in each of our cells to help the DNA function properly. Many of these structures (such as histones and ribonucleic acid, or RNA) exist in the chromosomes discussed earlier in this chapter. Chemical reactions occur with our DNA and these structures throughout our lives. Our DNA also reacts with other internal body molecules and external substances that enter our bodies. These reactions and interactions can change how the DNA functions. How the DNA is used and manipulated to create different types of proteins and other molecules is called epigenetics (*epi-* meaning "around" or "on the outside"). Although each cell of the body has similar DNA, each cell type, such as a heart muscle cell or a skin cell, has different epigenetics at work, producing very different types of cells with very different functions (a heart muscle cell is very different from a skin cell though they have the same DNA). Think of cooking: you can use the same ingredients (genes) to produce very different foods (muscle cell or nerve cell) depending on the cook, the utensils, the cooking methods, and so on (epigenetics).

Sometimes epigenetic changes can cause the DNA to produce unwanted results. For example, chemicals from smoking, bad gut bacteria, or ultraviolet light can cause chemical structure changes in DNA, causing the DNA to act and function in such a way as to cause lupus (if the DNA contains lupus-related genes). Other epigenetic changes can involve the histones and RNA.

People with lupus commonly develop autoantibodies (like anti-dsDNA and anti-histone, chapter 4) against these structures with epigenetic abnormalities. Examples of autoantibodies against the RNA component include anti-SSA, anti-RNP, and anti-Smith (chapter 4).

Many things (such as diet, aging, hormones, drugs, and cigarettes) can cause epigenetic changes. In lupus and other autoimmune diseases, these influences on epigenetics are called triggers. They can trigger lupus-related genes to become active and cause the person to develop lupus. Epigenetic changes can last a person's entire life and even be passed down to future generations. For example, someone born with the lupus-related genes could get sun exposure and smoke cigarettes: these actions can cause epigenetic changes and potentially turn on the lupus genes, but they don't always. While that person's epigenetics may be affected, that person may never develop lupus. But suppose they have children: the altered epigenetics can be passed on to the child, increasing the child's risk of lupus.

Environmental influences on our DNA, through epigenetics, help explain why, even though identical twins have the same genes, both twins do not necessarily develop lupus. Instead, something occurs in one of the twins (such as mononucleosis, smoking, or a low vitamin D level), which alters the DNA through this process of epigenetics and, in turn, causes lupus to develop.

Ultraviolet Light (UVB and UVA-2)

Developing lupus shortly after a sunny vacation is not unusual. Prolonged sun exposure or getting several bad sunburns before the age of 20 increases the chances of getting SLE. In Europe, Northern Ireland, the United Kingdom, and Finland have the lowest rates of SLE, while Spain and Italy, which are closer to the equator, have higher rates.

Sun exposure increases the risk for lupus due to its ultraviolet (UV) light. Ultraviolet light is so named because its wavelength frequency is higher (*ultra-* is Latin for "beyond") than that of the color violet. Ultraviolet light is not visible to humans, but it can cause chemical reactions in them.

There are three major types (called "bands") of UV light: UVA, UVB, and UVC rays (see chapter 38). UVA light is further broken down into UVA-1 and UVA-2 band spectrums. UVA-2 and UVB rays are the most important in causing lupus or lupus flares. The sun is the major source of UVA and UVB rays. Indoor lighting from incandescent and fluorescent (but not LED) light bulbs also emits UVA and UVB light. UVC light does not make it through the atmosphere, so it is not a factor. In contrast, some doctors think that UVA-1 light could be beneficial in lupus.

UVA-2 and UVB rays damage the skin cells and are a reason that sunburns, skin aging, and skin cancer occur. In people with lupus-related genes, these UV rays, including those given off in lower amounts by indoor lighting, continuously interact with and damage the skin cells. The damaged cells then release their contents, including their nuclei, into the surrounding fluids (either lymph or blood; chapter 9). These nuclear proteins (also called nuclear antigens) from the damaged cells can interact with lupus autoantibodies, such as antinuclear and dsDNA antibodies, encouraging the immune system to become more active and causing inflammation and damage. This immune system activation causes not only lupus rashes (such as the butterfly rash or a sun-sensitive rash), but also problems in other parts of the body, such as the joints (arthritis), lungs (pleurisy), and kidneys (lupus nephritis). All people with lupus should protect themselves from UV light (see chapter 38 for details).

Infections

SLE may first develop during or soon after a flu-like illness or viral syndrome. When a person contracts a viral infection, the body produces increased antibodies, specifically targeting the infecting virus. Some studies have shown that a higher number of people

---

LUPUS IN FOCUS

LED bulbs

Did you know that LED bulbs do not have UV light? People with lupus should consider changing the bulbs in their homes and workplaces to LED bulbs to minimize UV light exposure.

with lupus are positive for antibodies to some viruses than people without lupus, suggesting that these viral infections may play a role in causing SLE.

Epstein Barr virus (EBV) has some of the most convincing research as a possible trigger or cause of lupus. EBV is the virus that causes mononucleosis (commonly called mono). Earlier studies showed that people with lupus have higher EBV antibody levels in their blood than people without lupus. People with SLE have more EBV-infected cells and higher levels of the actual virus in their blood than healthy people. In addition, EBV is seen more often in people with other autoimmune diseases and may play a role in their development. These include rheumatoid arthritis, juvenile diabetes type I, multiple sclerosis, juvenile idiopathic arthritis, inflammatory bowel disease, Sjögren's disease, and celiac disease (gluten-sensitive enteropathy).

Thus far, a vaccine for EBV has been studied in four clinical trials. The vaccines have not prevented EBV, but they have decreased how sick people get from EBV. If an effective vaccine is developed in the future, we could see if it could potentially lower the risk of getting lupus.

There have also been reports of people with lupus having actual parts of viruses in their body tissues. Researchers have found larger amounts of EBV, parvovirus, cytomegalovirus (CMV), human papillomavirus (HPV), Dengue virus, human T-cell lymphotropic virus, and herpes virus particles and antibodies in people with lupus compared to those without lupus. These findings suggest that viral infections may play a role in developing SLE. In addition, the medical literature reports cases in which people develop SLE or lupus-like diseases after infections such as EBV, CMV, and parvovirus. (The latter can cause an illness that can look exactly like lupus but disappears over time.) I (Donald Thomas, MD) have two patients who developed classic SLE after having well-documented parvovirus infections. Their lupus has persisted many years after their parvovirus infection.

HPV is especially of interest. SLE patients are more likely to be infected with HPV when diagnosed and have increased rates of developing cancer (such as cervical cancer) due to the HPV infection. Some vaccines (such as Gardasil, chapters 22 and 23) can decrease the risk of HPV infection and HPV-associated cancers. Young people should consider getting vaccinated against HPV (especially while young, before sexual activity) to reduce these risks.

There is an important connection between viral infections, genes, and SLE. Some genes identified as causing lupus also produce an immune system substance called interferon, which helps our body fight viruses such as the flu, EBV, and the common cold. When viruses infect us, our immune system produces interferons. These interferons then cause the white blood cells of our immune system to attack and get rid of the virus. In the process, they may also help cause the fever, body pain, and severe fatigue that we commonly feel during viral infections. After the immune system defeats the virus in our body, interferon production decreases. We then begin to feel much better as the fevers, pain, and fatigue go away.

Some lupus-related genes produce higher amounts of interferon than usual. If a person who has these lupus genes becomes infected by a virus such as EBV, the genes turn on appropriately. But then after the infection is under control, rather than turning off (which is the action taken by normal interferon-producing genes), these genes continue to be active and produce too much interferon. The continued excessive interferon production may cause fatigue, fever, and pain in this person, who then develops SLE. Eighty percent of people with moderate to severe lupus have very high levels of interferon (see anifrolumab, chapter 34).

Abnormal Microbiome

The entire collection of microorganisms that live in and on us is known as our microbiome (*micro-* referring to their microscopic size, and *-biome* referring to a community of organisms occurring together). We hope to have many good microorganisms in our microbiome to help keep us safe from those that can cause bad infections and disease, but imbalances between beneficial and harmful microorganisms can occur.

Antibiotics used for infections, such as pneumonia or a urinary tract infection, can kill off too many beneficial bacteria. If this happens in the mouth or vagina, for example, a bad fungus called *Candida albicans* can grow out of control. Usually this fungus is kept in check by beneficial bacteria, but if the beneficial bacteria have disappeared due to antibiotics, a person can end up having a fungus or yeast infection of the mouth (called thrush) or vagina (called candidal vaginitis).

Our microbiome is huge. While adult bodies contain about 40 trillion cells, adult microbiomes have around 100 trillion microbes (those inside and on us). We have over twice as many bacteria, viruses, and fungi in our bodies as we do our own cells.

In addition, different parts of our body have their own microbiomes. Our intestines, for example, have more than half of all the white blood cells of the immune system that produce antibodies (B cells). The gut microbiome constantly interacts with these immune system cells. Beneficial organisms in the gut microbiome promote a healthy immune system, while harmful organisms may cause immune system abnormalities that can increase the risk for diseases related to the immune system, such as autoimmune disorders and cancers. This harmful interaction between the gut microbiome (or food) with the intestinal immune system has been termed "leaky gut syndrome" in lay publications.

Microbiome research on lupus mice and humans with SLE shows that they typically have lower numbers of beneficial bacteria and higher numbers of bacteria that result in an abnormal intestinal microbiome. This abnormal intestinal microbiome interacts with the intestinal wall immune system, potentially causing immune system abnormalities. Microbiome research studies have shown that this can result in the production of autoantibodies (such as anti-ds DNA and anti-SSA), as occurs in SLE.

The best studies that we have so far about the microbiome and SLE are from animal research. In some species of mice, all the members usually get severe lupus, making them an especially useful study group. Research shows that it is possible to create bacteria-free lupus mice, expose them to different types of bacteria in their intestines, and see what happens to their immune systems and lupus. It also shows that certain types of bacteria increase lupus disease activity by causing the production of immune proteins and antibodies typically found in lupus.

For example, *Lactobacillus reuteri* (*L. reuteri*) has been found to cause increased interferon levels. At the Yale School of Medicine, lupus experts studied *L. reuteri* bacteria in lupus mice. They knew that increased short-chain fatty acids in the gut could increase good bacteria and reduce levels of *L. reuteri*. They also knew that if mice eat a poorly digested starch, called resistant starch, the starch remains in the gut, ferments, and produces those short-chain fatty acids. Therefore, they fed the lupus mice a resistant-starch diet and found that after six months, the mice on this diet lived longer, had much less lupus disease activity, and had normal interferon levels. It appeared that they could improve their lupus by simply changing their diet.

Changing the microbiome with diet could potentially have important benefits in humans with SLE. For example, a beneficial bacterium in the gut microbiome called *Clostridiales* is important in fermenting short-chain fatty acids, which are potentially good for the immune system (as seen in the lupus mice above). Humans with SLE have fewer Clostridiales and higher quantities of *L. reuteri*. Therefore, the question arises of whether people with SLE could correct this condition—increase the good Clostridiales and decrease the bad *L. reuteri*—by including resistant starches in their diet. We need good studies in humans to see if dietary changes could improve the microbiome and help decrease disease activity, as it did in the lupus mice research.

The New York University Langone Medical Center Lupus Center showed that their lupus nephritis patients have five times the amount of a bacteria called *Ruminococcus gnavus* (RG) and fewer beneficial bacteria in their gut microbiome. Those patients with the most severe lupus nephritis had the highest numbers of RG. Patients with more RG also had higher anti-ds DNA levels and lower C3 and C4 complement levels (high anti-ds DNA and low C3/C4 occur in more active lupus).

Our skin is another important microbiome location. Organisms in and on the skin interact with the skin's immune system. Bacteria called *Cutibacterium acnes* (previously called *Propionibacterium acnes)* on the skin increase immune system activity, resulting in the production of anti-SSA autoantibodies, which are important in lupus and Sjögren's disease.

Another important microbiome region is the mouth, which is discussed in the next section of this chapter.

One challenge, though, is that doctors don't know if an abnormal microbiome may cause lupus or if lupus may cause the abnormal microbiome that we see in lupus. In other words, which came first, the chicken or the egg? However, these studies provide more evidence that an abnormal microbiome may alter the immune system in people genetically predisposed to lupus. Many factors can cause the microbiome to become abnormal, including diet, infections, antibiotics, sex, stress, and other environmental exposures (cigarettes, pollutants, toxins, other medications). If we can identify the factors that alter the microbiome in genetically predisposed people, and if these factors can be avoided or corrected, then it may be possible to decrease the risk of developing lupus or reduce disease activity if someone already has lupus.

Poor Dental Health

Dental plaque is the collection of bacteria and the substances that connect the bacteria (called the biofilm) to our teeth. It is part of our natural mouth microbiome. However, if we do not floss and brush our teeth regularly, this plaque can cause an infection called gingivitis, which can damage surrounding gum (or gingiva). Periodontal disease, which involves the infection, inflammation, and deterioration of the gums and bone disease (*perio-* means "around" and *-dontal* refers to the teeth), occurs almost twice as often in people with SLE. Dental plaque may play a role in developing lupus and make it worse when it does. The plaque bacteria and its biofilm easily interact with the immune system within the gum's soft tissues and by entering the bloodstream during gum bleeding.

Periodontal disease has been shown to cause increased autoantibody formation (such as anti-SSA and ANCA, discussed in chapter 4) and inflammation throughout the body. The Oklahoma Medical Research Foundation showed that SLE patients with higher dsDNA antibodies and lower C3 and C4 levels (which occur during higher disease activity in lupus) produced higher antibody levels against the bacteria in dental plaque than patients with better disease control.

Several studies have even shown that the treatment of periodontal disease in lupus can improve overall disease activity. One study looked at SLE patients with severe disease who also had periodontal disease. One group of the patients received excellent periodontal treatment by dentists, and their SLE was treated with a chemotherapy drug called cyclophosphamide plus prednisone. A similar group of SLE patients with periodontal disease were treated with these medications but did not receive periodontal disease treatment. Those who received periodontal disease treatment ended up having their lupus do better than the group that did not receive periodontal disease treatment. It would be prudent for people at risk for SLE or who have lupus to floss daily, brush regularly, and see a dentist regularly for dental cleanings and dental problems.

Vitamin D Deficiency

Vitamin D, a hormone manufactured by skin cells, has an important role in maintaining normal calcium levels and keeping the bones strong. It is also essential for healthy immune system function since white blood cells need vitamin D to work properly. (These cells have vitamin D receptors within their cellullar contents to which vitamin D attaches.)

The lack of vitamin D may increase the chance of developing SLE. Although some controversy surrounds this view, studies show that low vitamin D levels cause immune system abnormalities that could promote SLE. For example, low levels cause decreased levels of a type of T cell (a type of white blood cell, chapter 2) called Tregs that helps keep the immune system calm and not overactive. Low vitamin D is also associated with overactive B cells (see chapter 2) and higher interferon levels. Lower numbers of Tregs along with increased B cells and interferon levels are associated with increased lupus disease activity.

One study looked at people who had family members with SLE and had genes that interfere with how the body handles vitamin D. When these individuals developed low vitamin D levels, they had a higher chance of going from a healthy state to having SLE.

There is even a theory linking low vitamin D levels with Epstein Barr virus (EBV) infections, which is thought to be a possible trigger for developing SLE. Low vitamin D levels can cause low levels of a type of white blood cell called CD8+ T cells, which are important for our body to fight off viral infections such as EBV. If a person with low vitamin D levels and reduced CD8+ T-cells becomes infected with EBV, the infection could become more severe and infect more B cells (the cells responsible for producing lupus autoantibodies). These infected B cells can become more active and make the autoantibodies (such as ANA) causing lupus.

Studies show that newly diagnosed SLE patients have significantly lower vitamin D levels than healthy people from the same geographic location. An Egyptian study demonstrated this difference. The study also showed that the newly diagnosed SLE patients with lower vitamin D levels had higher levels of autoantibodies, more immune system inflammatory molecules, and worse lupus disease activity.

Given all these findings, vitamin D deficiency has to be entertained as a possible cause or trigger for lupus to develop in someone born with the predisposing genes.

Low vitamin D levels have also been associated with worse disease activity in people who already have SLE. A 2012 study showed that when light-skinned people with SLE developed low vitamin D levels in winter months, they were more likely to have lupus flares than when their vitamin D levels increased during sunny months. The researchers noted that the measured levels of vitamin D correlated so well with lupus disease activity that vitamin D levels could be followed to monitor the severity of lupus in some patients.

Several studies have shown that vitamin D can help lower lupus disease activity when given to SLE patients who have low levels (see chapter 35). Many lupus experts consider vitamin D an important treatment in most SLE patients.

The UV Light and Vitamin D Conundrum

You may have realized by this point that there seems to be a disconnect among the interactions of UV light, lupus, and vitamin D. UV light contact with the skin is needed to produce vitamin D. However, UV light also increases lupus disease activity. Well, if UV light increases vitamin D levels, then this should help decrease lupus disease activity (or lupus onset). Yet, UV light does just the opposite (it makes lupus worse).

A way to think about this is that when UV light contacts skin and causes the skin cells to produce vitamin D, this process is separate from how UV light makes lupus worse. It makes lupus worse by causing skin cell damage. Someone can have one of these processes occurring while the other process is not as active. For example, if someone is inside most of the time and has dark pigmented skin (which reduces UV penetration into the skin), that person has a greater chance of becoming deficient in vitamin D. This reduced vitamin D could potentially trigger that person's lupus immune system to become dysfunctional and more active, causing increased lupus disease activity. A lot of UV light is not necessary for this person to develop worsening lupus.

Another theory is that people can get sick with lupus and realize that sun exposure makes them feel sicker, so they get into the habit of staying indoors. This lack of sun exposure could be another reason for the low vitamin D levels that we see in so many newly diagnosed lupus patients and in people with known lupus who are flaring up.

But then not everyone who gets lupus or whose lupus flares has low vitamin D levels (although this is a common situation, as discussed in the previous section). While someone with light colored skin could regularly get enough light exposure to have great vitamin D levels, this UV light could also be the trigger that causes the person to develop SLE as a new diagnosis or to develop a lupus flare in the person who already has SLE.

Someone else with lupus could have dark skin, stay indoors most of the time, have a great vitamin D level by taking a supplement, yet still get enough UV light to increase lupus immune system activity. Most indoor light bulbs (other than LED bulbs) give off continuous low levels of UV light. Though it is not a lot all at once, it adds up over time. Even just a little bit damages skin cells, causing them to release their inner contents into the body, leading to increased lupus immune system activity (as discussed above).

Everyone's lupus is different, and most people are likely to have different thresholds for how sensitive they are to different lupus triggers.

In the end, though, UV light prevention can be more difficult to control than correcting vitamin D deficiency. Vitamin D deficiency can be easily tested for and corrected. If someone with lupus avoids the sun, uses sunscreen religiously, and then develops a vitamin D deficiency, taking a vitamin D supplement is a ready solution (see chapters 35 and 38).

Cigarette Smoking

In 1980, a report described a 25-year-old lab technician who came into regular contact with a chemical called hydrazine. She developed an illness like SLE, with sun sensitivity, fatigue, joint pain, and a red rash on the face. Tobacco contains hydrazine. Many studies have shown that smoking tobacco increases the risk of developing systemic lupus, cutaneous lupus, and other autoimmune diseases (such as rheumatoid arthritis). Tobacco also has many other dangerous chemicals, such as cadmium, polycyclic aromatic hydrocarbons, and insecticides, which may increase the risk of developing SLE. Cigarette smoking is well known to cause the epigenetic changes we discussed earlier and may thus increase the risk of developing SLE or having lupus flare. With all these chemicals present in cigarettes, it is not surprising that exposure to secondhand smoke may also increase the risk. A 2014 study showed that adults who were exposed as children to secondhand smoke in the home were almost twice as likely to develop SLE than those who had not.

Medications

As discussed in chapter 1, certain medications can cause drug induced lupus (DIL). The first report of a drug causing a lupus-like disease was in 1954. A 44-year-old woman took hydralazine (Apresoline) for high blood pressure and then developed very low blood cell counts. This is the first case of DIL. Many lupus-causing drugs have since been identified, as discussed in chapter 1. Fortunately, DIL disappears when the patient stops taking the drug.

In rare cases, some vaccines can cause SLE. In my practice, I have one patient who developed SLE immediately after receiving the yellow fever vaccine. The medical literature also reports cases occurring after COVID, influenza (flu), hepatitis B, and HPV vaccinations. We know it can happen, but fortunately, it is rare. Research studies that evaluate groups of lupus patients report that vaccines do not cause lupus. However, these studies are unable to identify rare events like this.

One medication deserving special attention is the sulfonamide (sulfa) antibiotic trimethoprim-sulfamethoxazole (co-trimoxazole, Bactrim). Many people with SLE will have a flare of their disease or develop an allergic reaction when taking this antibiotic. Therefore, we recommend that people with lupus never take this antibiotic. Make sure you carry an allergy list with you (along with an updated medication list, see chapter 5) at all times that includes the phrase "intolerant of sulfonamide antibiotics." This could save you from a severe lupus flare. If you become sick from an infection, it is hard to remember everything to tell doctors.

Given the role of sex hormones, such as estrogen, in causing lupus or making it worse, it makes sense to wonder if SLE may occur more often or worsen in women who take estrogen-containing medications. Birth control pills with very small estrogen doses probably do not cause lupus to occur or to flare. The 2019 American College of Rheumatology Reproductive Guidelines state that it is safe to take low estrogen birth control. By contrast, medications taken to decrease the effects of menopause, such as hot flashes, have higher amounts of estrogen. They appear to increase mild lupus flares and therefore should be avoided by most postmenopausal women (unless they greatly improve quality of life by decreasing hot flashes). In addition, anyone who is positive for antiphospholipid antibodies (see chapters 4 and 9)—which is anywhere between 30% and 50% of women with SLE—should avoid estrogen-containing medications. They increase the chances of developing blood clots.

Food

There have been case reports of eating alfalfa sprouts and developing SLE. Research studies in macaque monkeys showed that a high L-canavanine diet (including alfalfa sprouts) caused severe lupus in several of them. Alfalfa and mung bean sprouts contain high levels of L-canavanine. This amino acid protein stimulates the immune system. It is probably prudent for people with SLE to avoid alfalfa sprouts and mung bean sprouts. Legumes, fava beans, and onions also have L-canavanine. However, there are no reports of lupus being caused by eating them.

Coffee may be helpful in lupus. A study from Colombia found that coffee drinkers were less likely to develop SLE. A 2020 Italian research study showed that SLE patients who drank less than three cups of coffee per week (low intake) had higher lupus disease activity (lupus nephritis, nerve disorders, low blood counts, high anti-dsDNA, and low complements).

Green tea may also be beneficial. Though most green tea studies were small, a larger 2017 Iranian study showed that daily green tea consumption significantly lowered lupus disease activity.

Moderate alcohol use may also have benefits for those who are genetically predisposed to developing SLE. This is because alcohol may reduce systemic inflammation and cause lupus-preventing epigenetic changes. Alcohol consumption lowers levels of an inflammation-causing immune molecule called IL-6 (interleukin 6). SLE patients often have high levels of IL-6. Another immune system molecule, stem cell factor (SCF), appears important for SLE onset. Women who drink alcohol have lower levels of SCF. Beer has lots of niacin (a vitamin) and substances called humulones (found in hops). Both can decrease inflammation. Wine (especially red wine) has resveratrol, a substance that has anti-inflammatory properties.

A 2014 paper from Harvard summarized the different studies on alcohol and SLE development and concluded that together the results "suggest a possible protective effect of moderate alcohol consumption on the development of SLE." Since then, a study evaluating 59,000 Black women in the United States and another study that followed 204,055 women (> 90% were white) also showed lower risks for developing SLE among those who drank moderate amounts of alcohol.

Chapter 38 defines what constitutes moderate alcohol consumption. It varies by sex, age, and type of alcohol. It is always difficult to recommend alcohol because drinking even a little too much can lead to devastating liver damage, heart damage, brain and nerve damage, fatal car accidents, and alcoholism.

Silica and Other Minerals

Silica is a mineral found in quartz, sand, rocks, and soil. Silica has direct effects on the immune system, and many studies show that silica exposure can lead to lupus and other autoimmune diseases (such as rheumatoid arthritis and scleroderma). Increased exposure to silica can occur in various occupations, including mining, dental hygiene, highway construction, stone masonry, dry cleaning, and janitorial work, among others. Silica can cause lupus in laboratory research animals. The more silica someone is exposed to (higher amounts at a time along with longer periods of exposure), the higher the chances of developing SLE.

Uranium increases autoimmune diseases in animals. However, it has recently been implicated in causing lupus. Uranium miners in a study conducted in 2000 were found to have elevated levels of autoantibodies. More recently, a study showed a direct link between high levels of uranium exposure and SLE. The study took place in Fernald, Ohio, which had a uranium processing plant that closed in 1988, but high levels of uranium persisted in air and water samples. Twenty-five out of over 4,000 exposed people (workers or those who lived nearby) developed SLE. Those who had high levels of exposure were four times more likely to develop SLE.

Cadmium can cause lupus-like disease and lupus nephritis in rats. Its presence in cigarettes (known to increase lupus) could be another potential explanation for why smoking can cause lupus in genetically predisposed people.

Lupus inflammation and damage on body organs involves a chemical process called oxidation. Beneficial enzymes that prevent oxidative damage are called anti-oxidative enzymes. Selenium is an important component of anti-oxidative enzymes. SLE patients tend to have lower blood levels of the mineral selenium. Also, selenium may be protective against lupus damage. Selenium occurs in meats, seafood, liver, grains, seeds from selenium-rich soils, and in lentils as well as in other legumes (like beans and smooth peanut butter). Therefore, it may be important for people from families with an autoimmune disease to ensure they get enough selenium through selenium-rich foods.

The Environmental Protection Agency ranks mercury as a top-three priority pollutant. We are exposed to mercury through contaminated seafood and dental fillings. It is found in thermometers and fluorescent lightbulbs. Workers with increased exposure to mercury include those who manufacture mirrors, fluorescent lights, and x-ray machines. Dental assistants, as well as workers in the paper and pulp industries, also have increased exposure. Mice exposed to mercury are more likely to be ANA positive and develop lupus-like disease. One study showed that those in the dental profession were seven times more likely to develop lupus. Those in other mercury-associated jobs were close to four times more likely. Studies from Brazil of people living near portions of the Amazon River with high mercury levels, and those who fished there, were more likely to be ANA positive.

Xenoestrogens

Xeno- comes from the Greek word meaning foreign. Xenoestrogens are chemicals that imitate estrogen. Xenoestrogens could play a role in lupus since estrogens can increase lupus onset and disease activity. Examples of xenoestrogens include phthalates, bisphenol A, and polycyclic aromatic hydrocarbons.

In 2003, researchers reported that phthalates caused worse lupus and high anti-dsDNA (chapter 4) levels in lupus-susceptible mice. Other researchers have reproduced these results. This is of concern because phthalates exist in many products (such as lipstick and many others noted below), which could increase the occurrence of autoimmune disorders such as SLE. Researchers are investigating this possibility.

A 2008 study suggested that wearing lipstick more than twice weekly increased the risk of developing SLE. Those who started using lipstick at an earlier age and used lipstick most often had the highest rates of SLE. Lipstick contains phthalates and many other chemicals and dyes. It also contains eosin, which has been shown to cause inflammation and increased light sensitivity. One study is not enough to say that lipstick causes lupus; more studies are needed.

If a lupus patient wishes to minimize their exposure to phthalates, they would have to use as many naturally occurring products (especially plant-based) as possible and avoid manufactured plastics, cosmetics, paints, rubber, toys, paints, and cleaners. Look for the words "phthalate-free" on cosmetics and "VOC-free" in paints. You can use glass products instead of plastic, eat fresh and frozen foods instead of canned, and avoid fabric softeners (dryer sheets and liquids) and many air fresheners. Another source is the enteric coating on pills, which delays the release of drugs into the intestinal system. Enteric-coated pills decrease stomach upset, but they are high in phthalates.

That being said, there is not enough evidence to warn patients to avoid phthalates. Doing so would be difficult since they are commonplace. But it is worth bearing in mind that phthalates are a possible lupus trigger.

Bisphenol A (BPA) is a xenoestrogen widely found in epoxy resins (common in paints and adhesives) and plastics. BPA can increase interferons (discussed previously) and white blood cell activity. Mice with lupus exposed to BPA developed more lupus auto-antibodies and disease activity. BPA effects on humans and lupus need to be studied.

Polycyclic aromatic hydrocarbons (PAHs) are pollutants with xenoestrogen properties and include over 100 chemicals in coal, oil, dyes, plastics, pesticides, and cigarettes. Residents of Hobbs, New Mexico, who were exposed to high PAH levels developed many more cases of lupus than those living in non-exposed surrounding communities. In another study, a Black community in North Georgia exposed to high industrial emissions had a markedly increased number of people with SLE.

Likewise, some of the components of air pollution, such as polycyclic aromatic hydrocarbons and some trace elements, may increase the risk of developing SLE. In one study, cities with pollution, primarily from diesel cars, had much higher SLE rates than less polluted rural areas. Another survey from Crete confirmed that people living in urban areas were twice as likely to have SLE than those in rural areas.

Stress and Lack of Sleep

Many studies show that stress may trigger lupus (chapters 4 and 38). Stress and trauma have significant effects on the immune system.

After the 9/11 attacks on New York City's World Trade Center, nearby residents who developed posttraumatic stress disorder (PTSD) were three times more likely to develop systemic autoimmune disease.

A study showed that veterans with PTSD returning from Iraq and Afghanistan were twice as likely to develop SLE than veterans without PTSD. The time from a PTSD diagnosis to onset of SLE was often short. SLE occurred in these veterans with PTSD an average of seven months after the PTSD event. A 2017 Boston study further showed that women with PTSD or a traumatic event history (like sexual assault, severe accidents, or even witnessing accidents) were three times more likely to develop SLE. In 2018, the Nurses' Health Study (a large study following over 67,000 American nurses) showed that women with high levels of physical and emotional abuse as children were three times more likely to develop SLE.

In addition to these American studies, a study from Japan showed that daily psychological stress doubled the risk of SLE.

A lack of adequate sleep may also contribute to developing lupus. A lack of sleep may increase inflammation. Two studies from Taiwan showed that women diagnosed with sleep problems had higher SLE rates than other women. Conversely, a Japanese study suggested that sufficient sleep may reduce the chances of getting SLE. A 2018 US study following 436 relatives of SLE patients over an average of 6 years showed that those who slept less than 7 hours a night at the start of the study were 3 times more likely to develop lupus. Of the 436, 56 developed SLE.

Other Environmental Triggers

Silicone implants have been used in medicine since the 1960s, most notably in the form of breast implants. Although silicone implants have been suggested as a possible cause, there is no evidence of a direct link to SLE.

Echinacea is an herbal supplement to help colds and the flu. Echinacea can increase immune system activity. Since lupus is a disease where the immune system is overactive, people with SLE should not take substances that further boost the immune system.

Some doctors have also recommended that people with autoimmune diseases not take melatonin. This is based on the theory that melatonin may increase immune system activity. However, melatonin has not been shown to be harmful in lupus. Several studies in mice with lupus have shown that female mice receiving melatonin developed less inflammation, less auto-antibody production, and less kidney inflammation. One study using melatonin in people with a related autoimmune disease, rheumatoid arthritis, showed that melatonin had no bad effects. A group of scientists presented evidence in 2014 and 2019 that melatonin increased the numbers of Tregs (discussed earlier), which help reduce autoimmunity. They argued that melatonin should be investigated as a potential treatment for autoimmune diseases. Therefore, we do not ask our patients to avoid melatonin.

Pesticides may also increase the risk of SLE. The Women's Health Initiative (a large, ongoing study of women looking at multiple health issues) showed an increased risk for autoimmune diseases (including lupus) in women who worked with insecticide chemicals. A separate US agricultural study also showed that women who worked in pesticide production were at higher risk of SLE. In contrast, those who applied pesticides to crops did not. They explained that those who manufactured pesticides had significantly higher exposure doses than those who spread it on crops. A 2018 Boston study looked at women who had had an exterminator in their home for ant, cockroach, or termite problems. They were twice as likely to develop SLE. A difficult aspect of investigating pesticides and SLE is that many different chemicals are used in pesticides. We do not know which agents could be the potential cause.

Hair dyes have a compound called para-phenylenediamine (PPD) that has been shown to increase the immune system and inflammation in animal studies. It is found in the highest concentration in darker-colored hair dyes. A 2001 American research study showed that using hair dyes for six or more years increased the risk of SLE.

"If I Have Lupus, Will My Children Develop It, Too?"

Some experts believe that if a mother has SLE, her daughters have up to a 10% chance of developing SLE, while only 2% of her sons will. Researchers at the Lupus Clinic at Johns Hopkins Hospital think that if a mother has SLE, her child has only a 2% chance. A 2017 study suggested that the actual numbers could be higher.

However, the answer to this question involves much more than just assigning a number. Much of it depends on genetics. Some families have many lupus-related genes (a high genetic load), increasing the likelihood of having a child with lupus. A family with a low genetic load may have a very low risk.

Should the children of people with SLE be evaluated for lupus? Most rheumatologists do not recommend doing so. Depending upon the study, anywhere between 25% and 67% of children born to women with SLE are ANA positive (the screening test for lupus). Most of them never develop SLE, and being ANA positive could cause needless

Chances of family members getting SLE

In a 2017 study of 409 people who had at least 1 relative with SLE over an average of 6 years, 11% of them developed SLE. Having inflammatory arthritis, a rash from sun exposure, anti-RNP or high levels of anti-SSA (Ro) increased the chances. In addition, 11% of those who were initially ANA negative eventually developed SLE (in other words, being ANA negative does not guarantee you won't develop SLE). It is easy to forget about the parents of SLE patients, but it is notable that 6% of parents in the study also developed SLE over the study period.

A 2020 Brazilian study showed that when people with juvenile-onset SLE have children, those children have a higher risk of SLE than children born to parents with adult-onset SLE. People with juvenile-onset SLE tend to have genes that are more likely to cause lupus, and they tend to have a higher number of those genes. In other words, they have a higher genetic load of genes that can cause lupus.

Table 3.1   How Children of SLE Patients Can Try to Prevent Lupus

- Abide by ultraviolet light–protection measures (chapter 38).
- Get vaccinated against HPV (preferably at 11–12 years old).
- Floss and brush teeth daily to help prevent periodontal disease.
- Have your vitamin D level monitored; take a vitamin D supplement if it is low.
- Never smoke cigarettes; avoid second-hand smoke.
- Avoid sulfa antibiotics (add to allergy list).
- Do not eat alfalfa sprouts nor mung bean sprouts.
- Consider healthy use of moderate alcohol drinking when old enough (see chapter 38).
- Eat a diet rich in omega-3 fatty acids (flaxseed, cold-water fish, chia seed, walnuts, etc.; chapter 38).
- Consider eating "resistant starches" regularly (legumes, peas, overnight oats, etc.; chapter 38).
- Ensure adequate dietary intake of selenium (seafood, whole grains, lentils, beans, and smooth peanut butter).
- Consider decreasing exposure to phthalates (lipstick, plastics, cosmetics).
- Learn to cope with stress; do daily breathing exercises; practice mindfulness (chapter 38).
- Get at least 7 hours of sleep each night.
- Avoid the herbal supplement Echinacea.
- Avoid exposure to pesticides.
- Avoid using hair dyes.

anxiety. Repeated testing over their lifetime to see if they develop SLE could be time-consuming and expensive.

Also, being ANA negative does not mean that one will not develop SLE. In the 2017 study of relatives of SLE patients mentioned above, some who ended up developing SLE were ANA negative when the study started. Tests showing children to be ANA negative could create the false hope that they may never develop SLE.

The children of parents with SLE should learn the symptoms of SLE, such as joint pains, rashes, mouth sores, hair loss, and fatigue. If any of these symptoms ever occur, they should see their physician for proper testing. They should also avoid SLE triggers (table 3.1). A 2021 Harvard study showed that vitamin D and omega-3 fatty acid supplements lowered the risk of developing autoimmune disease in close to 26,000 subjects followed from 2011 to 2017. Vitamin D3 in doses of 2,000 IU daily reduced the risk by 22%, and 1,000 mg daily of an omega-3 fatty acid lowered the risk by 18%. It is helpful to know that preventing a potential lupus trigger (low vitamin D levels in this case) could reduce the risk of developing an autoimmune disease like lupus.

KEY POINTS TO REMEMBER

1. As with other autoimmune diseases, SLE occurs in people born with lupus-related genes. But having these genes alone does not necessarily mean they will develop SLE.

2. The more of these genes someone is born with, the higher the chances that person has of developing SLE. Some genes are more likely to cause lupus than others.

3. Some ethnic groups, such as non-white Hispanics, Black people, and Native Americans, have an increased risk of developing SLE.

4. Certain environmental triggers may interact with these genes to turn them on, causing SLE. Examples of triggers include sun exposure, occupational exposure to silica (such as working with pottery and ceramics), some medications, infections (such as Epstein Barr virus and parvovirus), eating alfalfa sprouts, having low vitamin D levels, stress, and smoking tobacco.

5. Women are much more likely to develop SLE than men due to the influence of sex hormones on the immune system. Some lupus-related genes are found on the X-chromosome.

The Meaning of All Those Lab Tests

Ashté Collins, MD, FASN (Non-Immunology Labs), and Sean A. Whelton, MD, FACP, FACR (Immunology Labs), *Contributing Editors*

This chapter explains the laboratory tests that doctors use to diagnose and monitor SLE. It can be helpful for people with lupus to understand what their test results may (or may not) mean. Some lab results can point out potential problems with their lupus; others may not be significant.

We do not list "normal" lab values for most lab test results. Normal lab test values usually appear on the lab results and vary between laboratory sites. We cover only the most important parts of a test for people with SLE.

Some lab tests are performed primarily to help diagnose SLE (table 4.1) and ensure that other disorders are not present. Doctors first use most of the tests described in the section called "Immunological Tests" for diagnostic purposes rather than to monitor disease activity. Table 4.2 lists tests doctors use to check disease activity and see how SLE responds to treatment. Doctors also use some tests to ensure that there are no side effects from drugs used to treat lupus.

This chapter does not need to be read in its entirety unless you want to learn about SLE comprehensively. Rather, this chapter best serves as a reference source to interpret specific tests. Whenever you notice abnormal labs, look them up in this chapter (or use the index to find the page quickly). You can usually tell if any of your labs are abnormal if you see "high" or "low" printed on your results. Sometimes they will be highlighted in bold font or in a different color (like red). You can also compare them to the expected normal values under the label "reference range" or "normal."

You may also want to consider asking your doctor what antibodies were positive during the evaluation of your lupus and look them up under the "Immunological Tests" section of this chapter. This could give you some clues as to what kinds of problems you may be at increased risk for from lupus. Different laboratories often have slightly different names for the same tests. We have included alternate names for tests in parentheses after test names.

Urine Tests

Urinalysis

Doctors use urinalysis in SLE patients to see if there is evidence of nephritis (kidney inflammation). They also use it to watch patients with known kidney problems to see how they respond to therapy. The test can potentially pick up other issues such as

Table 4.1 Lab Tests That Help Diagnose SLE

Test	How It Is Helpful
Anti-ds DNA	Positive in 40% to 80% of SLE patients; indicates increased risk of kidney inflammation (nephritis); uncommon in people who do not have SLE
Anti-Smith	Positive in 15% to 30% of SLE patients; rare in people who do not have SLE
Antinuclear antibody (ANA)	Positive in almost all SLE patients
Antiphospholipid antibodies (lupus anticoagulant, anticardiolipin antibodies, anti-beta-2 glycoprotein I, and false-positive tests for syphilis, e.g., RPR and VDRL)	Present in 30% to 50% of SLE patients; increased risk for blood clots and miscarriages
BC4d	Seen primarily in SLE (available only via the Exagen AVISE test). Rare in people who do not have SLE.
C3, C4, and CH50 complement levels	May be decreased in SLE patients; low C3 or C4 may be due to a genetic deficiency in complement causing SLE
Complete blood cell count (CBC)	
Hemoglobin	May be decreased in SLE
Lymphocyte count	May be decreased in SLE
Neutrophil count	May be decreased in SLE
Platelets	May be decreased in SLE
WBCs	May be decreased in SLE
Direct Coombs' antibody	May be positive in SLE; indicates increased risk of hemolytic anemia
EC4d	Seen primarily in SLE patients (available only via the Exagen AVISE test)
Ribosomal-P antibody	Found primarily in SLE patients. Rare in people who do not have SLE.
Urinalysis	Presence of cellular casts, elevated protein, or increased RBCs or WBCs could mean kidney inflammation (nephritis)

Table 4.2 Lab Tests That Help Follow SLE Disease Activity

Test	How It Is Helpful
Anti-ds DNA antibody	May increase during increased SLE activity and decrease with successful treatment
C1q antibody	May increase when SLE is active, especially when there is kidney inflammation; may decrease when lupus gets better
C3, C4 complement levels	May decrease during increased SLE activity and improve with successful treatment; levels do not change with disease activity in some people
Complete blood cell count (CBC)	
Hemoglobin	May be decreased when SLE is active; often improves when SLE responds to treatment; a doctor should rule out causes, like iron deficiency)
Lymphocyte count	May be decreased in SLE
Platelets	May be decreased when SLE is active, and should improve when SLE responds to treatment; can be useful for monitoring disease activity in some patients with elevated platelets (higher with more active disease)
WBC	May be decreased when SLE is active
CRP	Not reliable in most patients, but can fluctuate with disease activity in some
EC4d	May increase when SLE is active and decrease when SLE disease activity improves (available only from Exagen AVISE test)
ESR (sedimentation rate)	Not reliable in most patients; fluctuates with disease activity in some
Gammaglobulin level on SPEP	May be higher during increased SLE activity and lower with successful treatment
Random urine protein/creatinine	Elevated level could mean lupus nephritis; level should decrease with successful treatment when due to lupus nephritis
Urinalysis	Cellular casts, elevated protein, or increased RBCs or WBCs could mean lupus nephritis; these should improve with successful treatment

urinary tract infections, diabetes, kidney stones, drug side effects, or kidney/bladder cancer.

How to Do It: You urinate into a cup provided by the laboratory. Suppose a doctor wants to look for a urinary tract infection. In that case, they will order a urine culture and ask you to urinate into a sterile cup, which you will then cover with a lid. It is crucial to ensure that bacteria do not contaminate the specimen from sources outside the bladder. For example, bacteria from the fingers or the skin surrounding the urethra (the tube through which urine flows out of the body) could contaminate the specimen if not collected correctly. There can even be bacteria inside the urethra, contaminating the urine sample.

To avoid contamination, obtain a "clean-catch midstream" sample. To do this, first wash your hands. Next, remove the lid from the cup (making sure not to touch the inside of the container or cover) and put it down near you with the inside section facing up. Place the cup on an easy-to-reach surface. Pull apart the labia (if you have labia) or retract the foreskin (if you have one) with one hand. Using your other hand, wipe the urethra three times with three sterile wipes (front to back if you have a vagina). Keep the labia or foreskin retracted with one hand and grab the cup with the other. Urinate the first couple of seconds into the toilet (this gets rid of any bacteria from the urethra). Then urinate into the cup to the fill line (the "midstream" portion of the urine collection). Empty the last part of your urine into the toilet. Immediately put the lid securely on the cup, making sure not to touch the inside of the cover or the container.

If your doctor requests a regular urine sample without a culture, you should follow this same procedure. It avoids other contaminants, such as white blood cells, red blood cells, and proteins, which could produce inaccurate results. You will probably get a nonsterile container without a lid.

How to Find It on Your Lab Results Slip: Look for "urinalysis," "macroscopic urinalysis," or "microscopic urinalysis."

What It Looks For: The urinalysis usually has two major parts. The first part (the macroscopic urinalysis by some labs) uses a thin strip of test paper called a dipstick. The lab technician dips it into the urine, removes it, then looks at it. The dipstick has multiple small sections that change color to show a particular result. These include urine color, character (clear versus turbid), specific gravity, pH, protein, glucose, ketones, occult blood, urobilinogen, bilirubin, leukocyte esterase, and nitrite. In the next few sections, we discuss only urine protein, glucose, occult blood, leukocyte esterase, and nitrite. These are the most important tests for lupus patients.

The second major part of the urinalysis is the microscopic urinalysis, which is not always performed. The laboratory technician places a urine drop on a slide and evaluates it under the microscope ("microscopic") to see if there are increased cells or other abnormalities (such as bacteria).

Urine Macroscopic Exam
Urine Protein. An elevated amount of protein in the urine is usually the first sign of inflammation in the kidneys from lupus.

There are several ways to measure urine protein. The most common is the dipstick method. Normally, very little protein passes through the kidneys into the urine. The

> **LUPUS IN FOCUS**
>
> **Most urine protein dipstick abnormalities are not due to kidney problems**
>
> Common causes of positive dipstick protein results that are not due to kidney problems include exercise, fever, infection, dehydration, emotional stress, afternoon or evening urine collection, and pregnancy. Your doctor will order other tests to ensure a positive result is not due to kidney lupus inflammation.

result is reported as either negative, trace (or 10 mg/dL), 1 + (30 mg/dL), 2 + (100 mg/dL), 3 + (300 mg/dL), or 4 + (> 2,000 mg/dL). A normal result would be either "negative" or "trace." A result of 1+ may or may not be important, but 2+ or higher usually means something is causing too much urinary protein.

If the score is high, your doctor should order a urine protein-to-creatinine ratio (UPCR, discussed below). It is one of the best and easiest tests to determine whether patients have active lupus nephritis. Most lupus experts order a UPCR with every urine sample because someone can have active lupus nephritis and have a negative urine protein dipstick result, yet the UPCR is elevated (and therefore, more reliable). Doctors can also watch the UPCR over time to see if a patient with known kidney disease improves or worsens.

Urine Glucose. Glucose generally does not pass into the urine unless the blood glucose levels are higher than 180 mg/dL. High glucose levels occur mainly in people with diabetes.

Blood (Occult Blood). Hematuria is a condition in which red blood cells are in the urine. Lupus nephritis can cause hematuria, so we monitor this regularly. However, hematuria is more commonly due to menstruation, urinary tract infections (UTIs), or kidney stones. Other kidney diseases, bladder cancer, and kidney cancer can also cause hematuria, but fortunately these are uncommon.

Leukocyte Esterase. This looks for white blood cells in the urine. It checks for an enzyme called leukocyte esterase that white blood cells release. The most common reason for elevated leukocyte esterase levels is a UTI. Leukocyte esterase can also be elevated in other conditions like lupus nephritis and other kidney diseases. Mucus or cells from the surrounding skin could also contaminate the urine due to improper collection. In this case, the leukocyte esterase result is not useful.

Nitrite. Nitrite can be positive from bacteria, either due to a UTI or contamination from not collecting the urine sample properly.

Urine Microscopic Exam
Red Blood Cells (RBCs). Elevated urine red blood cells, or hematuria, can be due to menstruation (blood getting into the urine by contamination from the surrounding vaginal tissues), a UTI, or kidney stones. Lupus nephritis, other kidney diseases, and kidney or bladder cancer can also cause an increase in urine RBCs. Any increase in RBCs is a reason for further investigation.

White Blood Cells (WBCs). An elevation of white blood cells in the urine can be due to a (UTI), lupus nephritis, or other kidney diseases. It can also be due to contamination from surrounding tissues if the specimen is not collected properly.

Squamous Epithelial Cells. Elevated urinary squamous epithelial cells usually mean that the patient did not properly collect the urine specimen. These are skin cells from around the urethra. This tells your doctor to interpret the rest of the urine test with caution. This contaminated urine sample could also have falsely elevated RBC, WBC, and bacteria counts.

Bacteria. Bacteria are not usually present in a properly collected urine specimen. If there are increased bacteria (not due to contamination), it might mean that you have a (UTI). If you have pain while urinating, discomfort in the lower abdomen, the urge to urinate more than usual, or back pain with fever, you might have a UTI.

Asymptomatic bacteriuria describes the presence of bacteria in the urine without these symptoms. Doctors usually do not treat it except during pregnancy or before urinary tract surgery.

Casts. The kidneys have many tiny tubes, called tubules, through which urine flows before entering the ureters (the larger tubes connecting the kidneys to the bladder). Sometimes substances in the urine (such as blood cells and proteins) can clump up in these tiny tubules. When these clumps break free and flow into the urine, they form microscopic tube-shaped clusters called casts. Examining the casts under the microscope is necessary to characterize the casts better and determine whether they are due to kidney disease.

Hyaline casts are common and are not indicative of kidney disease. However, red blood cell casts, white blood cell casts, epithelial cell casts, fatty casts, granular casts, and waxy casts can all be present in people with various forms of kidney disease, including lupus nephritis.

Urine Protein-to-Creatinine Ratio (UPCR, Protein/G Creat, Protein/Creat Ratio)

What It Looks For: The protein-to-creatinine ratio (UPCR) is one of the most useful tests for SLE. Many rheumatologists order this test for SLE patients at most office visits to ensure they do not have nephritis. The protein concentration (labeled as protein, urine) and creatinine concentration (labeled as creatinine, urine) appear separately on the lab slip. (See creatinine, or serum creatinine, in the "Metabolic Panel" section of "Blood Tests" that follows the urine test section for a definition of creatinine.) These two values are not helpful by themselves. They can vary greatly depending on whether you have been drinking a lot of fluids that day (the urine will be diluted) or may have been a little dehydrated (the urine will be concentrated). Pay attention only to the results of the UPCR.

Suppose the UPCR shows an excessive amount of protein (called proteinuria). In that case, your doctor will most likely investigate this further to find out the cause. They may order a 24-hour urine collection or even a kidney biopsy to see if there is any evidence of lupus nephritis.

Almost everyone with active lupus nephritis has elevated urinary protein. Besides lupus nephritis, there are other potential causes. One is an increased amount of blood because red blood cells have a lot of protein. Sometimes lupus medications, such as non-steroidal anti-inflammatory drugs (like ibuprofen and naproxen), can cause proteinuria. An unrelated kidney disease, such as from diabetes or high blood pressure, can be another cause.

Suppose someone has an elevated UPCR and has a negative urine dipstick protein. In that case, this often means that the patient has a protein in the urine that does not include albumin (the protein measured with a dipstick). These other proteins include immunoglobulins, beta2-microglobulin, retinol-binding protein, albumin breakdown products, myoglobin, and hemoglobin. We rarely need to identify exactly which proteins are involved. Immunoglobulins and albumin breakdown products are most likely in lupus patients.

There are many possible causes of an elevated UPCR with a negative dipstick urine protein. One is a condition called overflow proteinuria, in which the body produces too many proteins that end up in the urine and show up as proteinuria. This excessive amount of protein is "overflowing" into the urine. This can occur in multiple myeloma, rhabdomyolysis (severe muscle damage), and hemolytic anemia. Theoretically, "overflow proteinuria" could happen in SLE patients with hypergammaglobulinemia (especially if they have gammaglobulins called light chains and heavy chains).

Tubular proteinuria can also cause a normal urine protein dipstick result. This happens when inflammation or damage occurs to the renal tubules (microscopic-sized tubes in the kidneys). The renal tubules are essential for absorbing small proteins that are not usually measured by urine dipsticks. This problem can be seen in most kidney disorders that cause permanent kidney damage (including lupus). The most common causes are high blood pressure, diabetes, and hardening of the arteries.

Occasionally, a patient can have a negative urine dipstick protein and an elevated random UPCR if they drink a lot of fluids. This increased intake of fluids can cause the urine to be diluted, creating a false negative dipstick result. This is when getting a 24-hour urine protein is important to accurately measure the urine protein excretion.

How Doctors Do It: The urine sample for the UPCR test goes through a machine that measures the concentration of protein and creatinine. It then divides the protein measurement by the creatinine to obtain the ratio. Since creatinine is normally filtered into the urine from the kidney, your doctor can figure out if the protein excretion from the kidneys is abnormal compared to the amount of creatinine the kidneys would be expected to excrete. The higher the ratio above normal, the more protein is being lost.

It is best to do a random UPCR in the morning. A condition called orthostatic proteinuria can cause elevated levels later in the day, which is normal. If a patient has a mildly elevated UPCR, they will need to drink plenty of fluids to hydrate themselves, then repeat the urine test as their first or second urine void in the morning to ensure a better result. **It is a good habit to always collect your urine samples first thing in the morning after hydration.**

24-Hour Urine

How to Do It: The best way to measure protein leaking through the kidneys is with a 24-hour collection. You should choose a day when you can most easily collect all the

Causes of a normal dipstick protein but elevated urine protein/creatinine

The urine dipstick protein measures a type of protein called albumin. If other types of protein are being spilled excessively from the kidneys, you can have a normal dipstick result. This occurs especially with tubular proteinuria and overflow proteinuria. These are discussed in the main text.

urine you make in a 24-hour period, such as a day when you can stay home. Urinate into the toilet immediately after getting up on the morning of your collection. Write down the time you do this; then collect every drop of urine into the jug for the rest of the day. Store the plastic jug as directed by your laboratory (either in a basin lined with ice or in the refrigerator). If it is not possible to keep the jug cool, it can be kept at room temperature if it is returned as soon as the collection is complete. If you have a bowel movement, you must also collect the urine that comes simultaneously. Do not allow any feces into the urine jug, but if this happens, leave them in the urine jug and do not try to remove them. When you get up the following morning, urinate into the jug within 10 minutes of the time you marked down the day before. For example, if you marked down 6:55, you should collect this final urine sample between 6:45 A.M. and 7:05 A.M. If you need to urinate an hour or so before that time, collect that urine. Then, drink a full glass of water or more to ensure you can urinate within 10 minutes of the marked time. If you need to urinate within 20 minutes, try to hold it until it is time.

Return the jug to the laboratory within a day or two of the collection—the sooner, the better. If you have a creatinine clearance ordered (which is usually required), you will need to give a blood sample when you drop off your urine collection.

24-Hour Urine Protein

What It Looks For: This is the best way to measure how much protein is being spilled into the urine. It is valuable to diagnose kidney disease and to help check how someone responds to treatment.

24-Hour Urine Creatinine Clearance

What It Looks For: This measures how well the kidneys are working (how well the kidneys are filtering wastes from the blood). The medical term for measuring kidney function is the glomerular filtration rate (GFR). Calculating the creatinine clearance on a 24-hour urine collection is one way to measure kidney function (or GFR). The GFR can also be estimated (eGFR) by measuring the serum creatinine in the blood, discussed later in this chapter.

The higher the creatinine clearance results, the better the kidney function. For example, a creatinine clearance (or GFR) of greater than 90 mL/min (milliliters per minute) is normal. Anything less than 90 mL/min signifies that the kidneys are not functioning correctly. Complete kidney failure, also called end-stage renal disease, occurs when the level is below 15 mL/min.

Blood Tests

Most tests needed to monitor the organs, drug effects on the body, and how the immune system is doing are done through blood tests. The first section discusses the two most ordered blood tests—the metabolic panel and the complete blood cell count (CBC). The second section discusses other (miscellaneous) tests that do not assess the immune system (like thyroid function and vitamin levels). The third section discusses immune system tests.

Metabolic Panel (Chemistry Panel, BMP, or CMP)

How Doctors Do It: Blood is collected in a red-topped vacuum tube (called a Vacutainer). It is used to test the kidneys, the liver, electrolytes, blood sugar, acidity, and protein levels. We list only those tests most important for SLE.

Glucose. Glucose is a necessary sugar for body energy. However, too high a glucose level could be due to diabetes. This is of concern in SLE for a couple of reasons. People with SLE are at increased risk of heart attacks, hardening of the arteries, and strokes. Diabetes can cause these to occur earlier. Diabetes is discussed in chapter 21.

Blood Urea Nitrogen (BUN). Urea nitrogen is a body waste product. The BUN result (high or low) needs to be compared to the serum creatinine and eGFR (estimated glomerular filtration rate) in order to understand why it is high or low (discussed below). It can be elevated due to dehydration, fluid pills (diuretics), other blood pressure drugs (ARBs and ACE inhibitors, see chapter 12), congestive heart failure, gastrointestinal bleeding, severe liver disease, or the kidneys not working properly. It can also be high as a result of eating a high-protein diet, trauma, or taking steroids like prednisone.

On a side note, we will use the term "dehydration" throughout the book to simplify language for nonmedical personnel. However, the correct medical term would be "hypovolemia" or "volume depletion."

BUN-to-Creatinine Ratio (BUN:SCr). The BUN-to-creatinine ratio should be around 10:1. Suppose someone has decreased kidney function and the BUN-to-creatinine ratio is 20:1 or higher. Reduced kidney blood flow may be one reason for this, but dehydration, diuretics or other blood pressure pills, congestive heart failure, or severe liver disease can all cause this result. Another possibility for an increased BUN-to-creatinine ratio is if the person has significantly decreased muscle mass, which would lower that person's creatinine. This scenario becomes more common in people as they get older or have taken steroids.

Creatinine (Serum Creatinine or SCr). Serum (a blood sample) creatinine helps estimate kidney function. Creatinine is a muscle waste product. It can also come from ingested meat. The amount of creatinine entering the blood is a constant amount, and how well the kidneys filter it from the blood and excrete it into the urine helps measure how well the kidneys can remove waste products from the body. This process is called "kidney function."

Some drugs can increase creatinine levels

Bosutinib, cefoxitin, chloroquine, cimetidine (Tagamet), cobicistat, crizotinib, dolutegravir, dronedarone, flucytosine, gefitinib, hydroxychloroquine (Plaquenil), imatinib, IVIG, olaparib, pazopanib, sorafenib, rucaparib, and trimethoprim-sulfamethoxazole (Bactrim, Septra) can elevate creatinine levels, which can make it appear that there are kidney problems when there may be none. After stopping these medications, the serum creatinine test should be repeated to figure out the correct result.

If the kidneys do not function normally, serum creatinine increases. Elevated serum creatinine can be from kidney disease or other potential problems, such as dehydration, heart failure, medications, or liver failure. Creatinine levels can vary due to how muscular the person is, age, race, and gender. Doctors use the estimated glomerular filtration rate (eGFR), discussed below, to correct for some of these variables instead of relying only on serum creatinine measures.

How well the kidneys function as a filter of waste products is a separate issue from the amount of protein that leaks from the kidney filters and into the urine. Kidney function is measured by blood samples (eGFR), whereas the amount of urine protein is measured with a urine sample (urine protein to creatinine ratio, UPCR), discussed earlier. One can have lupus nephritis causing protein to leak into the urine, as noted by a high UPCR, yet still have perfect kidney function (filtering waste products from the body) as noted by a high eGFR (below). However, both can be affected by severe lupus nephritis. The more severe the inflammation and damage, the more likely it is to have poor kidney function (a low eGFR) as well as elevated urine protein. Mild, early lupus nephritis will have a high UPCR with a normal eGFR.

Estimated Glomerular Filtration Rate (eGFR). The medical term for measuring kidney function is "glomerular filtration rate" or "GFR." The GFR is approximated on the chemistry panel as the eGFR. It is not perfect and can be inaccurate in some people.

The eGFR should be 90 mL/min or higher. If it is less than 90 mL/min, the kidneys are not properly filtering the blood, and there may be some kidney damage. If the eGFR is less than 90 mL/min for three months or longer, then that person has chronic kidney disease. If the eGFR is less than 15 mL/min, they have kidney failure and may need dialysis.

Doctors can use the eGFR to determine if it is safe to use non-steroidal anti-inflammatory drugs. They should not be used if the eGFR is low.

Albumin. Albumin is an essential protein produced by the liver, and it is the most abundant blood protein. Inflammation can cause decreased albumin levels and is a common reason for low albumin levels in SLE. However, a markedly low albumin level could also be due to severe liver disease or malnutrition. Serum albumin can also be low if it is lost in the urine from kidney disease. A high albumin level is usually due to dehydration.

Alkaline Phosphatase (ALP). All tissues of the body contain the enzyme (a type of protein) ALP. Its job is to remove phosphate molecules from compounds. These changed compounds then perform various functions depending upon the tissue. For example, bone ALP is essential in building strong bones. ALP from bones and the intestines are the predominant types in the blood. Slightly elevated and low levels are common and usually not important. If significantly high (depending on the lab), additional blood tests can find if the elevation is coming from the bones or the liver and if the elevated level is an actual problem.

Alanine Aminotransferase (ALT, SGPT). This test is used to assess whether a person has possible liver and muscle problems. It is usually combined with the aspartate aminotransferase (AST) test, described next.

Aspartate Aminotransferase (AST, SGOT). AST (SGOT), alkaline phosphatase, ALT, and bilirubin are grouped under "liver function tests." AST is an enzyme found in multiple organs, especially the liver, muscles, kidney, brain, heart, pancreas, and red blood cells. Lower than normal blood levels can be due to low muscle mass and frailty. Elevated AST and/or ALT levels can potentially be caused by a variety of issues, including medication toxicity, liver problems, muscle disease, heart problems, and hemolytic anemia. AST is most significant when elevated in conjunction with an elevated ALT level.

ALT and AST are especially helpful in tracking people on certain medications that can potentially affect the liver (such as methotrexate, azathioprine, and leflunomide). Mild elevations usually do not indicate significant problems (such as liver damage). However, values two to three times over the upper limits of normal sometimes require a change in therapy (such as lowering the drug dose or stopping it).

Muscle inflammation or damage can also cause elevated AST and ALT. Doctors will often order muscle enzyme tests, such as creatine phosphokinase (CPK) and aldolase, in the setting of elevated AST and/or ALT to see if they are of muscle origin.

It is not uncommon to have mildly elevated AST levels without a definite cause when the ALT is normal.

Bilirubin, Total. Your body produces bilirubin when liver cells break down red blood cells that have reached the end of their lifespan. The liver secretes this bilirubin into bile and excretes the bile via the gallbladder into the intestines where it mixes with the feces. If a liver problem reduces bile excretion, the blood bilirubin level may increase. If it becomes very high, then bilirubin can cause a yellowish discoloration of the skin and whites of the eyes (jaundice).

Another cause of elevated bilirubin is lupus-induced hemolytic anemia (chapter 9). Hemolytic anemia is due to the body's immune system's destruction of red blood cells.

Complete Blood Cell Count (CBC)

The CBC evaluates the blood cells and includes multiple blood count test results. There are three major blood cell components: white blood cells, red blood cells, and platelets. All three can be affected by SLE or the medications used to treat SLE and are usually checked regularly. We list only those tests important in SLE.

How Doctors Do It: Blood is placed into a purple-topped tube, and then it is analyzed in a laboratory CBC machine.

White Blood Cells (WBCs). The medical term for white blood cells is "leukocytes." The WBC count includes the quantity of all white blood cells. The CBC measures different types of WBCs—neutrophils (also called granulocytes), lymphocytes, monocytes, basophils, and eosinophils. The first two are the more important in SLE (chapter 9).

Hemoglobin (HGB, or Hb). Hb is a red blood cell protein. It carries oxygen through the blood to body cells and tissues. The term for a lower-than-normal Hb is "anemia" (chapter 9).

Hematocrit (HCT, "crit"). Hct measures the proportion of blood volume composed of red blood cells (RBCs). Like Hb, a low Hct can also be used to diagnose anemia (chapter 9).

Mean Corpuscular Volume (MCV). MCV measures the average size of circulating red blood cells. It helps narrow down the causes of anemia (chapter 9). A low MCV could be due to iron deficiency, thalassemia (an inherited anemia), sickle cell disease, or lead poisoning (this last is rare). Iron deficiency anemia from monthly blood loss (menses), which can occur in women of child-bearing age, is one of the most common anemias in SLE.

A high MCV (larger than normal RBCs) could be due to vitamin B12 deficiency, folic acid deficiency, liver disease, medications, low thyroid hormone (hypothyroidism), or excessive alcohol. Methotrexate commonly causes a mildly elevated MCV due to its impact on the bone marrow cells that produce RBCs. Fortunately, a high MCV from methotrexate usually does not lead to other problems. Metformin can also increase MCV and is rarely a concern.

Lupus autoimmune hemolytic anemia can cause a high MCV due to an increased number of large, young red blood cells called reticulocytes.

The most common cause of anemia in people with SLE is "anemia of inflammation" (also called "anemia of chronic disease"), where the MCV is usually normal.

Platelet Count. Platelets (also called thrombocytes) are the smallest blood cells and are made up of cell fragments. They are considered cells but lack a nucleus (a cell component that contains our DNA). They are essential for forming the clots that keep us from bleeding. SLE can occasionally cause the platelet count to be lower than usual (thrombocytopenia) and is one classification criterion for SLE (see chapters 1 and 9).

The platelet count might be elevated (thrombocytosis) for many reasons, including infection, inflammation, and iron deficiency anemia (chapters 9 and 22).

Basophils (Absolute Basophil Count). Basophils are a type of WBC that help fight infections and participate in allergic reactions. The most common causes of an elevated basophil count (basophilia) are inflammation, infections, hypothyroidism, and allergic reactions. On rare occasions they can be elevated in a blood cancer called leukemia. Some SLE patients have lower than normal basophil counts. If the basophil numbers increase during lupus treatment, this can be a sign of reduced lupus disease activity and successful treatment.

Lymphocytes (Absolute Lymphocyte Count, ALC). Lymphocytes are a family of WBCs that includes B cells and T cells (also called B lymphocytes and T lymphocytes, see chapter 1 and 3). They identify foreign invaders by recognizing their foreign proteins, called antigens (chapter 1), and alert the rest of the immune system to fend them off. B cells produce antibodies, which identify and help eliminate foreign substances invading the body. The B cells produce the numerous autoantibodies (such as antinuclear antibody, anti-DNA, anti-Smith) of SLE.

Lymphocytes are often lower than normal (lymphopenia, chapter 9) in patients with SLE and are one of the SLE classification criteria (see chapter 1). Steroids, such as prednisone, can also lower the lymphocyte count.

Increased lymphocytes can be seen from infections, inflammation, or rarely from blood cancers such as leukemia.

Neutrophils (Absolute Neutrophil Count, ANC). Neutrophils are white blood cells that are important for fighting infections, especially bacteria. Some people with lupus can have low neutrophil counts (neutropenia) due to SLE or medications (chapter 9).

High levels can occur from steroids, infections, inflammation, or rarely from blood cancers such as leukemia.

Miscellaneous Tests

The metabolic test and CBC discussed above are the two most ordered non-immunologic blood tests. This section lists other non-immunologic tests.

Aldolase. Aldolase is an enzyme found in all cells. The highest amounts are in the muscles, brain, and liver. High levels can occur due to muscle damage or inflammation. Lupus-induced muscle inflammation (myositis, chapter 7) can produce high aldolase and other muscle enzyme (CPK, LDH, myoglobin, AST, and ALT) elevations. The aldolase should reduce or normalize if myositis treatment is successful.

ALKPHOS. See Alkaline Phosphatase under Metabolic Panel.

Calcitriol (1, 25 di-OH Vitamin D). See Vitamin D, 1, 25-Dihydroxy.

Cortisol. Cortisol is an important hormone released by the adrenal glands (chapter 26), which also secrete many other types of hormones. Adrenal insufficiency with low cortisol levels can occur in people who have taken steroids, such as prednisone. Blood draws to measure cortisol should be in the morning for best accuracy. Low levels are suggestive of adrenal insufficiency. Cortisol levels out during the day (highest in the morning). Blood drawn later in the day can give a falsely low value. Cortisol level tests should be repeated if normal and if there is a high degree of suspicion for adrenal insufficiency. Cortisol level tests are not helpful in people currently taking a steroid, such as prednisone, because the test cannot distinguish prednisone from body-produced cortisol.

The vitamin biotin interferes with the blood test results from some labs and should be stopped at least 72 hours before the test.

C-Reactive Protein (CRP). Elevated CRP sometimes indicates inflammation. Levels are sometimes, but not always, elevated when SLE is active. Very high levels can sometimes indicate possible infection. A special CRP measurement called high-sensitivity CRP can predict an increased risk for heart attacks, strokes, and atherosclerosis (chapter 21).

Both SLE flares and infections can cause fever, but they are treated differently, so it is important to quickly determine which one the patient has. Infection culture results can take three days or more. Erythrocyte sedimentation rates (ESRs, discussed below) and CRP values tend to be higher in many infections compared to how high they are in active SLE. However, lupus aortitis (vasculitis of the aorta), pleuritis (pleurisy), and pericarditis (chapter 11) can cause levels as high as we see during infections.

Many studies have tried to figure out formulas using CRP and ESR that may help differentiate between a lupus flare and infection, but no proven methods exist.

Creatine Kinase (Creatine Phosphokinase, CK, and CPK). CPK is found in many different tissues, but the largest amounts are in muscle. The amount of CPK in the blood is directly proportional to the amount of body muscle. Muscular people can have high CPK levels and have nothing wrong.

In others, high levels can occur from muscle damage or inflammation. Lupus-induced muscle inflammation (myositis, chapter 7) can produce high CPK and other muscle enzyme (aldolase, LDH, myoglobin, AST, and ALT) elevations. The amount of CPK should decrease or normalize if myositis treatment is successful.

Biotin supplement can artificially lower test results in some laboratories. Supplements having biotin (vitamin B7) should be stopped three days before blood work.

Creatine Phosphokinase. See Creatine Kinase.

Creatinine, Urine. See Urine Protein-to-Creatinine Ratio under Urine Tests.

LUPUS IN FOCUS

Biotin can interfere with blood test results

Biotin is a common vitamin for hair and fingernail growth. It is commonly found in vitamin B7, vitamin H, and vitamin B complex supplements, in prenatal and multiple vitamins, and in dietary supplements for skin, hair, and nails. Biotin can interfere with blood test results' accuracy by interfering with how the test's chemical interactions occur, especially at higher doses. It is best to stop biotin-containing supplements three days before blood work.

Blood work that can be incorrect due to biotin includes cortisol, brain natriuretic peptide, creatine phosphokinase (CPK), DHEA, dsDNA antibody (by multiplex immunoassay), estradiol, folate, FSH, growth hormone, LH, myoglobin, parathyroid hormone, TSH, thyrotropin receptor antibody, thyroxine (T4), triiodothyronine (T3), troponin, and 25-OH vitamin D. Biotin does not interfere with all labs; it depends upon the method used for testing.

CRP. See C-Reactive Protein.

Erythrocyte Sedimentation Rate (Sedimentation Rate, Sed Rate; ESR, Westergren). Most people with active SLE inflammation have an elevated ESR because of the inflammation. However, many do not. ESR elevations can also occur from anemia, obesity, older age, being female, pregnancy, and other inflammation causes (such as infection). See "C-Reactive Protein" for discussion.

ESR. See Erythrocyte Sedimentation Rate.

Folate, Hemolysate (Folate, Serum; Folate, Plasma; Folic Acid). Serum folate levels can vary significantly based on recent dietary intake and not reflect the body's actual folate level. Serum folate levels do not help find folate deficiency compared to checking RBC folate levels. See Folate, RBC.

Folate, RBC. Folate is another term for folic acid and vitamin B9. Low RBC folate levels are useful in diagnosing folic acid deficiency (chapter 9).

The supplement biotin can interfere with test results' accuracy, causing higher levels than expected. Supplements with biotin (vitamin B7) should be stopped three days before your blood work.

Folate, Serum. See Folate, Hemolysate.

Glucose-6-Phosphate Dehydrogenase (G6PD). G6PD is an enzyme inside red blood cells that helps protect them from damage. Some people have low G6PD (G6PD deficiency) due to abnormal genes they inherit from their parents. Some medications (such as dapsone, nitrofurantoin, and quinacrine) can cause severe anemia in those with G6PD deficiency, so doctors will usually check patients' G6PD levels before using these medications.

Haptoglobin. Haptoglobin is a protein that binds to hemoglobin after destroyed red blood cells (RBCs) release hemoglobin into the blood. RBCs can become damaged because they are too old or due to a condition called hemolytic anemia. Hemolytic anemia is an autoimmune form of anemia where the immune system attacks the RBCs. It occurs in approximately 10% of people with SLE and is one of the classification criteria (see chapter 1). The haptoglobin blood test does not measure haptoglobin that is bound to hemoglobin. It measures only the unbound haptoglobin (free haptoglobin). Thus, the value goes down as it gets used up during lupus-induced hemolytic anemia. Haptoglobin levels are decreased and may be undetectable during hemolytic anemia.

The liver makes more haptoglobin during inflammation. Some people with SLE have high haptoglobin levels during higher disease activity.

Hemoglobin A1c (Glycated Hemoglobin, Hemoglobin A1, Hb A1, and HbA1c). Hemoglobin A1c is a blood test used to diagnose and monitor diabetes and prediabetes (chapter 21).

Methotrexate Polyglutamate Level (MTXPG). This measures the polyglutamate form of methotrexate (MTX) in red blood cells. For rheumatoid arthritis (RA), MTX is most effective when the level reached is more than 60 nmol/L. Doctors sometimes measure MTXPG when RA is not under reasonable control. If the level is less than 60, then an MTX dose increase may be helpful. While there are no studies to assess the usefulness of this test in SLE patients, it may nonetheless be helpful in some real-world patients.

MTXPG levels can help assess drug adherence; very low levels can indicate that someone is not taking their MTX regularly.

Mycophenolic Acid Level (Mycophenolate Level, MPA level). The drugs mycophenolate mofetil (MMF, CellCept) and mycophenolic acid (MPA, Myfortic) are commonly prescribed for SLE. MPA levels do not help decide the correct dose of MMF or MPA in SLE patients. We do not know if we should aim for any particular levels to get a good result. However, MPA levels can help assess drug adherence; very low levels can indicate that someone is not taking their medicine regularly.

Myoglobin. Myoglobin is found in muscles. It holds oxygen and releases it to the muscle cell when needed. This function is what allows you to hold your breath and still move easily for a while (such as when you swim under water). Myoglobin enters the blood only after muscle injury, such as after trauma, exercise, or inflammation. Lupus-induced muscle inflammation (myositis, chapter 7) can produce elevated myoglobin and other muscle enzyme (aldolase, LDH, CPK, AST, and ALT) elevations. The myoglobin should reduce or normalize after the myositis treatment is successful.

Parathyroid Hormone, Intact (Parathyroid Hormone, PTH). The parathyroid glands are four tiny glands that sit behind the larger thyroid gland just below the Adam's apple region of the neck (most prominent in men). The parathyroid glands secrete parathyroid hormone (PTH) to regulate how much calcium and phosphorus are in the blood. PTH directs the kidneys to hold on to calcium instead of secreting it into the urine. It also signals the kidneys to make a more active form of vitamin D, which increases calcium absorption from the intestines. PTH also directs the kidneys to secrete more phosphorus into the urine. Low PTH levels are not common in SLE.

High PTH can occur due to low vitamin D levels, which are common in SLE (chapter 3). Low vitamin D triggers the parathyroid glands to produce more PTH. This increase in PTH causes the kidneys to produce more active vitamin D and release more calcium from the bones to support blood calcium levels. The resulting loss of calcium from bone can lead to bone weakness if severe enough (osteomalacia). This is particularly a concern due to the malabsorption of vitamin D after gastric bypass surgery.

PTH levels can also rise in people with lupus-related kidney disease. One complication of elevated PTH levels due to kidney disease is that excessive calcium is released from the bones, making them brittle (renal osteodystrophy, chapter 24).

Another common cause of elevated PTH is primary hyperparathyroidism (HPT). Overactive parathyroid glands secrete too much PTH in primary HPT. Sometimes the enlarged parathyroid gland should be removed surgically. People with lupus do not get HPT more than others.

Low PTH levels in patients with low calcium suggest hypoparathyroidism, but this is not related to lupus and is rare.

Biotin supplements can cause artificially low PTH levels in some laboratories. Supplements with biotin (vitamin B7) should be stopped three days before blood work.

Protein, Urine. See Urine Protein-to-Creatinine Ratio under Urine Tests.

PTH. See Parathyroid Hormone.

Reticulocyte Count. Young red blood cells (RBCs) released from the bone marrow are called reticulocytes. Measuring their number can indicate how many new RBCs the bone marrow is making. When RBCs are destroyed, as in hemolytic anemia, the bone marrow produces more reticulocytes. A very high reticulocyte count can be useful in diagnosing SLE hemolytic anemia. Bleeding can also cause an elevated reticulocyte count. This can occur from surgery, menstruation, or damage to the digestive system (such as from ulcers, polyps, or cancer). Most other causes of anemia (such as anemia of chronic disease, iron deficiency anemia, vitamin B12 deficiency, or folic acid deficiency) do not cause increased reticulocytes because the bone marrow has difficulty producing new RBCs due to these deficiencies and inflammation.

Sedimentation Rate. See Erythrocyte Sedimentation Rate.

Synovial Fluid Nucleated Cells (Synovial Fluid Polymorphonuclear Cells). Synovial fluid acts as a lubricant between the moving parts of joints, the hinges between bones that allow us to move (like the hips, knees, ankles, shoulders, and elbows). Joint inflammation or damage is called arthritis and can sometimes produce extra synovial fluid. Sometimes it is helpful for doctors to remove the liquid (usually when giving a cortisone injection) to help the joint feel better. The doctor may send a sample to the lab to figure out the cause of arthritis. Normal synovial fluid contains less than 200 cells/mL.

SLE can cause inflammatory arthritis, associated with increased white blood cells. The inflamed joints' synovial fluid typically has WBC counts (or synovial fluid nucleated cell count) greater than 2,000 cells/mL. Lupus can also cause arthritis with minimal inflammation and cell counts between 200 and 2,000.

Tacrolimus Level (FK506). Tacrolimus is a drug used to treat lupus, especially lupus nephritis (kidney inflammation). Small doses are usually used, so measuring tacrolimus drug levels is not generally necessary to monitor its effectiveness or safety. Sometimes we measure it to ensure we are not giving too much tacrolimus and sometimes to make sure someone is taking the drug.

Thiopurine Methyltransferase Activity (TPMT). Doctors often obtain this test in people before prescribing the drug azathioprine (AZA, Imuran, chapter 32). The enzyme thiopurine methyltransferase breaks down AZA in the body to harmless compounds to reduce the chances of AZA hurting the body. Approximately 11% of people make a lower-than-normal amount of TPMT and are at higher risk for AZA side effects, such as bone marrow suppression (causing low blood cell counts) and liver damage. If the TPMT is reduced, then a lower dose of azathioprine may be used (or not at all). Blood counts and liver enzymes are also usually checked more closely.

Thyroid-Stimulating Hormone (Thyrotropin; TSH, 3rd Generation). The pituitary gland in the brain produces thyroid-stimulating hormone (TSH) and releases it into the bloodstream. TSH directs the thyroid gland (located under the Adam's apple region in the neck) to release thyroid hormones. TSH is the most useful test in detecting an underactive thyroid (hypothyroidism) or an overactive thyroid (hyperthyroidism). If the TSH is abnormal, a doctor can then order other thyroid function tests (such as T3 and T4 levels) to figure out whether the cause of the thyroid dysfunction is a problem with the thyroid gland itself or whether it is due to the brain releasing an abnormal amount of TSH. See chapter 17.

TPMT. See Thiopurine Methyltransferase Activity.

Troponin (Cardiac troponin, Troponin T, Troponin I). Troponins are heart muscle proteins not normally found in blood. When someone has recent heart muscle damage, blood troponin levels can increase. Troponin is usually measured to see if someone has had a recent heart attack (chapter 21). However, it can be useful in SLE patients to see if there is heart muscle inflammation (lupus myocarditis, chapter 11).

Biotin supplements might cause falsely low troponin levels. Biotin (vitamin B7) should be stopped three days before blood work.

TSH, 3rd Generation. See Thyroid-Stimulating Hormone.

Vitamin B12 (Cobalamin, B12). Doctors measure vitamin B12 levels in people with anemia or nerve problems because vitamin B12 deficiency can cause either (chapter 9). Nerve damage from vitamin B12 deficiency can cause tingling, muscle weakness, difficulty walking, memory loss, and irritability. Vitamin B12 deficiency can also contribute to osteoporosis.

If a vitamin B12 level is borderline or low-normal, someone might still have a B12 deficiency. In this case, the doctor may order a methylmalonic acid level and a homocysteine level, which would be elevated in vitamin B12 deficiency.

Vitamin D, 1, 25-Dihydroxy (Calcitriol; 1, 25 di-OH Vitamin D). Calcitriol is the active form of vitamin D. The kidneys produce it from calcidiol (25-hydroxy). Vitamin D, 1, 25 di-OH does not last long in the bloodstream and is unreliable when watching most vitamin D problems.

Vitamin D, 25-Hydroxy (Calcidiol, 25-Hydroxycalciferol, 25-OH-D). This is the most useful blood test for diagnosing and monitoring vitamin D problems. We usually aim for a level around 40 ng/mL to help lupus disease activity. See chapters 3, 35, and 38.

Immunology Tests

This list includes the immunologic labs most often ordered for SLE patients. The laboratory performs all these tests on blood samples. The tests usually appear on a laboratory results sheet under their actual names, rather than under the general heading of "Immunological Tests."

Note that various laboratories use different names for tests. One lab may label an anti-double-stranded DNA test "dsDNA Antibody." Another may label it "Anti-dsDNA."

There are several ways to refer to autoantibodies. Some labs and doctors use "anti-" before the antibody name (as in "anti-dsDNA") while others use "dsDNA antibody." Both are correct and mean the same. Some even use "anti-dsDNA antibody," Although this is redundant since "antibody" is not needed after anti-dsDNA.

To simplify the list that follows, if a test name can be used with or without the "anti-" prefix, we include it without the prefix. In other words, if your lab test shows that you have a positive "anti-Sm antibody," look under "Sm antibody" in this chapter. Alternative names appear in parentheses after each lab entry.

Antinuclear Antibody (ANA, FANA). This test shows elevated levels in almost everyone with SLE. It is rarely negative in newly diagnosed people with SLE when evaluated by the immunofluorescence assay (IFA) lab method using HEp-2 cells (explained below). ANA positivity fulfills one of the SLE classification criteria, and it is an absolute requirement for the newest ACR/EULAR 2019 criteria (chapter 1). If the test is negative (before treatment), an SLE diagnosis is unlikely. Although people with SLE have different organ problems, this is a common thread uniting almost all. Those ANA-negative SLE patients are usually positive for other antibodies such as anti-dsDNA or anti-SSA, or they have SLE from a genetic deficiency in complement levels (chapter 3).

The nucleus is the center structure of the body's cells that holds the genetic DNA and other molecules needed for DNA processing. People with SLE make antibodies aimed at various proteins/antigens found within the nucleus (including DNA). Antinuclear antibodies represent many different antibodies instead of just one antibody. Many of these are found in people without SLE. Up to 20% of healthy people are positive for ANA (depending upon the study and the ANA test used). ANA levels increase with age, occurring in up to 37% of healthy people older than 65.

Other disorders, such as other autoimmune diseases, liver disease, infections, and cancers, as well as some medicines, can cause positive ANAs. Most ANA-positive people do not have lupus. When someone is positive for ANA, it is essential to conduct other tests, including those measuring different autoantibodies, which are more suggestive of particular diseases. This helps decide whether the person has lupus, has another condition, is taking a medication known to cause a positive ANA, or (most commonly) that the ANA is not due to any disease at all.

Some autoantibodies that make up a positive ANA (such as anti-Sm, anti-ds DNA, and anti-ribosomal-P, which are specific for SLE) indicate certain diseases and are helpful in

LUPUS IN FOCUS

ANA should not be called the "lupus test"

The most common systemic autoimmune disorder in people positive for ANA is Sjögren's disease (chapter 14), not lupus. Since ANA is seen much more commonly in healthy individuals and those with Sjögren's, it should not be called the "lupus test."

making disease diagnoses. Other autoantibodies that produce a positive ANA, such as anti-single stranded DNA, are so common that they are unhelpful. Still others may be so common in many different autoimmune diseases, such as anti-SSA and anti-RNP, that they are not helpful in narrowing down one diagnosis, yet they increase the chances that the tested person may have an autoimmune disease as the cause of their problems.

There are several methods for testing antinuclear antibodies. The first is performed by various techniques lumped together as "solid phase immunoassays," including the multiplex immunoassay and the enzyme-linked immunosorbent assay (ELISA). Many insurance companies prefer these methods because they are relatively inexpensive. Laboratories like them because they are less time-consuming than the immunofluorescence assay (IFA) method described below. This trend is unfortunate because they are the least accurate methods.

The antinuclear antibody test using IFA has around 150 or more antigens (types of proteins) that ANA can be attracted to. The multiplex immunoassays detect only about 10 antigens. Up to 35% of people with SLE test negative using the multiplex immunoassay. The way to spot this less accurate method on your lab slip is to look for the words "ANA-D," "ANA Direct," "Antinuclear Antibodies Direct," "ANAchoice® Screen," or "ANA Screen," followed by a simple numerical result not containing a colon (:), as well as the words "negative," "positive," or "equivocal," and without including a pattern (described below).

The IFA is the "gold standard" for screening for SLE. With the current IFA that uses HEp-2 cells, it is rare to have newly diagnosed SLE and be negative for ANA.

HEp-2 stands for "Human Epidermoid tumor cell-line #2." In 1951, while working at the Sloan-Kettering Institute for Cancer Research in New York, Dr. Helene Toolan took cancer cells from a 57-year-old man with cancer of the windpipe (a laryngeal human epidermoid cell tumor) and implanted them under the skin of rats. She successfully kept the cells alive for many generations, allowing them to be used for research. She labeled his cancer cell specimen "H.Ep. #2" because it was the second human epidermoid cancer cells that she described in her 1954 research paper (H.Ep. #1 came from a different patient). These cells kept multiplying in the lab, essentially becoming immortal. Subsequent studies showed them highly beneficial for ANA testing. Today, HEp-2 cells also contain cervical cancer cells due to laboratory contamination in the 1950s or 1960s. Nonetheless, they are the most useful test for ANA.

The IFA ANA test applies the person's serum (the transparent liquid part of blood separated from the blood cells) to some HEp-2 cells on a microscope slide. If ANAs are present in the person's blood, they bind to antigens in the HEp-2 cells. The technician adds liquid holding specially treated immunoglobulins that bind to the ends of antibodies. Each immunoglobulin has a chemical that glows (fluoresces) under certain lights. These immunoglobulins attach to the ends of any antibodies that may have attached to cells on the slide.

When HEp-2 cells are viewed under the microscope, a yellowish-green glow on the cells indicates a positive ANA. If it is, another series of tests is performed. These involve adding a fluid to dilute the person's serum in several steps, using more fluid each time. When the technician adds an equal part of the diluting solution to the serum, the result is a 1:1 mix (or titer). When the lab technician adds a second equal amount of diluting solution, the result is a 1:2 titer; and so on. This method is repeated until the serum no long fluoresces under the microscope. The last titer in which the technician sees fluorescence is the final titer result. The more dilutions that can be made, the higher the titer number and the higher the ANA concentration.

Most labs consider a titer of 1:40 or 1:80 and higher to be a positive ANA. The higher the titer, the greater the chances are that the ANA is due to a disease such as SLE. For example, a person with an ANA of greater than 1:1280 is much more likely to have a systemic autoimmune condition (such as SLE) than an ANA of 1:80.

The glowing ANA can form different patterns. These can supply clues as to what antibodies may be causing the ANA. These patterns usually contribute little to diagnosing patients. Still, we discuss them since they do appear in the lab results.

The two most common patterns are diffuse (also called homogenous) and speckled. They appear under the microscope just as they sound. The diffuse pattern has fluorescent green filling up the entire nucleus, while the speckled pattern has many separate dots. DNA and histone antibodies often cause the diffuse pattern. Smith, RNP, SSA, and SSB antibodies can cause a speckled pattern. However, diffuse and speckled are the most common patterns in healthy people and are not useful.

Nuclear-dense, fine-speckled pattern ANA is a special type of pattern that may be important in the future. Research suggests that someone positive for this pattern but negative for other autoantibodies (like anti-dsDNA and anti-Smith) is unlikely to have SLE. If this research is confirmed, this could be a helpful test in the future. It's not yet commercially available.

Nucleolar pattern is completely different. Some describe it as looking like "puppy dog feet." Although it can be seen in SLE, it is more common in people with scleroderma (also called systemic sclerosis, chapter 2).

The centromere pattern is due to centromere antibodies commonly seen in systemic sclerosis with limited cutaneous involvement. This is a type of scleroderma (chapter 2) often called CREST (which stands for Calcium deposits, Raynaud's phenomenon, Esophageal dysmotility, Sclerodactyly, and Telangiectasias). However, centromere pattern can also be seen in SLE (see Centromere Antibody).

ANA levels do not reliably fluctuate with disease activity and usually do not help monitor SLE treatment, except when they become negative on treatment as discussed in the next section.

ANA-negative SLE. ANA-negativity and having SLE can occur in some situations. A negative ANA IFA using HEp-2 is unusual in patients newly diagnosed with SLE. Cases of newly diagnosed ANA-negative SLE patients were much more common before 1988 when ANA testing did not include HEp-2. Before 1988, approximately 5% of new cases of SLE were ANA-negative. With IFA using HEp-2, it occurs in less than 2%. ANA-negative SLE patients tend to have milder disease with higher rates of arthritis and malar (butterfly) rash and lower rates of nephritis (kidney inflammation) and to be older and more often Caucasian than ANA-positive patients.

There are multiple reasons for potentially being ANA-negative (table 4.3). One of the biggest problems is wide variability in ANA test kits' accuracy. Dr. David Pisetsky (a rheumatologist at Duke University in North Carolina) and colleagues did several studies evaluating multiple ANA test kits. The results varied widely, with 0.6% to 28% of SLE patients testing negative for ANA. This is too much variability to be acceptable. We try to prevent this potential problem of missing a diagnosis of SLE by ordering an added ANA

Table 4.3 Causes of Negative ANA by IFA (Using HEp-2) in SLE

- Variation in quality of the lab doing the testing
- Setting a value too high for positive results (for example, requiring ≥ 1:160 rather than ≥ 1:80)
- Intermittent ANA positivity (ANA can fluctuate between positive and negative in one individual)
- Having antibodies to proteins outside of the nucleus (in the cell's cytoplasm); lab often reports these anti-cytoplasmic antibodies as negative on ANA testing
- Having antibodies to proteins that appear while the cell is dividing (called mitotic antibodies); lab reports these as negative on ANA testing
- Low immunoglobulin levels
- Successful treatment in an SLE patient who was previously ANA positive

test that uses a different lab method (ELISA, or bead-based multiplex). This approach is supported by a 2020 Belgium study, which showed that testing two ANA's in a patient using different methods decreases the risk of missing the diagnosis. We also order other autoantibodies (anti-dsDNA, anti-SSA, and antiphospholipid antibodies) and request the AVISE Lupus Test (discussed later) when we have a strong suspicion of SLE in a patient negative for ANA.

Patients with cutaneous lupus (skin lupus) are usually ANA-positive in the presence of systemic lupus. A 2019 study at the University of Pennsylvania showed that 37% of their cutaneous lupus patients were ANA-negative.

The most common reason for someone with lupus being ANA-negative is treatment. Medications that better control SLE can cause ANA to become negative 20% to 30% of the time. This can cause problems when they see a new rheumatologist because of insurance changes or moving to a different area. We have had several SLE patients under excellent control seen by new rheumatologists elsewhere, and when newly drawn labs showed negative ANAs, the doctors stopped their medicines and told them they did not have SLE. Unfortunately, they had disease flares, including one with new-onset pulmonary hypertension, another with a severe lupus stroke, and another who developed lupus pneumonitis (lung inflammation). Patients should keep records of their first lab results and doctor's notes, as mentioned in chapter 1, to show this information to new doctors and prevent this from happening.

One study showed that SLE patients who become ANA-negative on treatment have fewer lupus flares than persistently ANA-positive patients. The previous edition of this book stated that ANA tests need not be repeat in SLE patients. However, since a negative result is a good sign (predicting fewer flares), repeat testing can be helpful.

Acetylcholine Receptor Antibodies (AChR-Ab). AChR-Abs are highly specific for the autoimmune muscle disease called myasthenia gravis (MG).

Actin Antibody. See Smooth Muscle Antibody.

What can I do if I think I may have lupus, but I'm told my ANA is negative?

Due to variations in the quality of lab results between laboratories plus the fact that ANA-negative lupus is rare, if you strongly feel that you could have lupus, ask your doctor to order an ANA test by a different lab technique (in other words, make sure it was done by both an IFA method and an ELISA or multiplex immunoassay method) and check for SSA antibody, dsDNA antibody, antiphospholipid antibodies (lupus anticoagulant, cardiolipin antibody, and beta-2 glycoprotein I antibody), plus get the AVISE Lupus test (discussed later in this chapter). If all of these are negative, your doctors should search for an alternative reason for your symptoms.

ADAMTS13 Activity Level. ADAMTS13 is a shortening of "**A**-**D**isintegrin **A**nd **M**etalloprotease with a **T**hrombospondin type 1 motif, member 13." This blood test is used to help diagnose thrombotic angiopathies (chapter 9). It is ordered primarily on very sick hospitalized patients. ADAMTS13 is important for preventing too much blood clotting. Severely low levels (most often defined as < 10%) cause a potentially deadly thrombotic angiopathy called thrombotic thrombocytopenic purpura (TTP, chapter 9).

ANCA. See Neutrophil Cytoplasmic Antibodies.

Aquaporin-4-IgG Antibody (AQP4-IgG Antibody, Neuromyelitis optica-IgG Antibody, NMO-IgG Antibody). AQP4-IgG antibody occurs in a condition called neuromyelitis optica spectrum syndrome, which causes spinal cord and brain inflammation. This can manifest as longitudinal transverse myelitis, inflammation of the main nerve that goes to the eye (optic neuritis), and areas of brain inflammation. The antibody attacks an important protein called aquaporin-4, which is found on nerve cell surfaces and is important for water flow in and out of the cell. This antibody is positive in most patients with this nerve problem. Sometimes, it can be negative at first, so repeating the blood test in suspicious cases should be done. Levels of AQP4-IgG antibodies tends to fluctuate with disease activity and can become negative after successful treatment.

ß-2 Glycoprotein I Antibodies (Beta-2 Glycoprotein I Antibodies, Anti-ß-2 Glycoprotein I, and ß-2 GPI). Beta-2 GPI (ß is the Greek letter "beta") is one of the antiphospholipid antibodies (see cardiolipin antibody and chapters 9 and 18). Its presence in undifferentiated connective tissue disease (chapter 2) increases the chances of developing SLE. Beta-2 GPI fulfills one of the SLE classification criteria (see chapter 1).

C1q. Complements are essential immune system proteins important in fighting off infections. Each is given a number based upon the order in which it was discovered, starting with C1 complement in 1907. C1 is broken down into fragments during the fight against bacteria and foreign invaders; C1q is one of those fragments. Very low levels can sometimes indicate C1q deficiency, which can cause lupus and increased infections (chapter 3).

C1q Antibody (anti-C1q). Anti-C1q occurs in 25% to 50% of SLE patients (depending on the population studied). Up to 4% of healthy middle-aged people and 18% of those older than 70 can also be anti-C1q-positive. It can occasionally be seen in other systemic autoimmune disorders and hepatitis C infections. Its presence in undifferentiated connective tissue disease (chapter 2) increases the chances of developing SLE.

In SLE patients with hypocomplementemic urticarial vasculitis (HCUV, chapter 8), anti-C1q is always present. It is believed to cause the skin inflammation in HCUV.

The antibody can directly cause kidney inflammation (lupus nephritis), especially in the most severe forms of class III and class IV (chapter 12). Most lupus nephritis patients are positive for C1q antibody (close to 100% of class III and IV in one study). The combination of anti-C1q, dsDNA antibody, and low C3 or C4 complement levels is highly predictive of developing class III or class IV lupus nephritis. SLE patients who are positive for anti-C1q are twice as likely to develop lupus nephritis than anti-C1q-negative patients. The urine-protein creatinine ratio, anti-dsDNA, and C3 and C4 complement levels should be watched closely in anti-C1q-positive patients to look for possible lupus nephritis.

One of the best uses of the C1q antibody is in monitoring lupus nephritis. The level can increase two to six months before a lupus nephritis flare. Levels also tend to decrease significantly with successful lupus nephritis treatment. Although most rheumatologists monitor lupus nephritis with anti-dsDNA and C3 and C4 complement levels, some studies suggest anti-C1q may be more reliable.

C3. See Complement C3.

C4. See Complement C4.

C-ANCA. See Cytoplasmic ANCA.

Carbamylated Protein Antibody (Anti-CarP). Anti-CarP is present in about one-third of patients with rheumatoid arthritis (RA). While RA is easier to diagnose when patients are positive for rheumatoid factor or CCP antibody, some RA patients test negative for these and have a condition called seronegative RA. In these seronegative RA patients, 17% to 25% are anti-CarP-positive. Those who are tend to have worse arthritis (more bone destruction) and may be at increased risk for heart attacks and strokes.

Anti-CarP can be seen in 30% to 50% of SLE patients (depending upon the lab). Low blood cell counts and kidney inflammation (lupus nephritis) may be less common in anti-CarP-positive SLE patients. A 2018 Italian study found CarP antibodies in half of their SLE arthritis patients; it was much less common in those without SLE arthritis. Another large European study showed that CarP-positive SLE patients were more likely to have erosive arthritis (in which the arthritis is severe, causing bone destruction).

Cardiolipin Antibodies (Anticardiolipin Antibodies, ACA, ACLA). Cardiolipin is a fatty molecule (called a phospholipid) initially discovered in animal hearts in the 1940s.

Cardio- comes from the Greek word for "heart." Cardiolipin antibodies are a type of anti-phospholipid antibody (aPLA, chapter 9).

About 30% to 55% of people with SLE are ACA-positive. Cardiolipin antibodies appear as IgG, IgM, or IgA anticardiolipin antibodies. Close to 20% of SLE patients are positive for aPLAs for an average of 3 years (up to 7.5 years) before being diagnosed with lupus. These patients tend to have more severe disease with an increased chance for antiphospholipid syndrome (APS), lupus nephritis (chapter 12), and neuropsychiatric lupus (chapter 13).

Antiphospholipid syndrome (APS, chapters 9 and 18) is a condition in which aPLAs cause blood clots or recurrent miscarriages. Approximately 50% of SLE patients with antiphospholipid antibodies (such as ACAs) may get blood clots or have recurrent miscarriages due to APS. High IgG ACA levels are especially associated with blood clots, but they can also occur with IgM and IgA ACAs. A positive IgM ACA may also increase the risk of hemolytic anemia.

ACAs fulfill one of the SLE classification criteria(see chapter 1).

CarP antibody. See Carbamylated Protein Antibody.

CCP Antibodies. See Cyclic Citrullinated Peptide Antibodies.

Centromere Antibody (Anticentromere Antibody, ACA, anti-CENP). ACAs are commonly seen in a systemic autoimmune disease called systemic sclerosis (scleroderma), especially a form called systemic sclerosis with limited cutaneous involvement or CREST syndrome. They also occur in 2% of people with SLE; many of those patients do not show evidence of scleroderma.

CH50 (Total Hemolytic Complement, CH_{50}, 50% Hemolytic Complement Activity, Total Complement Activity). Complements are immune system proteins that work with antibodies and white blood cells to attack and destroy invading organisms (such as bacteria). CH50 measures how well nine complement proteins (C1–C9) work together. If any of these complements are significantly too low, or not working correctly, the CH50 will be low. The CH50 level can decrease in some people with active SLE and fulfills one of the SLE classification criteria (chapter 1).

Note: the "H" in CH50 stands for hemolytic. The test measures how well a person's complements (the "C" in CH50), as measured from a blood sample, destroy sheep red blood cells (RBCs) in the laboratory. The scientific name for the destruction of RBCs is hemolysis.

A low CH50 level can also be seen in an immune system disease called IgG4-related disease. This condition can cause autoimmune pancreatitis, lymphadenopathy (swollen lymph glands), inflammation of large arteries, pneumonitis (lung inflammation), nephritis (kidney inflammation), inflammation of the liver (hepatitis), and swollen parotid glands (salivary glands). Since SLE can also cause these problems along with a low CH50, doctors must consider the possibilities of both SLE and IgG4-related disease in these patients.

A genetic deficiency in producing complement proteins C2, C3, or C4 can sometimes cause SLE (see chapter 1). A normal CH50 level indicates that C2, C3, or C4 deficiency is not a cause of someone's SLE.

Chromatin Antibody (Anti-Chromatin Antibody; Nucleosome Antibody). Chromatin refers to the complex of DNA and other proteins within each chromosome in the nuclei of cells. Chromatin is like the yarn of wool in a sock (with the sock being the chromosome). If you were to unravel a long string of yarn from the sock, that is what the chromatin would resemble. About 60% to 70% of people with SLE are positive for anti-chromatin. Anti-chromatin-positive SLE patients may be at increased risk for kidney inflammation (lupus nephritis).

Anti-chromatin can occur in other systemic autoimmune diseases (especially drug-induced lupus, mixed connective tissue disease, and scleroderma), but much less often than in SLE.

Sometimes it can be difficult to tell if a patient may have SLE or Sjögren's disease when they first come to a rheumatologist. One study showed that if that patient is positive for chromatin and SSA antibodies, they most likely have SLE.

In some people with SLE, chromatin antibodies fluctuate with disease activity, decreasing in value when there is better control of lupus.

Complement C2 (Complement Component C2). Complements are immune system proteins that work with antibodies and white blood cells to attack and destroy invading organisms (such as bacteria). Doctors generally do not monitor C2 in SLE, although they may request the test to look for C2-deficiency, a genetic cause of SLE.

Complement C3 (C3, Complement Component C3). Complements are immune system proteins that work with antibodies and white blood cells to attack and destroy invading organisms (such as bacteria). The immune system of some people with SLE will use up C3 or C4 during the immune activation process. This can cause C3 and C4 blood levels to decrease. For example, in someone whose C3 or C4 levels consistently drop during disease flares and improve during disease control, it can be helpful to monitor these levels. It is especially useful in monitoring some people with lupus nephritis (kidney inflammation).

In most people with lupus, C3 and C4 do not change much with disease activity. C3 and C4 decrease during active lupus disease but can be replenished quickly by the body, causing the levels to become normal or even elevated even when SLE is very active. In these individuals, measuring a different type of complement called EC4d, a cell-bound complement activation product (discussed later in this chapter), may be more helpful. Low C3 and C4 fulfill one of the SLE classification criteria (chapter 1).

In patients who otherwise appear to be doing well, progressively decreasing C3 or C4 might signal a potential upcoming flare, especially if associated with rising anti-dsDNA. Low C3 or C4 in someone with undifferentiated connective tissue disease (chapter 2) increases the chances of developing SLE.

C3 and C4 can increase during nonspecific inflammation. However, high levels have not been shown to be helpful when treating lupus patients.

Increased estradiol (a female hormone) causes higher liver production of C3 and C4 during pregnancy. If these levels do not rise during pregnancy, that can be a sign of active SLE during pregnancy and can indicate an increased risk for pregnancy complications such as preeclampsia.

Low C3 and C4 can also be seen in an immune disease called IgG4-related disease. See CH50.

Complement C4 (C4, Complement Component C4). See Complement C3.

Cryoglobulins. Cryo- comes from the Greek word for "cold" and refers to immune system molecules (called immunoglobulins) that clump together (precipitate) when the blood becomes cooler. Cryoglobulins can form in people with SLE and high disease activity. Cryoglobulin-positive SLE patients tend to have an increased chance of lupus kidney inflammation (nephritis) and vasculitis (blood vessel inflammation). Cryoglobulins can be seen under the microscope inside the kidneys of lupus nephritis patients, suggesting they may directly play a role in kidney inflammation.

Cyclic Citrullinated Peptide Antibodies (Anti-CCP Antibody, CCP IgG Antibodies, CCP Antibody). Doctors most commonly use the CCP antibody test to diagnose rheumatoid arthritis. Up to 25% of people with SLE are also CCP-positive and are more likely to have arthritis and joint bone erosions (destroyed bone next to joints, visible on x-ray and ultrasonography). These findings are more typical of rheumatoid arthritis than lupus arthritis. CCP-positive SLE patients who have arthritis and bone erosions may have an overlap of rheumatoid arthritis and lupus (called "rhupus").

Cytoplasmic ANCA (c-ANCA, C-Anti-Neutrophil Cytoplasmic Antibody). ANCA are assessed in the lab using the IFA method, as is ANA IFA discussed earlier. However, neutrophils are used instead of HEp-2 cells. See Neutrophil Cytoplasmic Antibody for the definition of ANCA.

C-ANCA describes ANCA where the staining (or glow) seen under the microscope by the lab technician occurs throughout the cytoplasm (the area between the nucleus and the outer cell wall). It is usually caused by PR3-ANCA (but not always).

Dilute Russell's Viper Venom Test. See Lupus Anticoagulant.

DNA (Single-Stranded) Antibodies (Anti-ss DNA, ss-DNA Antibodies). DNA, or deoxyribonucleic acid, is the genetic code contained in the nuclei of the body's cells. It is composed of two strands of proteins twisted around each other, which form double-stranded DNA. If the two strands are separated, each one is called single-stranded DNA. Although antibodies that identify just the single strands (in other words, anti-single-stranded DNA) appear in 70% of SLE patients, they also appear in many other disorders, including non-rheumatologic conditions and healthy individuals. They are unhelpful in the care of SLE patients.

dsDNA Antibody (Anti-dsDNA Antibody, Anti-Double-Stranded DNA Antibody, DNA (DS) AB, Anti-Native DNA). DNA (deoxyribonucleic acid) is the genetic code contained in the nuclei of the body's cells. It is composed of two strands of proteins twisted around each other, which form double-stranded-DNA (also known as native DNA). Antibodies directed toward this DNA structure appear in 40% to 80% SLE patients (depending on the laboratory method and the patient population studied).

Anti-dsDNA is a specific blood test for SLE (meaning that a positive test is not common in people without SLE). Anti-dsDNA positivity fulfills one of the SLE classification criteria (chapter 1). However, it can occasionally be seen in other systemic autoimmune diseases (especially Sjögren's disease and drug-induced lupus). Its presence in someone with undifferentiated connective tissue disease (chapter 2) increases the chances of that person developing SLE.

In addition to helping diagnose SLE, it helps monitor treatment. In some people, anti-dsDNA may rise during periods of lupus activity and decline when the person is better. Some SLE patients can have a high anti-dsDNA months before lupus flares. A progressively increasing anti-dsDNA level might signal a potential flare in patients who otherwise appear to be doing well, especially if it is associated with a decreasing C3 or C4 level or increasing EC4d.

Some people can have elevated anti-dsDNA levels that do not fluctuate with disease activity. It usually takes some time for the doctor to determine whether monitoring these levels is useful in the individual patient.

Anti-dsDNA SLE patients are at increased risk of having lupus nephritis (kidney inflammation) or vasculitis (blood vessel inflammation). This does not mean that they will develop either. Instead, a positive result tells the doctor to pay closer attention to these possibilities.

There are several different ways to measure anti-dsDNA antibodies. These include ELISA (discussed earlier in the ANA section), Farr radioimmunoassay, chemiluminescence immunoassay (CIA), and the *Crithidia luciliae* immunofluorescence assay. ELISA anti-dsDNA is the least helpful because it can be positive more often in non-lupus disorders.

The Crithidia test is one of the most specific for SLE (in other words, it is rarely found in people who do not have SLE). However, it can miss some people with SLE (in other words, it can be negative in someone with SLE while another method for anti-dsDNA may be positive).

Anti-dsDNA by the CIA and Farr methods may be the best methods for monitoring lupus disease activity. However, patients vary greatly regarding which anti-dsDNA methods they are positive for and which method most predictably reflects their lupus disease activity. Therefore, I tend to measure several different methods for anti-dsDNA to assess how they fluctuate with the patient's disease over time and eventually choose the method that is most useful. Although, overall, ELISA anti-dsDNA may be the least helpful, I have patients who are negative for all the other anti-dsDNA tests but are positive for ELISA anti-dsDNA, which fluctuates predictably with their disease activity.

Anti-dsDNA levels are rarely seen in drug-induced lupus (DIL). Elevated levels might occur in DIL due to minocycline, propylthiouracil, quinidine, and tumor necrosis factor inhibitors (like adalimumab [Humira], etanercept [Enbrel], and infliximab [Remicade]).

Biotin supplements can interfere with test results' accuracy when anti-dsDNA is measured using some multiplex immunoassays. Biotin (vitamin B7) should be stopped three days before blood work.

ENA (Extractable Nuclear Antibodies). See Extractable Nuclear Antibodies.

Endomysial Antibody (IgA Endomysial Assay, Endomysium Antibody, EMA). This is useful in diagnosing an autoimmune disease called celiac disease, which is an allergic-type reaction triggered by dietary gluten. It can cause difficulty with intestinal absorption of nutrients. In patients with SLE, 5% to 14% are EMA-positive, but most do not have celiac disease. Testing for IgA tissue transglutaminase antibodies is a more reliable blood test for diagnosing celiac disease in SLE. See also Tissue Transglutaminase Antibody.

Extractable Nuclear Antibodies (Anti-ENA, Antiextractable Nuclear Antibodies, ENA). These are antibodies directed at the protein antigens in the extract of cells. "Extract" is a laboratory term used because salt extraction isolates the nuclear proteins these antibodies identify. Many different proteins/antigens in this extract can cause autoantibody formation. ENAs include anti-RNP, anti-Smith, anti-SSA, anti-SSB, anti-Jo 1, anti-Scl 70, and others. However, some laboratories reserve this term for anti-RNP and anti-Smith antibodies. See RNP Antibody and Smith Antibody.

False-Positive Syphilis Test. See Rapid Plasma Reagin Test and Venereal Disease Research Laboratory Test.

Fluorescent Treponemal Antibody Absorption Test (Treponema Pallidum Antibodies, FTA-Ab, FTA-ABS). This test identifies people infected with syphilis (a sexually transmitted disease). The screening tests for syphilis are usually the rapid plasma reagin (RPR) and venereal disease research laboratory (VDRL) tests. If either is positive, it is mandatory to conduct a confirmatory test such as the FTA-Ab.

If someone is positive for RPR or VDRL yet negative for FTA-Ab, this is called a false positive syphilis test, and the person does not have syphilis. False positive syphilis tests can occur in people with antiphospholipid antibodies as well as in SLE patients. False-positive syphilis tests fulfill one of the SLE classification criteria (chapter 1).

Gamma Globulins. See Serum Protein Electrophoresis.

Gastric Parietal Cell Antibody. See Parietal Cell Antibody.

Gliadin Antibody (Anti-Gliadin Antibody, Gliadin Antibody Profile). Anti-gliadin antibody is often used to help diagnose an autoimmune disorder called celiac disease, which causes the intestines not to absorb nutrients correctly. However, about 23% of SLE patients are positive for anti-gliadin antibodies without having celiac disease or other disease associations. Anti-gliadin does not help diagnose celiac disease in SLE patients. Tissue Transglutaminase Antibody IgA is the most reliable blood test.

H2a/H2b Antibody. See Histone Antibodies.

H3 Antibody. See Histone Antibodies.

H4 Antibody. See Histone Antibodies.

Histone Antibodies (Anti-Histone, H2a/H2b Antibody, H3 Antibody, and H4 Antibody). Histones are protein complexes that work with the DNA in your cells' nuclei (center). Anti-histone occurs in 50% to 70% of SLE patients. They also appear in other systemic autoimmune diseases but are mostly used in diagnosing drug-induced lupus (DIL; chapter 1). Anti-histone positivity does not mean that someone has DIL. It merely means that it is possible. SLE (not caused by a drug) is a more common cause of anti-histone than DIL.

A negative anti-histone does not necessarily mean that someone doesn't have DIL. Histone antibodies are seen in less than half the cases of DIL caused by minocycline, propylthiouracil, and quinidine.

Hydroxychloroquine, whole blood (HCQ, whole blood levels). Not taking hydroxychloroquine (HCQ, Plaquenil) regularly can result in low blood levels, worse lupus disease activity, more frequent flares, and progressive, permanent organ damage. This blood test can show us which patients are not taking their medication as prescribed. When nonadherent patients are found, we can determine what prevents them from taking their medication regularly and help figure out how to improve adherence. Studies show that when HCQ is taken regularly and the blood level improves, disease activity improves (in other words, the patient gets better), decreasing the need for steroids and stronger medicines.

The science in using HCQ levels optimally is in its infancy. Studies are being performed to determine the best blood levels to control lupus disease and prevent side effects. Levels of 1000 to 1200 ng/mL are optimal (but levels as high as 1500 to 2000 ng/mL may be acceptable).

IFE. See Immunoelectrophoresis.

Immunoelectrophoresis (IFE). This blood test is ordered when elevated suspicious immunoglobulins are detected on the serum protein electrophoresis (SPEP). If an elevation of one type of immunoglobulin is seen (called a monoclonal protein), the IFE can help categorize what type of monoclonal protein it is.

Immunoglobulin A (IgA). "Immunoglobulin" is another name for "antibody." The immunoglobulins are divided into five major classes (A, D, E, G, and M). IgA is essential for fighting off infections in the moist skin (called the mucosa) lining of the sinuses, nose, mouth, and inner ears down to the lungs. People with low levels can potentially have higher rates of infections in these areas. Low IgA levels indicate IgA deficiency and is an immunodeficiency (chapter 22). It can be genetic and occurs more commonly in people with autoimmune diseases, such as SLE. Immunosuppressants (table 22.1), especially rituximab and cyclosporin, can also cause IgA deficiency.

Immunoglobulin E (IgE). Immunoglobulins are discussed under Immunoglobulin A. Measuring IgE levels is not usually helpful in SLE. IgE is most important in allergic reactions. A high IgE level can be seen in people with allergies (such as to pollen, animals, and drugs), which often cause asthma, itchy eyes, runny nose, and hives.

Immunoglobulin G (IgG). Immunoglobulins are discussed under Immunoglobulin A. IgG is the primary immunoglobulin that helps fight infections from bacteria and viruses. High levels can be seen in SLE during immune system overactivity. IgG can decrease during periods of less disease activity. In patients with undifferentiated connective tissue disease, an elevated IgG increases the chances of its evolving to SLE or Sjögren's disease.

IgG can be low (hypogammaglobulinemia) in people with some immunodeficiency disorders, increasing infection risks. SLE patients are at increased risk of immunodeficiency disorders involving IgG, such as common variable immunodeficiency. However, some medicines used to treat lupus (especially steroids, hydroxychloroquine, immunosuppressants, and the medications used to treat seizures) can also reduce IgG.

Immunoglobulin G4 (IgG4, IgG subclass 4). Immunoglobulins are discussed under Immunoglobulin A. IgG4 is a subclass of IgG. Measuring IgG4 levels is most important to help diagnose a disorder called IgG4-related disease. This disorder can occasionally look like lupus in that it can cause pancreatic inflammation (autoimmune pancreatitis), lymphadenopathy (swollen lymph glands), vasculitis, pneumonitis (lung inflammation), nephritis (kidney inflammation), inflammation of the liver (hepatitis), and swollen parotid glands (salivary glands). IgG4-related disease can also cause low C3, C4, and CH50 complement levels. IgG4 levels are elevated in most but not all people with IgG4-related disease.

Immunoglobulin G subclasses (IgG 1, 2, 3, 4). Immunoglobulins are discussed under Immunoglobulin A. IgG is further broken down into four subclasses. Measuring these is primarily helpful in finding patients with normal total IgG levels but with recurrent infections due to a deficiency of one of the subclasses. IgG2 subclass deficiency may be more common in people with SLE.

Immunoglobulin M (IgM). Immunoglobulins are discussed under Immunoglobulin A. Low IgM can increase the risk for infections. Low IgM can be due to inherited immunodeficiency disorders such as common variable immunodeficiency and selective IgM deficiency (both occur more often in SLE). In addition, immunosuppressants (table 22.1), especially rituximab, can lower IgM.

Intrinsic Factor Blocking Antibody (IF-Blocking Antibody). IF-blocking antibody is used to diagnose pernicious anemia (PA), an autoimmune disease. PA reduces vitamin B12 absorption, leading to vitamin B12 deficiency and possible nerve and red blood cell problems (chapter 9). Although it is positive only in 60% to 70% of people with PA, a positive result is diagnostic.

La Antibody (Anti-La). See SSB.

Liver-Kidney Microsomal-1 Antibodies (ALKM-1). These antibodies are used to help diagnose patients with autoimmune hepatitis (AIH). It is not common in SLE unless the person also has AIH.

Lupus Anticoagulant (Dilute Russell's Viper Venom Test, PTT-LA with Reflex to Hexagonal Phase Return, dRVVT with Mixing Study, LAC, dRVVT, Kaolin Clot Time). LAC is one of the antiphospholipid antibodies (see Cardiolipin Antibody and chapter 9).

Approximately 30% of people with SLE are LAC-positive, and roughly half of them may develop blood clots. LAC fulfills one of the SLE classification criteria (chapter 1). A Mexican study showed that LAC-positive SLE patients who were also positive for anti-RNP had a higher risk of blood clots than anti-RNP-negative patients.

The term "lupus anticoagulant" is confusing because a coagulant is a substance that causes blood clots (coagulated liquid becomes thicker) and fewer bleeding problems. An *anti*-coagulant should do the opposite (decrease clotting and increase bleeding). However, LAC increases the risk of blood clots rather than excessive bleeding (opposite of how it sounds). The "coagulant" part of the name comes from how the antibodies function in the lab. People with a high result on a test called partial thromboplastin time (PTT) bleed too easily. In the 1940s and 1950s, doctors noted that some people with SLE had elevated PTT levels. However, instead of bleeding too easily, they had dangerous blood clots. LAC interferes with the PTT lab reaction, giving artificially elevated PTT results while increasing blood clotting problems.

Microsomal Antibody (Antithyroid Microsomal Antibody). See Anti-Thyroid Peroxidase Antibody.

Mitochondrial Antibody (AMA). AMA occurs in primary biliary cirrhosis, which is rare in SLE. Yet, AMA occurs in one-third of SLE patients and may be more common in lupus nephritis.

Monoclonal Protein (M-Spike, M Protein). On serum protein electrophoresis (SPEP), if one immunoglobulin type (or more precisely, a clone) is elevated, it is reported as an "M-spike." It denotes a monoclonal protein (monoclonal gammopathy; chapter 9).

LUPUS IN FOCUS

Russell's viper venom

A common method for detecting LAC is using Russell's viper (from India) venom. This venom is one of the deadliest in the world. It causes the blood to clot and kills more people in India than the venom from any other snake.

The lab technician mixes Russell's viper venom with the patient's serum and phospholipid. The venom requires phospholipids to clot. However, if the person has phospholipid antibodies (LAC in this case), they bind to the phospholipids and prevent the venom from using them to clot. Clotting takes longer than expected, making the test positive for LAC.

MPO-ANCA (Myeloperoxidase-ANCA). See Neutrophil Cytoplasmic Antibody.

MuSK Antibodies. MuSK antibodies are very specific for the autoimmune muscle disease called myasthenia gravis (MG), meaning that they rarely occur in people without MG.

Neutrophil Cytoplasmic Antibodies (ANCA, Anti-Neutrophil Cytoplasmic Antibodies). Anti-neutrophil cytoplasmic antibodies (ANCAs) detect proteins found outside the nuclei (in the cytoplasm) of neutrophils and monocytes (types of white blood cells). ANCAs are most often useful in diagnosing a group of diseases called vasculitis (especially two called granulomatosis with polyangiitis and microscopic polyangiitis). They also occur in 15% to 20% of SLE patients.

There are two major types of ANCA—PR3-ANCA (proteinase 3-ANCA) and MPO-ANCA (myeloperoxidase-ANCA). PR3-ANCA is most common in the vasculitis syndrome called granulomatosis with polyangiitis. The MPO-ANCA is most common in the one called microscopic polyangiitis. Both vasculitides (the plural of "vasculitis") have an increased chance of causing severe kidney disease.

ANCA-positive lupus nephritis (kidney inflammation) patients may be at increased risk of more severe disease than ANCA-negative patients. A 2019 Chinese study showed that lupus nephritis patients were twice as likely to be MPO-positive than PR3-positive. Those with MPO-ANCA had more severe kidney disease and were more likely to go into kidney failure requiring dialysis than PR3-ANCA-positive patients. An earlier study from India showed that PR3-ANCA-positive lupus nephritis patients also tended to have more severe kidney disease.

Although rare, ANCA positivity can be seen in drug-induced lupus, especially those with kidney inflammation (nephritis).

NMO-IgG Antibody (Neuromyelitis Optica-IgG Antibody). See Aquaporin-4-IgG Antibody.

Nucleosome Antibody. See Chromatin Antibody.

Parietal Cell Antibody (Gastric Parietal Cell Antibody, APCA). APCA is most often seen in patients with gastritis (stomach inflammation) or pernicious anemia (an autoimmune disease causing vitamin B12 deficiency due to decreased stomach absorption of vitamin B12). APCA does not occur more commonly in SLE patients.

Perinuclear ANCA (p-ANCA, Perinuclear-Anti-Neutrophil Cytoplasmic Antibody). ANCA is assessed in the lab using the IFA method, as is ANA IFA discussed earlier. However, neutrophils are used instead of HEp-2 cells. See Neutrophil Cytoplasmic Antibody for the definition of ANCA.

P-ANCA is the term used to describe ANCA where the staining (or glow) seen under the microscope occurs around the nucleus of the cells (and does not extend throughout the cytoplasm as in C-ANCA). It is usually caused by MPO-ANCA (but not always).

Phosphatidylserine Antibody (Antiphosphatidylserine Antibody). This is one of the antiphospholipid antibodies (chapter 9). It appears in one-third of people with SLE and 50% to 75% of patients with antiphospholipid syndrome (APS). However, this antibody is not as predictive for blood clots as lupus anticoagulant. As of 2023, it is not included in the classification criteria for APS.

Phospholipase A2 Receptor Autoantibodies (PLA2R Antibodies, Anti-PLA2R). Anti-PLA2R helps diagnose a kidney disease called primary membranous nephropathy. They have not been studied much in lupus, but a 2019 Spanish study did show that 5% of SLE patients were positive for anti-PLA2R and that 20% of patients with lupus membranous nephritis (chapter 12) were positive for this antibody. Anti-PLA2R levels decreased with treatment, but these patients did not respond as well to therapy as did PLA2R-negative patients. The PLA2R-positive patients also had an increased risk for kidney failure requiring dialysis. More studies are needed to assess the usefulness of anti-PLA2R in SLE.

PM-Scl Antibody (Anti-PM-Scl, Anti PM-1). PM-Scl antibody is seen mostly in polymyositis, dermatomyositis, and scleroderma patients. It is one of the potential causes of a nucleolar pattern ANA. A 2016 Spanish study showed that anti-PM-Scl-positive SLE patients were more likely to have Raynaud's phenomenon.

Interstitial lung disease (lung scarring or pulmonary fibrosis) is common in patients with anti-PM-Scl-positive disorders. It would be prudent to get a chest x-ray, pulmonary function tests, and a high-resolution chest CT in someone with positive anti-PM-Scl and pulmonary symptoms (cough, shortness of breath, or an abnormal lung exam on physical examination).

PR3-ANCA (Proteinase 3-ANCA). See Neutrophil Cytoplasmic Antibody.

PTT-LA with Reflex to Hexagonal Phase Return. See Lupus Anticoagulant.

Rapid Plasma Reagin Test (Nontreponemal Test, Serologic Test for Syphilis, RPR, STS). RPR and the Venereal Disease Research Laboratory Test (VDRL) are screening tests for syphilis, a sexually transmitted disease due to the bacteria *Treponema pallidum*. However, it is possible to be positive for these tests but not have syphilis. If the RPR or VDRL is positive, a doctor must do a confirmatory syphilis test, such as the fluorescent treponemal absorption antibody test (FTA-Ab) or the *Treponema pallidum* particle agglutination test (TPPAT). If the FTA-Ab or TPPAT is positive, then that person has been infected with syphilis.

If either is negative, the person does not have syphilis but has a false positive syphilis test. This occurs in 15% to 30% of people with SLE. False-positive syphilis tests occur in the laboratory due to antiphospholipid antibodies (chapter 9). A false-positive syphilis test fulfills one of the SLE classification criteria (chapter 1).

RF, RF IgA, RF IgG, or RF IgM. See Rheumatoid Factor.

Rheumatoid Arthritis Factor. See Rheumatoid Factor.

Rheumatoid Factor (Rheumatoid Arthritis Factor, RA Factor, RA Latex Turbid, RA Latex, RF Titer, RF, RF IgA, RF IgG, and RF IgM). Immunoglobulins are immune system proteins that identify foreign proteins or antigens and protect the body. Rheumatoid factor is an immunoglobulin that attaches to other immunoglobulins. Rheumatoid factor may play an essential role in the healthy immune system by clearing away unwanted immunoglobulins. Therefore, many healthy people are RF-positive. Doctors most commonly use rheumatoid factor to help diagnose rheumatoid arthritis (RA). Approximately 85% of people with rheumatoid arthritis are RF-positive.

Elevated RF occurs in many inflammatory diseases, including infections, cancers, liver diseases, lung diseases, and other autoimmune disorders such as SLE. Of people with SLE, 20% to 30% are RF-positive. Some reports suggest that high RF levels may decrease the chances of having lupus nephritis (kidney inflammation). RF positivity also appears to be more common in SLE patients with pulmonary hypertension, vasculitis, and serositis, and those with overlap syndrome with RA or Sjögren's. Very high RF is most often seen in Sjögren's disease, cryoglobulinemia, hepatitis C, and rheumatoid arthritis.

Ribosomal-P Antibody (Anti-P). Ribosomal-P antibody is the most specific blood test for SLE (more than Smith and dsDNA antibodies). In other words, ribosomal-P antibody–positive people rarely do not have SLE. Between 10% and 35% of people with SLE are anti-P-positive, but the percentage may be as high as 40% to 50% in Asians and pediatric SLE.

Anti-P-positive SLE patients are especially at increased risk of developing liver inflammation (lupus hepatitis). A meta-analysis study showed that anti-P-positive SLE patients have a 744% greater odds of having lupus hepatitis than anti-P-negative patients. However, most anti-P-positive patients do not develop hepatitis.

Although some anti-P-positive patients are at increased risk of severe depression and psychosis (hallucinations, delusional thoughts, and disorientation), most are not. There are various ways to measure anti-P in the lab. Many methods do not have an association with depression and psychosis, while others, such as those recognizing the C-terminal 22 peptide, do.

Other problems that may occur in anti-P-positive patients include malar (butterfly) rash, mouth sores, sun sensitivity, and lupus nephritis.

RNA Polymerase III Antibody (RNAP III, anti-RNAP3). Anti-RNAP3 is usually seen in scleroderma (chapter 2). Anti-RNAP3-positive scleroderma patients are at high risk for

LUPUS IN FOCUS

How someone with SLE can be mistakenly diagnosed with rheumatoid arthritis

RF occurs in 30% of SLE patients, and inflammatory arthritis is one of the most common lupus problems. SLE can initially cause arthritis that can look like RA (and no other problems initially) while also producing RF. The person could meet criteria for RA and be diagnosed with RA. Other issues that clue the doctor into realizing that the person has SLE instead may slowly emerge occur over time, leading the doctor to realize it was lupus all along. Another possibility is that the person may have both (rhupus).

severe kidney damage (scleroderma renal crisis). One small study showed that one of three anti-RNAP3-positive SLE patients had scleroderma-like features. However, anti-RNAP3 is uncommon in SLE.

RNP Antibody (Anti-Ribonucleic Protein, Anti-RNP, Anti-Sm/RNP, Anti-Mo, U1RNP antibody). This is not to be confused with anti-U3RNP (seen in myositis).

Anti-RNP is often included as one of the extractable nuclear antibodies (ENA) by some laboratories. It appears in 30% to 60% of SLE patients (depending on the study population and laboratory). Anti-RNP increases the risk of having esophageal dysmotility (chapter 15), myocarditis (chapter 11), Raynaud's (chapter 11), lung inflammation, pulmonary hypertension (chapter 10), brain inflammation, low white blood cell counts, arthritis, and myositis (chapter 7). RNP-positive SLE patients may have a lower risk of severe kidney inflammation (nephritis). Several cases of babies born with neonatal lupus to anti-RNP-positive women have been reported; however, this is rare.

Anti-RNP does not fluctuate consistently with disease activity and does not help see how SLE responds to therapy. RNP antibody can be positive in someone many years before they develop lupus. Anti-RNP-positive people who are thought to be healthy should be monitored regularly.

ANA positivity is common in relatives of patients with SLE. A 2017 study showed that RNP-positive relatives were more likely to develop SLE than those who were RNP-negative.

RNP antibodies are not indicative of any one disease. They also appear in rheumatoid arthritis, Raynaud's phenomenon, Sjögren's, and scleroderma. It is most useful in diagnosing a systemic autoimmune disease called mixed connective tissue disease (MCTD, chapter 2). These patients usually have high anti-U1-RNP antibodies (especially anti-RNP-70kDa) with negative anti-Smith antibodies. RNP antibodies can be further divided into IgM and IgG forms. Patients with SLE are more likely to have high levels of the IgM type (IgG is more common in MCTD). Some labs have begun to report on IgG anti-U1-RNP and anti-RNP70. This may help in distinguishing SLE from MCTD.

Ro Antibody (Anti-Ro). See SSA.

RPR. See Rapid Plasma Reagin Test.

Scl-70 Antibody. See Scleroderma Antibody.

Scleroderma Antibody (Anti-Scleroderma 70 Antibody, Topoisomerase I Antibody, Anti-Scl-70). Anti-Scl-70 most commonly appears in systemic sclerosis with diffuse cutaneous involvement. This is a type of scleroderma (chapter 2), a systemic autoimmune disease that causes skin thickening. Anti-Scl-70-positive scleroderma patients are at increased risk for severe lung scarring (called interstitial lung disease) and ulcerations (open sores) on their fingertips. This antibody is uncommon in SLE.

Serum Protein Electrophoresis (SPEP). SPEP detects different blood protein types. For example, it can measure the amount of albumin (an important blood protein). SPEP most helpfully measures immunoglobulins (see immunoglobulin A).

Immunoglobulins are produced by B cells (B lymphocytes, a type of white blood cell). In lupus, the B cells often produce too many immunoglobulins (IGs), called hypergammaglobulinemia, as part of the overactive immune system. When they produce many different types (or clones) of IGs, it is called a polyclonal gammopathy (also polyclonal hypergammaglobulinemia). If they produce one type (or clone), it is called a monoclonal gammopathy (chapter 9)

When the B cells produce a lower number of IGs than normal, it is called hypogammaglobulinemia. Hypogammaglobulinemia can occur because of immunosuppressants (table 22.1) or as a separate disorder related to genes that cause the person to have SLE. Hypogammaglobulinemia can increase the risk of infections (chapter 22).

Sm Antibody. See Smith Antibody.

Smith Antibody (Anti-Smith Antibody, Anti-Sm, Sm Antibody). Anti-Sm is included in the extractable nuclear antibodies (ENA) along with anti-RNP. It is present in 10% to 40% of SLE patients. It usually occurs along with anti-RNP. In other words, if anti-Sm is positive, anti-RNP is almost always positive. The most important thing about anti-Smith is that it is very specific for SLE. It rarely appears in individuals without SLE. Anti-Sm fulfills one of the SLE classification criteria (chapter 1).

It is more common in people of African ancestry. It is associated with an increased risk for pleurisy, nephritis (kidney inflammation), psychosis, seizures, lung disease, low white blood cell counts, arthritis, discoid rash, butterfly rash, vasculitis, pulmonary hypertension, mouth sores, and worse overall disease. It does not fluctuate with disease activity. This test is useful only for diagnosing lupus and not how lupus responds to therapy.

Note that anti-Sm/RNP is not the same as anti-Sm. Anti-Sm/RNP (Smith/RNP) detects the combination of Smith and RNP together. It is like the RNP antibody. It can be seen in autoimmune disorders other than SLE. See RNP antibody.

Sm/RNP Antibody. See RNP Antibody.

Smooth Muscle Antibody (Anti-smooth muscle, ASMA, Anti-Actin Antibody). ASMA helps diagnose autoimmune hepatitis (AIH). It can also be seen in another autoimmune liver disease called primary biliary cirrhosis. ASMA-positive SLE patients with elevated liver

LUPUS IN FOCUS

Origin of anti-Smith

Dr. Eng Tan and Dr. Henry Kunkel first discovered anti-Smith antibody in an aspiring artist and a talented painter named Stephanie Smith. After developing arthritis, rash, and pleurisy, she was diagnosed with SLE in 1959. She died of the disease in 1969 at 22 years of age. A copy of a still life that she painted for Dr. Eng. is at lupusencyclopedia.com/book-photos/.

enzymes should be tested for AIH (chapter 15). However, 18% of healthy people are also ASMA-positive.

SPEP: See Serum Protein Electrophoresis.

SSA (Anti-Sjögren's Disease A, Sjögren's Anti-SS-A, Anti-SSA, Ro Antibody). Anti-SSA and anti-SSB were discovered in 1961 in Sjögren's disease patients. Sjögren's disease (chapter 2) is a systemic autoimmune disorder that attacks the body's moisture-producing glands, causing dry eyes and dry mouth. The medical terms for them are "Sjögren's Syndrome-A" and "Sjögren's Syndrome-B" antibodies (or anti-SSA and anti-SSB for short).

In 1969, the laboratory of Dr. Morris "Moe" Reichlin described antibodies in SLE patients. He named them anti-Ro and anti-La. "Ro" and "La" were the first two letters of the last names of the patients with the antibodies. Researchers later showed that anti-SSA was the same as anti-Ro, and anti-SSB was the same as anti-La. These terms are now interchangeable, with anti-SSA meaning the same as anti-Ro and anti-SSB meaning the same as anti-La.

Of historical interest, the last name of the lupus patient with the newly discovered anti-Ro was Robert (pronounced roh-BAIR'). The last name of the patient with anti-La was Lane—personal communication with Dr. Hal Scofield, MD, an associate of Dr. Reichlin.

Between 60% and 75% of people with Sjögren's disease are anti-SSA-positive, but it can be present in any systemic autoimmune disease, as well as in nonautoimmune conditions such as cancer and infection.

Anti-SSA is more commonly positive in SLE patients than anti-SSB. SSA is positive in 20% to 60% of people with SLE (depending on the patient population and the laboratory method). Anti-SSA-positive SLE patients have an increased risk of rashes with sun exposure (especially subacute cutaneous lupus), lung inflammation (pneumonitis), shrinking lung syndrome, liver inflammation (hepatitis), pancreatic inflammation (pancreatitis), heart inflammation (myocarditis), low platelet counts (thrombocytopenia), low lymphocyte counts (lymphopenia), and an overlap syndrome with Sjögren's.

Although it is rare, some ANA-negative SLE patients are anti-SSA-positive. If someone is thought to have SLE, but their ANA is negative, doctors should check for anti-SSA.

Anti-SSA is one of the earliest autoantibodies to appear in many patients, even many years before their SLE or Sjögren's diagnosis. Anti-SSA-positive people who have no evidence for disease should be monitored regularly. We recommend that people in this situation learn about the symptoms of lupus (such as butterfly rash, joint pains, mouth sores, hair loss, and fatigue) and Sjögren's (dry mouth and dry eyes) and if any occur, see a rheumatologist. Note, though, some anti-SSA-positive people never develop any disease.

Anti-SSA can cross through the placenta, enter the fetus, and potentially cause tissue damage in the unborn baby's heart or skin (called neonatal lupus; chapter 18).

SSB (Anti-Sjögren's Disease B, Sjögren's Anti-SS-B, Anti-SSB, La Antibody, Ha Antibody). Anti-SSB antibodies occur in approximately 50% of anti-SSA-positive patients. They are detectable in 15% to 25% of people with SLE and 40% to 60% of people with Sjögren's, but they can also be present in any systemic autoimmune disease and nonautoimmune conditions such as cancer and infection. People with SLE who are positive for both anti-SSA and anti-SSB antibodies have a higher risk of subacute cutaneous lupus, sun sensitivity, pericarditis (inflammation around the heart), and seizures, but they are less likely to develop lupus nephritis (kidney inflammation). Anti-SSB-positive women are slightly more likely to have a child with neonatal lupus (chapter 18). Also, people with SLE who are positive for anti-SSA plus anti-SSB antibodies are at increased risk of developing Sjögren's disease. It is unusual to be positive for anti-SSB without being positive for anti-SSA (isolated anti-SSB), but this can occur. Isolated anti-SSB positivity (anti-SSA-negative) doesn't increase the risk for Sjögren's.

ss-DNA Antibodies. See DNA (Single-Stranded) Antibodies.

Thyroglobulin Antibody. See Thyroid Antithyroglobulin Antibody.

Thyroid Antithyroglobulin Antibody (AbTg, Antithyroglobulin Antibody, Thyroglobulin Antibody, and TgAb). TgAb is directed toward thyroglobulin, a protein produced by the thyroid gland. One out of three people with SLE will also have autoimmune thyroid disease (chapter 17). TgAb is primarily found in high levels in Hashimoto's thyroiditis but can appear in other autoimmune thyroid diseases such as Graves' disease. Up to 19% of SLE patients can be positive for AbTg.

Thyroid Microsomal Antibody (Antimicrosomal Antibody, Microsomal Antibody, and Anti-Thyroid Peroxidase Antibody). See Thyroid Peroxidase Antibody.

Thyroid Peroxidase Antibody (AbTPO, Microsomal antibody, Thyroperoxidase Antibody, TPO Antibody, TPOAb). TPOAb is directed toward an enzyme in the thyroid gland called thyroid peroxidase, which is essential to providing iodine during the production of thyroid hormones. One out of three people with SLE will also have autoimmune thyroid disease (chapter 17). Thyroid peroxidase antibody appears in especially high levels in a thyroid disorder called Hashimoto's thyroiditis. It can also occur in other autoimmune thyroid diseases such as Graves' disease. Up to 38% of SLE patients can be positive for AbTPO.

Thyroid Stimulating Hormone Receptor Antibody. See Thyrotropin Receptor Antibody.

Thyrotropin Receptor Antibody (Thyroid Stimulating Hormone Receptor Antibody, TSH Receptor Antibody, Thyrotropin-Binding Inhibitory Immunoglobulin, TSH Receptor-Binding Inhibitory Immunoglobulin, TRAb, TBII). Thyrotropin receptor antibody appears in people with an autoimmune thyroid condition called Graves' disease, which causes an overactive thyroid (hyperthyroidism) and an enlarged thyroid gland (goiter).

Biotin supplements can sometimes cause artificially high values. Biotin (vitamin B7) should be stopped three days before blood work.

Tissue Transglutaminase Antibody (Anti-Tissue Transglutaminase, Anti-tTG). Anti-tTG helps diagnose an autoimmune disease called celiac disease, which causes difficulty absorbing nutrients from the intestines. Anti-tTG can be IgG (immunoglobulin G) or IgA (immunoglobulin A). It is the IgA form that is highly specific for celiac disease. IgG anti-tTG occurs in around 2% of SLE patients and is not associated with celiac disease.

People with SLE are at increased risk of having celiac disease. If symptoms suggestive of celiac disease develop, anti-tTG should be tested while the person eats a diet containing gluten (chapter 15). A positive IgA anti-tTG can help diagnose celiac disease. However, a small intestine biopsy is the most accurate method.

Selective IgA deficiency (in some people with SLE) can cause a falsely negative test. It is important to measure an IgA level when measuring an IgA anti-tTG. If the IgA level is low, the IgA anti-tTG level is negative, and the suspicion for celiac disease is high, then a small intestine biopsy should be considered.

Topoisomerase I Antibody. See Scleroderma Antibody.

Treponema Pallidum Antibodies. See Fluorescent Treponemal Antibody Absorption Test
Treponema Pallidum. See Particle Agglutination Test.

Treponema Pallidum Particle Agglutination Test (TPPA). This is another confirmatory test for syphilis (see Fluorescent Treponemal Antibody Absorption Test) and is used similarly.

U1RNP Antibody. See RNP Antibody.

VDRL. See Venereal Disease Research Laboratory Test.

Venereal Disease Research Laboratory Test (VDRL). See Rapid Plasma Reagin Test.

Newer Specialty Tests

This section of the chapter is a new addition to this book and includes tests not performed by laboratories (such as LabCorp and Quest) commonly used by commercial and government insurance carriers. All the following tests are performed by a specialty laboratory called Exagen Inc. (located in California). I was hoping to include other laboratories specializing in lupus, but they will not have their tests commercially available during the production of this edition. Interferon gene signature testing (IFGS, see anifrolumab, chapter 34) did become available in some laboratories just prior to printing, but since we do not yet understand how to use IFGS properly in clinical practice, it is not included. Some labs done by Exagen (such as methotrexate polyglutamate levels, hydroxychloroquine levels, and antiphospholipid tests) are also performed by LabCorp and Quest, so those tests are described earlier in this chapter.

Cell-Bound Complement Activation Products (CB-CAPS). Although C3 and C4 complements are regularly measured in SLE, they have several problems.

1. C3 and C4 levels have a wide range of "normal" values in healthy individuals. These ranges overlap those of SLE patients' levels.

2. C3 and C4 are broken down into smaller fragments during lupus disease activity. The standard tests measure the C3 and C4 rather than their lupus-induced fragments.

3. The liver produces more C3 and C4 during inflammation (as happens during active lupus), which can counterbalance lower C3 and C4 levels. This often results in normal or high levels during active lupus inflammation.

4. Some SLE patients have a genetic deficiency in C4 production, causing low C4 levels not related to active lupus disease.

Thinking about the above problems with C3 and C4, it makes sense that it would be better to measure the C3 and C4 fragments produced during active lupus disease activity. While these fragments are short-lived when dissolved in the blood, during lupus inflammation, some C3 and C4 components attach to the outer membranes of blood cells and remain attached for the cell's lifespan. These "cell-bound" complement fragments (or activation products) are easier to measure than the C3 and C4 fragments in the blood. They are called cell-bound complement activation products, or CB-CAPs. The C4d (complement 4–derived) components that attach to B lymphocytes (BC4d), platelets (PC4d), and erythrocytes (EC4d) are particularly elevated in SLE while being very uncommon in people without SLE.

EC4d and BC4d elevations are around twice as common than low C3 or C4 in people with active SLE. This is important because measuring these may be more helpful in finding patients with SLE and checking how active their disease is and how well they respond to therapy.

BC4d (B Lymphocyte-Bound Complement 4–Derived). BC4d measures the amount of C4d fragments produced during lupus disease activity that attach to the outer membranes of B lymphocytes (B cells). BC4d is highly specific for SLE. It is very unusual to see elevated levels in people without SLE. In the studies performed thus far, a few patients with vasculitis (inflammation of the blood vessels) and some with Sjögren's disease had elevated levels, but most people with high levels have SLE. It is more specific for SLE than EC4d is. It is one of the test components used for the AVISE Lupus Test discussed below. A positive BC4d is so particular for lupus that having an elevated BC4d gives the largest number of points for the AVISE Lupus Test result, significantly increasing the chance for a positive result.

LUPUS IN FOCUS

CB-CAPS can help predict disease severity

A large 2020 American study showed that patients with normal CB-CAPS (EC4d and BC4d) and C3 and C4 complements (C3/C4) tended to have little active disease as a group (though there were some outliers). Those with elevated CB-CAPS but normal C3/C4 tended to have moderate disease activity. Patients with positive CB-CAPS and low C3/C4 tended to have severe (high) lupus disease activity.

EC4d (Erythrocyte-Bound Complement–4 Derived). EC4d measures the amount of C4d fragments produced during lupus disease activity that attach to the outer membranes of erythrocytes (red blood cells). EC4d is specific for SLE, meaning that it is unusual to see elevated levels in people who do not have SLE. However, it is not as specific as BC4d. It is also one of the components of the AVISE Lupus Test.

An advantage of EC4d is that it fluctuates with lupus disease activity and is used in the AVISE SLE Monitor Test discussed below.

PC4d (Platelet-Bound Complement 4–Derived). PC4d measures the amount of C4d fragments produced during lupus disease activity that attach to the outer membranes of platelets. PC4d is a part of the AVISE SLE Monitor Test. SLE patients with elevated PC4d are at increased risk for blood clots, especially in the veins (such as deep venous thrombosis, chapter 9). Around 20% of SLE patients are positive for PC4d, and it is rarely found in people without SLE. In 2019, the Johns Hopkins Lupus Center showed that patients with elevated PC4d and positive lupus anticoagulant and low C3 levels were particularly at high risk for strokes, heart attacks, and blood clots. We are awaiting more research to see if these results are reproduced in other studies.

AVISE Lupus Test. This tests for the likelihood of someone having SLE. AVISE is word play on the word "advise," referring to the test's ability to advise doctors on how to diagnose their patients better with lupus and related diseases.

The analysis is performed in two stages called Tier 1 and Tier 2. In Tier 1, the laboratory measures a person's levels of anti-Smith, EC4d, BC4d, and anti-dsDNA. Very high levels for any of these are likely due to SLE and are reported as a positive Tier 1 result. In studies, a few patients with Sjögren's disease had positive Tier 1 results. Hence, as with most tests for lupus, it is not perfect.

Suppose someone has a negative Tier 1 result. In that case, testing proceeds to the next stage (Tier 2). Other autoantibodies that are more commonly seen in other autoimmune diseases are measured. These antibodies include anti-CCP (seen more often in rheumatoid arthritis), anti-SSB (more common in Sjögren's disease), anti-CENP (more common in limited scleroderma), anti-Scl-70 (more common in diffuse scleroderma), and anti-Jo1 (more common in polymyositis). Since these antibodies are less common in SLE (though they can occur), each is assigned a negative numerical value if present. The labs that suggest possible SLE—antibodies (ANA, Smith, dsDNA) and the CB-CAPS (EC4d and BC4d) are given positive values. These numbers are plugged into a mathematical formula.

Any positive result is reported with the statement that "this assessment is associated with an increased likelihood of SLE." A negative number score is reported as a negative result. The greater a positive score value is, the more likely the patient is to have SLE. The greater a negative score, the less likely the patient is to have SLE.

One study performed by the lupus expert Dr. Daniel Wallace and the fibromyalgia expert Dr. Stuart Silverman showed that the AVISE Lupus Test was particularly helpful in distinguishing patients with SLE from patients with fibromyalgia (chapter 27).

A 2019 study showed that the AVISE Lupus Test could diagnose patients with SLE and "probable SLE" better than the usual commercial labs used by most rheumatologists. Another 2019 study showed that the AVISE Lupus Test could diagnose SLE more

How many with a positive or negative AVISE-Lupus Test will get SLE?

In 2020, the University of California, Los Angeles, published a study evaluating 117 people with symptoms suggestive of possible SLE and watched them for over 2 years. Of those with a positive AVISE-Lupus Test result, 65% developed SLE. Only 10% of those with a negative AVISE-Lupus Test developed SLE.

quickly, thereby significantly decreasing the cost of diagnosis. Using this test resulted in a savings of $2,256 per suspected SLE patient over four years. Most of the cost savings came from preventing the hospitalization of untreated patients.

Since the AVISE Lupus Test requires a doctor's office to prepare and ship it to the laboratory that reads the test (Exagen), many offices do not order it. However, there are laboratory drawing sites that can perform the test. Sites and instructions are found at www.avisetest.com/telavise-draw-site-locator. (Disclaimer—Dr. Thomas is on the Speakers' Bureau for Exagen).

AVISE SLE Monitor Test. It is essential to assess how active the immune system (inflammation) is in a patient with SLE to see how well treatment is doing. The more common lupus disease activity tests that doctors order are C3, C4, and anti-dsDNA. However, as described earlier, these are not helpful in most patients.

The AVISE SLE Monitor test includes EC4d levels and anti-C1q (discussed earlier) that are more helpful in many patients. It also involves measuring anti-dsDNA by a lab method called chemiluminescence immunoassay (CIA), which is more useful in most SLE patients than the methods commonly used by most laboratories (such as Quest and LabCorp). To be thorough, this test also includes the standard C3 and C4. The AVISE SLE Monitor Test also measures PC4d (discussed earlier).

KEY POINTS TO REMEMBER

1. SLE patients need to know how to collect a urine sample properly because one is necessary at most office visits.

2. People with SLE should regularly have labs to check potential lupus problems affecting blood counts, the liver, and the kidneys. The most common labs that are performed regularly include a complete blood cell count, metabolic chemistry panel, urinalysis, urine protein/creatinine ratio, C3, C4, and anti-dsDNA.

3. Many people with lupus also need labs drawn regularly to ensure that there are no drug side effects.

4. A doctor may order many different antibody tests. Doctors do not usually repeat these tests (other than anti-dsDNA) because most antibody levels do not fluctuate with disease activity.

5. It can be useful to know what antibodies you are positive for to understand how your doctor diagnosed your lupus and what problems from SLE you are potentially at an increased risk for.

6. Newer tests have appeared during the past decade to aid in diagnosing and monitoring SLE patients, including the AVISE Lupus Test and the AVISE SLE Monitor Test.

How Lupus Directly Affects the Body

General Effects on the Body

Jerik Leung, MPH, and Alfred Kim, MD, PhD, *Contributing Editors*

This book discusses the problems of SLE in two parts. Part II (chapters 6–20) covers those directly due to the immune system attacking the body (the direct autoimmune issues). Part III (chapters 21–28) highlights SLE complications due to other reasons. Some of the problems and complexities in part III occur indirectly because of permanent damage to the body from previous bouts of lupus flares and inflammation or due to the drugs used to treat SLE. There are other problems for which we do not have a simple explanation as to why they occur more often in lupus patients, including infections, heart attacks, strokes, osteoporosis, and fibromyalgia, which we discuss in part III.

The reason for separating these problems into two sections is that many issues are directly due to the immune system attacking the body (chapters 6–20). These respond to medications that target and calm the immune system (called immunomodulating drugs). The problems in part III are treated differently and not with immunomodulatory drugs.

This book discusses both common and uncommon SLE problems. One notable addition to this second edition is a result of feedback from some readers of the first edition saying they wanted to know about rare complications from SLE. It can be hard to find useful information regarding these rare problems. This edition fills that gap.

This chapter introduces how SLE can affect the body in general. It addresses the quality of life in lupus patients, how different labs can predict various lupus problems, and discusses flares and remission topics. Allergies are discussed at the end of the chapter.

Lupus Affects Everyone Differently

The problems and symptoms of lupus vary significantly from person to person. Sometimes a newly diagnosed person will say, "I can't have lupus. I don't have the butterfly rash and joint pain." But lupus affects everyone differently. For example, the butterfly rash is commonly shown in pictures to represent someone with SLE. However, the butterfly rash occurs in less than one-third of SLE patients. This rash is shown in photos because it is easy to recognize.

An important reason why every lupus patient is different is due to the many lupus-related genes and how the environment affects those genes (epigenetics, chapter 3). In 2013, the rheumatologist Dr. John Kolstoe demonstrated how genes cause so much variation in patients by calculating how many differences can occur. He estimated 27,405 different combinations among the 33 known lupus-associated genes. Interactions between a person's environment and their genes further increase the number of combinations and shape what that person's lupus could look like. Five times as many lupus-related genes (over 150) are now known, so the number of combinations is much higher than 27,405.

Sometimes we have clues that can predict lupus problems. For example, anti-SSA (labs discussed in chapter 4) increases the chance of getting dry eyes, dry mouth, and rashes with sun exposure. A high anti-dsDNA, low C3, low C4, high EC4d, or a positive anti-C1q increases the chance of developing lupus nephritis (kidney inflammation). Some labs predict less severe lupus problems. For example, anti-SSB-positive SLE patients have a lower chance of developing lupus nephritis.

Ethnicity, gender, and even income can play a role (chapter 19). SLE patients with lower incomes, non-white SLE patients, children with SLE, and men with SLE tend to have more severe disease.

Clues that can sometimes predict these potential lupus patterns are listed in table 5.1. Rheumatologists look carefully for these potential problems in people with abnormal lab tests or who fit the demographics in this table. Ask your rheumatologist what antibodies and lupus blood tests you are positive for so you can understand some of these variables that could potentially affect you.

Note, though, that none of these clues is set in stone. Just because you are positive for a blood test or fit a certain demographic does *not* necessarily mean you will end up with that associated lupus problem. For example, you can be anti-SSA-positive and never develop a skin rash or have elevated anti-dsDNA with low C3 and never develop nephritis. Some older adults have severe lupus with kidney disease, while most African Americans do not develop brain inflammation or lupus nephritis.

SLE Effects on Quality of Life (QoL)

"Quality of life" (QoL) is a broad term referring to how people perceive their enjoyment of life. It includes health (physical and mental), finances, independence, ability to participate in desired activities, living situation, safety, and many other aspects of life. Having a good QoL includes being healthy. If diagnosed with a disease such as lupus, a good QoL means not feeling sick from the disease, but also not having any problems related to medical treatments.

There has been a greater focus on QoL in lupus patients during the past few years. Many SLE patients have a lower QoL than average. This finding is not surprising since we know that SLE can affect any organ of the body and that it can range in severity from mild to life-threatening. In addition, treatments for SLE may disrupt a person's enjoyment of life and cause barriers to employment and social interactions. Although it is easy to imagine lupus problems such as arthritis pain, nerve damage, fatigue, and memory issues decreasing QoL, other lupus problems such as skin issues prove to be a bigger problem than previously thought. Cosmetic impacts such as hair loss and rashes can negatively affect self-image and reduce QoL. There are also age differences. For example, a study of children with lupus showed that arthritis substantially interfered with QoL while cutaneous (skin) lupus did not. In older age groups, by contrast, cutaneous (skin) lupus significantly decreases QoL due to appearance and self-esteem issues.

Table 5.1 Some Predictors of Possible Problems in SLE

Lab Finding or Demographic	SLE Problem
Antiphospholipid antibodies (beta-2 glycoprotein I antibody, lupus anticoagulant, cardiolipin antibodies, false-positive syphilis tests, phosphatidylserine antibodies)	Blood clots, strokes, heart attacks, low platelet counts, hemolytic anemia, livedo reticularis rash, kidney involvement (blood clots); memory problems; miscarriages; increased long-term organ damage
C1q antibody	Kidney inflammation (lupus nephritis)
Chromatin antibody	Kidney inflammation (lupus nephritis)
Low C3 and C4 complement	Kidney inflammation (lupus nephritis)
Coombs' antibody	Autoimmune hemolytic anemia
Cryoglobulins	Kidney disease, vasculitis
CCP antibody	Severe arthritis, rheumatoid arthritis (rhupus)
Double-stranded-DNA antibody	Kidney inflammation (lupus nephritis), blood vessel inflammation (vasculitis)
Ribosomal-P antibody	Liver, kidney, and skin disease; anxiety, depression, psychosis
RNP antibody	Raynaud's phenomenon, esophageal dysmotility, pulmonary hypertension, myocarditis; increased risk for polyimmunity (multiple autoimmune disorders)
SS-A (Ro) antibody	Sun-sensitive rash, Sjögren's , lung inflammation, low platelet counts, myocarditis, pancreatitis, hepatitis, subacute cutaneous lupus; neonatal lupus; increased risk for polyimmunity
SS-B (La) antibody	Sjögren's; neonatal lupus; likely to have kidney inflammation (lupus nephritis); increased risk for polyimmunity
African American race	Kidney inflammation (lupus nephritis), brain disease, pleurisy, discoid lupus
Men	More severe disease than in women
Children	More major organ disease, especially kidney inflammation (lupus nephritis)
Elderly	Less severe inflammation; fewer low blood counts; less Raynaud's, hair loss, butterfly rash, sun-sensitive rashes, lupus nephritis, and brain involvement than younger adults. Higher chances of Sjögren's disease, pleurisy, lung disease, and arthritis. Permanent damage more likely in aging organs.

LUPUS IN FOCUS

Dental problems are common in SLE

A 2017 Brazilian study showed that most SLE patients had tooth loss, dental cavities, inflammation, or mouth infections. Poor oral health made eating food difficult and caused a lower quality of life. SLE patients should be meticulous with their dental care to help decrease these problems (chapter 14).

Researchers now realize that it is essential to show QoL improvements with treatments for lupus and are directly measuring QoL more often in research studies to help search for treatments that improve QoL. To illustrate our point, a literature search for "lupus" and "quality of life" in the title of research studies shows that while there were only nine studies in 2010, there were 337 studies in January 2021.

There are many ways researchers measure QoL, including assessing fatigue, memory, physical health, mental health, and social functioning. These research measurements are called patient-reported outcomes (PROs).

SLE patients are often affected by problems (such as depression, anxiety, fibromyalgia) that are not directly due to the body's immune system damage. Nonetheless, these play a significant role in QoL issues and must be dealt with in addition to treating the lupus disease itself (see type II symptoms below).

A 2019 study from the Lupus Clinic at the Washington University School of Medicine in St. Louis, Missouri, highlighted QoL problems on which previous research had not focused. The researchers interviewed SLE patients and showed that other contributors to poor QoL included the unpredictable symptoms of lupus (being fine one day but not the next), poor communication with those around them (friends, family, and health care providers), feeling that others do not validate their problems (like unusual lupus symptoms, pain, and fatigue), and lacking an adequate social support system.

Problems with lack of social support and not being validated by others is due in part from lupus being an invisible disease. The person with SLE may look perfectly normal, yet fatigue, weakness, memory problems (lupus fog), and joint pain commonly occur and can greatly interfere with the ability to function and enjoy life. Many people with SLE suffering from these invisible symptoms often avoid activities, such as work, hobbies, entertainment, family commitments, and social gatherings. Not being able to participate in these activities may result in the loss of close relationships, leaving patients feeling isolated and misunderstood. Relationships (with loved ones, coworkers, and even health care providers) can be further damaged when others question the validity of the effects of lupus on the person. Figuring out how to provide better social support structures (involving friends, family, health care providers, and patient support groups) is necessary to improve QoL.

Some predictors of better QoL in SLE patients include exercising, maintaining muscle strength, taking antimalarial medications (such as hydroxychloroquine), not taking steroids, getting into remission or low disease activity with treatments, and participating in group psychotherapy. There do appear to be some gender differences. Men tend to have less social support than women, while women tend to have worse pain, worse lupus symptoms, and more problems with memory than men.

There are actions that patients can take to improve their QoL. Reading this book and putting its recommendations into action is an excellent start. We health care providers also need to learn to play a more active role in empathizing with patients by truly listening to them and genuinely trying to understand what is happening to them and how they feel. A 2016 study showed that when nurses actively improved their empathy skills while caring for SLE patients, those patients had significant improvements in their QoL compared to patients who received the usual medical care.

Type I and Type II Symptoms

The Lupus Clinic at Duke University in Durham, North Carolina, has developed a way for its doctors to provide better patient care. Rheumatologists are usually good at evaluating and treating lupus problems that are directly related to the immune system and inflammatory part of their disease; they call these type I symptoms. These include inflammatory arthritis, nephritis (kidney inflammation), lupus rashes, mouth ulcers, pleurisy, fevers, seizures, blood clots, Raynaud's phenomenon, and others. These problems have well-defined treatments and are discussed in part II of this book.

Type II symptoms are also troubling for patients, though they are not often addressed by doctors. These include fatigue, widespread pain, depression, sleep problems, and difficulties with memory and concentration ("lupus fog"). The doctors in the Lupus Clinic at Duke are trained to ask patients about type II symptoms. Getting into the habit of doing so forces them to solve more problems that are important to patients.

For example, suppose a patient with SLE is in remission from the immunologic and inflammatory part of their disease (type I symptoms) yet has memory and concentration problems that significantly affect quality of life. In that case, it is common for a doctor to respond that these are not due to their lupus, which is in remission. In an interview with *Rheumatology News* (a newspaper about rheumatologic issues), Dr. Jennifer Rogers (a rheumatologist at Duke) says that a better response would be something like, "Yes, this is your lupus. I believe you. But we don't need to give you [x] immunosuppressives for this. What you need to do is take your Cymbalta, work on your exercise," and so on.

Unfortunately, many health care providers focus only on type I symptoms. At the same time, you, the patient, may need more help with your type II symptoms. We recommend that you write down three problems you would like to address at each doctor's visit. Give this list to your doctor immediately at the start of the office visit. This will help your doctor be prepared to address them early rather than being pressed for time if given the list at the end of the appointment.

Fortunately, you yourself can start addressing many type II symptoms. This book gives much practical advice on those things that are in your power to improve. Go to the index and look up your problem (such as fatigue or memory loss). It will tell you the pages that give you the tools you need to address them.

The Patterns of Lupus Disease Activity

Three different disease activity patterns have been described in lupus patients: they are known as prolonged remission, relapsing-remittent, and chronic active. Lupus centers have evaluated how often these patterns occur in their patients. One comes from the Toronto Lupus Clinic in Canada, which reported in 2018 that approximately 70% were in the relapsing-remitting pattern. This means that they have intermittent periods of lupus flares (relapsing) and periods of feeling well (remitting). We also commonly say that their lupus is "waxing and waning." It is the most common pattern that many lupus centers see. Around 10% of Toronto's patients had a chronic active disease pattern (also called persistently active). These are patients who constantly have active inflammation with no periods of disease inactivity (remission). Only 10% of the patients were in a state of "prolonged remission."

Many of my patients are in the prolonged remission pattern because they regularly take their medications and follow the advice in "The Lupus Secrets." They often tell me, "I feel like I have nothing wrong with me," to which I reply, "Perfect, that is how I always want you to feel." But I also remind them to keep doing what they are doing, including taking their medications, even when they feel perfectly normal. Stopping usually ends up causing their lupus to flare up, sometimes severely.

Lupus Flares

A lupus flare is when a worsening of persistent lupus problems occurs, an issue under reasonable control comes back, or a new problem develops that was not present before. For example, if someone with SLE who is in low disease activity (defined below) with continuous painless ulcers on the roof of the mouth develops sores that become more numerous and painful, this would be a lupus flare. Or if someone is perfectly fine one day and then develops a fever, fatigue, and joint pains the next, this would also be a lupus flare.

The Lupus Foundation of America (LFA) defines a flare as "a measurable increase in disease activity in one or more organ systems involving new or worse clinical signs and symptoms and/or lab measurements. The increase must be considered clinically significant by the assessor (physician or clinical researcher) and in most cases should prompt the consideration of a change or an increase in treatment."

In addition to a person's description of how they are feeling, lab tests can help identify a flare. To return to the example of the patient with mouth sores: it would be important to check their lupus labs (such as a urine sample and blood work) to make sure something more serious is not going on with any internal organs, such as the kidneys, liver, and/or blood counts. The doctor may need to consider adjusting the patient's treatment regimen, depending upon the results.

Although many SLE patients have the same recurring problems, SLE can unexpectedly cause new problems. A rheumatologist would consider the occurrence of a new complication (based on symptoms or a new abnormal lab test) a flare. For example, suppose someone always has low complement levels and a high anti-ds DNA level with normal urine labs. In that case, that person is stable and does not have a flare. But suppose this same person suddenly develops excessive urine protein due to an onset of lupus nephritis. In this case, their rheumatologist will consider this result evidence of a lupus flare.

Preparing for flares and knowing what to do during a flare are important. Flares can potentially cause permanent damage to affected body areas. For example, an arthritis flare could cause joint damage, or a lung flare could cause permanent lung scarring. Any flare can potentially cause inflammation and damage to blood vessels, increasing the risk for heart attacks and strokes. Use the included "Lupus Flare Plan" (table 5.2) to learn how to prepare for any flares and how to have them dealt with appropriately. You can also download the original PDF form from the LFA website at www.lupus.org/FlarePlan.

Bring the form with you to your next rheumatology visit and ask for help answering the questions, including what you can do at home during flares to treat individual problems. For example, if you get painful mouth sores, having some prescription-strength dental steroid paste on hand can help. Or, if you have muscle or joint pains, applying hot or cold compresses may help.

Some treatments may involve medication. For instance, a doctor may prescribe a short course of steroids (such as a methylprednisolone Dose Pak) during flares. Sometimes, it is better to get a shot of steroids in the buttock than to take steroid pills as demonstrated by the FLOAT study (flares in lupus: outcome assessment trial) from the Johns Hopkins Lupus Center in Baltimore, Maryland. This can be a faster and potentially safer way to help with flares. You should find out if this is a good option for you and how to arrange to have it done quickly. My patients know they can call my medical assistant and come in immediately during flares to get this cortisone injection. It can make a huge difference by controlling lupus flares quickly before they get out of control. Moderate to severe flares should be dealt with directly by your doctor, so it is vital to learn what types of flares should be seen by your doctor.

Identifying the causes (triggers) of lupus flares is important. Most well-known triggers can potentially cause lupus flares in any patient. However, some triggers can be more important than others, depending on the person. Knowing and avoiding your triggers can lower your risk of flares.

Someone's lupus labs may be able to predict some triggers. For example, anti-SSA increases the risk for flaring from ultraviolet (UV) light exposure. Anti-SSA-positive patients should be especially diligent in protecting themselves from UV light exposure (chapter 38). Other potential triggers of lupus include low vitamin D levels, cigarette smoking, stress, lack of sleep, missing doses of medications, not wearing sunscreen daily, taking sulfonamide antibiotics, having an infection, and taking supplements that increase immune system activity (such as Echinacea).

Sometimes flares occur for no apparent reason. At other times, it may be easy to figure out the trigger (such as forgetting to wear sunscreen, missing medication doses, or being under stress). Getting into the habit of writing down when you flare can help you identify triggers and focus on that aspect of your medical care.

Even so, some triggers can be difficult to prevent. Stress is one example. Although reducing stress can be difficult (if you're experiencing increased pressure at work, for example), chapter 38 lists practical ways to reduce the ill effects of stress. As with stress and many other triggers: if there are actions that can prevent them, you should take them if you can.

You have no control over some triggers, such as hormone fluctuations during menstrual cycles. Weather conditions are another. The Johns Hopkins Lupus Center in Baltimore, Maryland, showed that lupus rashes and arthritis were most common in

Table 5.2 Your Lupus Flare Plan

Fill in with help from the doctor treating your lupus, who could be a rheumatologist, nurse practitioner, physician assistant, primary care provider, dermatologist, or immunologist.

1. If I think I have a flare, will my doctor want to see me immediately?	If yes, how do I make an appointment ASAP? What should I do if I'm told that the next appointment is more than a few days away?
2. What's the best way for me to explain my symptoms to my doctor?	Examples include "patient portal message to the doctor" or "tell symptoms to phone staff"
3. What will my doctor do to get my symptoms under control ASAP?	Examples include " start prednisone," "increase the dose of prednisone," or "go to the doctor's office for a cortisone shot in the buttock."
4. Should I have blood and urine tests with each flare?	If yes, how do I have the tests ordered and done quickly?
5. How will I recognize a flare?	Here is a list of common flare symptoms. Circle all that you have had in the past or you're currently having. Ask your doctor what you can do in the future if any of these occur with a flare. • Fatigue • Joint pain • Joint stiffness upon waking • Hair loss • Sores in mouth or nose • Chest pain that hurts upon breathing in • Fingers turn blue or white when cold (Raynaud's phenomenon, chapter 11) • Skin rash or sores—see a dermatologist who is familiar with lupus for any new rash • Fever. *If you have a fever, see a doctor immediately to find out if it is due to infection or lupus. Examples: primary care provider, rheumatologist, urgent care center, emergency room.)*
6. Since you were first diagnosed with lupus, these symptoms often repeat during flares. Ask your doctor if there are things you can do at home to help.	List symptoms you had when you were diagnosed: _____ _____ _____

Table 5.2 (*continued*)

7. Lupus problems that occurred after your diagnosis may recur during flares.	List recurring lupus problems: _____ _____ _____ _____
8. New lupus problems can occur during flares. A new symptom also could be due to something else (for example, a medication side effect or a viral illness).	Write new symptoms here: _____ _____ _____
9. There are certain triggers that are commonly experienced by SLE patients.	Circle all that you experienced before a flare: • Ultraviolet (UV) light exposure (tables 38.1 and 38.2). Stay strict about UV protection (tables 38.3 and 38.4). • Cigarette smoke (also secondhand smoke). Find help at smokefree.gov or call 1-800-QUIT-NOW. • Sulfonamide (sulfa) antibiotics such as trimethoprim-sulfamethoxazole (Septra® and Bactrim®). Tell all health care professionals that you must avoid sulfonamide antibiotics. Always carry an up-to-date list of your medications and allergies that includes sulfonamide antibiotics. • Echinacea herbal supplements (chapter 3). • Alfalfa sprouts & mung bean sprouts (chapter 3). • Stress. Learn to decrease stress (table 38.9). • Low vitamin D. Ensure your blood level is 40 ng/mL or higher (chapters 3 and 35) • Not taking medications as prescribed (see "adherence" in chapter 29).

Source: Modified and used with permission from ©The Lupus Foundation of America at lupus.org /s3fs-public/Doc%20-%20PDF/NRCL/Your%20Lupus%20Flare%20Plan_2020.pdf.

the summer in their patients, while kidney involvement was less common. Pleurisy (inflammation of the lining around the lungs) and low blood counts flared more often after hotter temperatures and higher humidity. Windier periods were more closely associated with arthritis, low blood counts, nerve problems, and lung inflammation flares. Periods of higher pollution saw flares of arthritis, rashes, pleurisy, and low blood counts. Surprisingly, barometric pressure changes did not predict lupus flares.

These findings reflect Baltimore's weather conditions and may not be accurate in other areas. It's possible, though, that these trends occur elsewhere, and research is ongoing.

The role of pollution is receiving more notice. A Canadian study showed that some lupus lab abnormalities (notably elevated anti-dsDNA and casts in the urine, which can indicate kidney inflammation) tended to occur during increased pollution. A 2019 Chinese study showed increased hospital admissions for lupus flares during increased pollution. These data suggest that when organizations such as the US National Weather Service put out alerts on pollution (such as an unhealthy Air Quality Index) for people with chronic illnesses, SLE patients should also heed these warnings.

Doctors have long suspected that infections may trigger lupus flares. A 2018 Mexican study showed that many SLE patients had a severe lupus flare after a bacterial bloodstream infection. Infection with *Streptococcus pneumoniae* (also called pneumococcus) was the most common cause, particularly in those with low C4 levels. This also provides additional evidence that lupus patients need to be vaccinated to prevent pneumococcus infections (chapter 22).

Permanent Organ Damage

There are two potential outcomes when lupus causes inflammation in the body's organs (such as the kidneys, skin, joints, lungs). If the inflammation is mild and brief, the area may heal with no residual damage after the inflammation goes away. This inflammation resolution can occur spontaneously since lupus can come and go naturally (called "waxing and waning"). Or, more commonly, the inflammation can go away due to the medications used to treat lupus. If the body can completely heal the area, the organ can go back to its original good health. However, if mild inflammation occurs for a long time or if moderate to severe inflammation occurs for even a short time, permanent damage may occur. In lupus pneumonitis (lung inflammation), parts of the lung can be permanently destroyed, decreasing the ability of the bloodstream to absorb oxygen. In lupus nephritis (kidney inflammation), part of the kidney can be damaged, decreasing the ability to filter the blood properly. Discoid lupus of the scalp could permanently damage hair follicles, leaving permanent hair loss.

One of the essential goals of lupus treatment is to avoid permanent organ damage and achieve remission. Over the years, some of our patients have been reluctant to accept necessary therapy, stating, "I don't feel too bad." However, they often don't realize that even mild and persistent inflammation can permanently damage organs such as the kidneys, heart, lungs, and blood vessels. Many patients will recite their fear of the medications, not fully understanding that the permanent organ damage usually far outweighs any potential side effects from the medicines. Patients and doctors need to discuss patient experiences and perceptions of medication to find the best approach to ensure adherence.

Steroids, such as prednisone, are the exception. Though they initially can be lifesaving and improve quality of life, in the long run, they increase (rather than decrease) organ damage. Even low prednisone doses for prolonged periods cause ongoing organ damage. Some organ damage (such as cataracts of the eyes and thinning bones) is from the steroids themselves. Other areas of damage, such as to the blood vessels, can lead to heart attacks, strokes, and blood clots. Doctors need to try to get lupus into remission using non-steroid drugs, while trying to get patients off steroids.

Remission and Low Disease Activity

Our goal in treating SLE is to strive for remission (this includes stopping flares) to prevent any ongoing damage to the body from type I symptoms. Suppose you cannot identify any correctible triggers listed in the Lupus Flare Plan, such as not missing any doses of your medicines (table 5.2). In that case, you should ask your doctor if your treatment should be adjusted.

Not everyone who has SLE develops recurrent flares. Many respond so well to treatment that their symptoms and problems come under control and never or rarely recur. Doctors label this "clinically quiescent" or "remission." Quiescent means that something is in a state of inactivity. If someone with SLE is clinically quiescent, this means that their disease has been calmed down sufficiently with medications. Although rheumatologists often use "remission" and "clinically quiescent" interchangeably, lupus experts are now leaning more towards using "remission."

Being in remission or clinically quiescent does not mean that the lupus is gone. It merely means that it is under reasonable control from treatments that calm the immune system. This is different from how "remission" is used when talking about cancer; in that case the cancer is gone, and the person needs no more medication. Someone in remission from SLE must continue to take their medications and regularly see the doctor to ensure that the SLE stays under proper control. Unfortunately, some SLE patients stop taking their medicines and seeing their doctors when they feel well and are in remission. Usually, they show up in a rheumatologist's office later with a flare. These flares can even be severe or life-threatening.

Note that type II symptoms discussed above may not get better on some lupus medicines. These symptoms usually require other forms of treatment, which should be discussed with your rheumatologist to determine your best options.

It is rare for SLE patients to go into complete remission and not require treatment. A 2005 Canadian study showed that only 12 patients out of 703 were in remission for 5 years or longer while not taking any medications. Forty-six patients could stay off medications for at least a year during the study. The vast majority flared and required treatment. The worry with stopping treatment in SLE patients is that flares increase the risk for developing permanent damage to body organs. Because of this, lupus experts agree that all SLE patients should be on treatment, especially an antimalarial (such as hydroxychloroquine), which has been shown to reduce flares.

In 2021, a task force on the Definitions of Remission in Systemic Lupus Erythematosus (DORIS for short) defined remission in plain language as having no active lupus inflammatory disease. Yet, complement levels could be low, and anti-dsDNA could be high. Medicines that calm the immune system are allowed (and expected) for a patient to qualify as being in remission. It is best not to be taking steroids to be considered to be in remission. But very small doses are allowed by DORIS.

Lupus doctors realize that not all SLE patients can go into remission on the medications that we currently have available. In that case, the next best goal is to get them into low disease activity. In research studies, this is often called low disease activity state, or LDAS.

Researchers continue to work on defining LDAS. One definition states that someone is in an LDAS if they do not have lupus nephritis and have a score of four or less on a disease activity measurement called the SLEDAI (SLE Disease Activity Index). You can view the SLEDAI form at http://www.sledai-2k.com/sledai2k.pdf. If the person is on steroids, the dose has to be in the low range (such as prednisone less than 7.5 mg daily). Their doctor also must agree they are in low disease activity. This is important, because the SLEDAI does not measure some important lupus problems, such as lung inflammation. If someone has more going on than LDAS, they would be considered to have moderate disease activity or higher.

How to Prevent Lupus Flares and Permanent Organ Damage

Achieving complete remission (on an antimalarial with no active lupus and having normal serologies) is the best way to prevent organ damage. Being in complete remission on treatment, but without the need for steroids, also appears to prevent organ damage. Patients can be on other immunosuppressants (table 22.1). These patients (complete remission or complete remission on treatment but without steroids) are the least likely to have ongoing permanent organ damage and lupus flares. Working with your rheumatologist to achieve one of these remission types should be a top priority. Also, do your part by putting "The Lupus Secrets" described in chapter 44 into practice.

Some SLE patients are unable to achieve those two types of remission. The next best goals are to be in remission on steroids (less than 6 mg prednisone daily), in remission with positive serologies (low C3, low C4, high EC4d, high anti-dsDNA, or high anti-C1q), or in low disease activity. These groups appear to have more flares and additional permanent organ damage over time. However, the flares and damage are much less than patients with moderate active disease and worse.

So how do you achieve remission or low disease activity? We have some good news. You, the patient, have more control than you may think, and giving you that control is the main reason for this book. It is also why I put together a list called "The Lupus Secrets." I use the word "secret" not to mean that they should be kept a secret, but because most lupus patients and many doctors do not know them. As a group, my patients who learn, memorize, and put the "Lupus Secrets" into practice do the best in the long run. Make sure to go to the last chapter of this book to see the "Lupus Secrets." Make sure to put them into practice in your own life, and you can significantly improve your chances of controlling your lupus better.

Of course, every SLE patient is different. Some have such severe SLE that they can do everything in the Lupus Secrets yet still have active disease. If you are one of these people, I guarantee that if you do everything in that list, you will do better than someone who is in your situation but not putting them into practice. Also, if you are one of these people who has active lupus disease and are practicing all the Lupus Secrets, make sure to see your lupus doctor (usually a rheumatologist) regularly and ask at each visit what can be done differently with your treatment and medications to get better disease control.

Studies show that patients who practice self-care and learn to manage their lupus improve and have a better QoL than patients who do not. If you are reading this book and have come to this chapter—congratulations! You have already shown that you are motivated to do what you can to learn to control lupus and not let lupus control you. We wish you the very best in achieving this goal.

KEY POINTS TO REMEMBER

1. SLE can cause many problems that differ from person to person.

2. Some issues are directly due to inflammation (such as nephritis and arthritis). Rheumatologists use anti-inflammatory and immunomodulating medicines (medicines that calm the immune system) to treat these. The following chapters of part II discuss these issues in detail.

3. Other problems (such as fibromyalgia and osteoporosis) commonly seen in people with SLE are not directly due to the inflammation of lupus. They may be caused by medications, long-term damage from SLE, or other reasons. Doctors treat these problems with therapies other than immunomodulating medicines. Part III covers these.

4. Blood abnormalities, age, gender, or ethnicity may increase the chances of developing specific lupus problems (table 5.1).

5. SLE can have periods of quiescence (remission) and periods of increased activity (flares). It is essential to see your doctor during flares to ensure that other problems (such as nephritis) are not occurring.

6. Do not stop taking your medications when you are feeling well. You will put yourself at risk for lupus flares that can sometimes be severe and even life-threatening.

7. Prepare ahead of time for possible flares. Fill out the Lupus Foundation of America's "Lupus Flare Plan," discuss it during your next doctor visit, and then use it during any future flares.

8. Abide by and put into practice everything in "The Lupus Secrets" (the last chapter of this book) to improve your chances for remission and low disease activity.

Allergies in SLE Patients

SLE patients have more allergies and intolerances to antibiotics such as penicillin, cephalosporins, sulfonamides, and the antibiotic erythromycin than other people. The most important antibiotic intolerance is to the sulfonamide (often called "sulfa") antibiotic group. The most prescribed sulfonamide antibiotic is trimethoprim-sulfamethoxazole (Bactrim and Septra). Around one-third of SLE patients have reactions to Bactrim, which can cause lupus flares as well. These reactions are more common in Caucasians, those with low lymphocyte counts (lymphopenia), and anti-SSA-positive patients. Still, they can occur in any lupus patient and cause fevers, sun-sensitive rashes, and low blood cell counts. Sometimes these flares can be severe. Many other antibiotics are now available, and sulfonamide antibiotics can usually be avoided.

We recommend that all lupus patients always carry an up-to-date medication list. It should include an allergy list that includes sulfa antibiotics. This can protect you if you ever get sick and end up in the emergency room, where it can be hard to remember your entire medical history.

Note that the sulfa intolerance in lupus patients pertains only to sulfonamide antibiotics. It is OK to take sulfates, sulfites, and non-antibiotic sulfonamides such as furosemide, hydrochlorothiazide, acetazolamide, sulfonylureas used for diabetes, and celecoxib.

While lupus patients are more likely to be intolerant of the antibiotics penicillin, cephalosporins, and erythromycin, these do not generally cause lupus flares. The vast majority of SLE patients tolerate them well. Therefore, they do not need to be avoided.

LUPUS IN FOCUS

Sulfur versus sulfonamides versus other sulfa drugs and lupus

The element sulfur exists in all of us, so none of us is allergic to sulfur. Many different molecules contain sulfur, including sulfates, sulfites, and sulfonamides. Lupus patients have an increased risk of lupus flares when treated with sulfonamide antibiotics (specifically trimethoprim-sulfamethoxazole, or Bactrim). Non-antibiotic sulfonamides (furosemide, hydrochlorothiazide, acetazolamide, sulfonylureas used for diabetes, and celecoxib) are different from Bactrim and do not cause lupus flares. They are generally safe for lupus patients (unless they just happen to have an allergy to that particular drug). Sulfates and sulfites are not associated with lupus flares.

Allergies to pollen, animals, foods, and medicines, among other things are widespread in the general population. Approximately one out of three SLE patients also have environmental allergies (pollen, animals, dust mites, and others). Whether these types of allergies occur more commonly in lupus patients is unknown, and more extensive study is needed.

Allergy shots (called immunotherapy) are a common treatment for allergies. While guidelines suggest that these shots are safe for lupus patients who are in remission, patients should be monitored closely to ensure that immunotherapy does not cause flares. Allergy shots should be avoided for patients not in remission. Some guidelines, such as that of the European Academy of Allergy and Clinical Immunology, state that patients who have cutaneous lupus (without having SLE) can get allergy shots if the disease is "stabilized." Additional considerations are that immunosuppressants (table 22.1) may cause allergy shots to not work well. However, hydroxychloroquine (Plaquenil) and chloroquine likely do not interfere with allergy shots.

KEY POINTS TO REMEMBER

1. Most true allergies probably do not occur more frequently in lupus patients.

2. All SLE patients should avoid sulfonamide antibiotics (Bactrim and Sulfa). It is OK to take sulfates, sulfites, and non-antibiotic sulfonamides such as Lasix, hydrochlorothiazide, acetazolamide, sulfonylureas used for diabetes, and celecoxib.

3. SLE patients in remission may be able to safely get allergy shots.

The rest of part II is devoted to the full range of lupus problems. The next chapter discusses symptoms such as weight loss, fevers, and fatigue (called constitutional symptoms). Those following discuss problems in each organ system separately, the medical tests used to diagnose them, and how they are treated.

Constitutional Symptoms

Maria Chou, MD, *Contributing Editor*

Constitutional symptoms affect the whole person due to disease. Malaise, fatigue, fever, and weight loss are among those experienced by SLE patients. These can occur any time the disease is active, or they can occur due to problems other than SLE.

Malaise

Malaise is a feeling of being unwell. It is not always easy to pin down. Some common descriptors of malaise include vague feelings of discomfort and overall weakness (different from actual muscle weakness). It is the kind of feeling you get at the beginning of a cold or flu when you feel that something is wrong, but don't know exactly what since you don't yet have a cough, sore throat, or runny nose. Fatigue can be part of the feeling of malaise, but someone can have malaise without feeling fatigued. Malaise often affects one's quality of life and ability to perform critical daily activities.

Fatigue

Fatigue is a general loss of physical and mental energy. It is not the same as weakness or drowsiness (see chapter 40). Mild fatigue, which can affect people who are trying to do something active, goes away once they rest. Severe fatigue continues even when someone is resting. Fatigue affects over 80% of SLE patients. Obese SLE patients are more likely to have fatigue than patients of normal body weight. Numerous studies show that weight loss and exercise improve energy in overweight SLE patients.

Many rheumatologists and their patients consider fatigue to be one of SLE's most frustrating symptoms. Patients regularly report fatigue to be the number one cause of keeping them from doing normal daily activities and the number one cause of having a poor quality of life. It can be challenging to find a reason for the fatigue, and it can be tough to treat. Fatigue is sometimes a direct result of inflammation occurring throughout the body from active SLE. If so, it usually responds well to treatment with medications that calm the immune system, such as steroids, belimumab (Benlysta), anifrolumab (Saphnelo), or hydroxychloroquine (Plaquenil).

Fatigue may be due to many other problems. Depression, fibromyalgia, stress, sleep disorders, anemia, postural orthostatic tachycardia syndrome (POTS, chapter 11), thyroid disease, poor lifestyle habits, pain, and medications can cause fatigue. Therefore, when a person with SLE has significant fatigue when the SLE is well controlled, the doctor must consider these possibilities. If you have substantial fatigue, ask your doctor to check you for these. Consider taking some home surveys such as the ones for depression and anxiety (tables 13.3 and 13.5), obstructive sleep apnea (OSA, table 6.4), and fibromyalgia (chapter 27). A high score suggests that you may have that disorder.

Another common cause of fatigue is adrenal insufficiency (a condition that can occur while steroid doses are being decreased). If you notice that you are becoming more fatigued as you take lower doses of steroids, read chapter 26, and discuss this possibility with your doctor.

Some partners of patients with severe fatigue state that the effects of the fatigue spill over into their relationship, negatively affecting their daily lives. A 2015 study from The Netherlands addressing this issue showed that those couples who worked harder on communication skills and acceptance and understood more about SLE ended up with higher satisfaction rates in their relationships.

It is essential to realize that fatigue is often due to multiple factors and rarely has a simple cure. Vitamins, for example, rarely help unless the person has a significant vitamin deficiency. Still, there are things you can do to improve your energy level. If you have considerable fatigue, review table 6.1 to find possible causes and learn to better manage the fatigue.

Inadequate good quality sleep is one of the most common causes of fatigue in SLE. Problems with sleep include not getting enough hours of sleep, having trouble falling asleep, waking up in the middle of the night and being unable to get back to sleep. Difficulty with memory, poor coping skills, depressed mood, and obesity are all health problems tied to lack of sleep. Most sleep experts recommend eight or more hours of restful sleep for most people. Unfortunately, today's fast-paced lifestyle means that a

Table 6.1 How to Increase Energy Levels

- See your doctor to look for specific causes of fatigue.
- Take the home surveys on anxiety and depression (tables 13.3 and 13.5), obstructive sleep apnea (table 6.4), and fibromyalgia (chapter 27). Let your doctor know if you score high on any of these tests.
- Work on sleep hygiene techniques (table 6.2).
- Take DHEA up to 200 mg a day if your lupus is active and approved by your doctor (chapter 35).
- Take vitamin D supplements if your vitamin D level is low.
- Go on a low-calorie or low-carbohydrate diet to lose weight, if overweight.
- Ask for an antidepressant if depression symptoms exist (insomnia, difficulty concentrating, moodiness, loss of interest in enjoyable activities, loss of sexual interest, or if you have feelings of guilt or low self-worth).
- Learn your limits; pace yourself.
- On bad fatigue days, do not do more than one important activity. Try to do more on better days.

large percentage of people do not get enough sleep. If you do not get enough sleep at night or do not feel well-rested when you get up, you should work on your sleep habits, or "sleep hygiene" (table 6.2).

Many people sabotage their sleep by unconsciously getting into habits that disrupt the sleep cycle. Review table 6.2 about sleep hygiene several times and commit yourself to everything listed.

Some patients have difficulty incorporating sleep hygiene techniques in their lives. They may find that a more formal approach works better, especially when dealing with a "racing mind" that keeps them from sleeping. In these instances, another option is cognitive behavioral therapy for insomnia, or CBT-I. The American Academy of Sleep Medicine and the National Institutes of Health recommend CBT-I as the best, initial therapy for insomnia. You can contact your local sleep centers (especially those affiliated with major medical centers) or find CBT-I courses online, such as at www.cbtforinsomnia.com. The American Board of Sleep Medicine and the Society for Behavioral Sleep Medicine can supply a list of doctors specially trained in CBT-I.

In 2020, a large group of sleep experts reviewed the best studies about treatments for insomnia. They came up with a list of those therapies with the best evidence for being helpful and safe and those that should be avoided. They recommended CBT-I, along with other therapies (table 6.3).

More than half of SLE patients have a sleep disorder that causes fatigue. These sleep disorders include obstructive sleep apnea (OSA), periodic limb movement disorder (PLMD), and restless legs syndrome (RLS). Most can be diagnosed using a test called a polysomnogram (sleep study). Each sleep disorder requires different forms of therapy, but all include working on sleep hygiene techniques, as discussed before.

OSA is a condition in which the neck's soft tissues cause the breathing passages to narrow while someone sleeps, leading to disturbed sleep. Some common symptoms of OSA are fatigue, falling asleep easily while at rest (such as while watching TV), snoring, having difficulty concentrating, being moody, and waking up with a headache or dry mouth. It is more common in overweight people and people with a larger than average neck size. Doctors tend to underdiagnose OSA in women, which means that many women with SLE who have OSA do not know they have it. Not only can OSA cause fatigue, but it also increases the risk of heart disease and high blood pressure when untreated. There are many ways to treat OSA, including weight loss and wearing a mouth guard to open the airway while sleeping. A mask that is connected to a machine and forces air into the lungs to keep people breathing correctly while they sleep is another option. The CPAP (Continuous Positive Airway Pressure) machine is the most used device. For those who have difficulty using CPAPs, incorporating CBT-I makes it easier to do so. In some cases, surgery is performed to remove excessive tissue within the throat, allowing the person to breathe properly. Proper treatment can make a big difference in energy levels and quality of life.

If you have any of the symptoms seen in OSA, take the simple questionnaire in table 6.4. If you answer "yes" to two or more questions, you have an increased risk of having OSA. If you do not answer "yes" to two or more of the questions, ask yourself if your body mass index (BMI) is over 30 (chapter 21), you are over 50, or your neck circumference is 16 inches or larger if you are a woman or 17 inches or larger if you are a man. If you answer "yes" to any of these, you should let your doctor know. OSA is easy to diagnose with a sleep study performed at a sleep center or home.

Table 6.2 Sleep Hygiene Techniques

- The most important thing: participate in an online "cognitive behavioral therapy for insomnia" course such as at www.cbtforinsomnia.com or www.sleepio.com; or use the app CBT-I Coach.

- Maintain a regular sleep schedule; get up and go to bed at the same time daily.

- Reduce stress (table 38.9).

- Exercise daily; mornings and afternoons are best. Don't exercise right before bed.

- Avoid naps late in the afternoon or evening.

- Finish eating 2 to 3 hours before bed; a light snack is fine, but avoid foods containing sugar, which can stimulate the mind and interfere with falling asleep.

- Limit fluids before bed to keep from getting up to urinate.

- Avoid caffeine 6 hours before bed.

- Do not smoke. If you do, don't smoke for 2 hours before bed; nicotine is a stimulant.

- Avoid alcohol 2 to 5 hours before bed; alcohol disrupts the sleep cycle.

- Avoid drugs that are stimulating (ask your doctor).

- Avoid mind-stimulating activities a few hours before bed (reading technical articles, listing tasks to do, trouble-shooting, paying bills, etc.).

- Have a hot bath 1 to 2 hours before bed; it raises your body temperature, and as your temperature decreases afterward, you will get sleepy.

- Keep indoor lighting low for a few hours before bed.

- Establish a regular, relaxing bedtime regimen (aromatherapy, drink warm milk, read, listen to soft music, meditate, pray, relaxation/breathing exercises).

- Ensure your sleeping environment is quiet and comfortable (comfortable mattress and pillows; white noise such as a fan; pleasant, light smells).

- If pets wake you, keep them outside of the bedroom.

- Use the bedroom only for sleep and sex; never eat, read, or watch TV in bed.

- Never keep a TV, computer, or work materials in your bedroom.

- Go to bed only when sleepy.

- If you can't sleep within 15 to 20 minutes in bed, go to another room, read something boring under low light, meditate, pray, listen to soft music, or do relaxation/breathing exercises until sleepy.

- If your mind races, preventing you from sleeping, perform mindfulness (chapter 38) for 5–10 minutes before bed. Use an app such as Relax Lite or Headspace.

- If you have dry mouth, use a mouth lubricant like Biotene Mouth Spray, or use xylitol lozenges (such as Xylimelts) before bed.

- Avoid "blue light" (smartphones, computer screens) 1 hour before bed.

- Get exposure to light first thing in the morning to set your biological clock. Consider using a non-UV light, like Philips goLITE BLU or Miroco UV Free Lux Brightness light.

Table 6.3 Insomnia Treatments

Strongly Recommended Treatment

Cognitive-behavioral therapy, including sleep hygiene

Other Possible Treatments

Brief behavioral therapy for insomnia (BBT-I:)

Auricular acupuncture with seed and pellet

Prescription drugs, brief periods only: doxepin, zaleplon, zolpidem, eszopiclone

Treatments That May Also Be Effective

Mindfulness meditation (chapter 39)

Other types of acupuncture (auricular has the best evidence)

Aerobic exercise, strength training, tai chi, yoga, qigong

Prescription drugs, brief periods only: ramelteon, suvorexant

Source: Adapted from the U.S. Department of Defense, *Clinical Practice Guidelines: The Management of Chronic Insomnia Disorder and Obstructive Sleep Apnea* (2019).

Table 6.4 STOP Questionnaire for Obstructive Sleep Apnea

- Do you *S*nore loudly (louder than talking or loud enough for people to hear through closed doors)?
- Do you often feel *T*ired, fatigued, or sleepy during the daytime?
- Have you ever had anyone *O*bserve you stop breathing while you sleep?
- Are you being treated or have you received treatment for high blood *P*ressure?
- If you answer "yes" to two or more of the above, then you should get a sleep study.

Another therapy that may help fatigue is the steroid hormone DHEA (dehydroepiandrosterone). Many people with SLE have low DHEA levels. Some studies have shown that taking DHEA may help increase a sense of well-being and decrease fatigue in people with mild to moderate disease activity when they take 200 mg daily. (Note, though, that acne and unwanted hair growth are potential side effects.) If your doctor tells you that your SLE is under reasonable control, then DHEA will most likely not help. The role of DHEA and fatigue in SLE has been questioned by many doctors.

Although you can obtain DHEA over the counter without a prescription, be careful. Many over-the-counter products do not have the correct amounts of DHEA since the FDA does not supply quality controls on over-the-counter supplements. It is best to get a prescription from your doctor and have a compounding pharmacist supply a high-quality product instead.

Studies suggest that vitamin D deficiency may contribute to fatigue in some SLE patients. Vitamin D levels lower than 30 ng/mL are associated with fatigue in SLE. Those with the lowest levels (< 10 ng/mL) have the worst energy levels. A 2016 research study on young people with SLE showed that fatigue and SLE disease activity improved when low vitamin D levels were treated. This combination of the lowest vitamin D levels being associated with the worst fatigue and then energy levels improving once vitamin D levels were improved with treatment is good evidence for low vitamin D being a cause of fatigue in SLE.

Losing weight through dieting can also improve energy. A 2012 study showed that women with SLE had significant improvements in energy after losing weight over six weeks. Half the women used a low-carbohydrate diet, and the other half used a standard low-calorie diet. The amount of weight loss and energy increase was similar in the two groups.

Two of the most common causes of fatigue in people with SLE are depression and fibromyalgia (chapters 13 and 27). These two conditions are related to an imbalance of chemicals in the body's nerves involved with mood, sleep, energy levels, memory, and pain. Exercise is an important treatment for both disorders. Treatment also includes medications (such as antidepressants) that try to normalize these chemical imbalances. Studies also suggest that a significant number of people who have unexplained fatigue can improve with the use of antidepressants, even if their symptoms do not qualify as depression. Some experts recommend their use in people with fatigue if a definite reason for fatigue is not clear. They consider the potential benefits of the medication to outweigh the potential risk for side effects.

A 2018 study from Rush University in Chicago, Illinois, showed that fibromyalgia, depression, and stress were more commonly the causes of fatigue than lupus inflammation. To help deal with fatigue, SLE patients should learn to manage stress as much as possible (chapter 38).

Doctors cannot overemphasize the importance of regular exercise to treat fatigue. Many of the problems causing fatigue in SLE (such as depression, fibromyalgia, OSA, and insomnia) can improve with regular exercise. True, it is difficult to force yourself to move and exercise more when your body tells you not to, but there are ways to encourage yourself, such as joining a fitness program or walking with friends. Interactive exercise programs are another option. One study used Nintendo's Wii Fit, a program that you can plug into your television. Fifteen sedentary (non-exercising) women with SLE who had moderate to severe fatigue exercised using Wii Fit 3 days weekly, 30 minutes at a time. At the end of 10 weeks, they had significant reductions in fatigue. This is not an advertisement for Wii Fit. However, it is a good illustration of how SLE patients who are physically inactive (due to life-altering fatigue) can improve their energy levels after exercising regularly. A 2016 study that evaluated non-drug treatments of fatigue in SLE patients concluded that exercise, acupuncture, and other interventions such as sleep hygiene and stress reduction helped. However, aerobic exercise had the best evidence as a treatment.

Learning the importance of not overdoing things and understanding your limitations is also helpful for dealing with fatigue. A popular tool for gauging your limits was developed by an SLE patient, Christine Miserandino, who described her "Spoon Theory" in a 2003 blog post. One day, when a friend asked her what it was like to have SLE, Christine handed her some spoons. Each one represented a unit of energy, she explained. Each day, she started out with a limited number of spoons. Every activity that she did that day took away one or more spoons. This way of thinking about her activities helped her ration her energy expenditure each day so as not to go over her energy stores. Hence the "Spoon Theory," which is popular with many SLE patients. Many people who practice the Spoon Theory call themselves "spoonies" and connect on social media using #spoonies.

Fever

Normal temperature varies a lot from person to person, ranging from 96.0°F to 100.8°F when taken orally (thermometer placed under the tongue). It also varies based on the time of day. Body temperature is usually lowest at 6:00 A.M. and highest at 6:00 P.M. You have a fever if your oral temperature in the early morning is higher than 98.9°F or your late afternoon temperature is higher than 99.9°F.

Of people with SLE, 50% to 70% will develop fever as a problem. Fever due to lupus inflammation generally responds well to acetaminophen (Tylenol) and non-steroidal anti-inflammatory drugs (NSAIDs) such as ibuprofen or naproxen, and steroids (chapter 7).

However, you should never automatically blame a fever on SLE. It is crucial to consider infection as a possible cause because people with SLE are at increased risk of infections (chapter 22). Infections in people with SLE may require antibiotics and medicines that decrease fever. People with SLE who have a fever, especially if on immunosuppressants such as prednisone, should always see their physicians right away to ensure it is not due to an infection. It can be a mistake to wait and see if the fever resolves on its own. Illnesses due to a minor infection such as colds are frequent and may not require antibiotics. However, it is better to leave this decision to a health care provider, especially since infection is one of the leading causes of death in SLE.

Weight Loss

Weight loss occurs in up to half of SLE patients. Weight loss can occur for many reasons, including decreased food intake from malaise, abnormalities in taste (chapters 13 and 15), and reduced appetite (anorexia). In some SLE patients, absorption of nutrients from the intestinal tract decreases (chapter 15). Lupus inflammation and fever cause the body to use up more calories. In addition, muscle loss (sarcopenia, chapter 7) can contribute to weight loss.

However, other things can also cause weight loss. Drugs, such as hydroxychloroquine and many immunosuppressants, can sometimes cause a loss of appetite as a medication side effect, and thus weight loss. If the weight loss due to drug side effects is substantial, the doctor will usually want to change therapy (reducing doses or changing the drug).

Other conditions that can cause weight loss include depression, an overactive thyroid, gluten hypersensitivity (chapter 15), reduced eating due to gastroesophageal reflux or peptic ulcer disease (chapter 28), and even cancers. Therefore, if a person with SLE has weight loss and their SLE appears inactive, doctors must consider other possible causes.

When weight loss is due to the lupus inflammation, it can generally be reversed with treatment of the disease (such as with hydroxychloroquine and immunosuppressants, table 22.1).

Lupus cachexia

An important cause of weight loss is cachexia. It comes from the Greek for "bad things" (*kakos*) and "state of being" (*hexus*). In lupus cachexia, inflammation increases metabolism, resulting in loss of muscle and weight out of proportion to the amount of food eaten. Decreased muscle strength, fatigue, and low appetite commonly occur.

A 2020 Johns Hopkins Lupus Clinic (Baltimore, Maryland) study showed that 56% of their SLE patients had cachexia. (Note that Johns Hopkins typically sees sicker than average SLE patients.) They generally had a lot of systemic inflammation, especially involving the serosae (chapter 1), kidneys, bone marrow, and blood vessels (vasculitis). After treatment of their lupus, 80% recovered their weight, while 20% did not. Those who had persistent cachexia had a high rate of ongoing organ damage. The researchers were surprised to note that cachexia occurred as often in their lupus patients as it does in cancer patients.

KEY POINTS TO REMEMBER

1. Constitutional symptoms (malaise, fever, fatigue, and weight loss) occur commonly in SLE. However, they can be caused by other disorders as well.

2. If you have a fever, it is crucial to see your doctor right away. Although fevers occur with SLE, you must consider infection first.

3. Fatigue is one of the most common and frustrating problems in SLE.

4. If fatigue is due to lupus inflammation, energy levels should improve when the SLE is treated with steroids or other medicines such as hydroxychloroquine (Plaquenil) that calm the immune system.

5. There are other problems to consider as causes of fatigue, such as abnormal thyroid function and anemia. The doctor can check for these with blood tests.

6. If these tests are all normal, you need to consider other possibilities as the cause of fatigue. Take the tests for depression and anxiety (tables 13.3 and 13.5), OSA (table 6.4), and fibromyalgia (chapter 27). If you score high on any of these tests, let your doctor know for proper evaluation and treatment.

7. If you have significant fatigue, make sure to follow the advice in table 6.1 and work hard on improving your sleep hygiene (table 6.2).

8. Problems other than SLE can cause weight loss, including depression, gastrointestinal issues (such as gluten hypersensitivity or gastroesophageal reflux), and an overactive thyroid. Even hydroxychloroquine (the medicine most used for SLE) can cause weight loss.

The Musculoskeletal System

Jemima Albayda, MD, *Contributing Editor*

The musculoskeletal system is comprised of the muscles (*musculo-*), bones ("skeletal"), joints, and adjacent structures (such as tendons). The joints are the hinges between the bones that allow movement.

Approximately 90% of SLE patients have joint or muscle pain at some point due to their lupus. Because the musculoskeletal system is the most common part of the body to be affected by SLE (causing aches and pains, or rheumatism), rheumatologists became the specialists dedicated to diagnosing and managing SLE patients.

Osteoporosis (fragile bones that can break) and avascular necrosis (where a section of bone dies) are also musculoskeletal problems that occur in SLE. However, these are usually not due to the inflammation of lupus itself and are discussed in part III.

Inflammatory Arthritis

Most people with SLE develop arthritis with joint inflammation (inflammatory arthritis). On physical examination, an arthritis diagnosis is appropriate if the doctor finds evidence of inflammation, such as soft tissue joint swelling and decreased range of motion. Joint x-rays can be useful in making sure there are no other reasons for joint pain.

Lupus inflammatory arthritis often causes morning joint stiffness that can take 30 minutes or longer to loosen up. Arthritis that is not due to inflammation (noninflammatory arthritis) typically causes mild and brief morning stiffness (if at all).

The most common noninflammatory arthritis is osteoarthritis. Osteoarthritis is often called degenerative joint disease, or "wear and tear" arthritis. It occurs due to the aging process or trauma (joint injury). While someone with lupus arthritis will typically say, "My fingers and elbows are so stiff in the mornings that it can take an hour for them to loosen up," someone with osteoarthritis will typically say, "My joints are stiff when I get up, but loosen up by the time I'm done with my shower." The amount of time it takes to loosen up can help determine the difference between the two. Most SLE patients will develop osteoarthritis as they get older (due to the aging process). It is important to distinguish between lupus arthritis and osteoarthritis since they are treated very differently.

Lupus arthritis most commonly affects the elbows, wrists, knuckles, middle joints of the fingers, knees, ankles, and the joints where the toes connect to the foot. When a person with SLE develops pain in the neck, shoulder muscles, back, and sides of the hips, it is usually caused by something other than SLE. Examples include bursitis, tendonitis, degenerative arthritis, pinched nerves, and fibromyalgia (chapter 27). Doctors treat fibromyalgia differently than lupus arthritis. Moreover, lupus does not typically cause "pain all over," which is more commonly due to something else such as fibromyalgia or depression. Overall body pain is considered one of the type II symptoms discussed in chapter 5.

Fortunately, the arthritis of lupus is usually not crippling or deforming. This is different than the related autoimmune disorder, rheumatoid arthritis, which commonly causes joint deformities if not treated.

Some people with lupus arthritis develop joint deformities. One type is called Jaccoud's (pronounced yah COOZ) arthropathy, which usually affects the fingers. It is a reversible deformity in that the doctor can straighten them out during physical exam (called reversible deformities), but it is not permanently reversible. After the doctor releases the affected fingers, they revert to their deformed shape. When Jaccoud's worsens over time, the joints can lose their mobility, leaving the person with "fixed deformities" that cannot be straightened out.

An example of Jaccoud's arthropathy is figure 7.1. This is an SLE patient of mine who gave me permission to publish her ultrasound and hand photos.

Note how the end joints of the fingers are bent (flexed), and the middle joints are bent in the opposite direction (extended). This type of deformity is called a swan-neck deformity (it is the shape of a swan's neck). When the opposite occurs (the end joint is extended and the middle joint is flexed), it is called a boutonniere deformity. When these deformities occur in the thumb joints, they are called Z-thumb deformities because the thumb looks like the letter Z.

Another potential problem is that some people with SLE will have an overlap syndrome (chapter 2) with rheumatoid arthritis (RA) called rhupus (a combination of **rhe**umatoid arthritis and **lupus**). These patients typically have a lot of joint swelling on examination, morning stiffness lasting an hour or longer, and evidence of damage on x-rays (called erosions), as well as usually being RF or CCP antibody–positive (chapter 4).

In SLE, it is also very common to have inflammatory joint pain (without definite arthritis). While the condition has no formal definition, it is typically characterized by experiencing 30 minutes or more of morning stiffness and tenderness of the joints (even in the absence of joint swelling and loss of range of motion).

Both inflammatory joint pain and inflammatory arthritis are SLE classification criteria (chapter 1).

"Arthralgia" is an umbrella term meaning "joint pain." Many lupus patients will have joint pains without having inflammation. In that case, they are said to have arthralgias rather than inflammatory arthritis or inflammatory joint pain. Arthralgias are common in other conditions, such as depression, fibromyalgia, thyroid problems, and sleep apnea. Therefore, having joint pain without actual joint inflammation is not part of the SLE classification criteria (chapter 1).

Many rheumatologists use ultrasound to help diagnose joint inflammation. It is one of the most accurate ways to tell if there is active inflammation from lupus. An ultrasound picture of a joint with active lupus inflammatory arthritis is shown in figure 7.2. The large white square in the photo is the area where inflammation can be identified using an ultrasound technique called "color Doppler." Note the very bottom thicker white line closest to the bottom of the large square. That is the edge of wrist bone. The

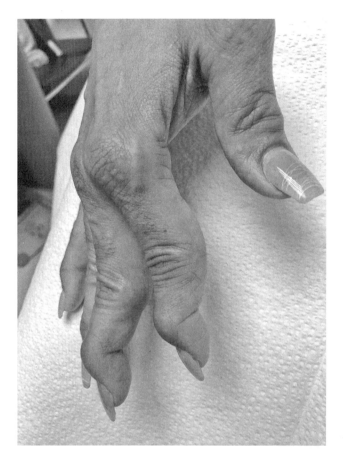

Figure 7.1 Swan neck deformities of fingers due to Jaccoud's arthropathy

dark (blackish) oval-shaped area above it represents increased fluid and swelling of the wrist joint due to lupus arthritis. On the outer left rim of the dark area is an oval-like area with a thin black rim. There is another similar area attached to its bottom left, and another is a separate area to its upper right. These are areas of lupus inflammation in the wrist joint, confirming that this patient has lupus inflammatory arthritis. On the ultrasound machine, these areas would show up as orange, red, or blue (depending on the Doppler technique). The color version of this photo is online at www.lupusencyclopedia .com/book-photos. The orange-colored areas in the online color version are the regions of active inflammation. Normal joints should not have these areas of orange.

Ultrasound exams show that 25% to 75% of lupus patients previously diagnosed with noninflammatory arthralgia actually have joint or tendon inflammation (discussed below). This is an important distinction for two reasons. First, a correct diagnosis (using ultrasound) of arthritis rather than of arthralgia can lead to a faster SLE diagnosis. Second, lupus arthritis requires medications to calm inflammation rather than just pain medicines.

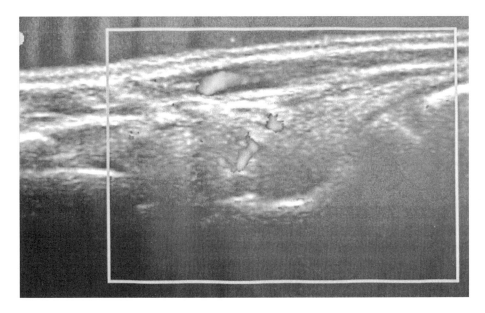

Figure 7.2 Ultrasound of lupus arthritis of the wrist (see main text for description)

Rheumatologists treat lupus arthritis with non-steroidal anti-inflammatory drugs (NSAIDS, such as ibuprofen and naproxen) and hydroxychloroquine. Sometimes doctors also prescribe stronger immunosuppressants (table 22.1).

Some rheumatologists use tumor necrosis factor inhibitors (TNFi) for patients with SLE. TNFi include etanercept (Enbrel), adalimumab (Humira), infliximab (Remicade and Inflectra), golimumab (Simponi), and certolizumab (Cimzia). While this group of medications has been associated with drug-induced lupus, it has not been shown to worsen lupus in patients who already have SLE. Also, many SLE patients do well with TNFi therapy, especially those with lupus and rheumatoid overlap syndrome (rhupus).

The goal in treating lupus arthritis is to get it into remission such that there is no active inflammation on physical or ultrasound examination. This differs from previous recommendations, where a common goal was simply to decrease pain. That resulted in too many SLE patients ending up with permanent joint deformities from Jaccoud's arthropathy.

An essential part of the treatment regimen of people with arthritis and arthralgias is exercise. Due to pain, many people cannot be as active as they were before developing lupus. They usually lose muscle mass, strength, and joint flexibility, which not only prevents them from doing activities they previously could but can also lead to muscle weakness and more pain. This becomes a vicious cycle such that the pain leads to less activity, less activity causes loss of function and more pain, and so on. Many studies show that people with arthritis who force themselves to exercise regularly end up with less pain, develop more muscle mass, do more activities, and have a better quality of life. Not only does exercise help with pain and function, but it has other benefits such as keeping weight under better control, decreasing the chances of strokes and heart attacks (chapter 21), and helping with mood in those with depression.

Regular exercise is an important treatment for everyone with SLE. If you do not know how to exercise or are afraid you may injure yourself considering your health condition, ask your doctor to refer you to a physical therapist (PT). A PT can thoroughly evaluate your physical health and design a safe exercise regimen for you.

Tendonitis and Tenosynovitis

Tendonitis (tendinitis) and tenosynovitis are also common in SLE. The tendons are sinewy, inelastic fibrous tissues that connect the muscles to the bones. When muscles contract, the tendons enable the muscles to move the much stronger bones. Just as lupus can cause joint inflammation, it can also cause tendon inflammation (tendonitis). Tendonitis usually causes pain around and between the joints. The joint pains seen in SLE are often due to tendonitis rather than arthritis.

A lubricating sheath surrounds some tendons. This sheath is called the tenosynovium, and it helps tendons glide more smoothly and stay in place. When these become inflamed, the condition is called tenosynovitis.

A typical example of tenosynovitis occurs in the tendons of the palm. These tendons help bend the fingers, such as when gripping something. Someone with this kind of tenosynovitis can have pain while bending the fingers, and the finger can even get stuck in a flexed position. The affected person may need to use the other hand to straighten out the finger. This type of tenosynovitis is often called trigger finger.

Tenosynovitis inflammation can go away on its own or after successful SLE treatments. However, scar tissue (permanent damage) may be left between the tendon and its surrounding sheath. The scar tissue is a result of the healing process, and it can cause ongoing pain and trigger finger.

A lupus tenosynovitis ultrasound is shown in figure 7.3. Review the description of figure 7.2 earlier to know how inflammation appears in these black-and-white ultrasound photos. This (figure 7.3) is an image of the tendon that bends the index finger of the woman's hand pictured in figure 7.1. In the center of the large white square, running from left to right, are a bunch of parallel white and black lines. They fill up the middle one-third of the square. These are tendon fibers. At the top of these lines, toward the left, is a thicker white line, then two oval areas with black rims, then another thick white line above those. The space between the thick white lines is the lubricating surface between the tendon and its tendon sheath (thin piece of tissue) that surrounds it. The purpose of the tendon sheath is to keep the tendon in place and provide a lubricated surface for it to glide smoothly while bending the finger. Normally there is little to no separation between these lines on ultrasound of a normal tendon. The space here represents increased swelling from lupus inflammation. The two round areas with black rims are areas of lupus inflammation. They are red- and blue-colored on the actual ultrasound and are easily seen in the online photo at lupusencyclopedia.com/book-photos.

The tendon sheath inflammation causes pain when she bends her finger. Since I could see that she had active inflammation (the red and blue dots on the ultrasound) and not just scar tissue, I knew I needed to adjust her medicines to calm down the immune system better. If I had not seen the inflammation, I would have supposed that her pain was probably from scar tissue and treated it with pain relievers, exercise, and cortisone injections (see chapter 31).

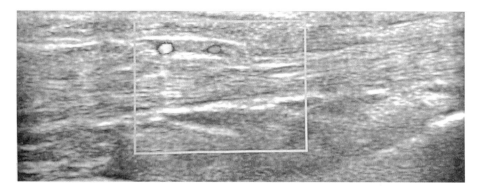

Figure 7.3 Ultrasound of inflammatory tenosynovitis due to lupus (see main text for description)

Some other examples of tendonitis include rotator cuff tendonitis (at the shoulder), epicondylitis at the elbow (commonly called tennis elbow and golfer's elbow), Achilles' tendonitis (back of the ankle), and plantar fasciitis (bottom of the heel).

Just as with arthritis, the tendonitis of SLE is treated with NSAIDs and hydroxychloroquine (Plaquenil), while stronger immunosuppressants (table 22.1) are used for more severe cases. Resting the tendon to allow the body to heal is important. If you have tendonitis (or arthritis), ask your doctor or physical therapist about joint protection measures. An injection with a corticosteroid (a cortisone injection) is one of the safest and quickest ways to treat tendonitis and tenosynovitis. Using an ice pack as needed can also help to decrease pain severity.

Enthesitis

The location where any ligament or tendon attaches to a bone is called an enthesis. Inflammation of an enthesis is called enthesitis. Enthesitis usually does not cause joint swelling. On physical examination, tenderness is found on the bony sides of the joints, away from the joint line. Enthesitis explains why many SLE patients with joint pain do not have joint swelling.

These entheses (the plural of enthesis) also occur in the areas of tenderness that doctors push on to help diagnose fibromyalgia. This could help explain why so many SLE patients are diagnosed with fibromyalgia. We have had SLE patients with secondary fibromyalgia improve dramatically with immunosuppressants. This makes us wonder if some of our SLE patients with fibromyalgia may have had lupus enthesitis instead. This is another good reason for using ultrasound to figure out what is causing the pain in SLE patients.

Chondritis

Chondritis refers to cartilage inflammation. Cartilage is a firm, flexible tissue that helps support areas that require flexibility. For example, the firm area above your ear lobes is the cartilage of the outer ear, as are the firm parts of your nostrils. Inflammation of these areas (chondritis) causes redness and pain. Other areas of cartilage that can also be involved include the windpipes (trachea and bronchi), voice box (larynx), and the joints.

Chondritis is primarily seen in a systemic autoimmune disease called relapsing polychondritis. Chondritis rarely occurs in SLE (less than 1% of patients). It is unknown if this is primarily a direct problem from lupus or if these patients have an overlap syndrome with relapsing polychondritis.

The most important thing for doctors to consider in an SLE patient with chondritis is that there is no trachea inflammation. If there is, the windpipe can become soft (instead of firm) and collapse, making it very difficult to breathe. Chondritis is treated with immunosuppressants.

Myositis

Myositis refers to muscle inflammation due to a direct attack by the immune system; it occurs in up to 10% of SLE patients. This inflammation may cause muscle weakness or pain (myalgia). Although many people with SLE can develop myalgias, most do not have actual myositis.

SLE patients can also have an overlap syndrome with the autoimmune diseases polymyositis or dermatomyositis (PM and DM, chapter 2). PM and DM cause similar problems with muscle weakness, pain, and test findings. However, PM and DM can have positive autoantibodies that distinguish them from lupus myositis.

Lupus myositis most commonly affects the muscles closest to the shoulders, hips, and thighs. Symptoms include having difficulty raising the arms to brush the hair or standing up from a chair without using the hands. On examination, the doctor may find these muscles weak and find an elevation in muscle enzymes in the blood work (such as CPK, aldolase, LDH, and AST levels; chapter 4). Often there is enough evidence from these findings to warrant treatment, but sometimes more specialized tests are required.

One of these tests is an electromyogram (EMG for short). This test, done in a doctor's office or a hospital, measures muscle electrical activity. It is not a very comfortable test because a technician inserts tiny needles into the muscles. The person then moves specific muscles when instructed. A doctor usually does not order this test unless they think it is vital to make a correct diagnosis. Typically, a doctor will order a nerve conduction study at the same time as the EMG to determine whether there is evidence of nerve damage causing the muscle weakness. The technician applies sticky electrodes to the skin, creating a tiny electrical shock between the electrodes to see how well the nerves respond. This test is also uncomfortable. However, it can provide critical information regarding nerve health.

If the doctor suspects myositis, they can also order muscle magnetic resonance imaging (MRI). MRI is usually done with the person lying down on a table, then entering a narrow tube where magnetic waves take pictures. Since this procedure does not use radiation, there is no risk of cancer. Sometimes MRIs are not helpful if there is significant metal in the body (such as having a metal hip replacement when evaluating the hip muscles). They can be dangerous if someone has a pacemaker or other implanted electronic device. Therefore, alert the technician or doctor if this applies to you.

Claustrophobic people often have difficulty getting through the test since the tube they must go into is narrow and loud noises are emitted. If you are claustrophobic, you may want to ask your doctor for medication to calm your nerves before the test. You could also ask to have it done in an MRI machine called an open MRI, which does not enclose a person in a tight tube. However, a regular MRI provides higher-quality results.

If there is still the possibility of myositis or the doctor needs to consider other causes of muscle problems after the above tests, a muscle biopsy may be required. "Biopsy" is the medical term for taking a small piece of tissue from the body for examination under a microscope. A muscle biopsy is usually taken from the large muscle in front of the thigh or the deltoid muscle in the upper arm. During a biopsy, which is typically performed as an outpatient procedure, a surgeon numbs the area with an anesthetic and then makes a cut in the skin (an incision) down to the muscle. A small piece of the muscle is removed and sent to the laboratory. The doctor then closes the incision with sutures.

If an SLE patient has myositis, doctors usually treat it with immunosuppressants, such as steroids, methotrexate, azathioprine, mycophenolate, rituximab, or tofacitinib (Xeljanz). Intravenous immunoglobulin (IVIG, chapter 35) can also help.

Achy muscles (myalgias) without actual muscle inflammation (myositis) are treated with pain relievers, such as acetaminophen (Tylenol), NSAIDs (such as ibuprofen and naproxen), or other analgesics such as tramadol (Ultram and Ultracet).

Just as with arthritis and arthralgias, regular exercise is essential for those with myositis and myalgias. Strengthening exercises are especially important. It can be beneficial to see a physical therapist to learn which exercises are most helpful.

A challenge with muscle weakness in lupus patients is that some drugs can cause muscle inflammation (myositis) or damage (myopathy). For example, the steroids used to treat myositis can themselves cause myopathy. The condition is called steroid myopathy (chapter 31). Steroid myopathy is treated by reducing the steroid dose.

Antimalarials (chapter 30), like hydroxychloroquine (HCQ) and chloroquine, are the drugs of choice for treating SLE. They can also cause muscle damage (antimalarial myopathy); however, this is very rare. Most cases described in the medical literature are from chloroquine, rather than HCQ. Antimalarial myopathy causes shoulder and hip weakness, and muscle enzymes (like CPK, chapter 4) are usually normal or only slightly elevated. A muscle biopsy is required for diagnosis, and it is treated by stopping the antimalarial. Antimalarial myopathy slowly improves after the drug is discontinued.

Since lupus increases heart attacks and stroke risks, cholesterol-lowering drugs called statins are often needed. These, too, can cause muscle damage (statin myopathy), although rarely. The appearance of symptoms, including muscle pain, weakness, or elevated muscle enzymes on blood tests, can take anywhere from just a few weeks to up to four years after starting the statin. After stopping the statin, it takes an average of two months for the muscle symptoms to improve but can take as long as a year.

Very rarely, an immune-mediated reaction to a statin can lead to true muscle inflammation (myositis). In those cases, muscle enzymes are generally very high, patients become very weak, and these conditions persist even after the statin medication is stopped. Blood tests can look for statin-induced antibodies (anti-HMGCR antibody). If confirmed, it is treated with immunosuppressants.

Other potential causes of muscle weakness include metabolic problems such as diabetes, hyperthyroidism, and hypothyroidism.

1. Arthritis exists when there is joint inflammation (determined on physical examination or ultrasound).

2. Arthralgias are joint pains that may or may not be due to actual inflammation or damage.

3. Arthritis and inflammatory joint pains (but not arthralgias) are included as an SLE classification criterion (chapter 1).

4. Arthralgias in SLE patients can be due to lupus, fibromyalgia, depression, or completely unrelated issues such as osteoarthritis.

5. Lupus arthritis (other than Jaccoud's) usually does not cause permanent joint damage and deformities. X-rays of affected joints usually appear normal.

6. The goal of treating lupus arthritis is remission—no evidence of inflammation on physical examination or ultrasound.

7. Doctors usually treat lupus arthritis with NSAIDs and hydroxychloroquine. Stronger immunosuppressants (table 22.1) may be necessary.

8. Tendonitis and tenosynovitis are common causes of joint pains in SLE patients.

9. Enthesitis can cause lupus pain and is difficult to detect without ultrasound.

10. Ultrasound helps identify inflammation as the cause of pain in SLE.

11. Chondritis is rare in SLE.

12. Myositis is usually painless, but occasionally muscle pain occurs.

13. Weakness, especially of the upper arms (causing difficulty raising the arms) and the hips (causing trouble standing up from a chair), is the most common symptom.

14. Some people with myositis are diagnosed with an overlap syndrome with polymyositis or dermatomyositis (chapter 2).

15. Myositis is diagnosed by finding muscle weakness on physical examination and elevated muscle enzymes in the blood (CPK, aldolase, LDH, and AST levels).

16. Sometimes, an EMG test or muscle biopsy is necessary.

17. Doctors usually treat myositis with immunosuppressants.

18. Myalgias (achy muscles), and arthralgias (achy joints) without actual inflammation (myositis and arthritis, respectively) are treated with pain relievers such as acetaminophen (Tylenol), NSAIDs (such as ibuprofen and naproxen), or other analgesics such as tramadol (Ultram and Ultracet).

19. All lupus patients who have joint pains, myositis, or myalgias should exercise regularly

How to Treat Your Pain

Your doctor can use prescription drugs or cortisone injections to help joint and muscle pains. However, there are things you can do on your own to help your pain (table 7.1).

Joint Protection

Joint protection is essential in dealing with pain. When you rest a painful joint or tendon, you help decrease inflammation, damage, and degeneration. The techniques described below should be used for all types of arthritis. Whenever you develop pain in any part of your body, practice the following general joint protection measures and the joint protection recommendations for that part. Overuse of a joint, incorrect use of a joint, and improper posture all contribute to injury and pain. If you take the recommended actions quickly enough in cases such as overuse tendonitis and arthritis, you may be able to stop the pain (lupusencyclopedia.com/joint-protection).

Whenever pain persists, it is vital to consider the possibility that you may be overstressing your joints and tendons. Think carefully about what you do at your job, at home, and while engaging in other activities and whether any of these may be aggravating your condition. For example, a person may keep getting wrist pain and then realize that this seems to occur the day after they crochet and knit. Repetitive tasks such as crocheting, typing on a computer, and texting on a cellphone are some of the most common contributors to joint and tendon damage. It is essential to identify activities that exacerbate your joint pain and do them less and for shorter periods. Using splints or braces to help reduce stress on affected tendons can also help.

Personality can play a significant role in causing and managing pain. Compulsive workers and perfectionists may have the attitude of "I'm going to finish this job if it kills

---

Table 7.1 How to Decrease Lupus Pains

- Protect painful joints (see lupusencyclopedia.com/joint-protection)
- Exercise:
  - Range-of-motion and stretching exercises
  - Low-impact aerobic exercise
  - Strengthening exercise
- Use over-the-counter medicines
- Try other treatments:
  - Heat and ice
  - Meditation and prayer
  - Yoga
  - Biofeedback
  - Acupuncture
  - Stress reduction
  - Practicing mindfulness (such as breathing exercises)

---

me." They need to learn to respect their pains, pay attention to what their body tells them, and recognize their potentially self-destructive behavior. It can be important to learn how to change your expectations and not be a perfectionist. Learning to avoid certain tasks can be just as important as learning to perform a job in a way that puts less stress on the joints. Ask your rheumatologist or physical therapist for specific joint protection advice. Also, go to lupusencyclopedia.com/joint-protection.

Exercise

Exercise is crucial for people with arthritis since it improves function, preserves the joints, strengthens the muscles, and decreases pain. Recommended exercises vary depending on the exact problem and the affected body parts. Ask your doctor for advice regarding specific activities or ask them to send you to a physical therapist for proper assessment and instruction.

We discuss some exercise basics. The broad categories are range-of-motion, stretching, aerobic, and strengthening. A good, well-balanced exercise program should include each these.

More recent studies point to the importance of avoiding prolonged sitting. Staying in a stationary position for extended amounts of time contributes to many health problems such as weight gain, heart attacks, strokes, diabetes, cancer, and early death. Getting into the habit of alternating between sitting and standing every 30 minutes can make a big difference. Devices such as smartphones and fitness watches, which vibrate or give other alarms to alert the user to get up and move around if they sense prolonged periods of not moving, can be helpful.

Range-of-Motion and Stretching Exercises
Joint range of motion refers to how far a joint can move in all directions. Over time, arthritis and pain can cause a loss of range of motion and a loss of function. Maintaining as much range of motion as possible is essential. You should move painful joints through their full range of motion every day. Use the hand of the opposite side of the body to move the painful joint gently as far as it can go without causing pain. Repeat this in every direction in which that joint can move.

You can do stretching exercises while you do range-of-motion exercises. They should be a regular part of the exercise regimen before or after aerobic or strengthening exercises. Stretching helps to keep the joints, muscles, and ligaments flexible. While there are many types of stretching exercises, it is vital to concentrate on staying relaxed while doing any of them. Each joint or muscle stretched should be held at a point where stretching is felt without pain. If it is painful, then you should relax the stretch slightly. You should hold the stretch for 15 to 30 seconds; breathe deeply and slowly to help relax your muscles.

Aerobic Exercises
Another term for aerobic exercise is "endurance exercise." Aerobic exercises work large muscle groups continuously to keep the heart rate elevated. Examples include brisk walking, stationary bicycling, high- and low-impact aerobic exercises, swimming, dancing, and using a treadmill or an elliptical exercise machine. However, other continuous activities, such as mowing the lawn, can also count. Studies show that aerobic exercise decreases arthritis pain, helps with weight loss, lessens stress and depression, improves muscle strength and function, helps control diabetes and high blood pres-

LUPUS IN FOCUS

How much should you exercise?

We recommend getting at least 150 minutes of moderate aerobic exercise per week and 2 days a week of moderate muscle strengthening exercises for all major muscle groups as per the Physical Activity Guidelines for Americans produced by the U.S. Department of Health and Human Services.

sure, helps prevent heart attacks and strokes, and increases lifespan. You should exercise to the point where you breathe harder than usual but can still speak in full sentences. It can also be helpful to aim for a target heart rate (which depends on your age). You can ask your doctor what target heart rate they recommend. Or visit the Mayo Clinic's site, mayoclinic.org/healthy-lifestyle/fitness/in-depth/exercise-intensity/art-20046887.

It is best to do aerobic exercise for 20 to 45 minutes 4 to 5 days a week. Avoid injuring joints, tendons, and muscles by starting with 5 to 10 minutes of light exercise and gradually increasing to the recommended goal of at least 150 minutes a week.

Strengthening Exercises

When you have pain or arthritis, the muscles around the painful joints weaken, tighten up, and get smaller (they atrophy). This begins a vicious cycle because as the muscles lose function, this in turn causes even more pain and disability. Research shows that weakness occurs more often in lupus patients. Weakness in the large muscles of the thigh contributes to thigh and knee pain, while weakness in the muscles of the lower legs and feet contributes to foot and ankle pain. All these areas of weakness cause difficulties with walking, standing, and running.

The importance of regular strengthening exercises cannot be overemphasized. They are vital to increasing muscle strength, improving function, and retaining a good quality of life. Muscles help absorb stress and strain away from the joints' more fragile ligaments and tendons. When your muscles get weaker, your ligaments and tendons are more likely to develop ongoing permanent damage and degeneration. The US Department of Health and Human Services recommends that everyone perform strengthening exercises of all major muscle groups two to three days a week as part of a healthy exercise regimen.

You can go to a gym and learn what exercises to do from a personal trainer or staff member. Consider getting exercise equipment to use at home as well. If you have more significant health problems, especially arthritis and joint pain, you should ask your doctor for advice or a referral to a physical therapist who can teach you what exercises to do. Today, there are various exercise classes designed specifically for people with arthritis. These classes are educational and give you the opportunity to exercise with people with similar problems.

Over-the-Counter Medicines

Some pain medications are available over-the-counter (OTC). While this chapter provides recommendations regarding when and how to use them, it is also important to read the package instructions thoroughly. Also, always check with your doctor first to ensure a given medication is safe for you. Otherwise, there is always the potential risk for drug interactions.

Acetaminophen (Tylenol, Many Other Brand Names)

Acetaminophen is one of the safest drugs for pain, aches, and fever. It is the drug of choice for osteoarthritis (also called degenerative joint disease).

Generic available: Yes. Often says "Pain Reliever" on the bottle. Look for "acetaminophen."

How acetaminophen works: Not fully understood.

Dosage: The maximum recommended daily dose is 2,000 to 4,000 mg a day (table 7.2). Ask your doctor how much you can handle safely. If significant pain relief does not occur by taking it on an as-needed basis, you should try taking it regularly around the clock. It can take up to a week to get the full effect when taken this way. This would be the equivalent of taking 500 mg tablets (Tylenol Extra Strength) two pills at a time, four times daily.

If you have a history of drinking alcohol to excess, don't exceed 2,000 mg to 3,000 mg a day and have your doctor monitor your blood liver enzymes (ALT and AST).

Acetaminophen and NSAIDs appear reduce pain through different mechanisms. Acetaminophen can help reduce pain more if you are already taking an NSAID. It is generally safe to take along with an NSAID.

Do not take if

- you have kidney disease, liver disease, have had severe hepatitis resulting in permanent liver damage, or have drunk alcohol excessively in the past. But ask your doctor—it may be OK to take in smaller doses.

- you drink more than two servings of alcohol in any 24-hour period.

- you are taking any prescription drugs that already contain acetaminophen.

Alcohol/food/herbal interactions: Do not drink more than two servings of alcohol a day while taking acetaminophen. See chapter 38 for alcohol serving recommendations.

Acetaminophen is absorbed best when taken on an empty stomach.

Avoid Echinacea, kava, willow, meadowsweet, and St. John's wort.

What to monitor while taking acetaminophen: blood liver enzymes (ALT and AST) if you have had a history of excess alcohol use.

Potential side effects of acetaminophen (table 7.3): Significant side effects from acetaminophen (table 7.3) are minimal if you do not take a higher dose than normal and as long as you do not drink too much alcohol. It is the safest pain medicine available. Even so, always check with your doctor before taking anything over the counter.

While taking acetaminophen, contact your doctor immediately if you develop jaundice (yellowed skin and whites of eyes).

Table 7.2 Acetaminophen (Tylenol) Maximum Recommended Doses

acetaminophen 650 mg (Tylenol Arthritis)	2 tablets 3 times a day
acetaminophen 500 mg (Tylenol Extra Strength)	2 tablets 4 times a day
acetaminophen 325 mg (Tylenol Regular Strength)	3 tablets 4 times a day

Table 7.3 Potential Side Effects of Acetaminophen

	Incidence	Side Effect Therapy
Nuisance side effect		
Rash	Rare	Stop taking it. Use cortisone creams or antihistamines.
Serious side effect		
Liver failure when taking more than 4,000 mg daily or if drinking too much alcohol	Rare	Seek medical attention immediately if you purposefully overdose (ingest more than 7,500 mg in a short period)

Table 7.4 Over-the-Counter NSAIDs

Generic	Brand
aspirin	Ascriptin, Bayer, Ecotrin
ibuprofen	Addaprin, Advil, Dyspel, Genpril, I-Prin, Motrin, NeoProfen, Provil
naproxen	Aleve, Flanax, Mediproxen

Pregnancy and breast-feeding: Major birth defects have not been seen, but it may increase the risk of asthma or undescended testes in a newborn baby. Since fever can cause birth defects, it is recommended to use acetaminophen for fever to protect the unborn baby.

Acetaminophen is considered safe while breast-feeding.

Geriatric use: No dose adjustments are needed unless there is significant chronic kidney disease, liver disease, or a history of alcoholism.

Non-Steroidal Anti-Inflammatory Drugs

Non-steroidal anti-inflammatory drugs (NSAIDs) are the largest group of medications used for aches and pains. Many OTC brands are available (table 7.4). It is crucial to ensure that you are not taking any prescription NSAIDs before considering an OTC NSAID. It is generally safe to take an NSAID along with acetaminophen to reduce pain. See complete information in chapter 36.

Other Modalities

You and your doctor can consider many other modalities to reduce pain.

Topical treatments: Topical medicines are therapies that you place on the skin over painful areas. They come in many forms, such as creams, gels, and patches. Effective ingredients include lidocaine, methyl salicylate, menthol, camphor, diclofenac, and capsaicin (same as capsicum). None of these is proven better than the others. Some appear to work better in some people than in others, so a trial-and-error approach to different types may be needed.

If you try capsaicin, be aware that one of the critical ingredients is chili peppers, so you must be careful not to get it in your eyes or on other mucous membranes (such as the nose, mouth, genitals).

Some topical treatments (such as capsaicin, diclofenac, and lidocaine) are best used regularly around the clock and not just as needed. They can also take several weeks to get the full benefit. We like to say that "it needs to build up in your system."

Heat therapy (thermotherapy): Muscle pain, muscle spasms (knots in the muscles), trigger points, and sore muscles after exercise can benefit from heat therapy. Heat can be applied in many ways, including a hot shower or bath, jacuzzi, steam room, warm whirlpool, heating pad, heat wrap, hot water bottle, heated gel pack, or heated bean bag. Applying heat for approximately 15 to 20 minutes is common.

Do not apply heat on joints affected by inflammatory arthritis, areas of infection, or areas where you have used capsaicin. If you have neuropathy (nerve damage), be careful as you could burn your skin if the heat source is too hot (you may not feel it) and do not use it for more than 20 minutes at a time.

Cold therapy (cryotherapy): Icing can be helpful for injuries, tendonitis, bursitis, and inflammation (such as lupus inflammatory arthritis). Ice therapy can be applied in many ways, including raw ice (like an ice cube), ice frozen in a Styrofoam cup, commercial ice or gel wraps, ice packs, or frozen bags of peas. Do not use bare ice for more than 1–3 minutes. Follow the rule of thumb "when you're numb, you're done." Cold compresses with a barrier between the ice and the skin (such as cups, wraps, and packs) may be applied longer.

Do not apply ice on areas of broken skin. If you have neuropathy (nerve damage), be careful as you could freeze your skin if the ice source is too cold (you may not feel it), and make sure not to use it for more than 1–3 minutes.

Complementary therapies: These include mindfulness, relaxation techniques, breathing exercises, acupuncture, massage therapy, yoga, and tai chi. See chapter 39.

KEY POINTS TO REMEMBER

1. Ask your rheumatologist or physical therapist for joint protection advice.

2. Exercise regularly with a combination of range-of-motion, stretching, aerobic, and strengthening exercises. Consider asking your doctor to send you to a physical therapist to learn how to exercise correctly.

3. Aim for at least 150 minutes a week of moderate aerobic exercise and 2 to 3 days a week of muscle-strengthening exercises.

4. Acetaminophen (Tylenol) is the safest medicine to take for pain but be careful if you drink excessive amounts of alcohol or have liver problems. Make sure your prescription drugs do not contain acetaminophen.

5. Over the counter NSAIDs include naproxen and ibuprofen. They have many potential side effects and drug interactions. Always ask your doctor before taking them and take only one NSAID at a time.

6. Over-the-counter topical pain relievers can help. Some need to be used regularly around the clock, and some may need to be taken for several weeks to get the full benefit of reduced pain.

7. Heat can be helpful for muscle spasm pain. Ice can be beneficial for inflammation pain.

8. See chapter 39 for mindfulness, acupuncture, and massage therapies.

Skin and Mucous Membranes

Ginette A. Okoye, MD, FAAD, Cheri Frey, MD,
and Divya Angra, MD, *Contributing Editors*

Around 80% of people with SLE develop problems of the skin or the mucous membranes inside the mouth or nose (collectively called mucocutaneous involvement). After joints, the skin and mucous membranes are the next most involved body parts in SLE. Although these problems are rarely life-threatening, their impact on appearance and self-esteem can be tremendous (chapter 5).

The skin is one of the body's organs. Lupus that affects the skin is called "cutaneous lupus." If someone has only cutaneous lupus, and no other organs are involved, they have only cutaneous lupus and not systemic lupus. If lupus affects additional organs, it is said to be "systemic" and is called SLE. In someone with SLE, cutaneous lupus can be one of that person's SLE manifestations. Cutaneous lupus occurs in most, but not all, SLE patients. Cutaneous lupus can also be a manifestation of the other forms of lupus: drug-induced lupus and neonatal lupus (chapters 1, 18, 41).

Two large groups of skin problems occur with SLE. The first, which is discussed in the following section, is comprised of lupus-specific rashes, meaning that they are seen only in lupus patients. They are also known as cutaneous lupus. The second group of rashes can be seen in many disorders other than just lupus and are discussed in later sections of this chapter.

Lupus-Specific Rashes (Cutaneous Lupus)

Doctors usually diagnose lupus rashes by the way they appear on physical examination. However, sometimes a skin biopsy is necessary. In this procedure, the doctor numbs the skin, snips out a small piece to be sent to a laboratory to be examined by a pathologist, and then either sews up the area with sutures (surgical thread) or uses glue or surgical adhesive tape. The doctor may sometimes need to order a particular type of biopsy study called immunofluorescence to make a proper diagnosis. In this study, the pathologist looks for deposits of immunoglobulins (a type of immune system protein) between the upper (epidermal) and lower (dermal) skin layers.

Lupus-specific rashes are so named because their biopsies share similar abnormalities under the microscope.

The lupus-specific rashes (synonymous with cutaneous lupus) are divided into acute cutaneous lupus erythematosus (ACLE), subacute cutaneous lupus erythematosus

Table 8.1 Cutaneous Lupus (Lupus-Specific Rashes)

Acute cutaneous lupus erythematosus (ACLE)

    Localized ACLE (the malar or butterfly rash)

    Generalized ACLE

    Toxic epidermal necrolysis-like ACLE

Subacute cutaneous lupus erythematosus (SCLE)

    Annular (also called polycyclic) SCLE

    Papulosquamous (also called psoriasiform) SCLE

Chronic cutaneous lupus erythematosus

    Discoid lupus erythematosus (DLE)

        Localized DLE

        Generalized DLE

    Lupus panniculitis (also called lupus profundus)

    Lupus erythematosus tumidus

    Chilblain lupus

    Hypertrophic (also hyperkeratotic and verrucous) DLE

(SCLE), and chronic cutaneous lupus erythematosus (CCLE) (table 8.1). Lupus-specific rashes are included as SLE classification criteria (chapter 1).

"Acute," "subacute," and "chronic" distinguish among types of cutaneous lupus in terms of the time frame. Thus, in ACLE, rashes often come on suddenly (acutely), last for a relatively brief period, and go away quickly either on their own or with treatment, usually leaving the skin with a normal appearance. On the opposite extreme, CCLE tends to last a long time. After treatment, it leaves behind areas of permanent skin damage and scarring that never go away (chronic). SCLE lies somewhere in the middle in that it does not develop as rapidly as ACLE or leave permanent scarring the way that CCLE does.

Virtually everyone with ACLE and bullous lupus erythematosus (described later) also has SLE. Around 10% to 15% of SCLE patients can develop SLE, while up to 20% of those with CCLE will. On the other extreme, people with lupus tumidus (described later) rarely develop the systemic form.

Acute Cutaneous Lupus Erythematosus

ACLE is divided into two patterns, localized and generalized. Localized ACLE is most commonly known as the butterfly (or malar) rash and occurs only on the face. Generalized ACLE involves skin above and below the neck.

ACLE is very sensitive to ultraviolet (UV) light (chapter 38), especially the sun. ACLE typically has a reddish or pinkish coloration that becomes more prominent with sun exposure. It can cause a warm sensation and be itchy (pruritic), and it can resolve after a few hours or last up to several weeks (an "acute" period of time).

When this kind of rash resolves with treatment, it does not cause permanent scarring. It can, however, occasionally leave some dark-colored areas called post-inflammatory

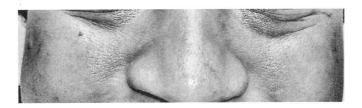

Figure 8.1 Malar rash in a person of color with SLE (see color versions of all photos at lupusencyclopedia.com/book-photos)

hyperpigmentation, which is a response of the skin to the inflammation, causing skin cells to produce more melanin (dark pigment), and which occurs more often in dark-skinned individuals.

It is important not to overlook lupus rashes in people of color. Lupus rashes, especially erythema (the medical terms for redness), can be difficult to recognize on darker skin tones, as compared with light skin tones. While the erythema appears bright red in the latter, it may look dark purple or dark brown on darker skin. If it is overlooked, there may be a delay in diagnosing people of color with lupus and providing them with essential treatments.

A butterfly rash (figure 8.1) is a reddish- or pink-colored rash occurring on areas of the face exposed to the sun (the cheeks and bridge of the nose). Sometimes, the rash may look swollen or scaly. This rash is often mistaken for sunburn. It is called a butterfly rash because in severe cases, if you were to draw an outline around the rash, the red cheeks would look like butterfly wings, and the rash on the bridge of the nose would look like its body. Other terms for this are "malar rash" and "malar erythema" ("malar" refers to the cheek area, "erythema" means "redness"). In those with SLE, the butterfly rash occurs in around 45% of Hispanics and Asians, 33% of Caucasians, and 25% of those with African heritage.

Not all facial redness in people with lupus is due to malar rash. Other possibilities include acne rosacea (figure 8.2) and seborrheic dermatitis (a type of scaly skin inflammation). Oral steroids can also cause facial redness. Rosacea is commonly mistaken for the malar rash. It is essential to know the difference because the treatment of malar rash is very different from that of rosacea.

Dermatomyositis (chapter 2) can also cause a rash mistaken for the lupus malar rash (especially in children). It is essential to check for muscle weakness on physical examination and high muscle enzymes (such as CPK and aldolase) in the blood work. These findings would suggest a diagnosis of dermatomyositis.

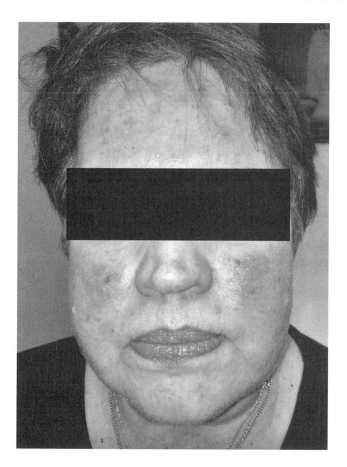

Figure 8.2 Steroid rosacea in an SLE patient taking prednisone. This is often mistaken for the SLE butterfly (malar) rash.
However, prednisone can make rosacea worse, while prednisone usually helps the lupus butterfly rash. Clues to this being
rosacea are the dilated blood vessels underneath the skin
(telangiectasias) and you can see a white bump (pustule) on
the left side of the photo on the person's cheek.

It often takes the help of a skin doctor (dermatologist) to correctly diagnose and treat
rashes in people who have lupus.

Generalized ACLE (with or without blisters) occurs on areas of skin above and below the neck. It typically causes a reddish-colored rash on parts of the body exposed to
UV light, such as the cheeks, forehead, chin, lips, ears, upper back, chest, and top parts
of the hands and forearms. When the photosensitive rash occurs on the hands, it usually occurs between the joints of the fingers (instead of directly over the joints). It may
also cause a reddish discoloration of the skin next to the fingernails. It sometimes involves skin covered with clothing, often in people who are particularly sick with severe
SLE. They often have fevers, joint pains, and other problems. In those who have SLE,

Caucasians and Hispanics have a higher chance of sun-sensitive rashes (approximately 40% chance) than those with Asian and African heritage (about 25% chance).

Toxic epidermal necrolysis-like ACLE is rare. "Toxic" refers to being dangerous; "epidermal" refers to the top layer of skin cells (the epidermis), and "necrolysis" refers to the death (*necro-*) of skin cells. It usually occurs in patients with severe SLE that affects major organs such as the kidneys, brain, and lungs. It is a diffuse red rash that can involve the entire body, especially sun-exposed areas, the lips, and inside the mouth. It is usually painful with blisters, and the skin can slough off. This exposes tissues under the skin to the environment, greatly increasing the risk of infection. Toxic epidermal necrolysis is a medical emergency requiring hospitalization, often in the burn unit of large hospitals. It can sometimes be initiated by a medication, so any recently started drugs should be discontinued. Treatment requires high doses of steroids and other immunosuppressants. Sometimes, intravenous immunoglobulin (IVIG) and plasma exchange therapies are needed (chapter 35). Most patients survive. However, there is an increased risk for death.

Subacute Cutaneous Lupus

Subacute cutaneous lupus erythematosus (SCLE) occurs in two major forms. One appears as red, scaly patches, almost like psoriasis, and is called psoriasiform SCLE (also called papulosquamous SCLE, figure 8.3). The other form of SCLE appears as reddish rings and is called annular SCLE. When SCLE heals, it can leave some discoloration on the skin, though it does not usually cause the severe skin scarring and hair loss that occurs in chronic cutaneous lupus. SCLE is most prominent in sun-exposed areas such as the back, chest, and arms. However, it can extend to other areas, such as the buttocks. Face and scalp involvement rarely occurs.

Although most patients with SCLE have it by itself with no other organs involved, 15% to 50% of SCLE patients (depending on the study) also have SLE, with additional organ involvement, which is usually musculoskeletal (chapter 7), rather than severe and associated with the brain or kidneys.

More than 80% of SCLE patients are positive for anti-SSA (anti-Ro) antibodies. Most patients with a related autoimmune disease called Sjögren's are also positive for anti-SSA. They can develop a rash similar to SCLE.

SCLE often worsens with sunlight exposure. It is more common in white people than in people of color.

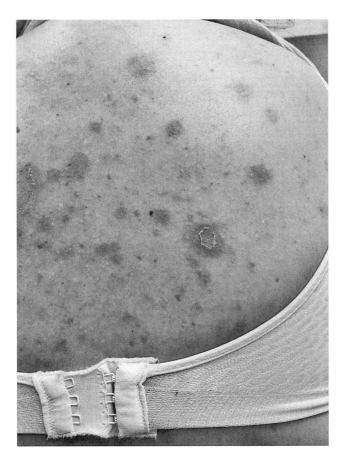

Figure 8.3 SCLE (psoriasiform or papulosquamous form) on the upper back of an SLE patient. Her SCLE got worse after she took the anti-ulcer medicine called lansoprazole (Prevacid). Her SCLE got markedly better after stopping the drug.

LUPUS IN FOCUS

Subacute cutaneous lupus can be a good sign in SLE

Around 10%–15% of SLE patients who also have SCLE can develop severe SLE problems such as brain or kidney inflammation (nephritis). This is much lower than in other SLE patients, up to 45% of whom get nephritis.

Around a third of the cases of SCLE are due to taking medication; the condition is called drug-induced SCLE (DI-SCLE; see table 8.2, and figure 8.3). If a person started any of the medicines that cause DI-SCLE even years before the rash began, the drug should be stopped to see if the rash disappears. Depending on the drug, the rash can start as quickly as 3 days after starting the medication, or as long as 11 years to develop.

Table 8.2 Drugs That Can Cause or Worsen Subacute Cutaneous Lupus Erythematosus

acebutolol

adalimumab (Humira, Amjevita, Cyltezo, Hadlima)

anastrozole (Arimidex)

angiotensin-converting enzyme inhibitors (ACEi)

bortezomib

bupropion (Aplenzin, Forfivo XL, Wellbutrin)

calcium channel blockers

capecitabine

captopril

carbamazepine

checkpoint inhibitor immunotherapy

cilazapril

cimetidine

diltiazem

docetaxel (Taxotere)

doxorubicin (Adriamycin)

D-penicillamine (Cuprimine, Depen Titratabs, D-Penamine)

etanercept (Enbrel, Erelzi, Eticovo)

fluorouracil agents (especially in Japanese)

gemcitabine (Infugem)

glyburide (Glynase)

golimumab (Simponi)

griseofulvin

hydrochlorothiazide

infliximab (Remicade, Renflexis, Inflectra, Remsima)

interferon (Intron A)

ipilimumab

lamotrigine (LaMICtal, Subvenite)

lansoprazole (Prevacid)

leflunomide (Arava)

leuprorelin (Eligard, Lupron)

minocycline (Minocin)

naproxen (Naprosyn, Aleve)

nifedipine (Adalat, Procardia)

nivolumab

omeprazole (Prilosec)

pantoprazole (Protonix)

pembrolizumab

phenytoin (Dilantin, Tremytoine)

Table 8.2 (*continued*)

piroxicam (Feldene)
pravastatin (Pravachol)
procainamide (Procan SR)
proton pump inhibitors (one of the most common causes)
ranitidine (Zantac)
simvastatin (FloLipid, Zocor)
spironolactone (Aldactone, CaroSpir)
statins
tamoxifen (Soltamox)
taxanes
terbinafine (LamISIL)
ticlopidine
tumor necrosis factor inhibitors (TNFi)
verapamil (Calan SR, Verelan)

Some of the most common causes of DI-SCLE include calcium channel blockers, thiazides, minocycline, and proton pump inhibitors (such as pantoprazole and omeprazole). Antifungal treatments, in particular, can cause DI-SCLE within a few weeks, while thiazides and most calcium channel blockers take much longer (months to years).

DI-SCLE goes away or gets much better after stopping the culprit medicine, although it can take an average of seven weeks to improve. Most cases of DI-SCLE get better with the use of medications that calm down the immune system (immunomodulators). However, DI-SCLE due to proton pump inhibitors (PPIs, used to treat heartburn and ulcers) usually does not improve with immunomodulators; instead, PPIs should be stopped.

SCLE can rarely be caused by cancer. SCLE can occur up to four years before cancer appears. The most commonly associated tumors are lung and breast cancers. However, it has also been seen in other cancers. SCLE usually improves with cancer treatment. When SCLE appears in someone without SLE, they should be evaluated for cancer. This should especially be done in those at high risk, such as smokers and the elderly.

Chronic Cutaneous Lupus

Chronic cutaneous lupus erythematosus (CCLE) is the most common type of cutaneous lupus. CCLE tends to last for a long time and often leaves permanent skin damage and scarring. We describe the more common varieties.

By far the most common form of CCLE is discoid lupus erythematosus (DLE). While most DLE patients never develop SLE, about 15% of SLE patients have DLE as one of their lupus problems.

Smokers have a higher risk of DLE than nonsmokers. DLE is more common in dark-skinned people. Women are three to nine times more likely to develop DLE than men.

The rash is called discoid because it looks like a disc. It usually begins with small red or pink scaly bumps. The red area then spreads outward. The center, where the DLE initially appeared, develops a scarred area with pigment changes (figures 8.4 and 8.5). When it occurs on the scalp, it can cause areas of permanent hair loss (figure 8.8), known as scarring alopecia ("alopecia" means "hair loss"). A common place for DLE is just outside the ear canal (called the conchal bowl), especially in people of African ancestry. The person may not notice anything except that the skin just outside the ear canals feels scaly.

Due to the disfigurement and scarring that DLE causes, it is vital to have it examined and treated by a doctor as fast as possible to decrease the possibility of permanent skin damage.

In people with only DLE, the amount of skin involvement predicts their chances of developing additional organ involvement (in other words, SLE). If the rash appears only above the neck (localized DLE), the person has about a 10% chance of developing SLE. If DLE occurs above and below the neck (generalized DLE), the chances are around 25%.

Children with DLE have a higher chance of developing SLE. As many as 25%–30% of children with DLE will progress to SLE within a few months or years (even those with localized DLE).

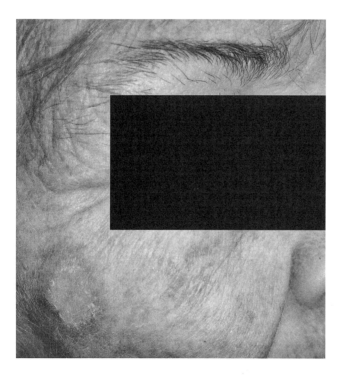

Figure 8.4 DLE on the cheek. The center is light-colored, scarred skin, while the border is red with some slight scaling. The red border is the area of active inflammation. If not treated adequately, it would grow larger, causing more permanent scarring in the center. The patient responded to hydroxychloroquine, leaving a small area of light-colored scar tissue. If she had had a darker skin tone, any permanent skin scarring would have been much more noticeable.

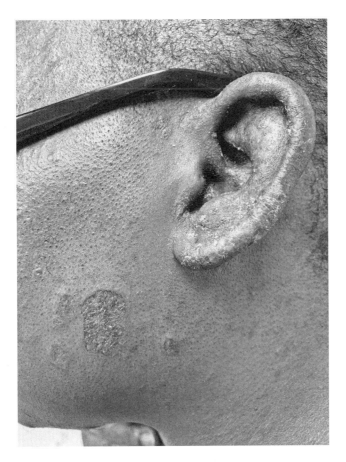

Figure 8.5 DLE on the cheek and ear of a person of color. In the online version, the redness is not as easily seen as in figure 8.4, while the dark pigment changes are more pronounced. DLE can cause significant, permanent skin color changes that can be cosmetically distressing. These changes can cause decreased quality of life and should not be minimized. Photo courtesy of Dr. Ginette Okoye, Howard University

DLE patients should be checked regularly with labs to pick up SLE early if it were to occur. Recommended labs include antinuclear antibodies, complete blood cell count, and a urinalysis. If the ANA is positive, labs such as anti-dsDNA, anti-Smith, antiphospholipid antibodies, C3/C4/CH50 complement levels, and direct Coombs' antibody should be checked.

Having DLE at the onset of SLE may be a good sign. These patients have a lower probability of developing severe SLE, such as kidney involvement (lupus nephritis). This is the opposite of those with the malar (butterfly rash), who have a higher chance of having more severe SLE.

Skin cancer (particularly squamous cell carcinoma) can occur within DLE lesions, especially in those with thin skin and light in color. Smoking, prolonged sun exposure, and being male increase the risk for cancer. Regularly using sunscreen (including on DLE lesions) and avoiding UV light lower the risk. The lips are the area most affected by skin cancer, but it can also affect the scalp, ears, and nose. If an open sore or lumpy (nodular) swelling develops in a DLE rash and doesn't improve with lupus treatments, a biopsy should be done. The treatment is surgical removal.

Lupus profundus (also called lupus panniculitis) is another type of CCLE. It is due to inflammation of fat underneath the skin ("panniculitis" means "inflammation of fat") and causes firm, tender areas under the skin, especially on the face, scalp, upper arms, buttocks, and upper thighs, to develop. When it occurs on the breasts, it is called lupus mastitis. The overlying skin can vary from being normal to having discoloration, scaling, and scarring (figure 8.6). Sometimes lupus panniculitis can be quite painful,

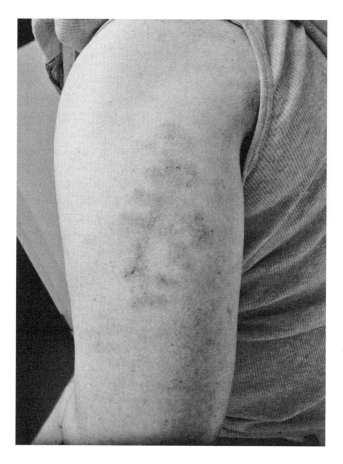

Figure 8.6 Lupus profundus (lupus panniculitis) on the upper arm. Lupus profundus can be readily identified by the deep, firm swelling felt underneath the skin where fat inflammation (panniculitis) is occurring.

unlike most cutaneous lupus. If left untreated, lupus panniculitis can cause tissue loss (especially fat) under the skin, leaving permanent skin indentations.

Another form of CCLE is lupus erythematosus tumidus (LET, "tumidus" means "swollen"). LET (also called tumid lupus) lesions are pink to purple raised (swollen) areas of skin and do not have scaling or open sores. They are highly sensitive to UV light and appear mostly on sun-exposed areas (figure 8.7). Although LET tends to be chronic, individual lesions can go away on their own within days to weeks of their first occurrence. In other words, they can appear intermittently. Unlike most chronic cutaneous lupus rashes, when they go away, they do not leave damage or scarring of the skin.

Due to the intermittent nature of LET, many dermatologists (particularly in Europe) put it under its own category of cutaneous lupus called "intermittent cutaneous lupus

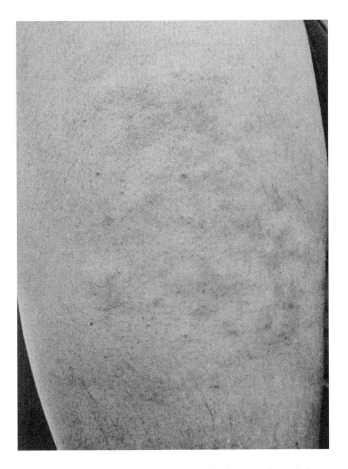

Figure 8.7 Tumid lupus in a person of color. Not the subtle darker colored areas of the tumid lupus compared with the surrounding normal skin. If you were to run your fingers lightly over the tumid lupus, it would feel firmer than the surrounding soft skin and would have raised areas intermixed with deeper areas. Photo courtesy of Dr. Ginette Okoye, Howard University

erythematosus." However, other groups, such as the Systemic Lupus International Collaboration Clinics (chapter 1), list it as a type of chronic cutaneous lupus, as we have done here.

LET patients rarely have SLE. Smokers appear to have a higher risk for lupus tumidus than nonsmokers.

LET tends to respond to steroids and antimalarials (such as hydroxychloroquine, chloroquine, and quinacrine).

Chilblain lupus (also called pernio, perniosis, and chilblains) causes reddish-colored areas on the fingers or toes due to inflammation from cold exposure, leading some dermatologists to nickname it "frostnip." *Chil-* comes from the word "chill," and *-blain* means "inflammatory swelling or blister." Chilblain lupus can be painful or itchy. Treatment includes medications that calm down inflammation (such as steroids and hydroxychloroquine) and increase blood supply to the fingers and toes (such as nifedipine).

Do not be confused by the term "lupus pernio," which is different from "pernio," meaning chilblain lupus when used alone. "Lupus pernio" refers to skin lesions on the face due to a disease called sarcoidosis. The term "lupus pernio" is a remnant from the days when lupus referred to skin lesions that could be due to either sarcoidosis, tuberculosis (an infection), or lupus (the autoimmune disease). Before modern medicine, it was not possible to tell the difference between these three. "Pernio" comes from the Latin word for ham. It refers to the pinkish-red color of the skin lesions (the color of sliced ham).

Cutaneous Lupus Treatments

Cutaneous lupus treatments vary depending on the severity of the rashes. If they are mild and cover a small area, cortisone cream (chapter 31), pimecrolimus cream (chapter 32), or tacrolimus ointment (chapter 32) can help.

It is important to use cortisone creams properly. When used too much, they can cause side effects, such as skin thinning and permanent areas of blood vessel formation (telangiectasia). Cortisone injections into localized rashes can be beneficial for some. Most people with cutaneous lupus should be treated with an antimalarial medication. If someone has only cutaneous lupus without other organ involvement (in other words, doesn't have SLE), taking hydroxychloroquine (HCQ, Plaquenil) regularly can help reduce the risk of progression to severe SLE. HCQ is the most used antimalarial. However, the antimalarials quinacrine and chloroquine can also be used.

The goal with treatment is remission (usually meaning no red, pink, or tender areas). If hydroxychloroquine is insufficient, doctors will often add quinacrine or stop hydroxychloroquine and change it to chloroquine (chapter 30). These treatment changes sometimes work better than hydroxychloroquine.

LUPUS IN FOCUS

Quinacrine

Quinacrine was not available for several years due to manufacturing problems. As of 2022, it became available again through compounding pharmacists. Complete information about quinacrine can be found at www.lupusencyclopedia .com/quinacrine.

If remission (or low disease activity) is not achieved with an antimalarial, a more potent medication such as isotretinoin, acitretin, dapsone, or an immunosuppressant (table 22.1) is usually added.

Mycophenolate mofetil (MMF), methotrexate (MTX), and azathioprine (AZA) are three of the most commonly used immunosuppressants for cutaneous lupus. However, MMF and MTX appear to work better than AZA. Leflunomide (LEF) has mixed results. On rare occasions, LEF can also cause drug-induced subacute cutaneous lupus.

Although seldom used, sulfasalazine can be useful in some patients. SLE patients are instructed to avoid antibiotic sulfonamides (sulfa drugs) since they occasionally cause lupus flares. However, this does not appear to occur with non-antibiotic sulfonamides, such as sulfasalazine.

Although rituximab (RTX, Rituxan) can be helpful for many SLE problems, its success rate in cutaneous lupus is not impressive. Only about half of patients with acute cutaneous lupus improve with rituximab. Lupus dermatologists recommend avoiding RTX for subacute cutaneous lupus and chronic cutaneous lupus.

One of the most effective treatments is thalidomide (Thalomid). However, it is usually reserved for the worst cases due to its potential for severe side effects such as birth defects and irreversible nerve damage.

Anifrolumab (Saphnelo) has impressive results in many patients with cutaneous lupus. It often works after only one or two treatments.

It is essential to not smoke. Smokers do not respond as well to antimalarials, and smokers tend to have worse lupus skin involvement. Smoking cessation can significantly help improve cutaneous lupus.

When cutaneous lupus doesn't respond to the standard treatments, other potential treatments include intravenous immunoglobulin (IVIG), apremilast (Otezla), clofazimine (an antibiotic with anti-inflammatory properties), lenalidomide (Revlimid, a cancer treatment), auranofin (gold), ustekinumab (Stelara), phenytoin (Dilantin, an anti-seizure medicine), cefuroxime (an antibiotic), danazol, extracorporeal photopheresis, pulsed dye laser treatments, and low doses of long-wavelength ultraviolet A1 light treatments. Note that UV A1 light does not worsen lupus (chapters 3 and 38).

Vitamin D is an essential treatment in many cutaneous lupus patients. Several studies have shown decreased systemic and cutaneous lupus disease activity with vitamin D treatment.

Nearly all lupus patients develop increased immune system activation and inflammation from UV exposure, even if they never notice it. All patients with cutaneous lupus need UV protection (chapter 38). Wearing sunscreen daily on exposed areas of skin,

LUPUS IN FOCUS

Photosensitivity that does not cause a rash

Some SLE patients develop problems other than a rash with UV light exposure. These include itching, stinging, or a burning sensation with no rash, as well as joint pain, weakness, fatigue, and headaches from UV light. Reactions can occur within minutes to a week after the exposure.

wearing clothing with UV light protection, and wearing a wide-brimmed hat whenever going outside are the minimum recommendations.

A supplement that may help with UV light protection is Polypodium leucotomos. It is a fern extract that may improve some UV-sensitive rashes.

If a rash has left some post-inflammatory hyperpigmentation (dark-colored areas), a dermatologist can prescribe lightening creams to decrease dark pigmentation.

KEY POINTS TO REMEMBER

1. Lupus-specific rashes (cutaneous lupus) occur only in people who have lupus.

2. Usually, lupus-specific rashes are easy to diagnose by their appearance, but sometimes a skin biopsy is necessary.

3. Most cutaneous lupus rashes can worsen with UV light. All lupus patients should protect themselves from UV light (chapter 38).

4. Almost all people with acute cutaneous lupus have additional organ involvement, meaning that they have SLE. Most of those with chronic cutaneous lupus erythematosus (CCLE, such as discoid lupus) do not have SLE (although 15%–20% of CCLE patients evolve to SLE over time).

5. One third of subacute cutaneous lupus erythematosus (SCLE) (table 8.2) is caused by or worsened by medicine. If you develop SCLE, let your doctor know if you started any of these drugs within the past few years.

6. CCLE can cause permanent scarring, pigment changes, and hair loss. Contact your doctor for treatment if it flares with redness, increased size of rash, or tenderness. Added damage is less likely if treated quickly.

7. The most common form of CCLE is DLE.

8. Treatment includes antimalarials (such as hydroxychloroquine), vitamin D, not smoking, UV light protection, cortisone injections, and topical creams/ointments like steroids, pimecrolimus, or tacrolimus. Severe cutaneous lupus may need stronger drugs.

9. All lupus patients are sensitive to UV light, even if they do not notice it themselves.

Nonspecific Rashes Seen in SLE

Some skin problems that occur with SLE can also occur with other conditions. These nonspecific rashes are described below.

Mucosal Ulcers and Mucositis

Ulcers are open sores that occur when overlying skin has eroded away, leaving exposed tissue beneath the skin surface. Mucosal ulcers are those that occur on lubricated skin surfaces (mucosae, plural for mucosa) such as inside the mouth, nose (nasal ulcers), and vagina. Mucosal ulcers in the mouth are also called oral ulcers and aphthous ulcers.

Table 8.3 Nonspecific Rashes in SLE Patients

Alopecia (hair loss)

Bruises

Calcinosis cutis

Changes of skin color

    Anti-malarial hyperpigmentation

    Post-inflammatory hyperpigmentation

    Quinacrine-induced yellow skin coloration

    Vitiligo

Cutaneous mucinosis

Dry skin

Erythema multiforme

Erythema nodosum

Erythromelalgia

Livedo reticularis

Nail changes

Neutrophilic dermatoses

Oral, nasal, and vaginal mucosa ulcers

Palmar erythema

Periungual erythema

Sclerodactyly

Subcutaneous nodules

Telangiectasias

Ulcers of skin

Urticaria (hives) and angioedema

Vasculitis of the skin

    Palpable purpura

    Urticarial vasculitis

    Vasculitic ulcers

However, most people with aphthous ulcers do not have lupus (that is, there are other causes of aphthous ulcers).

Oral and nasal ulcers are SLE classification criteria (chapter 1). Up to 45% of people with SLE develop oral or nasal ulcers. Oral ulcers can occur anywhere inside the mouth but most commonly on the roof (palate). They are usually painless, though not always. Another term used for mucosal ulcers, especially when the inflammation is widespread, is "mucositis." Sometimes these sores can spread to the lips. This occurs primarily in SLE patients with major organ involvement (such as the kidneys) and is often accompanied by fever.

A common cause of lip sores (often called canker sores, fever blisters, or cold sores in laypersons' terms) is infection from the herpes simplex virus. Herpes lesions tend to recur throughout a person's life. They are not due to lupus. The sores tend to occur more commonly in people on immunosuppressants (table 22.1). Taking antiviral medications usually helps decrease the severity of these outbreaks.

Nasal ulcers typically occur on the septum (the wall dividing the right and left nostrils) or mucosal skin covering the thick center cartilage of the nose. These can be painful. Vaginal ulcers are rare and occur only in 1%–2% of SLE patients. Genital herpes infection is often the cause, and herpes cultures of the ulcers should always be done during outbreaks.

Antimalarial drugs and immunosuppressants usually help reduce severity. However, local applications of steroids (as in triamcinolone in dental paste) can be useful, and, if applied right away and then used every few hours, they can heal the sores faster. Over-the-counter topical anesthetics, such as benzocaine, can reduce pain. Likewise, steroid nasal sprays (such as fluticasone, Flonase) can help nasal ulcers, and mild steroid creams can be used for vaginal ulcers.

Alopecia

There are two major forms of alopecia (the medical term for hair loss) in SLE. We described the first form, scarring alopecia, briefly in the section on DLE; it is illustrated in figure 8.8. Scarring alopecia is an area of permanent hair loss usually due to DLE. It is best treated aggressively and quickly to prevent permanent hair loss. Cortisone creams and cortisone injections can help. However, to prevent ongoing, permanent hair loss, it is best to be on an antimalarial drug with or without an immunosuppressant.

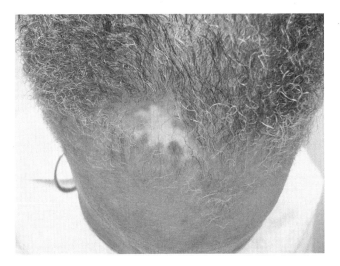

Figure 8.8 DLE causing scarring alopecia (permanent hair loss). Note the central white area with permanent hair loss. In the online version at lupusencyclopedia.com/book-photos /#scarring, the pink-colored border is active inflammation that can spread outward, causing more scar tissue and hair loss unless treated better.

The other form of alopecia is non-scarring alopecia, consisting of thinning of the hair (figure 8.9A). Another common term for it is "lupus hair." Strands of hair are often fragile and break easily, leaving short, coarse hairs and a stubby appearance. Non-scarring alopecia can occur throughout the scalp but is most common at the frontal hairline above the forehead. This type of hair loss is due to the hair follicles resting during increased lupus disease activity (called telogen effluvium). The hair stops growing to save energy for more critical body functions than growing hair. This condition is usually reversible, and the hair grows back when treatment brings the SLE under control (figure 8.9B). Non-scarring alopecia is one of the SLE classification criteria (chapter 1).

Subacute cutaneous lupus and lupus tumidus rarely affect the scalp, but they can cause nonscarring alopecia when they do. Successful treatment usually results in hair regrowth.

One out of ten SLE patients will have alopecia areata (AA) as a cause of non-scarring alopecia. AA is a separate autoimmune disorder in which the immune system attacks the hair follicles, causing decreased hair production. Typically, small circular areas of complete hair loss occur, although there may be some hairs within these areas that are much shorter than usual.

If AA first occurs while a patient is on belimumab (Benlysta), it could be due to the medication. An Israeli group reported 3 patients who developed AA while on belimumab within 4 to 12 months. In two patients, the AA resolved after belimumab was stopped. Another patient developed severe AA but continued belimumab since it controlled her SLE so well. The AA resolved with treatment directed at the alopecia areata. We really don't know if belimumab causes AA unless we see more cases reported in the medical literature.

There can be many other causes of hair loss in lupus patients. Figuring out the exact cause of hair loss is important because the treatments differ.

Thyroid disorders, iron deficiency, and stress can sometimes cause hair loss (these are treatable and reversible). Medications such as steroids, methotrexate, leflunomide, and cyclophosphamide can also cause hair loss. After people stop taking the drug or lower the dose, the hair grows back. Other types of alopecia occur commonly in lupus patients but are not due to lupus. These can be difficult for non-dermatologists to identify yet can mimic lupus alopecia. Three of the most common include androgenetic alopecia, traction alopecia, and central centrifugal cicatricial alopecia (CCCA).

Androgenetic alopecia is also called female pattern hair loss and male pattern hair loss. Genetics probably plays a role. Topical minoxidil (such as Rogaine) used twice daily can help. The regrowth of hair is typically very slow. It is essential to give most hair loss treatments 6 to 12 months of use before concluding whether they are working or not. Other treatments that can help are spironolactone (a fluid pill or diuretic) and low-dose minoxidil pills (such as 2.5 mg daily)

Traction alopecia occurs from tension on the hair follicles due to hairstyles, such as tight braids. This tension damages the hair follicles, and they stop producing hair. It may be aggravated by chemical hair relaxers, which can also cause painful pimples and scalp stinging sensations. Traction alopecia is usually worse at the hairline, and the hair shafts may be more delicate than in the past due to hair follicle damage. Treatment includes avoiding chemical hair relaxers and hairstyles that pull on the hair. Topical minoxidil (Rogaine), low-dose minoxidil pills, steroids, or antibiotics may help.

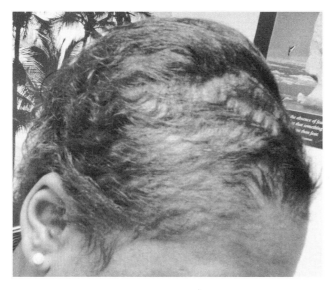

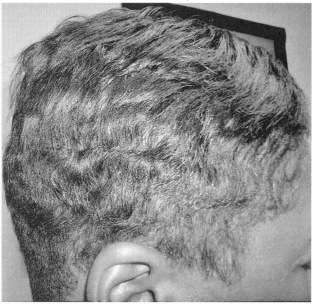

Figure 8.9 Non-scarring alopecia during a severe lupus nephritis flare, before (A) and after (B) treatment. Notice how the hair loss is most prevalent at the front part of the scalp (A). After treatment (mycophenolate, prednisone, and hydroxy-chloroquine), the hair grew back to the point where it could be styled (B).

It can be reversible if treated early. However, if it has gone on for a long time, the hair loss can be irreversible.

CCCA has also been called hot comb alopecia and chemical-induced cosmetic alopecia. CCCA occurs mainly in the center and top of the scalp. It typically starts in the center, expands outward over time, and can feel tender and itchy. Potential causes of CCCA include using hot combs or chemical relaxers or wearing hairstyles that involve braids and weaves. Some people may also have a genetic component (it is much more common in Black women).

CCCA can be very difficult to treat. Patients who respond to treatment best include those with active hair loss, scalp tenderness or discomfort, and evidence of inflammation on physical exam or biopsy. Those with long-standing hair loss who are not actively losing hair are less likely to respond.

Treatment with steroid creams, cortisone injections, anti-dandruff shampoos, minoxidil (pills and topical), or antibiotics can sometimes help. Some of the medicines used to treat lupus can also help, including hydroxychloroquine (Plaquenil), mycophenolate mofetil (CellCept), topical tacrolimus, and cyclosporine.

Other less common causes of hair loss that are not due to lupus include frontal fibrosing alopecia and lichen planopilaris. A fungal infection called tinea capitis can cause hair loss, though rarely. When it does, it is probably due to immunosuppressive drugs, which increase the risk of fungal infections.

There is a wide range of potential causes of hair loss. Unless a patient has classic discoid lupus or definite "lupus hair" that's easily recognized by a rheumatologist, it is best to see a *medical dermatologist* to figure out the diagnosis. But note that not all dermatologists are skilled in evaluating and managing lupus patients, so it is essential to find one who does. Properly evaluating lupus patients takes more time and knowledge than is usually needed for most routine dermatologic situations. You should generally avoid dermatologists who primarily perform cosmetic dermatology.

Bullous Lupus Erythematosus (BLE)

BLE is a nonspecific lupus rash. However, it occurs only in SLE patients. You cannot have BLE if you do not also have SLE. It is labeled "non-specific" because the biopsy looks very different under the microscope than that seen in the lupus-specific (or cutaneous lupus) rashes. BLE biopsies have lots of neutrophils (a type of white blood cell), while lupus-specific rash biopsies show lots of lymphocytes (a different white blood cell). Therefore, a different part of the immune system is causing the problem (not lupus-like). We do not know why this phenomenon occurs in some SLE patients.

"Bullous" is the medical term referring to fluid-filled skin blisters.

Although BLE occurs in people with SLE, it doesn't necessarily fluctuate with SLE disease activity. It can be very active while the rest of the person's lupus is under excellent control, or it can be in remission while other organs have active inflammation. Between 50% and 90% of BLE patients (depending on the study) have an increased risk for kidney involvement (lupus nephritis). Low blood counts, especially leucopenia (low white blood cell counts), also occur in most patients.

BLE usually responds well to therapy. Dapsone (chapter 35) is the drug of choice. If dapsone does not help, other options include colchicine, hydroxychloroquine, chloroquine, methotrexate, mycophenolate, or rituximab.

Urticaria and Angioedema

"Urticaria" is the medical term for "hives." Urticaria can occur when a person is exposed to something they are allergic to, such as cats. Urticaria can also occur in SLE patients due to their lupus inflammation. The hives often worsen with sun exposure, as in other forms of cutaneous lupus.

A related problem is called angioedema, which causes inflammation and swelling of the tissues below the skin surface. Angioedema often occurs on the face, particularly around the eyes or on the lips. The swollen areas may or may not be uncomfortable or tender. Urticaria and angioedema typically improve when the systemic inflammation of SLE is treated.

Vasculitis of the Skin (Cutaneous Vasculitis)

"Vasculitis" means "blood vessel inflammation." Vasculitis can occur in any of the body's blood vessels. If it causes decreased blood flow to the body area that the blood vessels supply, pain and tissue damage can occur. The blood vessels can also leak, causing swelling and bleeding into the surrounding tissues.

Cutaneous vasculitis occurs in up to 20% of SLE patients and can appear in many forms. The most common is palpable purpura. "Purpura" is a medical term for bruising; "palpable" means that the bruised areas are slightly raised and can be felt (palpated) with your finger. Your doctor may also call it leukocytoclastic vasculitis. This usually occurs on the lower legs and looks like many tiny areas of bruising. It is caused by small amounts of blood leaking from the inflamed blood vessels beneath the skin surface. The ankles can swell as a result.

When cutaneous vasculitis causes palpable purpura, it usually does not cause much of a problem beyond the cosmetic appearance and occasional swelling. On rare occasions, though, cutaneous vasculitis can be severe and result in large areas of painful dead skin and open ulcers. These most commonly occur on the legs, and treatment requires immunosuppressants.

Urticarial vasculitis is a less common form of vasculitis in SLE. Urticarial vasculitis looks like hives (urticaria)—hence the name. The skin lesions are slightly raised and tender. When they heal, they often leave color changes. Usually, a skin biopsy is needed for diagnosis. Urticarial vasculitis can occur either with normal or low complement levels in the blood work.

If blood complement levels are low in someone with urticarial vasculitis, it is called hypocomplementemic urticarial vasculitis (HUV). Blood work shows low levels of C4 (and sometimes C3) and high anti-C1q antibody levels (chapter 4). SLE patients with HUV are at increased risk of lupus nephritis, arthritis, eye inflammation (especially scleritis and episcleritis), and angioedema.

Some vasculitis patients are positive for cryoglobulins (chapter 4). *Cryo-* comes from the Greek word for "cold," while "globulins" refer to antibodies. Being positive for cryoglobulins is called cryoglobulinemia (*-emia* comes from the Greek for "blood"). One of the effects of cryoglobulins in an SLE patient is shown in figure 8.10 (a condition called erythromelalgia). We do not know completely how cryoglobulins cause erythromelalgia. Cryoglobulinemia is treated with immunosuppressants or plasmapheresis (chapter 35).

Occasionally, vasculitis of the skin can occur along with vasculitis in other body organs, such as the kidneys, so if you develop the symptoms of cutaneous vasculitis, it is essential that you see your doctor at once. Most of the time the internal organs won't be involved. Still, your doctor must check you thoroughly.

Skin Ulcers

An ulcer is an area of skin that has opened, allowing the tissues underneath the skin to become exposed. This is a potentially dangerous situation. The skin acts as a barrier, protecting the underlying tissues from infections and other contaminants.

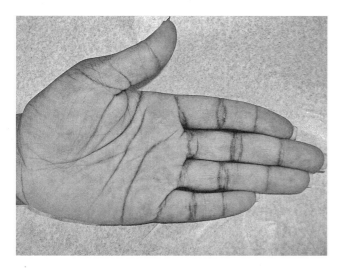

Figure 8.10 Erythromelalgia in an SLE patient. Note the splotches on the palm and fingers. She had very painful palms that felt worse with warmth and better when she stuck her hands under cold water. Blood tests showed that she was positive for cryoglobulins. This resolved with low-dose aspirin, steroids, hydroxychloroquine, and mycophenolate.

SLE patients can develop skin ulcers from several possible causes. One is vasculitis (blood vessel inflammation), as discussed above. Another is related to peripheral neuropathy (chapter 13), which causes decreased sensation, mainly in the feet. People with numbness of the feet from peripheral neuropathy should inspect their feet daily, especially the bottoms of their feet, to make sure there are no early signs of an ulcer.

Livedoid vasculopathy is a rare cause of skin ulcers. Livedoid vasculopathy starts with a rash on the arms or legs that can look like livedo reticularis (described below), hence the term "livedoid." It is caused by an abnormality of the small arteries (vasculopathy) within the skin, causing reduced skin blood flow and painful ulcers, especially on the feet. If the person is positive for antiphospholipid antibodies, it is treated with blood thinners such as aspirin.

Circulation problems involving leg veins and arteries can also lead to ulcers. When the veins of the legs are unable to drain fluid adequately, fluid and blood can pool in the lower legs (due to the pull of gravity). This can damage the skin and cause an ulcer. This vein problem is called venous insufficiency. It can be diagnosed with an ultrasound examination of the leg veins. The wearing down of the valves in the veins (commonly due to aging and genetics) is the most common cause.

Decreased blood flow through the arteries of the legs can also cause ulcers, most commonly in the feet and toes. This occurs because SLE patients can develop hardening of the arteries earlier than healthy people (accelerated atherosclerosis, chapter 21). Clogged arteries from antiphospholipid syndrome can also cause this (see chapter 9).

It is important to see a foot specialist (podiatrist) or go to a wound care clinic as soon as possible when foot ulcers occur. Some basic treatment strategies include keeping pressure off the ulcer, keeping it clean, and covering it regularly with a sterile bandage or dressing.

Skin ulcers can become infected. Signs of infection include pus within the ulcer or redness, tenderness, and warmth surrounding the ulcer. It is treated with antibiotics.

Bruises

Bruising (also called purpura) occurs when small blood vessels underneath the skin break open, causing the black and blue marks that we are familiar with after an accident. Over time, as the bruised area heals, purple, yellow, or red discoloration can occur. There are several causes of bruising in SLE. Each is treated differently.

As discussed above, lupus cutaneous vasculitis can cause palpable purpura. Although palpable purpura is usually seen in the ankles and lower parts of the legs, lupus vasculitis can also appear on the arms, upper legs, torso, and face in severe cases.

Low platelet counts (thrombocytopenia, chapter 9) can cause bruising in SLE. Platelets are essential for blood clotting. Reduced platelets can make it easier for the small blood vessels under the skin to bleed even after minimal pressure or trauma. Platelets are measured in the complete blood count blood test (CBC, chapter 4). If there is a new onset of bruising, a CBC should be obtained. Platelet counts are usually around $140 \times 10^3/\mu L$ and higher. People usually do not begin to bruise easily or bleed unless the platelet count goes below 30 to $50 \times 10^3/\mu L$. Easy bruising from lupus thrombocytopenia is treated with immunosuppressants. Other rarer causes of bruising in SLE are discussed in chapter 9.

By far the most common cause of bruising in lupus patients is medications such as prednisone, aspirin, nonsteroidal anti-inflammatory drugs (such as ibuprofen and naproxen), coumadin, and other blood thinners. Turmeric, vitamin E, omega-3 fatty acid supplements, and fish oil can also cause bruising. These bruised areas can be especially prominent on the arms and tops of the hands, making them easily noted and cosmetically troubling. The only treatment is to stop or lower the dose of the drug. This is often impossible for essential medications such as blood thinners needed to prevent blood clots (such as in patients with the antiphospholipid syndrome, chapter 9). Also, patients with SLE are at high risk for heart attacks and strokes, so taking low-dose aspirin is often essential.

Erythema nodosum (an unusual type of rash that may be seen in lupus) causes bruised areas as it heals (see erythema nodosum, below). Other less common causes of bruising, such as liver disease, severe infection, and vitamin deficiencies (such as vitamin C), are beyond the scope of this book.

Livedo Reticularis

Livedo reticularis (figure 8.11) is a rash caused by decreased blood flow in small blood vessels beneath the skin. It forms net-like areas of reddish or purplish discoloration, especially on the arms and legs. It rarely causes significant problems and usually does not cause permanent scarring. It can be more noticeable during periods of stress and cold. People with livedo reticularis sometimes (but not always) are positive for antiphospholipid antibodies (see chapters 4 and 9). People with antiphospholipid syndrome (APS, chapter 9) can develop livedo reticularis, as well as a more extreme example of livedo called livedo racemosa. If livedo reticularis occurs in someone with a stroke, it is called Sneddon syndrome. Sneddon syndrome is sometimes, but not always, due to antiphospholipid antibodies.

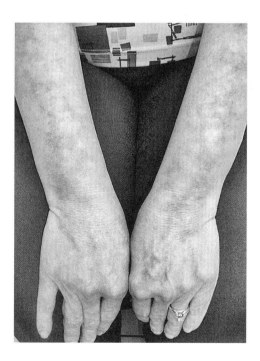

Figure 8.11 Livedo reticularis on the arms

Telangiectases (or Telangiectasias)

Telangiectases (figure 8.12) are areas of tiny, dilated blood vessels under the skin. They are usually blanchable ("blanch" means "pale"). This means that if you press on them, they temporarily lose their reddish or purplish coloration (become pale) due to the blood being squeezed out of the blood vessels. However, the coloration quickly returns when the blood refills the blood vessels. They are most common on the hands, face, lips, tongue, around the fingernails, and inside the mouth. They are usually permanent and do not improve with treatment.

Periungual Erythema

Peri- comes from the Greek word for "around," while *-unguis* is Greek for "nail." When dilated blood vessels under the skin (similar to telangiectases) occur in the skin next to the fingernails (the nail fold), that area of skin can redden. Periungual erythema is also called "periungual telangiectases." Similarly, dilated blood vessels can occur on the edges of the eyelids, causing them to appear reddish. SLE patients with periungual erythema commonly have antiphospholipid antibodies (see chapter 4). Like telangiectases, these dilated blood vessels are usually permanent and often do not improve with treatment.

Palmar Erythema
Reddish discoloration of the palms occurs in approximately 4% of SLE patients due to increased blood flow in the blood vessels of the skin of the palms. If the reddish color is net-like in appearance (as in livedo reticularis), it could be due to antiphospholipid antibodies. It is rarely a significant problem and is not treated. However, it usually improves with SLE treatment.

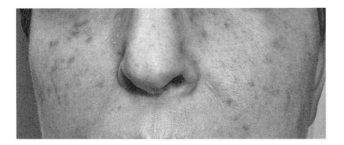

Figure 8.I2 Telangiectases on the cheeks of an SLE patient with scleroderma overlap. What makes these red marks different from other red lupus rashes is that they occur below the skin surface and do not cause any bumps that can be felt. If you apply pressure with your finger to one of the red splotches, the red color temporarily goes away because the blood is squeezed out of the underlying dilated blood vessels. The redness returns as the vessels fill up with blood again after lifting up the finger.

Erythromelalgia

Erythromelalgia (figure 8.10) refers to when the hands and/or feet become intensely red, hot, and painful from dilated or inflamed blood vessels. The affected areas feel better with cold and worse with warmth. This is the opposite of Raynaud's phenomenon. I have had several SLE patients with erythromelalgia. Two of them behaved the same way due to its discomfort. When I entered the exam room, these patients were standing at the sink, running cold water over their hands to help them feel better. Both were visibly miserable from the pain. Both responded well to high doses of steroids and aspirin. Fortunately, this lupus complication is rare.

Erythema Nodosum (EN)

"Erythema" is a medical term for redness, and "nodosum" means nodules or lumps. EN typically occurs on the legs around the shins, but can also occur elsewhere. EN first appears as small, tender, red, nodular (lumpy) areas underneath the skin. They are due to panniculitis (fat inflammation). When they heal, they typically leave a bruised-looking area. The appearance of EN is usually easy to identify and rarely needs a skin biopsy. It usually improves or resolves after successful treatment of SLE.

Cutaneous Mucinosis

Cutaneous mucinosis is rare in SLE. It is due to deposits of mucin in the skin. Mucin is a lubricating substance that your mucous membranes (such as the ones inside your mouth) typically produce. Doctors do not know why it deposits in small collections under the skin of some SLE patients. It typically appears as small areas of purplish bumps. A skin biopsy is usually needed for diagnosis. The lesions can get smaller and less discolored with successful SLE treatment.

Subcutaneous Nodules

Subcutaneous nodules are firm, round, rubbery feeling lumps that may occur under the skin in 5–10% of SLE patients. They appear most commonly on the fingers but can also occur on the feet, arms, and legs. They are very similar to the skin nodules that appear in rheumatoid arthritis patients. Most SLE patients with subcutaneous nodules have inflammatory arthritis (chapter 7) with significant joint swelling, and they are often positive for rheumatoid factor (RF, chapter 4). Many of these patients with subcutaneous nodules, arthritis, and RF have an overlap of SLE and rheumatoid arthritis (also known as rhupus). The nodules often get smaller with successful SLE treatment. Cortisone injections can reduce the size and pain of large or tender nodules.

Sclerodactyly

Sclero- comes from the Greek word for "hard" while *-dactyly* means "finger." Sclerodactyly is also called acrosclerosis (*acro-* from the Greek for "tip" or "extremity"). Typically, the skin that covers the fingers moves smoothly over the bones. If you pinch some skin between the joints of the fingers, it should wrinkle easily. Sclerodactyly causes the skin to be harder than usual. It is difficult to move it around the fingers' bones or pinch and wrinkle it. This skin hardening is called scleroderma (*-derma* from the Greek word for skin). Sclerodactyly occurs due to the immune system causing scar tissue throughout the fingers' skin and small blood vessels. Most people with sclerodactyly also have Raynaud's phenomenon (chapter 11), where the fingers turn white or blue with cold or stress. In the earliest stages of sclerodactyly, many SLE patients will experience finger puffiness or swelling (finger edema). SLE patients with RNP antibodies are especially prone to sclerodactyly. Sometimes, they have mixed connective tissue disease (chapter 2). Most lupus patients with sclerodactyly have it because of their SLE. However, in some SLE patients, an overlap syndrome with systemic sclerosis (chapter 2) causes the sclerodactyly. While the early stages of "puffy fingers" can respond to immunosuppressants, sclerodactyly may not respond very well.

Digital Gangrene

"Digits" refer to the fingers and toes, while "gangrene" means "tissue death." If someone loses blood flow to the fingers or toes, the tissues that rely on that blood flow no longer have the necessary oxygen and nutrients to stay alive. The person will usually notice coolness of the affected digit at first, along with pain and numbness. The skin then turns dark at the tip. This complication is devastating. When it occurs, the person will lose part of the digit. Sometimes the end of the finger or toe will slowly die and disappear (called self-amputation). At other times, surgery is done to clean out the dead tissue and amputate it. Fortunately, this is rare, occurring in only 1% of SLE patients and only in those who have had SLE for many years.

There are many reasons why the arteries leading to the digits may become blocked. These include hardening of the arteries (atherosclerosis, chapter 21), vasculitis (chapter 11), cryoglobulinemia (chapter 11), severe Raynaud's phenomenon (chapter 11), and the antiphospholipid syndrome (APS, chapter 9). It can even be due to a rare complication from using the blood thinner warfarin (used to treat APS).

Digital gangrene is a medical emergency. The longer it takes to get treatment, the more extensive the dead tissue becomes, which could lead to the loss of a more substantial amount of the involved digits and even to amputation. Effective treatment depends upon the cause. Since the exact cause is often not known immediately, treatment is usually aimed at several possibilities to increase the chances of a good outcome. These include using medicines to open the arteries (such as nifedipine), high doses of steroids to calm down inflammation, pain killers (these help relax and open the blood vessels), blood thinners, and sometimes anti-cholesterol medicines (statins). If cryoglobulinemia is present, plasma exchange or apheresis may be needed (chapter 35).

After the attack and treatment, the affected person is usually left with toes or fingers entirely or partially gone. This can be very distressing and significantly affect the quality of life. Usually, there is no lingering pain, although occasionally there is.

Calcinosis Cutis

Calcinosis cutis is when calcium deposits occur under the skin. They appear as hard lumps under the skin, often pale in color in dark-skinned individuals. They occur most commonly in areas prone to pressure, such as the hands, knees, tendons, and fingertips. Repetitive pressure causing tissue damage is thought to play a role in their formation. Doctors diagnose this condition from x-rays (the deposits appear as bony-looking structures). Calcinosis cutis is uncommon in SLE.

The form of calcinosis cutis described above is also known as calcinosis circumscripta. *Circumscripta* is Latin for "circumscribed," meaning limited or restricted. It refers to small areas of calcium deposits under the skin. This is in contrast to calcinosis universalis, where there are large areas of extensive calcification, especially in the skin of the buttocks, arms, and legs. It can cause muscle pain, joint pain, and decreased ability to move. Calcinosis universalis is rare in SLE. When it occurs, it is in patients with persistently active SLE inflammation. It is more common in the systemic autoimmune disease called dermatomyositis (chapter 2).

When calcinosis cutis occurs, your doctor will check your calcium, phosphorus, vitamin D, and parathyroid hormone levels. If your doctor labels your calcinosis as "dystrophic calcinosis," this means that you have normal calcium and phosphorus levels. Cancer screening tests (such as mammograms, PAP smears, and chest x-rays) should also be done to ensure no evidence of cancer, which can also cause calcinosis.

Possible therapies include intravenous sodium thiosulfate and surgical removal.

Xerosis

"Xerosis" is the medical term for dry skin. It is common in SLE, especially in those who also have Sjögren's disease (chapter 14). It is often due to decreased lubricating oils from the skin's oil glands (sebaceous glands). One of the most common symptoms of dry skin is itchy skin. If you have itchy skin (especially during winter), dry skin is one of the most common causes. For dry skin treatment, see lupusencyclopedia.com/dry-skin-in-lupus.

Neutrophilic Dermatosis

Skin biopsies of lupus-specific rashes (such as malar rash, subacute cutaneous lupus, and discoid lupus) typically show inflammation due to lymphocytes (a type of white blood cell, WBC). In contrast, neutrophilic dermatoses show inflammation due to neutrophils, a different type of WBC. There are several kinds, including Sweet syndrome, pyoderma gangrenosum, amicrobial pustulosis of the folds, neutrophilic cutaneous lupus erythematosus, neutrophilic urticarial dermatosis, and Sweet-like neutrophilic dermatosis. Most of these require treatment with immunosuppressants. We include these to be complete, but due to their rarity, we will not go into detail.

Erythema Multiforme

Another rare skin problem is erythema multiforme (EM). The combination of lupus (either the systemic form or one of the cutaneous types) and EM is called Rowell syndrome (first described by Dr. Neville Rowell in 1963). As of 2020, there were only about 100 cases in the medical literature. EM lesions are described as "target lesions"; they have a pattern like the rings on an archery target. A central dark area or blister is surrounded by a clear area, which is in turn surrounded by a pinkish-red circular area. The number of circular rings varies. Patients with Rowell syndrome tend to be positive for antinuclear antibody, rheumatoid factor, anti-SSA(Ro), or anti-SSB(La) antibodies. These patients have an increased chance of having chilblain lupus (described above). They usually respond to typical treatments for cutaneous lupus, such as hydroxychloroquine, UV light protection, and immunosuppressants (for severe cases).

Nail Changes

Quite a few changes can occur in the nails in SLE. Nail surfaces may develop hard lines or ridges, while the edges of the nails may lift off the underlying skin at the end of the nails. Indentations or pits may occur, as well as areas of unusual dark or reddish discoloration. These do not necessarily improve with SLE treatment.

"Melanonychia" is the term used when the fingernails or toenails are black (*melano-* means "black" and *-nychia* means "nail"). Most of a nail may be black, or there can be one or more lines of black starting from the nail bed. Although many experts think this is rare in SLE, a South African study showed that one out of three Black SLE patients had melanonychia when first diagnosed. In that study, the patients with melanonychia ended up having milder lupus problems overall and a lower frequency of kidney involvement.

Hydroxychloroquine (HCQ) can cause melanonychia, just as it can cause skin pigmentation (discussed next). If areas of skin darkening are present in someone with melanonychia who has taken HCQ a long time, HCQ is the probable cause.

Skin Color Changes

Vitiligo is an autoimmune disease of the skin that causes the loss of pigment (figure 8.13). The immune system attacks the cells of the skin that produce melanin (responsible for pigmentation of the skin). There may be only a few small areas involved, or in extreme cases, a large percentage of the skin can have vitiligo. There is usually a

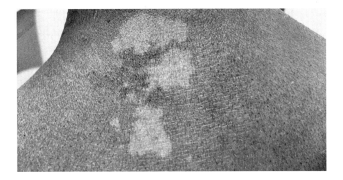

Figure 8.13 Vitiligo on the upper back of a person of color with SLE

sharp boundary between the patches of lighter color and normal skin coloration. They become more prominent if the surrounding skin becomes tan during summertime. Vitiligo may cause cosmetic concerns in some people, but fortunately, it is not a dangerous condition. There is no cure for vitiligo. Treatments such as steroids and tacrolimus ointment can help reduce spreading but usually do not bring pigmentation back. Recently, JAK inhibitors (such as baricitinib and tofacitinib, chapter 32) have shown promising results on bringing pigmentation back to vitiligo lesions.

Discoid lupus erythematosus (DLE) commonly causes permanent light and dark skin discoloration. As DLE lesions enlarge, permanent scar tissue forms in the center. This scarred area has no hair and is often lighter in color than the person's natural skin color (figure 8.8). This lighter-colored area is often surrounded by varying degrees of pink, red, or darker than normal skin coloration. Unfortunately, these color changes are permanent. Therefore, it is essential to treat DLE as soon as possible to stop the progressive inflammation and prevent permanent scarring.

Sometimes, when areas of vasculitis or antiphospholipid syndrome ulcers heal in the lower legs and around the ankles, they can leave permanent white or light-colored areas. These are called atrophie blanche.

After cutaneous lupus inflammation resolves, sometimes the skin cells will produce more pigment (melanin) in those areas. The medical term for this is "postinflammatory hyperpigmentation." Unfortunately, this can be permanent. Dark patches of skin can appear, particularly on the cheeks, forehead, nose, and ears. Prescription strength lightening creams and strict sun avoidance can help. Not everyone improves with lightening creams.

One of the potential long-term side effects of antimalarials (hydroxychloroquine, chloroquine, and quinacrine) is dark-colored skin patches (figure 8.14). They often

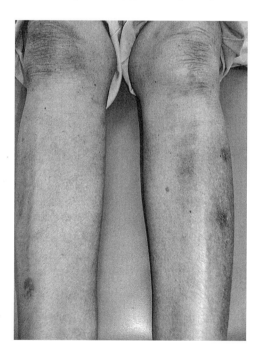

Figure 8.14 Dark patches of skin due to hydroxychloroquine around the shins of an SLE patient.

appear brown, black, or black and blue. They tend to develop on the legs (especially around the shins), neck, and face. Increased pigmentation can also occur inside the mouth (such as the upper palate) and nails and especially in areas where bruising occurs easily. Taking blood thinners (such as aspirin and warfarin) increases the risk. The coloration may decrease when the dose of the medicine decreases, but it is usually permanent. Since antimalarials have so many benefits in SLE (chapter 30) and are the safest SLE drugs, it is preferable to continue treatment and put up with the skin discoloration instead of risking a lupus flare by stopping the medicine.

Quinacrine can cause an unusual yellowish color of the skin, nails, and whites of the eyes in around 25% of people. The yellow tint does improve after the dose is decreased or after the person stops taking it. Patients and doctors should be aware that the condition can be mistaken for jaundice, prompting unnecessary procedures to evaluate the liver.

Rashes Due to Drug Reactions

Some of the most important causes of rashes are medications. All drugs can potentially cause reactions involving the skin. Sometimes, they can mimic acute cutaneous lupus, and it is important to be able to tell the difference. The treatment for a drug reaction is to stop the medication, while the treatment for cutaneous lupus is to increase immunosuppressants. The one exception is when medicine causes cutaneous lupus (most commonly SCLE), and the treatment is to stop the medicine. We have seen many patients treated inappropriately with steroids by well-meaning doctors, who presume, incorrectly, that they have a "lupus rash." I insist that my patients who develop rashes see a dermatologist in addition to myself, so that we can reach a proper diagnosis and treatment plan.

Treatments used for lupus, such as hydroxychloroquine (HCQ) and chloroquine, are also common causes of rashes. Around 10% of lupus patients will develop a skin reaction to HCQ. We usually stop HCQ until the rash resolves. If the rash was severe (life-threatening or requiring hospitalization), the patient should stay off HCQ. If the outbreak was not severe, HCQ can often be resumed using a technique called desensitization. Desensitization is a method of dealing with a medication that causes a side effect by prescribing it in tiny doses at first to get the body used to it. The daily dose is then slowly increased to a tolerable level (usually lower than the dose that caused the reaction).

There are several different desensitization techniques for HCQ. The easiest one consists of starting with just 40 mg a day, then slowly increasing the dose. The only way to obtain 40 mg of HCQ is to get it from a specialized pharmacist called a compounding pharmacist. Compounded drugs are expensive, and it can be difficult for patients to find a compounding pharmacist. Therefore, we prefer to use the standard 200 mg hydroxychloroquine tablets and have patients cut them. A good pill cutter can cut them into four pieces containing approximately 50 mg each. The patient can take one-quarter of a tablet a day for a week. This is followed by one-quarter of a tablet twice a day for a week, followed by one-quarter of a tablet three times a day for a week, then one-half tablet twice a day, at which point the total daily dose of 200 mg has been reached. Use a lower dose if this is not tolerated. Discuss desensitization with your doctor before trying it. Also, go to lupusencyclopedia.com/top-tips-on-taking-hydroxychloroquine-for-lupus.

An uncommon skin side effect of HCQ is the worsening or new onset of psoriasis. Psoriasis rashes are red, scaly lesions that commonly occur on the elbows, knees, and scalp. However, they can occur on any body part, including the palms and soles. They usually resolve after stopping the HCQ.

The most common side effect of the antimalarial quinacrine is quinacrine dermatitis, which typically occurs four to six weeks after starting the medicine. We ask all our patients who take quinacrine to stop it at once if they develop a rash. On rare occasions a rash can occur just before the quinacrine causes severely low blood counts (aplastic anemia) as a side effect. Aplastic anemia previously occurred when high doses were prescribed. It has not been seen with the current lower doses of quinacrine that we use. Quinacrine dermatitis usually goes away soon after the patient stops taking it. However, severe cases, described as lichenoid dermatitis by dermatologists, can take months to go away and can leave permanent scarring.

Shingles

Shingles (herpes zoster) is due to infection from the chickenpox virus and is a common problem in SLE patients. It causes a blistering, excruciatingly painful rash, usually on one side of the body. It is important to seek medical attention as soon as possible because the quicker an antiviral medicine is taken, the better the outcome. See chapter 22.

Skin Cancer

Although skin cancer is discussed in chapter 22, it is essential to mention it here. Other than the rare occurrences of squamous cell carcinoma (SCC) within discoid lupus, as discussed above, lupus itself does not cause skin cancer. But studies do suggest that some of the medicines we use to treat lupus may increase the risk for SCC and basal cell carcinoma (BCC). These medicines include tumor necrosis factor inhibitors (TNF inhibitors, Humira, Enbrel, Remicade, Simponi, Cimzia), methotrexate, azathioprine, mycophenolate, tacrolimus, cyclosporine and JAKi (chapter 32). If you take one of these medications long-term, it is a good idea to see a dermatologist once a year for a "skin cancer screen," in which your entire body is checked. If you get any new skin sores that won't go away, or if you have any sores that heal, then come back, make sure to show these to your doctor.

General Skin Care Advice

If you avoid UV light (chapter 38), use sunscreen religiously every day, never smoke cigarettes, and drink plenty of water daily, you will most likely have healthy, good-looking skin. But if you have cutaneous lupus and have skin pigment changes, hair loss, or excessive hair growth (which can happen with some medicines), a dermatologist's help can be invaluable. And it's advisable to see one in addition to your rheumatologist.

Lupus rashes can negatively affect one's quality of life. There are many strategies available to help improve their appearance. Those with lupus may use clothes and cosmetics to cover regions of permanent skin damage. Cosmetic camouflage is a type of makeup that can cover pigmented skin changes or skin contour changes and comes in different shades to match all skin colors. Cosmetic camouflage can be used daily or as needed, such as for social, leisure, or work activities. Alternatively, using a green-tinged primer for foundation makeup can decrease the redness of lupus rashes. Only a small amount of these green primers should be used. Ideally, this type of makeup should not clog pores or have fragrance. Some types of cosmetic camouflage and green primers also have SPF-rated sunscreen.

A recent study showed that cosmetic camouflage for facial skin damage improves female lupus patients' health-related quality of life. Study participants noted improvement in mood, self-image, physical functioning, depression, anxiety, and self-esteem by the end of the study. Therefore, cosmetic camouflage can be invaluable.

Consider getting a makeup consultation at a makeup counter if you can afford it. Large department stores often hire makeup artist associates who can help you learn to achieve your desired look.

Since hair loss can occur with lupus, many women with SLE rely on hats and wigs.

Tattoos and Lupus

It is not a good idea for SLE patients to get tattoos. Although many tattoo artists use proper sterile techniques, infections can occur. These include hepatitis B, hepatitis C, *Staphylococcus aureus* (a skin bacterial infection), endocarditis (heart infection), and HIV. If someone is on an immunosuppressant drug (table 22.1), the occurrence of one of these infections could be dangerous.

Some people can develop cutaneous lupus at the tattoo site. These cutaneous lupus lesions follow the pattern of the tattoo. Cutaneous lupus can even occur on tattoos placed well before the person had lupus. The medical term for these skin lesions occurring at tattoo markings (or other areas of skin damage) is the "Koebner phenomenon," or "Koebnerization." Tattoos can even be the target of attack from reactions to drugs used to treat lupus (figure 8.15).

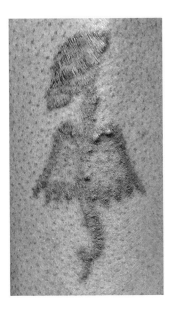

Figure 8.15 Drug-induced skin reaction within a tattoo. Note the bumps in this tattoo. These occurred due to a lichenoid drug reaction from hydroxychloroquine. The bumps were very itchy. Similar problems in tattoos can also occur from DLE and SCLE. Photo courtesy of Aubrey Wagenseller, MD, dermatologist, Silver Spring, Maryland

A 2019 Spanish study suggested it may be safe for lupus patients who are in remission (or who have low disease activity) and who are not on steroids or immunosuppressant drugs to get tattoos. However, this was a small study. It would be nice to have a more extensive research study to confirm these results before telling our patients that tattoos are safe.

KEY POINTS TO REMEMBER

1. Nonspecific rashes may occur in SLE patients. They appear in other disorders as well.

2. Oral and nasal ulcers are among the most common cutaneous (skin) manifestations of SLE. They are usually painless but occasionally painful. Steroid creams can be helpful.

3. Non-scarring alopecia improves and the hair grows back with successful SLE treatment.

4. You should show any skin problem to your doctor, so they can figure out whether it is due to SLE or an unrelated issue.

5. Let your doctor know if you begin to develop dark areas of skin in areas not previously affected by lupus. They may be due to hydroxychloroquine (Plaquenil).

6. Lupus skin problems can be devastating and negatively affect the quality of life. Consider reaching out to other lupus patients or a dermatologist to help to live with cutaneous lupus.

7. See a medical dermatologist regularly, in addition to your rheumatologist, to ensure that you are getting the best skin care advice possible.

8. Cosmetics (especially green-tinted primer to hide redness), hats, and wigs can help with concerns about appearance. Ask a dermatologist about cosmetic camouflage.

9. Consider getting annual skin cancer screening by a dermatologist yearly if you take TNF inhibitors (Humira, Enbrel, Remicade, Simponi, Cimzia), methotrexate, azathioprine, mycophenolate, tacrolimus, cyclosporine, or JAK inhibitors (like tofacitinib or baricitinib, chapter 32).

Blood and Lymph Systems

Emma Weeding, MD, *Contributing Editor*

Blood and lupus are intricately entwined. With its army of white blood cells (WBCs), the immune system is what causes lupus. Diagnosing SLE requires a variety of blood tests because this is where the antibodies are found. Most people with SLE have low blood counts, so finding low blood counts can help diagnose SLE. Low blood counts can occasionally cause problems such as infections (from low WBC counts), bleeding (from low platelets), or fatigue (from low red blood cell counts, also known as anemia).

There are three different types of blood cells—WBCs, red blood cells (RBCs), and platelets (plts)—and all three can decrease in SLE. Production of the blood cells begins primarily in the bone marrow, especially in the largest bones (arms, legs, pelvis, and spine). The bone marrow is continuously churning out new blood cells to take the place of old cells. A blood test called the complete blood count (CBC, chapter 4) evaluates the numbers of each type. These numbers help doctors figure out what is happening in the blood and bone marrow.

The lymph system is a network of lymphatic channels (tubes) attached to round or oval rubbery swellings called lymph nodes. The spleen, a large organ found in the left upper abdomen, is part of the lymphatic system. The lymphatic system is an essential part of the immune system and can be affected by SLE.

A vital characteristic of the blood is its ability to clot. The plts and many essential proteins stick to injured blood vessels when you get a cut. These plts and unique proteins clog the blood vessels and stop the bleeding. But not all blood clots are beneficial. Some people have antiphospholipid antibodies that make their blood thicker than usual. This can cause blood clots, causing problems like strokes. The medical term for this is "antiphospholipid antibody syndrome."

All of these problems are discussed in this chapter.

WBC Problems

WBCs are called leukocytes (also spelled leucocytes)—*leuko* coming from the Greek word for "white" and *-cyte* from the Greek word for "cell." These cells are the soldiers of the immune system. They find and fight infections, foreign objects (such as a splinter or bee sting), and cancer cells. SLE can sometimes reduce the WBC count. This is called leukopenia—*penia* means "decreased or less." Leukopenia occurs in approximately one out of every three SLE patients.

There are several types of WBCs, each with its own unique function. The most important for SLE are the neutrophils and the lymphocytes. Neutrophils are especially crucial for fighting off bacterial infections. Lymphocytes play many roles, including fighting off viral infections and ensuring proper overall immune system function. The medical term for a decrease in neutrophils is "neutropenia." The name for reduced lymphocytes is "lymphopenia." Lymphopenia (also called lymphocytopenia) is the more common finding, occurring in up to 80% of SLE patients. Neutropenia occurs in around one-third.

Note, though, that neutropenia can sometimes be considered "normal" due to genetics. Sub-Saharan African ancestry often causes this. If an SLE patient with African ancestry has neutropenia, we are not always sure if it is from SLE (representing lupus activity) or if it is a normal finding from genetics.

Leuokocytopenia can potentially cause infections. However, this is not always the case. In SLE, it is unclear if having a low WBC count, neutrophil count, or lymphocyte count increases this risk. Some studies show no increased risk from leukocytopenia while others suggest an increased risk.

How can a low number of WBCs not cause infections? The WBCs in your blood are just a small fraction of your body's total amount. Most are in the bone marrow, thymus, spleen, lymph nodes, and intestinal walls. When infection occurs, the immune system mobilizes these WBCs. They go into the blood and then to the infection where they are needed.

However, severely low blood counts, defined as an absolute neutrophil count less than 0.5×10^9/L (or less than 500) or an absolute lymphocyte count less than 0.35×10^9/L (or less than 350), most likely increase the risk for infections.

Doctors usually do not treat low WBC counts in SLE patients because they are usually not problematic. Also, low WBC counts do not improve with SLE treatment in many patients. On the other hand, steroids such as prednisone usually increase WBCs (especially neutrophils), but this is considered a drug side effect, rather than an intended treatment result. Steroids actually increase infections, even though they increase WBCs. The higher WBC count seen with steroids decreases as the steroid dose is reduced.

On the other hand, steroids typically reduces lymphocytes. This can be confusing since lymphopenia also occurs from SLE inflammation. When steroids cause lymphopenia, the lymphocyte count usually improves with lower steroid doses.

Finding leukopenia, neutropenia, or lymphopenia on the CBC can help diagnose SLE. They are part of the SLE classification criteria (chapter 1). The CBC can also help

LUPUS IN FOCUS

Granulocytopenia

Granulocytes are a family of white blood cells that includes neutrophils, eosinophils, and basophils. Another term for lower than normal neutrophils is "granulocytopenia." There are two other types of granulocytes: eosinophils and basophils. Although strictly speaking, "granulocytopenia" should mean a low number of neutrophils, eosinophils, and basophils, the term is commonly used just to refer to reduced neutrophils.

check the degree of lupus disease activity. The WBC counts (especially lymphocytes) can decrease during periods of increased disease activity and improve during better disease control. In addition, drugs can cause low WBCs, so we commonly monitor the CBC to ensure our patients tolerate their medicines.

Sometimes a doctor can link low WBCs from SLE directly to recurrent infections, but this is unusual. In my practice, I have a patient with recurrent boils (skin infections) due to severe SLE neutropenia. When she developed nephritis (kidney inflammation), and I needed to treat her with a strong immunosuppressant drug called mycophenolate mofetil (MMF, CellCept), I was cautious because MMF can cause low WBCs and greater infection risks. However, MMF improved her neutrophils because it was treating her lupus. Her skin infections disappeared.

Occasionally, an enlarged spleen (splenomegaly) can reduce the WBCs (discussed later in this chapter). Splenomegaly can also cause low plts and anemia.

Drug-Induced Low WBC Counts

Immunosuppressants (table 22.1) and other drugs can sometimes lower WBCs. The total WBC count (WBC), absolute neutrophil count (ANC), and absolute lymphocyte count (ALC) are the most important for monitoring WBC numbers on the CBC. Low levels due to medicine are called drug-induced leukopenia, drug-induced neutropenia, and drug-induced lymphopenia, respectively.

When one of the WBC counts becomes lower than normal because of a drug, it can sometimes increase the risk of infection. That is, while mildly decreased levels may not increase this risk, severely low levels can. It is OK to allow WBCs to be slightly lower than normal (lower than the patient's baseline) if the medicine is helping the person and not causing infections. It is standard to stop the offending drug if the counts drop into the severe category.

Other factors are important when deciding infection risks. These include older age (especially over 65), other diseases (such as diabetes, kidney/heart/lung disease, and immunodeficiency), and taking steroids. Take, for example, an 80-year-old diabetic who is on dialysis for kidney failure and takes prednisone—they have many infection risk factors. The offending immunosuppressant may need to be stopped, or the dose lowered even if the WBC count is only mildly low. Conversely, a relatively healthy young person whose SLE is in remission from an immunosuppressant may do best by continuing the drug if the WBCs are not severely low.

LUPUS IN FOCUS

Dealing with low white blood cell counts in people with African heritage

Many SLE patients already have low WBC, neutrophil, or lymphocyte counts due to SLE or due to their African heritage. In these patients, we use the lowest values that the patient had before being on any drugs and consider these their baseline values. If the counts do not drop significantly below the baseline values, it is acceptable to continue drugs that can cause low blood counts.

A normal WBC count is around 4.0×10^9/L (varies from lab to lab) or higher. Unless the WBC count goes below 3.0×10^9/L, the doctor might not stop the medicine or lower the dose.

A normal absolute neutrophil count (ANC) is around 1.5×10^9/L (or 1500/microL) and higher. An ANC less than 0.5×10^9/L (less than 500/microL) is called severe neutropenia. Many doctors allow ANC levels of 0.6 to 1.4 on a medication (without stopping or lowering the dose), if the patient is doing well and their infection risk factors are low.

The most severely low level of neutrophils is called agranulocytosis, which means the absence of granulocytes (the same thing as neutrophils). There is no commonly accepted definition for agranulocytosis. Some experts reserve its use for an ANC less than 100, while others use it for an ANC less than 500. No matter, agranulocytosis indicates a high risk of infection.

Lymphopenia is a little more complicated. Drug-induced lymphopenia usually occurs along with drug-induced neutropenia. In this case, the neutrophil count result usually decides what to do. Occasionally, drug-induced lymphopenia can occur while the neutrophil count is normal. Other situations can reduce lymphocytes, including older age, exercise, stress, and infections. A normal absolute lymphocyte count (ALC) is around 1.0×10^9/L and higher. Still, it can be normal for healthy people over 60 to have lymphocyte counts as low as 0.5×10^9/L (also noted as an ALC of 500).

The definition of severe lymphopenia can vary. A common cut-off value is an ALC less than 350. The decision to lower the dose of a medicine causing lymphopenia or stop it is similar to that for drug-induced neutropenia discussed above. Severe lymphopenia can increase the risk for infections such as a bacteria called *Pneumocystis jiroveci* (previously known as *P. carinii*). Some rheumatologists give patients with persistently severe lymphopenia antibiotics to prevent this infection. Trimethoprim-sulfamethoxazole (Bactrim) is the most used antibiotic to prevent *P. jiroveci* infection in non-lupus patients. However, it should be avoided in SLE because it can potentially cause lupus flares. Usually, dapsone or atovaquone is used instead.

If a medication needs to be stopped due to drug-induced low WBCs, it takes on average two weeks for the WBCs to return to normal (or to the patient's baseline). The actual time depends on how long the offending drug's effects on the immune system last. It can sometimes take as long as a couple of months. In rare cases the WBCs can remain low.

When severe neutropenia occurs, a group of drugs called granulocyte colony-stimulating factor (G-CSF) drugs can be used to increase WBCs and lower infection risk. Two G-CSF medications are Neupogen (filgrastim) and Leukine (sargramostim).

LUPUS IN FOCUS

Why does my doctor write my absolute neutrophil count as 1,500 instead of 1.5?

Lab results reported by laboratories are usually given using measurements similar to 1.5×10^9/L. This is read as "1.5 billion cells per liter." It is customary for doctors to convert this to its equivalent cells per mm^3 (cells per cubic millimeter). Health care providers usually note "the ANC is 1,500" (dropping the per volume designation) in the patient's records.

Early reports showed that SLE patients could be successfully treated with these. However, later studies showed that G-CSF could cause lupus flares, including severe lupus nephritis (kidney inflammation) and cutaneous vasculitis (blood vessel inflammation). Therefore, some experts recommend avoiding them.

Occasionally, a bone marrow biopsy (BMBX) is needed when evaluating low WBCs, since the bone marrow is the tissue inside the bones that produces most WBCs. BMBXs are usually done by hematologists (blood specialists). The biopsy can also examine issues with RBCs and plts. BMBXs are usually outpatient procedures, and the pelvic bone is the usual source. Once the biopsy area is anesthetized, the doctor inserts a biopsy needle into the bone and removes a piece of bone and marrow. Since it is challenging to anesthetize the bone itself, there usually is some discomfort. If you are afraid of pain, ask your doctor for sedation. The doctor then sends the biopsy to a lab for evaluation under a microscope by a doctor called a pathologist. It can take several days to weeks to get the results.

Monoclonal Gammopathy

Monoclonal gammopathy occurs in about 5% of people with SLE. It is helpful to review the immune system to understand it.

Plasma cells are a type of WBC (specifically B cells or B lymphocytes) that produce antibodies (immunoglobulins). These antibodies are normally directed toward potential invaders such as viruses and bacteria. One plasma cell makes only one type of immunoglobulin. When a foreign invader is present, the immune system alerts the proper plasma cells to multiply so that a large amount of that type of antibody is produced to fight the enemy. For example, if pneumococcal bacteria invade the lungs, the plasma cells that produce pneumococcal antibodies are alerted. Prior to the infection, there would have been very few of these plasma cells, but during the infection, their numbers greatly increase. Once the infection is gone, these plasma cells are no longer needed in such large numbers. They retire and die through a process called apoptosis (programmed cell death; see belimumab, chapter 34).

The immune system carefully regulates plasma cells to ensure that no one type gets out of control. If it does, it may start to reproduce too much, making too many of its own antibody type. Too many copies of one antibody type are unhealthy.

Immunoglobulins can be classified medically as a type of gamma globulin. Gamma globulins are heavier blood proteins than others when measured on a laboratory test called a serum protein electrophoresis (SPEP, chapter 4). "Gammopathy" denotes an abnormal production of gamma globulins, especially immunoglobulins, by the plasma cells (-opathy comes from the Greek word for "abnormality").

A large number of one plasma cell type (all making the same immunoglobulin or gamma globulin) is considered a clone of that particular plasma cell. The term "monoclonal" means "one clone" of one specific plasma cell, making the same gamma globulin. Therefore, when one type of plasma cell exists in large numbers and makes too much of the same immunoglobulin (or gamma globulin), it is called a monoclonal gammopathy (too many plasma cells making one clone of one type of gammaglobulin).

The problem with monoclonal gammopathy is that if these plasma cells multiply too much, they can take over the bone marrow and replace normal cells. The bone marrow is then unable to produce normal amounts of plts, RBCs, and other WBCs. Bone pain is common; the bones can become brittle and break, and the person is at risk of dying from severe bleeding (loss of plts) or infections (lack of WBCs). When one type of abnormal cell replaces normal cells, it is called cancer. When a monoclonal gammopathy becomes cancerous like this, it is called multiple myeloma (MM).

Suppose someone has a monoclonal gammopathy, but not MM. In that case, they are said to have a monoclonal gammopathy of undetermined significance (MGUS). It can be hard to tell which people with an MGUS will develop MM, which is why "undetermined significance" is used. In MGUS patients who do not have SLE, about 1% will develop MM per year. People with SLE appear to have a greater risk for MM. Studies suggest it may be around three times greater. (Note, this is different from the first edition, which states a lower risk for MM in SLE.) Doctors closely monitor MGUS as it is essential to find MM early to give proper treatment.

I have noted that many of my patients treated with belimumab (Benlysta), and rituximab (Rituxan) have had their MGUS resolve. This makes sense since overactive B cells cause MGUS and these drugs lower B cell activity. Could these two drugs possibly decrease the risk of developing MM in SLE patients with MGUS? We do not know, but it is possible.

Polyclonal Gammopathy

Polyclonal gammopathy (*poly*- means "many") is a condition in which an excess of many different clones of gamma globulins is produced. This is found on a serum protein electrophoresis (SPEP) blood test. In polyclonal gammopathy, the SPEP shows an increased amount of gamma globulins (called hypergammaglobulinemia) composed of many different types (or clones) of gamma globulins. This occurs due to the lupus immune system causing overall B cell overactivity. In some patients, it can help show how they respond to treatment. The numerical value of gamma globulins can be high during increased lupus disease activity and lower when doing better. Polyclonal gammopathy is especially common in those with Sjögren's disease.

Hemophagocytic Lymphohistiocytosis (Macrophage Activation Syndrome)

This is a rare condition. We previously referred to this as macrophage activation syndrome (MAS). More recent terminology favors hemophagocytic lymphohistiocytosis (HLH). HLH is the larger group of disorders that MAS is grouped under. HLH can be divided into primary HLH and secondary HLH forms. Primary HLH is probably genetic and most commonly occurs in small children. Secondary HLH occurs in people with problems that trigger it. Common triggers include rheumatic diseases (especially SLE and a condition called Still's disease), cancer, infection, and immunodeficiency disorders. Some with secondary causes seem to also have a genetic susceptibility. When secondary HLH occurs in SLE, it is commonly called HLH-MAS. However, many physicians stick to the older terminology and simply call it macrophage activation syndrome.

What is MAS? One might think of it as the immune system going crazy, causing uncontrolled inflammation and destroying organs. Macrophages are a type of WBC that plays a crucial role in SLE. Lupus macrophages identify parts of the person's body (such as double-stranded DNA), think they are foreign, and alert the rest of the immune system to attack those parts. In MAS, the macrophages become overactive, inciting the rest of the immune system to cause worse body inflammation and damage. The macrophages even swallow other cells to destroy them. The medical term for this is "phagocytosis."

This is where the word "hemophagocytic" originated from. *Hemo-* refers to blood, *-phago-* means "to eat," and *-cytic* refers to cells: the macrophages swallow other blood cells. The WBCs also release many immune system messengers (cytokines) that tell other WBCs to become more active. When the overactive macrophages produce huge amounts of dangerous, inflammation-causing cytokines, it is called a cytokine storm.

A person with HLH/MAS usually has fever over 101°F and is very sick. Bone and joint pains, severe diarrhea, shortness of breath, rash, bleeding, headache, seizures, and difficulty thinking are common. During intense inflammation, the liver can produce high amounts of ferritin (a protein that stores iron for the body). Therefore, high ferritin blood levels can indicate active inflammation. It is unclear why the liver produces so much ferritin during inflammation. Labs during HLH/MAS usually show high ferritin levels and low blood cell counts. Elevated liver enzymes and kidney failure are also common.

Untreated, it is fatal. Most patients respond to high doses of steroids and other immunosuppressants, such as cyclophosphamide. Plasma exchange (chapter 38) may be needed by some. An immunosuppressant not typically used for SLE called anakinra (Kineret) can be beneficial. With treatment, 75% to 95% of patients survive.

KEY POINTS TO REMEMBER

1. Low WBC counts (leukopenia), low lymphocytes (lymphopenia), and low neutrophils (neutropenia or granulocytopenia) are common in SLE.

2. Although WBCs are essential for fighting infections, lupus usually does not cause levels low enough to cause infections.

3. SLE medications often do not improve the numbers of WBCs.

4. Most immunosuppressants (table 22.1) can reduce WBCs, thereby increasing infection risks. Sometimes, the dosage needs to be reduced or the drug needs to be stopped.

5. Sometimes, a bone marrow biopsy is needed to figure out the cause of low blood counts.

6. Monoclonal gammopathy of undetermined significance occurs in roughly 5% of SLE patients. It can rarely progress to a cancer called multiple myeloma.

7. Polyclonal gammopathy with hypergammaglobulinemia can fluctuate with disease activity. The level of gammaglobulins can be higher when lupus is more active and lower when less active.

RBC Problems

Red blood cells (RBCs) are called erythrocytes. *Erythro-* comes from the Greek word for "red." Erythrocytes contain hemoglobin (Hb), a protein that carries oxygen. Low numbers of erythrocytes is called anemia. Doctors diagnose anemia by finding a low Hb level and a low hematocrit (chapter 4) on the CBC.

Since RBCs are essential for carrying oxygen throughout the body, anemia can cause problems. Mild anemia (where the hemoglobin is 10 mg/dl or higher) usually causes no problems. The lower the Hb, the greater its chances of causing issues. Symptoms of anemia may include feeling tired and short of breath with exertion. More severe symptoms, such as chest pain, shortness of breath at rest, lightheadedness, and feeling faint, may occur in people with heart or lung problems.

How quickly anemia occurs is also important. For example, someone with anemia for a long time could have a very low Hb, yet feel fine. Since their body has become used to being anemic, the body has learned to compensate in other ways. On the other hand, someone may become anemic quickly, such as by losing blood from a stomach ulcer. This abrupt onset can cause problems even though the anemia is mild.

There are many reasons why people with lupus can become anemic. It is important to figure out the exact reason for the anemia in order to treat it properly. That is why a doctor usually asks a patient to come in for more blood work (anemia workup) when they discover anemia. We discuss the more common reasons for anemia in SLE below in order of relative frequency.

Anemia of Inflammation

Anemia of inflammation (AI) is the most common anemia in SLE. This is also called anemia of chronic disease. It is due to the systemic inflammation of SLE, which causes the bone marrow to produce fewer RBCs.

One hint that someone may have AI is from the size of the RBCs. Although the bone marrow produces fewer RBCs during AI, those RBCs are normal sized. We measure RBC size (or the volume of each individual RBC) by their mean corpuscular volume (MCV) on the CBC. Anemia with normally sized RBCs (normal MCV) is called a normocytic anemia ("normo-" means "normal-sized"; -*cytic* refers to cell). Anemia of inflammation is a common cause of normocytic anemia.

If the RBCs are smaller than normal (low MCV), it is called a microcytic anemia (*micro-* means "small"); if they are larger than normal, it is a macrocytic anemia (*macro-* means "large"). For example, iron deficiency commonly causes a microcytic anemia, while vitamin B12 deficiency commonly causes a macrocytic anemia. There can always be exceptions, but the MCV helps narrow down the possibilities.

AI can occasionally cause a microcytic anemia, and iron deficiency can occasionally cause a normocytic anemia. Iron studies help figure it out. Recall from the HLH/MAS section above that the liver produces more ferritin during inflammation, so ferritin levels are often (but not always) increased in AI. Since ferritin is the protein that stores iron, iron deficiency causes low ferritin levels. Another iron study test is called the total iron-binding capacity (TIBC). The TIBC is usually low in AI, while it is usually high in iron deficiency.

AI generally improves, but not always, as SLE improves. If AI is causing problems such as fatigue and shortness of breath, a group of medications called erythropoiesis-stimulating agents (such as Aranesp, Epogen, and Procrit) can help. These medications are given by injection in a doctor's office.

People with AI usually do not need iron supplements. Most have plenty of iron in their body. The problem is that they cannot use it correctly to make enough RBCs (due to the effects of inflammation). Giving more iron to someone who already has a lot of iron will not help. However, if someone has iron deficiency and AI, then iron supplements are important. This is common since many SLE patients are menstruating women. Systemic inflammation can reduce iron absorption from the intestinal tract, reducing the effectiveness of oral iron supplements. We give iron by infusion in this case.

Iron Deficiency Anemia

Iron is a mineral and a vital part of the oxygen-carrying Hb found in RBCs. People without enough iron cannot make enough Hb for RBCs and can become anemic. The entire purpose for RBCs is to carry as much Hb as possible to supply oxygen to the body; think of RBCs as sacks of Hb. Therefore, when there is less Hb from iron deficiency anemia (IDA), the RBCs are not only fewer in number (anemia) but also smaller in size (microcytic, with a low MCV).

The most common reason for IDA is blood loss since the hemoglobin-containing RBCs contain a large amount of the body's iron. The most common cause of blood loss is menstruation. Since SLE commonly occurs in menstruating women, they often have IDA.

It is also common for women with SLE to have abnormal periods (chapter 18). A 2019 UK study showed that SLE patients were twice as likely to have heavy menstrual cycles (menorrhagia).

The second most common reason for IDA is bleeding from the gastrointestinal tract. For example, stomach ulcers may slowly leak blood. Polyps, which are stalks of abnormal tissue inside the intestines, may bleed. Colon cancer can slowly leak blood and cause iron-deficiency.

Identifying GI tract bleeding requires an endoscopy, in which a fiberoptic scope is inserted through the mouth to look into the esophagus and stomach (esophagogastroduodenoscopy, or EGD) or through the anus to look into the colon (colonoscopy). These procedures are usually recommended for anyone with IDA who is not menstruating and does not have another identifiable reason for losing blood (such as recent surgery or trauma). Endoscopies are important because cancers and other digestive system problems can be caught early.

A less common cause of IDA is malabsorption, where someone does not absorb iron sufficiently from food. Celiac sprue (gluten hypersensitivity) is one malabsorption disease. This is a problem in which gluten (found in some grains such as wheat) causes an allergic-type of reaction inside the intestines, which in turn causes the intestine's lining to change and prevents it from absorbing nutrients properly. The treatment for this is avoiding gluten-containing foods.

Iron studies in IDA are discussed in the previous section on anemia of inflammation (AI). Sometimes it can be difficult to tell the difference between IDA and AI. Another way to distinguish between them is to take iron supplements every day and measure the blood reticulocyte (immature RBC) count 7 to 10 days later. Iron supplementation causes the reticulocyte count to increase if there is IDA, but not in AI. A bone marrow biopsy is sometimes needed. In AI, there will be normal amounts of iron present in the biopsy. In contrast, bone marrow iron amounts will be low in IDA.

The treatment for IDA is to take iron supplements, which you can buy over the counter. Iron absorbs best when taken on an empty stomach. Iron is absorbed best in an acidic environment, and stomach digestive fluids are more acidic in the absence of food. It is also best to take an iron supplement with vitamin C, which increases stomach acidity. Infusions of iron are sometimes needed if someone does not tolerate iron supplements or if their anemia does not improve on them. The latter can occur especially in people with malabsorption (such as having celiac disease or after gastric bypass surgery) or in the setting of systemic inflammation, which causes decreased iron absorption.

Autoimmune Hemolytic Anemia

When the immune system attacks and destroys the RBCs directly, it causes autoimmune hemolytic anemia (AIHA). This is the only type of anemia that is one of the SLE classification criteria (chapter 1). It may occur in up to 10% of people with SLE. It can

LUPUS IN FOCUS

Do not take iron supplements without a doctor's guidance

If your body already has enough iron but you regularly take an iron supplement anyway, you can develop something called iron overload. Iron overload can damage the liver, heart, and joints and cause diabetes.

LUPUS IN FOCUS

Some people with iron deficiency crave eating strange things

"Pica" is the medical term for craving and eating non-food items. Some patients with an iron deficiency develop an urge to eat clay, stones, dirt, chalk, soap, paper, or, more commonly, ice (called pagophagia).

also occur in people without SLE. Typical blood-work findings for AIHA include a decreased haptoglobin level, an elevated reticulocyte count, increased LDH and bilirubin levels, and a positive Coombs' antibody (chapter 4). Also, the doctor may examine the blood under the microscope where they may see rounder than normal RBCs (called spherocytes).

AIHA with low plt counts is called Evans syndrome. Someone can have Evans syndrome by itself, or as a part of their SLE. Some people initially develop Evans syndrome and over time develop other organ involvement, consistent with SLE.

AIHA is not nearly as common as anemia of chronic disease or iron deficiency anemia. However, it is usually more severe and requires treatment with immunsuppressants. Rituximab (Rituxan, chapter 33) appears to have a high rate of success and tends to work quickly. IVIG (intravenous immunoglobulin) and danazol (chapter 35) are other options. Removing the spleen surgically (splenectomy) is another treatment choice. Patients undergoing splenectomy are at increased risk for infections and should abide by the recommendations in chapter 22 in the asplenia section.

Severe AIHA may require RBC transfusions. This can be complicated because many SLE patients have antibodies directed toward RBCs. It is best to look for these antibodies to find a compatible blood transfusion source, but since reactions to incompatible blood are typically mild enough to treat, giving a blood transfusion for severe AIHA even with unknown compatibility is recommended. It is much better to manage a mild blood transfusion reaction than to withhold a life-saving transfusion.

Pure Red Cell Aplasia

Pure red cell aplasia is rare. It occurs when autoantibodies in SLE attack the RBC-producing cells in the bone marrow. The clue to this diagnosis is severe anemia (low hemoglobin and hematocrit) along with an extremely low reticulocyte (baby RBCs, chapter 4) count. Before blaming lupus for pure red cell aplasia, it is crucial to ensure nothing else is causing it, such as infections (especially parvovirus) or medications. Any potential causative drug should be stopped. Successful treatment can occur with immunosuppressants, danazol, and IVIG. RBC transfusions may be needed for severe anemia. Most patients respond well to treatment.

Anemia of Chronic Kidney Disease

Anemia is common in people whose kidneys do not work correctly. Permanent kidney damage is called chronic kidney disease (CKD, discussed in chapter 12). If the damage is bad enough, the kidneys become less effective at removing toxins from the blood.

LUPUS IN FOCUS

Take folic acid if you have ongoing or recurrent autoimmune hemolytic anemia

In AIHA, the continuous need to make additional RBCs, which requires folic acid, causes folic acid depletion. Therefore, it is important to take 1–5 mg of folic acid supplements daily. If extra folic acid is not taken, people with AIHA can develop an additional anemia called megaloblastic anemia.

This is called renal insufficiency. Doctors diagnose renal insufficiency by finding a lower-than-average estimated glomerular filtration rate (eGFR) on blood work or a decreased creatinine clearance on a 24-hour urine sample (chapter 4).

The most common causes of CKD are diabetes, high blood pressure, atherosclerosis (hardening of the arteries, chapter 21), and aging. Around 40% of SLE patients will develop kidney inflammation (lupus nephritis), which can also cause CKD.

The kidneys secrete a hormone, erythropoietin, which stimulates the bone marrow to make RBCs. (Erythro- is Greek for "red," and -poietin means "maker" or "producer.") When someone develops CKD, the kidneys can make less erythropoietin, causing less RBC production and anemia. The severity of anemia tends to correlate with the severity of the CKD. Worse anemia tends to occur in those with worse CKD (those with lower eGFR).

If the hemoglobin level on the blood tests is 10 g/dL or lower, erythropoiesis-stimulating drugs (such as Aranesp, Epogen, and Procrit) can help, especially if problems such as fatigue are present. These medications are injected in a doctor's office.

Vitamin B12 Deficiency

Vitamin B12 is essential for blood cell formation and proper nerve function. Vitamin B12 deficiency can lead to anemia and nerve damage. With this kind of anemia, the RBCs usually become larger (called a macrocytic or megaloblastic anemia), as can be identified by an elevated MCV on the CBC (chapter 4). Other blood tests show either a low vitamin B12 level or a high methylmalonic acid level. Prompt treatment is necessary to prevent nerve damage.

One potential cause of vitamin B12 deficiency is an autoimmune disorder called pernicious anemia (PA). For adequate absorption in the intestines, the vitamin B12 we ingest needs to bind to a substance called intrinsic factor (IF). IF is produced by cells in the stomach lining called parietal cells. PA occurs when the immune system attacks the parietal cells in the stomach lining (resulting in low IF production) or produces antibodies to IF, preventing it from binding to vitamin B12. Both mechanisms cause a reduction in IF binding to vitamin B12 and therefore decreased vitamin B12 absorption by the intestines.

IF antibodies are diagnostic of PA. Gastric parietal cell antibodies can also help diagnose PA (but they can also be seen in some people who do not have PA).

Other causes of vitamin B12 deficiency include eating a vegetarian diet, alcoholism, or malabsorption (such as after gastric bypass surgery). Some medications, such as proton pump inhibitors (PPIs, chapter 28) and the diabetic medicine metformin can reduce vitamin B12 absorption.

Most people with a vitamin B12 deficiency, including pernicious anemia, do well taking over-the-counter vitamin B12 (also called cyanocobalamin), at doses of 1,000 mcg (micrograms) to 2,500 mcg each day. However, some people need vitamin B12 injections, which can be given in the doctor's office or at home. There is also a vitamin B12 nasal spray called Nascobal that can be used weekly.

Folic Acid Deficiency

Folic acid (also called folate) deficiency is usually due to a diet lacking in green, leafy vegetables or folate-enriched cereals or due to drinking too much alcohol. The medication methotrexate can also cause it. Like vitamin B12 deficiency, it causes macrocytic anemia (megaloblastic anemia) with larger-than-normal RBCs on the CBC (a high MCV). It is diagnosed with a low RBC folic acid level on blood testing. It is usually easy to treat by eating foods rich in folic acid, taking a folic acid or folinic acid (also called leucovorin) supplement, and decreasing alcohol consumption.

Folic acid deficiency can also create a problem in newborn babies called a neural tube defect. Therefore, doctors recommend that pregnant women take folate supplements.

Anemia Due to Medications

Many of the immunosuppressants (table 22.1) can also cause anemia, usually a macrocytic anemia with a high MCV. They do so by preventing the bone marrow from producing enough RBCs. Methotrexate is prone to causing anemia by interfering with how the body handles folic acid. To prevent low blood counts, everyone taking methotrexate should also take daily folic acid or weekly folinic acid (leucovorin). When a medication causes mild anemia, it is usually continued if it is helping the patient's lupus. However, if the anemia is causing any problems or the hemoglobin level is less than 10 g/dL, the drug may need to be stopped or the dosage lowered. Sometimes, erythropoiesis-stimulating agents (such as Aranesp, Epogen, and Procrit) are useful.

KEY POINTS TO REMEMBER

1. Doctors diagnose anemia by finding a low Hb level or Hct on the CBC.

2. The specific cause of anemia must be determined to know how to treat it.

3. Mild anemia (hemoglobin above 10 mg/dL) usually does not cause major problems.

4. Possible symptoms of anemia include fatigue, shortness of breath, lightheadedness, chest pain, and heart palpitations (fluttering sensations). Iron deficiency can cause a craving to eat ice (pagophagia).

5. The most common anemias in SLE are iron deficiency anemia (treated with iron supplements) and anemia of inflammation (treated by treating the lupus itself).

6. Autoimmune hemolytic anemia is due to the immune system attacking the RBCs and destroying them. It can be severe, and its treatment is with immunosuppressants. It is the only type of anemia in the SLE classification criteria (chapter 1).

7. Vitamin B12 and folic acid deficiencies can cause macrocytic (larger than normal RBCs) anemia and are treated with vitamin supplements.

8. A doctor can treat anemia of inflammation, anemia due to CKD, and drug-induced anemia with injections of erythropoiesis-stimulating agents such as Aranesp and Procrit.

Platelet Problems

Low Platelet Counts (Thrombocytopenia)

Platelets (plts, also called thrombocytes) are the third cellular component in blood. Thrombocytes are fragments of bone marrow cells called megakaryocytes. *Thrombo-* comes from the Greek word meaning "clot." Plts are important for blood clotting. If a blood vessel gets cut or leaks, the job of the plts is to stick together in clumps, form a clot, clog up the blood vessels, and prevent bleeding.

Just as with the WBCs and the RBCs, the lupus immune system can attack plts and reduce their number. A low plt count is called thrombocytopenia. When thrombocytopenia occurs due to an autoimmune process (the immune system attacks the plts), as in SLE, it is called immune thrombocytopenia (ITP). A normal plt count on the CBC should be around 140,000/microL to 450,000/microL (depending upon the lab). ITP occurs in 10% to 50% of people with SLE (this varies widely depending on the research study).

ITP can exist by itself, as an organ-specific autoimmune disease (chapter 2). Over time, around 5% to 10% of people with ITP will eventually develop other organ involvement, evolving into SLE (where the ITP is part of that person's SLE). This most commonly occurs within the first five years in ITP patients. However, most SLE patients with thrombocytopenia first develop thrombocytopenia at the time of their SLE onset or after they have already been diagnosed with SLE.

A very low plt count can cause someone to bleed and bruise more easily. However, plts are usually very effective and function normally in most patients with thrombocytopenia, even thought there are fewer plts than normal. SLE thrombocytopenia is most commonly found during routine blood testing, and the person does not feel anything wrong (no bleeding or bruising). However, sometimes it is diagnosed after someone goes to the doctor with excessive bruising, a bloody nose (called epistaxis), or blood in their stool. Fortunately, most people with SLE and thrombocytopenia do not have these problems because their plt counts are not low enough.

People with SLE and thrombocytopenia tend to develop more severe lupus than average. They should be vigilant in taking medications regularly, using sunscreen religiously, and having labs periodically checked.

Before a low plt count is assumed to be due to lupus, it is important to make sure it is truly low, since it is not uncommon to get a falsely low plt count (pseudothrombocytopenia; *pseudo-* means "false"). This occurs if the plts clump together in the test tube, and the laboratory machine that measures them counts a bunch of plts (one clump) as only one plt. To ensure someone doesn't have a falsely low plt count, the lab can examine the blood under the microscope to see if plt clumping is occurring. Another method is to remeasure the number of plts in a different blood tube having sodium citrate (called a purple top tube), which prevents plt clumping.

Other reasons such as infections and drugs should also be considered before blaming SLE. Some medicines that can cause a low plt count include immunosuppressants, antibiotics, anti-seizure medication, and heparin. A clue to medication being the cause of low plts is that this usually occurs very soon after the patient starts the drug.

Another cause of thrombocytopenia in SLE is the antiphospholipid antibody syndrome (APS, explained later in this chapter). Around one out of every three APS patints have low platelets, typically in the 100,000/microL to 140,000/microL range. Doctors believe this occurs due to the plts being used up in tiny areas of increased clotting. In this situation, the low plt count doesn't cause bleeding problems. On the contrary, these APS patients tend to be at increased risk of blood clots.

An enlarged spleen (splenomegaly, discussed later in the chapter) can cause thrombocytopenia, anemia, and leukopenia. When this occurs, the plts are usually just mildly decreased.

Thrombotic angiopathy (discussed later in this chapter) and macrophage activation syndrome (discussed previously) are other rare causes of thrombocytopenia in SLE.

Most people do not have bleeding problems unless the plt count drops below 25,000/microL. Patients are usually treated with medications if the plt count gets below 20,000/microL to 30,000/microL (different doctors use different thresholds). If, however, someone has bleeding problems with a level higher than 30,000/microL, medical treatment is needed. High-dose steroids, IVIG, and rituximab (Rituxan) are the most commonly used treatments. IVIG works fastest (within one to three days) followed by steroids, which can take two days to two weeks to work.

For severely low plt counts and active bleeding, intravenous (IV) transfusions of plts may be needed, but their effects last only a few hours, so they may have to be repeated while waiting for IVIG or steroids to help. IVIG raises the plt count in 80% of patients. However, it usually lasts for only two to six weeks, so other therapies are also needed.

Sometimes medications may not help reverse severely low plt levels, and people may need their spleen removed (discussed later in this chapter).

If the above treatments are inadequate, a group of medicines called thrombopoietin receptor agonists (also called thrombopoietin mimetics) can be used. These drugs stimulate the bone marrow to make plts. Three medications are available: romiplostim (Nplate), eltrombopag (Promacta, Revolade), and avatrombopag (Doptelet). All three have been used with success in SLE thrombocytopenia. However, SLE patients with antiphospholipid antibodies may be at higher risk for blood clots from these medicines, so caution is recommended.

A newer drug to treat ITP called fostamatinib (Tavalisse) was FDA-approved in 2018. However, as of 2023, it had not been studied in lupus-associated ITP.

Other treatments found useful in some SLE patients, but not used as often, include mycophenolate, azathioprine, cyclosporine, and cyclophosphamide.

Thrombotic Microangiopathy

Thrombotic microangiopathy is a rare but potentially deadly SLE problem. "Thrombotic" refers to blood clot production. *Micro-* means "small," and *-angiopathy* refers to blood vessel damage. Thrombotic microangiopathies cause abnormalities on the insides of tiny artery (arterioles) and capillary (the blood vessels that connect arterioles to your veins) blood vessel walls. These abnormalities then cause blood clotting and reduced blood flow. Involved organs become damaged since they cannot get enough blood supply from these clogged blood vessels. Plts are needed to make the blood clots,

---

LUPUS IN FOCUS

Why the lab result platelet number differs from what the doctor notes

As in the case of WBCs, doctors usually describe the number of platelets differently than on your lab slip. While the laboratory may report 150,000 platelets per microliter (mcL), doctors will often write the shortcut "150K," where the "K" means "1,000." 150K is the same as 150,000.

so the plt count lowers during this process. RBCs trying to get through the clogged blood vessels are damaged, causing a type of anemia called "microangiopathic anemia." Under the microscope, the RBCs look torn up.

There are several causes of thrombotic microangiopathy in SLE. Thrombotic thrombocytopenic purpura (TTP) is one. "Thrombotic" means that there is an increased amount of blood clotting. "Thrombocytopenic" means that the plt count is lower than usual; "purpura" is the medical term for bruising. The clots decrease blood flow to essential organs, causing kidney failure, neurologic problems (such as seizures and confusion), and fever, in addition to the low plt count and microangiopathic anemia. Finding an ADAMTS13 activity level of less than 10% on blood work or a positive ADAMTS13 inhibitor (chapter 4) can help confirm a TTP diagnosis.

Without treatment, this condition is fatal. However, high doses of steroids and plasmapheresis (also called plasma exchange and apheresis, chapter 38) greatly increase recovery chances. Rituximab (Rituxan), cyclophosphamide, eculizumab (Soliris), and caplacizumab (Cablivi) can also be used.

Other causes of thrombotic microangiopathy in SLE patients include medications or infections. These are treated by stopping the offending drug or treating the infection, respectively. Catastrophic antiphospholipid syndrome is another potential cause discussed later in this chapter.

High Platelet Counts (Thrombocytosis)

The most common causes of elevated plt counts in SLE are similar to those in people without lupus. They include inflammation (especially vasculitis), infection, iron deficiency, and anemia. Treatment is directed at the cause. In patients with SLE, a high plt count is rarely a reliable indicator of lupus disease activity. Still, it does occur in some. I have one patient whose plt count becomes very high when her lupus pneumonitis (lung inflammation) flares. It normalizes after successful treatment.

Another potential cause of high plts is the absence of a spleen (asplenia; *a-* comes from the Greek word for "without"). The spleen is essential for removing unwanted plts from the blood. When it is absent, the plt count can become elevated. Some people with SLE can develop a smaller spleen that doesn't work well (hyposplenism) or ceases to function at all (asplenia). A splenectomy is a surgical procedure where a surgeon removes the spleen. If the body destroys its own spleen (which can occur in SLE), it is called autosplenectomy (*auto-* meaning "one's self"). Some SLE patients have asplenia due to autosplenectomy. This probably occurs due to antiphospholipid antibodies causing blood clots and a loss of blood supply in the spleen. One study evaluated 17 SLE patients with high plts. Three of them had asplenia due to autosplenectomy as the cause, and all 3 were positive for antiphospholipid antibodies. See functional asplenia below, under "Spleen Problems."

Pancytopenia

Pan- means "all." Pancytopenia occurs when all three blood cells (white cells, red cells, and plts) are decreased. In SLE, the most common cause is lupus itself. As described previously, the evaluation and management are the same as evaluating each low blood cell type individually. Pancytopenia can especially happen in patients with an enlarged spleen (splenomegaly, discussed later in this chapter).

191

However, it is vital to ensure that there are no other reasons for pancytopenia. These include low vitamin B12 and RBC folate levels. If deficience are found, they are easy to treat with supplements. Immunosuppressants can also cause pancytopenia, just as they can cause a decrease in the individual blood cell types. In this situation, the medication dose should be decreased or stopped altogether, unless the pancytopenia is very mild. Severe infections can also cause pancytopenia, but this is usually obvious.

More dangerous causes of pancytopenia should also be considered. Macrophage activation syndrome is a potential cause (discussed earlier). Sometimes a bone marrow biopsy is needed to find the reason. The blood cells are produced in the bone marrow, so anything that may cause a decrease in the production of the blood cells may be diagnosed in this way. A bone marrow biopsy can also diagnose cancers (especially lymphoma and leukemia) and myelofibrosis (discussed next).

Autoimmune Myelofibrosis

Autoimmune myelofibrosis is a rare cause of pancytopenia. A group of rheumatologists and hematologists (blood experts) in Turkey found myelofibrosis in 20% of their SLE patients who underwent bone marrow biopsy for pancytopenia, while a group in Thailand found myelofibrosis in only 5%.

Myelo- comes from the Greek word for "marrow," and *-fibrosis* refers to scar tissue. In myelofibrosis part of the bone marrow is replaced by scar tissue. This scar tissue crowds out important cells that produce blood cells, causing low blood cell counts.

In people without lupus, myelofibrosis is due to blood cell cancers. This form is called "primary myelofibrosis." SLE myelofibrosis is called "autoimmune myelofibrosis." While primary myelofibrosis does not respond well to treatment, autoimmune myelofibrosis usually responds well to steroids and other lupus treatments (such as mycophenolate, IVIG, and rituximab). Surgical splenectomy can also help.

KEY POINTS TO REMEMBER

1. Thrombocytopenia in SLE is most commonly caused either by the immune system attacking the plts (decreasing their number) or from antiphospholipid antibody syndrome.

2. Bleeding problems usually do not occur until the plt count drops below 25,000/microL. So, doctors typically do not use more potent medicines unless the number decreases below 20,000/microL to 30,000/microL.

3. Removal of the spleen may be necessary in severe, resistant cases of thrombocytopenia.

4. Thrombotic thrombocytopenic purpura is a rare cause of low plts. It is always life-threatening and requires high-dose steroids and plasmapheresis.

Lymph Node Problems

The lymphatic system consists of organs that are important to lymphocytes. This includes where lymphocytes are produced (the bone marrow), where they are stored and mature (the thymus, lymph nodes, spleen, and tonsils), and the fluid (lymph) and connecting tubes (lymphatic vessels) in which they travel. Although lymphocytes also travel in the blood of our vascular (circulatory) system, blood is not considered part of the lymphatic system.

The lymph nodes (often called lymph glands) are small, oval-shaped, rubbery tissues connected by lymphatic channels. Circulating WBCs travel to them during periods of immune system stimulation. For example, if you get a Strep infection in your throat, the WBCs identify the infecting bacteria and travel to the cervical (neck) lymph nodes. They then communicate with other WBCs about the infection and cause more WBCs to go to the throat to kill the Strep bacteria. The number of WBCs filling lymph nodes can be enormous. This can cause your lymph nodes to swell and become uncomfortable (often noted as "swollen glands"). The medical term for swelling of the lymph nodes is "lymphadenopathy."

Roughly 50% of SLE patients will have lupus-induced lymphadenopathy, with swollen lymph nodes often noticeable in the neck, armpits, and groin. In some people, the lymph nodes swell during lupus flares. However, sometimes they can remain slightly swollen even when lupus appears to be well controlled.

A rare cause of lymphadenopathy in SLE is Kikuchi disease (also called Kikuchi histiocytic necrotizing lymphadenitis). Although this condition usually occurs alone, 3% to 13% of patients with Kikuchi disease develop SLE. It was initially described in 1972 among Japanese women. Since then, it has been found in people worldwide, but it is still more commonly seen in Asians. Kikuchi disease causes painful lymphadenopathy, especially in the neck. Approximately one-third of patients also have a fever, rash, joint pain, and a large spleen and liver. Less common problems include pleurisy, inflammatory arthritis, hepatitis, or brain and nerve inflammation. Since all of these things can be seen in SLE, it takes a skilled doctor to determine if someone has Kikuchi disease by itself or if it is occurring along with SLE.

LUPUS IN FOCUS

Lymphedema: a rare SLE problem

The lymphatic vessels are similar to our blood vessels (such as veins), except that they carry lymph fluid instead of blood. Lymph is made up of the fluid that surrounds the body's cells. This fluid flows into the lymphatic vessels, moving it to the blood that enters the heart to recirculate. In addition to this fluid, the lymph also contains lymphocytes and fats. If the lymphatic vessels become inflamed due to SLE (lupus lymphedema), fluid builds up in the extremities, most commonly in the feet and ankles, resulting in swelling.

Lupus lymphedema is rare, with only a few cases reported in the medical literature. These were treated with steroids. I have had only one patient with lymphedema at the time of her SLE diagnosis. It occurred when lupus inflammation was documented as active (positive EC4d, chapter 4). Fortunately, hers resolved with hydroxychloroquine. Steroids were not needed.

Kikuchi disease is diagnosed by a lymph node biopsy. The symptoms can improve with steroids and nonsteroidal anti-inflammatory drugs such as naproxen and ibuprofen. When it occurs by itself, it usually goes away within a few months, but it can recur. Since a small percentage of patients can develop SLE, Kikuchi disease patients should be monitored closely.

Sometimes, swollen lymph nodes in SLE patients can be from other problems such as infection or cancer, especially lymphoma (cancer of lymphocytes). SLE patients are three to five times more likely to develop lymphoma. If you develop persistently enlarged lymph nodes, your doctor may get a biopsy to figure out whether this is due to lupus or to lymphoma. A biopsy is also highly recommended if you are over 40 years old, have an enlarged spleen, or if the lymph node swelling occurs behind or just above the collar bone (clavicle).

Spleen Problems

The spleen is an organ found in the left upper abdomen, underneath the ribs. It is an essential part of the immune system because it removes things that have been tagged for removal by antibodies. The spleen also removes old blood cells so that they can be replaced by younger, healthy blood cells. The spleen enlarges in up to 50% of people with SLE, especially during periods of increased disease activity. Your doctor may find this on physical examination or when they do an ultrasound study or abdominal computerized tomography (CT scan) for other reasons. The medical term for an enlarged spleen is "splenomegaly." Sometimes the liver is enlarged as well; this is called hepatosplenomegaly. Splenomegaly does not usually cause major problems.

In rare cases (1% to 4%) SLE patients can have functional asplenia, also known as hyposplenism. Both terms are used to describe a spleen that does not function (see the earlier thrombocytosis section). Doctors can suspect this condition in patients with a high plt count. It can be confirmed by examining the blood under a microscope and using a nuclear medicine test called a liver-spleen scan (also called liver-spleen scintigraphy). This is often a permanent SLE complication. However, if the spleen problem is due to infection, spleen function can improve (called reversible functional asplenia) after antibiotics.

It is unknown whether SLE asplenia occurs due to antiphospholipid antibody clots, splenic blood vessel clogging due to large immune molecules (especially immune complexes), or a type of thrombotic angiopathy called disseminated intravascular coagulopathy (DIC). Because the spleen is an essential part of the immune system, people with a splenectomy (either surgical or from autosplenectomy) are at increased risk for infections. See chapter 22 for information on preventing and treating infections in people with hyposplenism and asplenia.

KEY POINTS TO REMEMBER

1. Enlarged lymph nodes (lymphadenopathy) and an enlarged spleen (splenomegaly) are common in SLE but rarely cause problems. Many people use the term "swollen glands" for lymphadenopathy.

2. If lymph nodes stay enlarged, a lymph node biopsy is sometimes needed to ensure no lymphoma (a type of cancer).

3. SLE can cause the spleen not to work properly. It is important to prevent infections when this occurs (chapter 22).

Antiphospholipid Antibodies and Antiphospholipid Syndrome

Between 30% and 50% of SLE patients have antiphospholipid (aPL) antibodies. These antibodies include anticardiolipin antibodies (ACLA), lupus anticoagulant (LAC), beta-2 glycoprotein I antibodies (anti-beta2GP-1), and anti-phosphatidylserine antibodies (chapter 4). Antiphospholipid antibodies can also be identified by the appearance of false positive syphilis tests (false positive RPR or VDRL, chapter 4).

Antiphospholipid antibodies can cause blood clotting. When this occurs, it is called antiphospholipid syndrome (discussed below). The pattern of aPL antibody positivity influences someone's risk of blood clots. The higher the antibody levels, the higher the risk. Persistently positive aPL antibodies (having a positive antibody every time it is checked) increase the risk more than having an occasionally abnormal antibody. If someone is positive for ACLA, LAC, and anti-beta2 GP-1, this is called triple positivity. People with triple positivity have a significantly higher risk for blood clots. Patients who are positive for LAC and PC4d (plt bound complement, chapter 4) and have low C3 complement levels are at high risk for heart attacks, blood clots, and strokes.

Problems other than lupus and APS can also cause aPL antibodies, the most common being infections. When infections cause positive aPL antibodies, they usually disappear after the infection resolves. Therefore, if someone has a positive aPL antibody, it is important to recheck it three months later (or longer) to see if it is still positive. A single positive aPL that is then negative on further repetitive testing is not important. This is one reason why a persistently positive test result is required as one of the SLE classification criteria (chapter 1) and the APS classification criteria.

LUPUS IN FOCUS

Repeatedly check beta-2 glycoprotein I antibodies (anti-beta2GP-1)

In 2020, the Lupus Center at Johns Hopkins Hospital showed that it is helpful to repeatedly check anti-beta 2 glycoprotein (anti-beta2GP-1) in SLE patients who have had blood clots. They looked for anti-beta2GP-1 about every four months for several years in their patients and found that if anti-beta2GP-1 was positive more than once yet negative at other times, the risk of blood clots increased. This is contrary to what doctors usually do, which is to repeat antiphospholipid antibodies three months after an initial positive result and, if that repeat test is negative, not to repeat it. The Johns Hopkins study showed that it is helpful to repeatedly check for anti-beta2GP-1. This ensures not missing the diagnosis of secondary antiphospholipid syndrome (APS).

Although it is rare to get blood clots from infection-related antibodies, blood clots have been reported in some infections. For example, the coronavirus responsible for the global COVID-19 pandemic has been associated with infection-induced blood clots from aPL antibodies.

When an aPL antibody–positive person gets blood clots, it is called antiphospholipid syndrome (APS). About 50% of APS patients have primary antiphospholipid syndrome, meaning that they have APS without SLE. The other 50% have SLE and APS (called secondary APS). One study showed that if someone has primary APS, they have about a 20% chance of developing SLE within 10 years.

Physicians need to exercise caution when deciding whether someone with APS also has SLE. SLE and primary APS can have similar effects. These include positive antinuclear antibodies, positive antiphospholipid antibodies, low plts, neurologic problems, and autoimmune hemolytic anemia. It is possible to have primary APS (without SLE) yet satisfy four or more SLE criteria. In 2018, a French group showed that one out of every four primary APS patients fulfilled the SLICC SLE classification criteria (chapter 1) despite not having lupus.

About 15% of SLE patients have secondary APS. Possible clotting problems from APS include blood clots in the legs called deep venous thrombosis (DVT), blood clots in the lungs called a pulmonary embolus (PE), blood clots in the arteries of the brain causing a stroke or transient ischemic attack (chapters 13 and 21), and blood clots in the arteries of the heart causing a heart attack. These antibodies can also cause pregnancy complications such as a miscarriage due to blood clots forming in the placenta (the organ that connects the fetus to the mother in the womb). These are discussed after the treatment sections below.

Most SLE patients with positive aPL antibodies do not develop blood clots and never develop APS. However, aPL-positive SLE patients tend to develop more organ damage than those without aPL antibodies, even in the absence of APS. Therefore, these antibodies must contribute to organ damage in ways other than just large blood clots. It is possible that they contribute to microscopic-level damage through other means.

Likewise, SLE patients with secondary APS tend to have worse lupus problems than those without APS. These include more organ damage, higher disease activity, and more significant organ involvement (such as nerve, brain, spinal cord, heart, lung, kidney, and eyes). They also have higher death rates.

Some APS patients have other APS complications such as skin ulcers, kidney involvement, diffuse alveolar hemorrhage (chapter 10), and low plt counts. Low plt counts from APS do not increase bleeding. A rash known as livedo reticularis (chapter 8) can occur due to clotting in small skin blood vessels. Small clots can also occur on heart valves (called Libman-Sacks endocarditis), causing difficulty with blood flowing properly through the heart.

Management of aPL Antibody–Positive Patients Who Do Not Have Blood Clots

While APS patients are treated with blood thinners (discussed in the next section), most aPL antibody–positive people who do not have blood clots do not require blood thinners. However, the European League Against Rheumatism (EULAR) recommends that SLE patients in this group consider taking low-dose aspirin (81 mg) daily if they have other problems that increase their risk for blood clots. But note that taking aspirin in this manner is controversial, since aspirin can increase the risk of internal bleeding (chapter 21). Discuss with your doctor before taking aspirin.

Another choice in preventing blood clots in people positive for aPL antibodies is statins. In addition to lowering cholesterol, statins reduce inflammation. A 2018 Japanese study showed that aPL antibody–positive patients who took a statin were much less likely to develop blood clots. More research is needed. But since there are many other reasons to consider statins in SLE (such as diabetes, high cholesterol, or other risk factors for heart attacks and strokes), it is good to have a low threshold for using statins in aPL antibody–positive patients.

Antiphospholipid Syndrome Treatment in SLE

People who develop APS blood clots are at high risk of them recurring and need lifelong blood thinners such as warfarin (Coumadin) or heparin. Those who take warfarin must get a blood test called a PT/INR (prothrombin time and international normalized ratio) at regular intervals to ensure their warfarin is dosed correctly. A normal INR (without warfarin) is about 1.0, and this measurement increases when someone takes warfarin. The higher above 1.0, the thinner the blood is. Usually, the doctor tries to keep the PT/INR between 2.0 and 3.0 for most APS patients.

For patients with blood clots in their arteries (arterial thrombosis), a higher INR of 3.0 to 4.0 may be recommended. Low-dose aspirin (81 mg) daily with warfarin at standard dosing (INR of 2.0–3.0) is an alternative for arterial blood clots. As of 2020, these recommendations were supported by the 16th International Congress on Antiphospholipid Antibodies Task Force, although some APS experts recommend an INR of 2.0–3.0 in all patients.

If the blood is too thin (has too high of an INR) due to warfarin, the person is at risk of bleeding, and the warfarin dose must be lowered. If the INR level is too low, the person is at risk of blood clots, and the amount needs to increase.

Fortunately, there are now devices that people can use at home to measure the INR and enable them to adjust their own warfarin. This has greatly simplified warfarin treatment. Most APS patients who take warfarin or heparin regularly have a much lower chance of developing recurrent blood clots. However, they are at increased risk of bleeding due to their medication and should take necessary precautions against this possibility.

It is essential for people taking warfarin to learn as much as they can about what can interfere with warfarin. For example, vitamin K-rich foods, such as many green vegetables, will keep warfarin from working correctly. A person on warfarin should therefore learn to control their vitamin K intake, since any change in vitamin K intake can affect the INR.

Ideally, a person on warfarin should not smoke cigarettes or drink alcohol since both affect warfarin levels. In addition, many drugs will either increase or decrease the INR, so it should be checked soon after any medication changes.

Taking warfarin for the rest of your life can be burdensome. Therefore, many patients ask if they can stop their blood thinner if they have not had a blood clot in a while. Several studies have addressed this question in patients with primary APS. These studies have had mixed results. Two studies showed a high risk for recurrent blood clots after warfarin was stopped, sometimes with dangerous effects such as catastrophic APS (discussed later in this chapter) and even death. Since SLE further increases the risk for blood clots, the decision to stop blood thinners in lupus APS patients should be approached cautiously.

The medication hydroxychloroquine (Plaquenil) may help APS. Hydroxychloroquine can reduce aPL antibody production and blood clots in SLE.

APS patients are more likely to have low vitamin D levels. Having SLE worsens vitamin D deficiency due to the need to use sunscreen and avoid ultraviolet (UV) light, which is necessary to produce vitamin D. Low vitamin D levels may increase the risk of blood clots, and some studies suggest that vitamin D supplementation may help lower this risk.

It is enticing to use newer blood thinners (instead of warfarin) that do not require frequent monitoring. These drugs are commonly called direct oral anti-coagulants (DOACs). They include rivaroxaban (Xarelto), dabigatran (Pradaxa), apixaban (Eliquis), and edoxaban (Savaysa). A study called TRAPS (Trial on Rivaroxaban in AntiPhospholipid Syndrome) was stopped midway through when 22% of the APS patients taking rivaroxaban developed dangerous blood clots; only 3% of those taking warfarin did. A 2020 French paper reported two patients who developed catastrophic antiphospholipid syndrome shortly after starting rivaroxaban. Therefore, DOACs should be avoided in APS.

Suppose, though, that someone has a venous (vein) blood clot, and the first blood test result shows one or two antiphospholipid antibodies (aPLAs). In that case, if the person was treated with a DOAC (a common treatment for venous clots) it is acceptable to continue the DOAC until a confirmatory blood test is done three months later. APS requires a repeatedly elevated aPLA, and false-positive results can occur. But if the repeat test is positive, confirming APS, the DOAC should be changed to warfarin.

If, however, the patient with the venous blood clot has triple-positivity (three different positive aPLAs), then heparin or warfarin should be used, rather than a DOAC. This is because triple-positivity is less likely to be a false positive and carries a high risk for blood clot recurrence if not taking heparin or warfarin. Even so, some patients with triple positivity might insist on taking a DOAC. In that case, a brain MRI is recommended to ensure no evidence of decreased blood supply or history of stroke. If any of these are present, warfarin or heparin should continue to be recommended, instead of a DOAC.

Some APS patients have low plt counts, but they do not increase bleeding. While it would be correct to stop warfarin in most people with low plts (low plts usually increase bleeding), warfarin is usually continued in patients with APS-associated thrombocytopenia.

While most people with APS do well on warfarin, aspirin, hydroxychloroquine, vitamin D, and statins, not everyone does. Some either do not tolerate warfarin or develop blood clots while taking it. Rituximab (Rituxan), IVIG, and even bone marrow transplantation are other treatment options.

There is mounting evidence that the complement system (chapter 3) is involved with blood clot formation in APS. Therefore, eculizumab (Soliris, a C5 complement inhibitor) can be considered for recurrent blood clots when standard therapies fail.

APS-induced blood clots can cause DVTs, PEs, heart attacks, strokes, spinal cord damage, and pregnancy problems (all described next). If any of the problems in the following sections occur in someone persistently positive for aPLAs, then that person

Your blood type may predict your risk for getting blood clots

Having a blood type of A, B, or AB (collectively known as non-O blood types) may increase the risk of getting blood clots. A 2018 study showed that men with a non-O blood type and positive for aPL antibodies were five times more likely to get blood clots than men with type O blood. This effect was not seen in women.

has APS. The only aPLAs used to diagnose APS are ACLA, LAC, and anti-beta2GP-1. We are unsure of the role of anti-phosphatidylserine antibodies.

Deep Venous Thrombosis

Thromb- means "blood clot," and *-osis* means "process" or "condition." Deep venous thrombosis (DVT) occurs when a blood clot forms in one of the deep veins of the arms or legs. It is much more common in the legs. Often the person will notice constant leg (or arm) pain and swelling, especially over the calf, sometimes with redness and warmth. This problem is considered a medical emergency. If the blood clot breaks loose from the blood vessel wall and travels to the lungs, causing a pulmonary embolism, it can be deadly. Anyone with symptoms suggestive of a DVT should go at once to the emergency room, where doctors will usually examine the veins with ultrasound, a medical imaging study that makes it possible to see what is occurring deep under the skin.

Pulmonary Embolus

"Pulmonary" refers to the lungs, and an embolus is a blood clot that travels through the bloodstream. Pulmonary embolus (PE), or pulmonary embolism, occurs when an embolus travels to the lung and clogs up an artery there. The most common source of PE is a DVT. If the embolus is large, it can block lung blood flow. This can reduce blood oxygen levels, which can be dangerous and even deadly.

Someone with a PE usually has shortness of breath and/or chest pains. A doctor can find evidence suggestive of a PE on an electrocardiogram (ECG), blood tests such as the D-dimer test, or chest x-rays. However, more definitive tests are needed. One of the best studies to diagnose pulmonary embolus is a chest computed tomography pulmonary angiogram (CTA). An x-ray called a ventilation/perfusion scan is necessary for places that do not have chest CTA.

Myocardial Infarction

A myocardial infarction (MI), commonly known as a heart attack, occurs when a blood clot blocks a coronary (heart) artery. This blocked artery causes a part of the heart muscle to die due to a lack of blood supply. The most common symptom is chest pain, often described as pressure in the chest, which can shoot to the arm, neck, or jaw. Sometimes nausea or shortness of breath can be the main symptom. A doctor may diagnose an MI by using an electrocardiogram along with blood tests that measure enzymes released from the heart muscle due to damage. Myocardial infarctions due to antiphospholipid antibodies are not common. However, MIs due to other problems associated with SLE are one of the most common causes of death in SLE (chapter 21).

Cerebrovascular Accident

If a blood clot occurs in a brain artery, there can be a loss of blood flow, causing that part of the brain to die. The term for this is a cerebrovascular accident (CVA), commonly called a stroke. You can think of it as a "heart attack of the brain." Sometimes, a blood clot in the brain can be temporary, causing brief symptoms and ultimately going away. This is termed a transient ischemic attack (TIA), or a mini-stroke. ("Transient" means "for a short time," and "ischemia" means "inadequate blood flow.") Although the outcome of a TIA is much better than the permanent problems seen in a CVA, it is nonetheless an urgent matter. Anyone with a TIA is at high risk of developing a full-blown CVA.

The symptoms of a CVA depend entirely on which part of the brain it affects. Symptoms can include difficulty talking, numbness, weakness, a droopy face, blurred vision, loss of vision, headache, and the inability to move correctly. Brain imaging studies, such as a CT scan or MRI, can diagnose a stroke. Aside from blood clots, strokes can occur for other reasons in people with SLE (chapters 13 and 21).

Myelitis

Myelitis occurs when there is damage to part of the spinal cord. *Myelo-* comes from the Greek word for "marrow." Before modern medicine, the spinal cord was referred to as the marrow of the spine.

In lupus, the cause is usually inflammation. It can also occur due to a clotted artery from APS. This is a devastating complication because it can cause permanent leg paralysis and may not improve with treatment. Usually, a combination of treatments is needed for myelitis in aPLA-positive patients, including blood thinners (heparin or warfarin), high doses of steroids, cyclophosphamide, or plasmapheresis (chapter 13).

Obstetrical Antiphospholipid Syndrome (Pregnancy Complications)

The placenta connects the fetus to the womb (uterus) of the mother. Some women with aPL antibodies develop blood clots in the placenta, leading to loss of blood flow to the fetus, causing a miscarriage. This can happen at any time during pregnancy. Doctors should check for aPL antibodies in women with recurrent miscarriages early in pregnancy or who have ever had any miscarriage in the second or third trimester. Giving blood thinners to pregnant women with APS (called obstetrical APS) dramatically increases the chances of a successful pregnancy.

Women with obstetrical APS should give themselves heparin shots during pregnancy (and often several weeks after delivery). Hydroxychloroquine (Plaquenil) and low-dose aspirin also help. By doing this, most women with APS can have a successful pregnancy.

Women with aPL antibodies can also have other pregnancy complications that can potentially result in the loss of the baby. These include preeclampsia (high blood pressure and protein in the urine), eclampsia (preeclampsia plus seizures), and HELLP syndrome. HELLP stands for hemolysis, elevated liver enzymes, and low platelets. Obstetrical APS is discussed in chapter 18.

Catastrophic Antiphospholipid Syndrome

A particularly severe antiphospholipid antibody syndrome is called the catastrophic antiphospholipid syndrome (CAPS). In CAPS, blood clots develop in multiple areas, causing many organs to fail. These people are very sick and usually end up in an intensive care unit. About 75% of patients with a CAPS episode have SLE with secondary APS, and roughly 50% of CAPS events are triggered by infection. The infection needs to be treated. Intravenous (IV) heparin should be used in all CAPS patients.

Many experts advocate using a triple therapy of IV heparin, high-dose steroids, and plasma exchange (or IVIG). A 2018 report from the International CAPS Registry showed that triple therapy worked best. Patients who do not respond to triple therapy can be treated with rituximab (Rituxan) or eculizumab (Soliris).

Unfortunately, 30% to 50% of CAPS victims die. Although it is a devastating complication, two-thirds of those who survive have no lingering problems from the episode. One-third of patients continue to have muscle weakness, loss of limbs due to the need for amputations, or permanent organ damage to the kidneys, heart, or brain.

Lupus Anticoagulant-Hypoprothrombinemia Syndrome

Lupus anticoagulant (LAC) can cause blood clots as a part of APS or be present in SLE, causing no problems. On rare occasions, though, it can be associated with excessive bleeding (instead of blood clots). This conditiom is called the lupus anticoagulant-hypoprothrombinemia syndrome (LA-HPS). Bleeding episodes can be mild to severe. The most common bleeding problems are bruises and nose bleeding. Others such as bleeding gums, heavy menstrual cycles, bloody urine, throwing up blood, or having bloody stools can also occur.

People with LA-HPS have other abnormal blood tests aside from a positive LAC. They also have prothrombin antibodies, low prothrombin activity, and elevated prothrombin time (PT). Prothrombin is an enzyme that is important for blood clotting. When lower levels occur due to lupus-induced prothrombin antibodies, abnormal bleeding can occur. These prothrombin antibodies are also responsible for activating lupus anticoagulant activity, but not blod clots.

LA-HPS is so rare that the best therapy is unknown. The most common treatments are high-dose steroids and blood product transfusions to help replace prothrombin (notably fresh frozen plasma and packed red cells). IVIG, cyclophosphamide, azathioprine,

---

LUPUS IN FOCUS

Can I donate blood if I have lupus?

In general, the American Red Cross allows SLE patients to donate blood if they are in remission or have low disease activity (ask your doctor). However, patients on blood thinners, mycophenolate mofetil (CellCept), thalidomide, or leflunomide (Arava), cannot donate blood. Aspirin is allowed. If unsure of eligibility, call the Red Cross at 866-236-3276.

and rituximab (Rituxan) have also been used successfully. LA-HPS appears to generally respond well to therapy, with only 2 deaths out of 92 reported cases as of 2018.

KEY POINTS TO REMEMBER

1. Between 30% and 50% of SLE patients are positive for antiphospholipid (aPL) antibodies (cardiolipin antibody, lupus anticoagulant, and beta-2 glycoprotein I antibody). Antiphospholipid antibodies can also potentially cause false-positive syphilis tests.

2. Up to 50% of people with these antibodies have antiphospholipid syndrome (APS), developing blood clots or miscarriages.

3. Some doctors recommend that patients with aPL antibodies take low-dose aspirin (81 mg a day) to help prevent blood clots.

4. People with APS usually need to be on hydroxychloroquine and blood thinners such as warfarin, aspirin, and heparin for the rest of their lives.

5. Patients can self-monitor warfarin INR levels at home and adjust their own dose.

6. Newer blood thinners such as Xarelto should not be used for APS unless the person is unable to take warfarin or heparin.

7. People with recurrent blood clots on standard therapy or people with catastrophic antiphospholipid syndrome may require high doses of steroids, apheresis (plasma exchange), IVIG, cyclophosphamide, or rituximab (Rituxan).

8. The treatment for obstetrical APS is usually hydroxychloroquine, heparin, and aspirin during pregnancy to increase the chances of a successful pregnancy.

9. Hydroxychloroquine, vitamin D, and statins may decrease blood clots risk in SLE patients with aPL antibodies.

10. Lupus anticoagulant-hypoprothrombinemia syndrome is a rare SLE complication and is not part of the antiphospholipid syndrome. Although patients are positive for LAC, they develop bleeding problems rather than clotting problems.

The Respiratory System

Nishant Gupta, MD, MS, *Contributing Editor*

The respiratory system is also called the pulmonary system (*pulmon-* means "lung"). It begins at the nose and mouth, where you breathe air in and out, and continues down the major windpipe (trachea), which further branches out into smaller windpipes called bronchi, and ends in the lungs. The last part of the lungs that the air reaches are tiny, microscopic sacs called alveoli. Alveoli have thin walls lined with small blood vessels called capillaries (see magnified view, figure 10.1). Oxygen from inhaled air is absorbed through the alveolar walls into the blood inside the capillaries. The blood entering the lungs by way of the pulmonary arteries, which come from the heart right ventricle (chapter 11), lacks oxygen. When inhaled oxygen is absorbed into these alveolar capillaries, the oxygen binds to hemoglobin (a protein that carries oxygen) in the red blood cells, causing the blood to become oxygenated. At the same time that oxygen is being absorbed, gases that the body does not need (such as carbon dioxide) are released. These unwanted gases travel from the alveolar capillaries into the air-containing portion of the lungs. When you breathe out, these gases leave the body.

Although SLE can affect any part of the respiratory system, the most common areas involved are lower respiratory areas (figure 10.1). This includes the alveoli, the interstitium (tissue in between the alveoli), the blood vessels, and the outer lung lining (the pleura). Pulmonary problems are so common in SLE that virtually all autopsies of SLE patients show lupus lung involvement. This chapter discusses the numerous ways SLE can affect the respiratory system.

Pleuritis (Pleurisy)

The pleura is the lining around the lungs. It consists of two thin layers of smooth, lubricated membranes. One layer envelops the lungs. The other attaches to the inside of the muscles and ribs around the lungs. Between these two layers is a light coating of lubricating fluid. When the lungs inflate and deflate during breathing, they lide smoothly under the rib cage.

Pleuritis is inflammation of the lung linings (pleura). Pleuritis occurs more often in men, in patients with positive RNP, Smith, and dsDNA antibodies, and in patients with coexisting Raynaud's (chapter 11). Patients with late-onset SLE (after 50 years old) also have an increased chance of developing pleuritis.

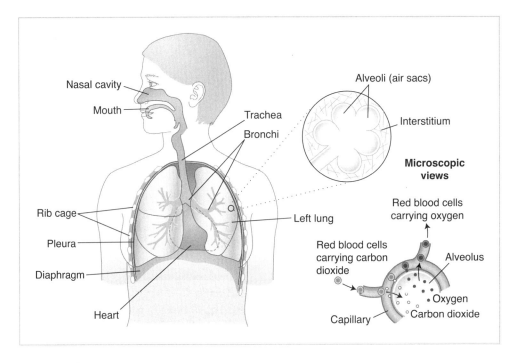

Figure 10.1 The respiratory system

LUPUS IN FOCUS

The importance of vaccines to prevent lung infections

Although all SLE patients are at increased risk for lung infections, those with lung disease are at particularly high risk. All SLE patients should get a yearly influenza vaccine (flu shot). We also recommend that all SLE patients get vaccinated against pneumococcal pneumonia and COVID-19 (chapter 22).

A similar type of lining exists around the heart (called the pericardium) and around the abdominal contents (called the peritoneum)—*peri-* means "around or about." The medical term for these linings (pleura, pericardium, and peritoneum) is "serosa." SLE can cause inflammation of the serosa, and the medical term for this is "serositis" (*-itis* means "inflammation of"). Serositis is part of the SLE classification criteria (chapter 1). When serositis occurs in the pleura, the medical term is "pleuritis" (or "pleurisy"). Similarly, the medical term is "pericarditis," when it occurs in the pericardium, and "peritonitis," when it occurs in the peritoneal lining.

Lupus serositis causes similar symptoms in these three areas. Healthy serosae (plural for serosa) allow the lungs, heart, and abdominal organs to move smoothly and effortlessly. During inflammation of the serosa, white blood cells enter the lining's space. The lubricating fluid loses its smoothness, and the layers rubbing against each other become roughened. This can cause pain when that organ moves. Normally people are not conscious of their breathing, but every breath is noticeable with pleuritis because of the pain.

When chest pain worsens with breathing, the medical term is "pleuritic chest pain." It is common in lupus pleuritis (and pericarditis, chapter 11). In addition to pleuritic chest pain, pleuritis can also cause shortness of breath, cough, and fever.

Other problems can also cause pleuritic chest pain (mimicking pleuritis). These include broken ribs, rib cartilage inflammation (costochondritis), sore ribs and muscles from poor posture, or other painful muscle problems such as fibromyalgia. A doctor must consider these other causes when evaluating chest pain that worsens with deep breathing.

To sort out these possibilities, we begin with the physical exam. Tenderness of the chest wall suggests other causes (such as costochondritis and fibromyalgia). Pleuritis can sometimes cause a rubbing sound, which occurs when the inflamed pleura layers or pericardium scrape against each other (it sounds like two pieces of sandpaper rubbing each other). We can hear this sound when we listen to the lungs and chest.The erythrocyte sedimentation rate and c-reactive protein (ESR and CRP; inflammation tests, chapter 4) are usually elevated. Very high ESR and CRP levels in SLE patients are most commonly seen during infections, pericarditis, pleuritis, and aortitis (discussed farther down in this chapter). If the ESR and CRP are normal, then other causes of chest pain are more likely.

A chest x-ray can look for fluid collection around the lungs. With pleuritis, the amount of extra fluid that occurs is often minimal, but sometimes there can be a large amount. This causes a pleural effusion ("effusion" is a medical term meaning "a collection of fluid").

The doctor often orders an ECG (electrocardiogram). This does not help diagnose pleuritis, but the ECG results may help diagnose pericarditis, the other type of lupus serositis that can cause pleuritic chest pain.

Pleuritis (pleurisy) is the most common SLE lung problem, occurring in 40% to 60% of patients. Yet, many SLE patients never notice they have it. We know this because autopsies of SLE patients show that up to 90% have had pleuritis at some point. Although pleurisy can be painful and cause shortness of breath, it rarely causes significant damage since it occurs outside the lungs.

If there is a pleural effusion, a doctor can sometimes drain the fluid (a procedure called thoracentesis). The doctor numbs up the chest wall muscles and skin, then inserts a needle through the numbed-up area and into the fluid to drain it out. Laboratory analysis helps determine the cause of the pleural effusion. This is typically not needed in SLE patients. Thoracentesis is most useful the first time someone has a pleural effusion and its cause is unknown. Other possible causes include other systemic autoimmune diseases (such as rheumatoid arthritis), infections, cancer, and kidney or liver failure. The pleural fluid will have different lab findings depending on the cause.

Sometimes, thoracentesis is needed for treatment, rather than for diagnosis. If someone has a large pleural effusion and trouble breathing, a thoracentesis can help them breathe much better.

Lupus pleuritis is usually treated with anti-inflammatory medicines. For mild cases, non-steroidal anti-inflammatory drugs (NSAIDs, chapter 36) such as naproxen may be used. Steroids may be necessary in more severe cases (in which the person has severe pain or when a large pleural effusion is present). Recurrent pleuritis attacks usually respond well to hydroxychloroquine. On occasion, stronger immunosuppressants (table 22.1) are necessary.

On rare occasions, pleural fluid may not respond to the above. In this case, pleurodesis (*pleuro-* from the Greek for "rib" or "side" and *-desis* from the Greek *desmos* for "bond") can be performed. Pleurodesis creates scar tissue within the pleura by injecting chemicals or talc or by scraping it. This scarring binds the outer lung surface to the inner ribcage, preventing fluid accumulation.

KEY POINTS TO REMEMBER

1. Pleuritis (also called pleurisy) is the most common lupus lung problem.

2. Most of the time, pleuritis causes no symptoms or problems.

3. The most common symptoms include pleuritic chest pain (pain with deep breathing), cough, and shortness of breath.

4. The initial treatments for are NSAIDs, steroids, and/or hydroxychloroquine (Plaquenil), but sometimes other immunosuppressants are needed.

5. If there is a lot of fluid around the lungs (pleural effusion), it may need drained by thoracentesis.

Pneumonitis

"Pneumonitis" is the term for any form of lung tissue inflammation. Pneumonia from infection is a type of pneumonitis. Around 1%–3% of SLE patients can have lung inflammation (pneumonitis) that behaves like pneumonia. It typically causes a cough, fever, chest pain, and sometimes shortness of breath. It can be difficult to distinguish infectious versus lupus pneumonitis. Lupus pneumonitis occurs when the immune system attacks the lungs' alveoli and interstitium (magnified view, figure 10.1). After it resolves, it may leave permanent lung scarring and damage. If this damage is mild, the person may not have any problems, but severe, the person may have difficulties breathing.

On chest x-ray (CXR), lupus pneumonitis shows infiltrates, which are fluffy white areas due to fluid collecting in either the interstitium or alveoli. The alveoli are the lungs' tiny air sacs that absorb oxygen. The interstitium is the connective tissue that supports the alveoli, holding them together. Lupus pneumonitis infiltrates look similar to infected infiltrates. Therefore, doctors usually prescribe antibiotics in this scenario (in addition to treating the lupus) just in case it is an infection.

Sometimes a high-resolution computed tomography (HRCT) scan is needed to see what is happening. HRCT uses more radiation than a CXR; therefore, doctors do not order it very often. Active inflammation from pneumonitis can have a ground-glass appearance on HRCT. This finding sometimes means there is fluid in the alveoli due to

Ground glass on CT scans

If a lung CT scan shows gray areas that look like frosted glass, it is called a "ground glass" findings. This is because ground glass findings look similar to frosted glass on CT, and frosted glass is produced by blasting fine, *ground glass* onto a glass surface. It is a non-specific finding but may help diagnose pneumonitis and interstitial lung disease. However, mild ground glass findings are also commonly seen in other conditions such as infections. In mild cases, physicians often repeat CT imaging in a few weeks to see if the findings resolve independently and decide if further tests are needed.

alveoloar inflammation (called alveolitis). However, ground-glass findings can also occur from infectious pneumonia, congestive heart failure, or other interstitial lung diseases discussed later in this chapter. Scar tissue in the interstitium from previous damage is another common HRCT finding in lupus pneumonitis.

Other tests, such as a bronchoscopy may be necessary. A bronchoscopy involves inserting a fiberoptic scope into the windpipe (through the nose or mouth) to look at the airways and lungs. This is typically performed under light sedation. The doctor can take pictures and collect fluid to send for cultures and other tests. In addition, a biopsy can help rule out other reasons for the lung problem, such as infection, cancer, or vasculitis (chapter 2). Under the microscope, a biopsy specimen of lupus pneumonitis shows lung tissue inflammation. If other causes of lung inflammation are excluded (such as infection), this can help diagnose lupus pneumonitis.

A surgical lung biopsy may be necessary if the above tests are unhelpful. In this procedure the surgeon makes a few small incisions into the chest wall and removes small pieces of lung tissue. Doctors usually reserve this for people with severe symptoms or whose treatment decisions require a biopsy. For example, lupus pneumonitis requires immunosuppressants, which would worsen an infection. In contrast, a lung infection is treated with antibiotics, which does not help lupus pneumonitis.

On rare occasions, some lupus treatments (such as methotrexate and cyclophosphamide) may cause pneumonitis. These may need to be stopped until the exact cause is determined.

Lupus pneumonitis usually requires high doses of steroids. Azathioprine (Imuran), mycophenolate (CellCept), rituximab (Rituxan), cyclophosphamide, and abatacept (Orencia) are other possible treatments. These can resolve inflammation, allow steroid dose reductions, and prevent pneumonitis recurrence. IVIG (intravenous immunoglobulin) or plasmapheresis (chapter 35) may be needed in complicated cases.

Lupus pneumonitis can be life-threatening. Around 40%–50% of patients do not survive severe bouts. Early detection and treatment are crucial. Approximately one-third of pneumonitis survivors will develop chronic interstitial lung disease (discussed later in this chapter).

1. Lupus pneumonitis occurs when lupus causes inflammation of the lung tissue.

2. The symptoms are like those of infectious pneumonia: cough, fever, shortness of breath, and chest pain.

3. CXR and HRCT scans for infectious pneumonia and lupus pneumonitis appear similar. Often, the person needs treatment for both possibilities (antibiotics plus immunosuppressants).

4. Some lupus drugs (such as methotrexate and cyclophosphamide) can cause lung inflammation. Doctors may need to stop these medications during pneumonitis.

5. HRCT scan can help diagnose lupus pneumonitis, assess its severity, and help make treatment decisions.

6. When lupus pneumonitis heals, it might leave some scar tissue or lead to the future development of interstitial lung disease.

7. Lupus pneumonitis has a high death rate.

Interstitial Lung Disease (Pulmonary Fibrosis)

The interstitium is the connective tissue supporting the alveoli and the lungs' small airway passages (see magnified view, figure 10.1). When this interstitium develops scarring or has inflammation, the condition is called interstitial lung disease (ILD).

If ILD consists primarily of scar tissue (fibrosis), it is called fibrosing lung disease or pulmonary fibrosis. Scarring occurs as a response to injury or inflammation. Often the body will form an excessive amount of connective tissue and collagen (scar tissue) after trying to heal inflammation. Think of the scar left after you get a skin cut. A similar process can occur in lung interstitium after episodes of inflammation. Scar tissue is not very flexible, so the lungs in ILD move less freely. Blood vessels (necessary for absorbing oxygen) cannot go through the scar, and the scar tissue compress the alveoli (essential for gas exchange). All these factors can cause inadequate absorption of oxygen and exhalation of carbon dioxide, leading to shortness of breath, chest pain, and cough.

After pleuritis, ILD is the second most common SLE lung problem, occurring in 5% to 20% of patients (depending on the study). A large Chinese study showed that SLE patients with ILD were more likely to have dry eyes, dry mouth, and anti-SSA (hallmark findings in Sjögren's, chapter 14). This suggests that SLE patients with Sjögren's disease may be more likely to have ILD than those without Sjögren's. ILD is also more common in SLE patients with Raynaud's, sclerodactyly (chapter 8) and anti-RNP (chapter 4) and in those who have had lupus pneumonitis.

A few common scenarios can lead to a diagnosis of ILD. One is after recurrent bouts of pneumonitis. Each episode can heal with scarring. A more common scenario testing in someone who has a progressive cough and/or shortness of breath leads to an ILD diagnosis. It is also possible for someone who feels fine and has no breathing problems to be diagnosed with ILD when the doctor hears something abnormal (called crackles

Rales and crackles on physical exam

"Rales" refers to a specific lung sound (usually at the bottom of the lungs, called the bases) heard through a stethoscope. They are almost always due to something wrong, such as ILD or heart failure.

Crackles is also most commonly heard at the lung bases and is typically present in patients with ILD. However, crackles can be heard in some situations without underlying lung disease. For instance, if a person has not been breathing deeply on a routine basis (such as an overweight person), the alveoli (tiny air sacs) in the lung bases can collapse. As the person breathes in deeply during their physical exam, the alveoli can fill back up, causing crackling sounds (crackles). However, after a few deep breaths, these crackles go away when all the alveoli are filled with air. These collapsed alveoli that open up with deep breathing are called atelectasis; it is not a significant problem.

or rales) on lung examination or based on chest imaging performed for unrelated reasons. It is not uncommon for patients to have mild ILD and not have symptoms.

Diagnosing ILD begins with a physical exam by the doctor. Often a doctor can hear changes in lung sounds with a stethoscope. A common description for these sounds is "Velcro crackles" because they resemble the sound of a Velcro strap being pulled apart. ILD in SLE typically affects the bottom of the lungs, so these crackles are usually most prominent at the lung bases.

A chest x-ray usually, but not always, shows scarring. The radiologist (a doctor who examines x-rays) may describe these as "increased interstitial markings" or "interstitial infiltrates." Often the doctor will order a chest HRCT, which shows the type and pattern of the lung changes. It is especially helpful to determine if there is active inflammation, which may appear as a ground glass. This can be useful in determining whether high doses of steroids or strong immunosuppressant medicines are indicated.

Pulmonary function tests (PFTs) are usually required to determine the disease severity and monitor it over time. These tests are conducted in a pulmonary lab at a hospital or in the office of a lung specialist (pulmonologist). Typically, PFTs in a patient with ILD reveal a restrictive pattern (called restrictive lung disease). A restrictive pattern means that the lungs do not expand normally due to the inelastic nature of the scar tissue in ILD. However, it is worth noting that ILD is one of many causes of restrictive lung disease. A more common cause is obesity (being overweight causes difficulty taking a full breath). Another is a rare condirion called shrinking lung syndrome (discussed later in the chapter).

Another part of the PFT helps determine the cause of the restrictive pattern—the diffusion capacity of the lung for carbon monoxide (DLCO). In this test, the patient breathes in air containing a small amount of carbon monoxide and holds it. Then the amount of carbon monoxide breathed back out is measured. The better the lungs absorb gases, the less carbon monoxide they will exhale. Healthy lungs absorb more carbon monoxide through the walls of the alveolar sacs into the blood vessels. If some condition (such as pneumonitis, ILD, or others) causes problems with either the alveolar sacs or the blood vessels (such as pulmonary hypertension, described below), the DLCO could be reduced. This is termed "decreased diffusion capacity." If the restrictive pattern is due to chest wall problems caused by obesity, the DLCO will be normal. In contrast, with ILD, the DLCO is usually reduced.

PFT results are helpful in monitoring ILD over time. If there is reversible inflammation in the lungs, successful treatment with medicines should cause PFTs to improve or stabilize. The numbers typically stay the same if the ILD was due to permanent scarring with no active inflammation. If the SLE medicines are not helping, and the lung disease worsens, the numbers may worsen.

It is important to figure out if ILD is due to permanent scarring or active inflammation. Finding ground-glass changes on HRCT can suggest possible alveolar inflammation (called alveolitis). A bronchoscopy can also help. So can a trial of steroids, since improvement following steroids can indicate that the patient had active inflammation. If there is active inflammation, steroids and other immunosuppressants (such as azathioprine, mycophenolate, rituximab, cyclophosphamide, or abatacept) can potentially prevent the lung condition from worsening, or it can improve the lungs.

If severe lung scarring (fibrosis) worsens (called progressive pulmonary fibrosis), it can lead to the need for oxygen treatment and lung transplantation. An FDA-approved drug called nintedanib (Ofev) has shown promise in slowing down the rate of decline in patients with progressive pulmonary fibrosis.

Everyone with significant ILD should participate in pulmonary rehabilitation (pulmonary rehab). Pulmonary rehab is a special physical therapy involving therapists highly trained in lung disease. They utilize equipment that monitors heart and lung function as patients exercise. This testing helps determine exercise ability, helping the therapist to develop the best exercise regimen. Participation in pulmonary rehab results in improved exercise capacity and better quality of life. In our opinion, this is an underused treatment in people who suffer from chronic lung disease. If you have symptomatic chronic lung disease, you should ask your lung doctor about pulmonary rehab.

A minority of people with lupus ILD will develop enough lung damage (respiratory failure) to require oxygen therapy. Some need to use it only while exercising, walking, or sleeping. The worst cases may need to use it all the time. Many patients resist using oxygen for many reasons, such as inconvenience and not wanting to appear sick to others. Even so, it is essential that people prescribed oxygen use it. Doing so can improve depression, memory, physical stamina, and quality of life.

Most patients with lupus-associated ILD do not develop respiratory failure. Some people never have any symptoms, while others may have varying degrees of breathing problems, chest pain, and cough. The most common symptom is shortness of breath during physical activity.

Lung transplantation may be needed in those with the most severe damage. A lung transplant can extend life span and improve quality of life. It is often recommended for patients in whom medical therapy is not helping and who have a high risk of dying within a few years. Some patients are not good candidates for lung transplantation due to chronic infection, a recent history of cancer, major damage to other organs (such as kidney failure or a heart disease), obesity, or other problems such as alcohol or cigarette smoke addiction.

Patients with ILD should take some important precautions. First, smoking cigarettes can worsen ILD and increase the chances of severe lung infections. No one with lupus should smoke (chapter 38). However, it is even more important for ILD patients not to do so.

Many SLE patients have esophagus (the tube connecting the mouth to the stomach) problems. One such problem is gastroesophageal reflux disease (GERD), where stomach contents back up into the esophagus (usually causing heartburn). Another problem is esophageal dysmotility (chapter 15). Here, the muscles do not normally push food down into the stomach. GERD and esophageal dysmotility can cause the acidic stomach contents to travel up the esophagus while someone is lying down or sleeping. This acidic fluid can drip back into the trachea (windpipe), go down into the lungs and cause damage. The person with GERD (or esophageal dysmotility) and ILD must be extra careful. They may need to take antacid medication every day. Measures to prevent acid contents from coming up from the stomach are covered in table 15.2.

The lungs are constantly under attack from germs you breathe in every day. Normal lungs and immune systems are very good at protecting people from these germs. However, SLE patients with ILD are at increased risk for lung infections, such as pneumonia. It is important to do everything possible to prevent lung infections. All patients should get the flu shot each year and vaccines against pneumococcal pneumonia (Pneumovax and Prevnar, chapter 22).

Although the information above is enough for many patients to understand ILD, there are specific types of ILD that lung experts (pulmonologists) look for. These are described next.

Nonspecific Interstitial Pneumonia (NSIP)

NSIP is the most common ILD in SLE. It causes lung inflammation and scarring. It has characteristic HRCT findings, so, a lung biopsy is usually not necessary. NSIP generally responds well to treatment with steroids and immunosuppressants like mycophenolate mofetil (CellCept), azathioprine (Imuran), rituximab (Rituxan), cyclosporine, cyclophosphamide, or abatacept (Orencia). Most patients achieve either improvement or stability of lung function decline with these treatments.

Lymphoid Interstitial Pneumonia (LIP)

LIP is a type of ILD in which inflammation affects the interstitium (the connective tissue between the alveoli) and the alveolar sacs. It is called "lymphoid" because the inflammation is due to lymphocytes (a type of white blood cell). It is not as common as NSIP. Chest HRCT often looks similar to NSIP but frequently contains pulmonary cysts (air-filled pockets) that help suggest LIP. A pulmonary cyst is a round, thin-walled region of air in the lung. Sometimes a biopsy is needed. LIP also usually resonds well to treatment.

Organizing Pneumonia (OP)

OP was formerly called bronchiolitis obliterans organizing pneumonia (BOOP). It causes inflammation, especially in and around the alveolar sacs. Chest x-ray is often

> **LUPUS IN FOCUS**
>
> **Honeycombing helps diagnose fibrotic lung disease**
>
> Honeycombing is a descriptive finding on CT scans of the chest, in which the larger holes in the honeycomb represent areas of destroyed lung tissue. Honeycombing is a sign of advanced lung fibrosis.

normal, and chest HRCT is often needed for diagnosis. OP can present symptoms that are similar to infectious pneumonia. It generally responds well to short–medium term courses (three to six months) of steroids, often with almost complete resolution.

Usual Interstitial Pneumonia (UIP)

UIP is a type of fibrotic (scarring) lung disease with very little inflammation. It has characteristic HRCT findings, so a lung biopsy is usually not necessary. Immunosuppressant drugs usually do not help UIP very much. UIP patients have a worse prognosis compared to other ILD patients. Treatment with Ofev may help slow down disease progression in UIP and other fibrotic ILDs. However, long-term studies of using Ofev in SLE patients are needed. Patients with UIP (and other ILDs) should get PFTs regularly to evaluate the lung function trajectory.

KEY POINTS TO REMEMBER

1. Interstitial lung disease (ILD) is a common problem in SLE.

2. ILD occurs due to lung inflammation and scarring.

3. A doctor can diagnose ILD with a chest x-ray, PFTs, and a CT scan of the chest. Occasionally, other studies, such as bronchoscopy and lung biopsy, may be necessary.

4. Most ILD patients do well with treatment.

5. The most common symptoms of ILD are shortness of breath during exertion and chronic cough, which may worsen over time.

6. If ILD worsens, steroids and potent immunosuppressants such as azathioprine, mycophenolate, cyclophosphamide, rituximab (Rituxan), or abatacept (Orencia) may be necessary.

7. If a person has GERD (or esophageal dysmotility) and ILD, it is crucial to treat the GERD aggressively (table 15.2).

8. People with ILD should never smoke.

9. Some immunosuppressants (such as methotrexate and azathioprine) can sometimes cause lung inflammation. Therefore, the doctor may need to stop them if they are unsure whether they contribute to the lung problem.

10. Nintedanib (Ofev) was FDA approved to treat chronic progressive fibrosing lung disease. It can be used in some SLE patients.

11. The various types of ILD (NSIP, LIP, OP, UIP) have different amounts of inflammation and scar tissue with varying responses to treatment and different long-term outcomes.

12. Patients with ILD should undergo periodic PFTs.

Diffuse Alveolar Hemorrhage (Pulmonary Hemorrhage)

"Hemorrhage" is the medical term for "bleeding." "Diffuse alveolar hemorrhage" (DAH) means "bleeding in the lungs." Other terms used to describe this lung problem include "pulmonary hemorrhage" and "hemorrhagic alveolitis." It is not the same thing as coughing up blood (medically known as hemoptysis). While commonly seen in patients with DAH, hemoptysis usually occurs due to other problems such as bronchitis.

DAH occurs in only 2% to 5% of SLE patients. SLE patients with antiphospholipid antibodies, low platelets, lupus nephritis (kidney inflammation), or low complements (chapter 4) are at increased risk for DAH. Most DAH patients also have lupus nephritis and low complements and are very sick.

DAH occurs when severe inflammation and damage in the alveolar air sacs cause blood leakage. The symptoms are usually similar to those of acute lupus pneumonitis—fever, cough, and shortness of breath (the same symptoms, by the way, that occur with infectious pneumonia). The most common lab abnormality is a drop in the red blood cell count (hemoglobin). Although SLE is one cause of DAH, it also occurs in other systemic autoimmune diseases (especially vasculitis), with infections, and from some medications. When it occurs in SLE, blood is in the sputum (saliva) about half the time. DAH often progress rapidly, leading to respiratory failure and the need for mechanical ventilation (an artificial breathing machine).

Since DAH can act very similar to infectious pneumonia, doctors place most patients on antibiotics. Chest imaging in DAH can look identical to lupus pneumonitis or infectious pneumonia, with chest x-rays showing alveolar infiltrates (fluffy white areas). Bronchoscopy is often necessary since it is almost impossible to tell whether someone has DAH, lupus pneumonitis, or severe infection. Cultures (for infection) and other labs can be done on the lung fluid obtained at bronchoscopy. The fluid shows a lot of blood in cases of DAH.

DAH therapy requires strong immunosuppressants (table 22.1). IVIG and a blood-filtering treatment called apheresis or plasmapheresis (chapter 35) are sometimes used.

DAH is a devastating SLE complication in which one out of three patients dies. Patients who do best include those who are younger, those who do not have a lung infection, and those who do not require mechanical ventilation. SLE patients who survive DAH continue to be at high risk for severe lupus complications and should be treated and monitored closely for the rest of their lives.

KEY POINTS TO REMEMBER

1. Diffuse alveolar hemorrhage (DAH) causes severe lung inflammation and bleeding.

2. DAH is rare and can be life-threatening.

3. Most DAH symptoms are similar to pneumonia (cough, fever, and shortness of breath), but sometimes there can be blood in the coughed-up sputum or phlegm.

4. DAH treatments include strong immunosuppressants, IVIG, apheresis, and plasmapheresis.

Pulmonary Embolism

The section on antiphospholipid syndrome (APS, chapter 9) discusses pulmonary embolism (PE), because in SLE patients PE is most commonly caused by APS. Another potential cause of PE is lupus membranous nephritis (Class V lupus kidney disease, chapter 12). In membranous nephritis, a large amount of protein is lost in the urine. When proteins that are important for preventing blood clots are lost, then blood clots can form. Up to 10% of SLE patients may develop a PE during their lifetime.

A PE most commonly comes from blood clots that first form in the large, deep veins of the leg (called a deep venous thrombosis, or DVT). A DVT can break away from the inner vein walls and travel to the lungs, where it clogs up a lung artery (pulmonary artery). Emboli (plural of embolus) and thrombi (plural of thrombosis) are types of blood clots. A thrombus is a blood clot that occurs where it first develops. An embolus is a blood clot that travels from somewhere else (it started out as a thrombus).

A PE blocks blood flow to a section of lung. The problems and symptoms the person develops depend on how large the blood clot is and how large and essential is the clogged artery that provides blood flow to the lungs. Shortness of breath and chest pain are the most common symptoms. Sometimes, but not always, the person may also have had discomfort and swelling in a leg, especially the calf area (typical of a DVT). If the clot is especially large, the PE can be life-threatening.

SLE patients are at higher risk of DVTs and PEs than people without SLE. They occur more commonly in bedridden patients due to their not moving the legs very much. Bedridden patients should consider taking blood thinners to prevent blood clots (after discussing this with a physician).

Doctors usually diagnose PE by either a V/Q (ventilation/perfusion, chapter 9) scan or a computed tomography pulmonary angiogram (also called a chest spiral CT). A D-dimer blood test can help. A normal D-dimer level can often (but not always) confirm that someone doesn't have a PE.

PE requires blood thinners such as warfarin (Coumadin) and heparin. Newer agents such as apixaban and rivaroxaban are convenient (don't require frequent blood monitoring). However, they should be avoided in APS (see chapter 9), which usually needs life-long warfarin therapy. If the PE is particularly severe and causes heart failure or low blood pressure, then surgery to remove the blood clot (called embolectomy) or the use of a potent blood-clot dissolver (thrombolytic therapy) may be needed.

Some patients cannot take blood thinners for various reasons (intolerance to the drugs or high risk for bleeding). These patients may require a filter in one of the large veins to prevent blood clots from traveling to the lungs. The most common type of filter is an inferior vena cava (IVC) filter.

1. A pulmonary embolism (PE) is a blood clot in the lungs' arteries that often originates from a leg blood clot.

2. PE can cause shortness of breath, chest pain, and fever.

3. Severe cases can be deadly.

4. In SLE patients, the most common causes of PE are antiphospholipid antibodies (chapter 9) and membranous nephritis (chapter 12).

5. The treatment for PE is blood thinners such as warfarin (Coumadin).

6. Antiphospholipid syndrome patients usually need life-long warfarin therapy.

Pulmonary Hypertension

The medical term "hypertension" means "high blood pressure." Pulmonary hypertension (PH) is when the pulmonary artery blood pressure is high. It is much less common than the everyday hypertension that many people have.

The pulmonary artery is the major artery (blood vessel) that carries blood from the heart to the lungs. The pulmonary artery then branches off into many smaller arteries. Their purpose is to take blood to the lungs (*pulmon-* means "lung") so that oxygen can enter the bloodstream and travel throughout the body.

The most common causes of PH are vasculitis (blood vessel inflammation), antiphospholipid syndrome, damage and scarring of the artery walls, interstitial lung disease, and heart failure. Autopsies show that the pulmonary artery walls in SLE patients are thicker and more scarred than normal. Pericarditis (inflammation around the heart), pleuritis, antiphospholipid antibodies, anti-RNP, Raynaud's phenomenon, and African ancestry increase the chances of developing PH. Elevated blood uric acid levels may also increase the risk.

Many people with mild PH do not have any symptoms. However, it can worsen, so it is important to watch closely. People with moderate to severe PH may have shortness of breath, chest pain, fatigue, heart palpitations, light-headedness, or swelling of the ankles. Unfortunately, severe PH has a high death rate.

To look for possible PH, doctors begin with the physical examination. The heart makes two distinct "lub-dub" sounds. If the second sound (the "dub") is louder than normal, this can be a sign for possible PH. Testing proceeds to an echocardiogram and PFTs.

An echocardiogram is a heart ultrasound (also called a sonogram or ultrasonogram). The technician applies gel to the chest and places a blunt instrument (a probe or transducer) on the gel. This probe sends sound waves (ultrasounds) into the body, where they bounce off the body's internal organs and back into the probe. Then, a computer forms a picture by reading these sound waves. An echocardiogram can find other heart problems such as excessive fluid around the heart, heart blood clots, infection, and heart valve and muscle problems. When looking for PH, the technician calculates the pulmonary artery pressure. This pressure result from an echocardiogram is only an estimate. A cardiac catheterization (described below) is much more accurate.

PFTs can also help. People with pulmonary hypertension usually have a decreased DLCO on PFTs. A low DLCO is often the first abnormality in someone with PH.

The next test is usually a right-sided cardiac catheterization. A long, thin tube (a catheter) is placed into a large vein in the neck or the groin after anesthetizing the area with numbing medication. The doctor carefully threads the catheter through the large vein until it enters the heart's right side, where it can measure the blood pressure there and in the pulmonary artery. This is the best way to determine whether someone has PH and how severe it is.

About 5% of SLE patients have PH when measured by cardiac catheterization. Echocardiograms suggest PH occurs in up to 24% of SLE patients. This is an overestimation due to echocardiograms not being highly accurate. The utility of doing echos is that they are noninvasive and they help reduce the chance of missing a diagnosis of PH.

Another common test is a six-minute walk test. During this test, people walk as far as they can for six minutes (to see if they get short of breath), and their blood oxygen levels are monitored. The six-minute walk is a reliable, easy test with results that mirror PH severity.

Heart failure with preserved ejection fraction (HFpEF) is a common cause of pulmonary hypertension in SLE. "Ejection fraction" refers to the percentage of blood the left side of the heart can squeeze out with each heart beat. The ejection fraction is measured on echocardiogram. Heart failure refers to when the heart is unable to push out enough blood to meet the body's demands. There are two main types of heart failure: one is decreased ejection fraction (where the heart muscle is severely damaged and unable to squeeze very well), and the other is HFpEF.

HFpEF used to be called diastolic dysfunction. Diastole is the phase when the heart muscle relaxes. In HFpEF, the heart muscle is stiffer than normal and does not relax enough to fill up with as much blood as it should. It is usually not very problematic when the person rests, but when they exert themselves or exercise, the heart may not be able to send enough blood for all the body's oxygen and nutrient requirements. This can cause fatigue and shortness of breath. It is most commonly seen in obese older patients with high blood pressure. It is treated with weight loss and by controlling blood pressure and reducing fluid overload with fluid pills (diuretics).

We have many SLE patients with PH due to HFpEF. A 2011 Spanish study that evaluated a large group of HFpEF patients showed that around 11% had systemic autoimmune diseases, including SLE. This association between autoimmune diseases and HFpEF could be related to early-onset hardening of the arteries and heart problems caused by autoimmunity (chapter 21).

In mild PH, no treatment may be necessary. The doctor will regularly monitor the tests (especially the echos and PFTs) to ensure it does not worsen.

In moderate to severe PH in which there is difficulty breathing, medications are prescribed to relax the pulmonary arteries and lower the pulmonary blood pressure. PH once had a high mortality rate, with 50% of SLE-related PH patients dying within two years. Today, 90% of patients are still alive after fifteen years. The life spans and quality of life of people with pulmonary hypertension have improved with early detection and better therapies. The wide variety of medications available to treat PH is beyond the scope of this book. Other therapies commonly used in PH patients include supplemental oxygen, blood thinners such as warfarin, diuretics (fluid pills), and exercise.

PH due to vasculitis (blood vessel inflammation) of the pulmonary arteries is often treated with high-dose steroids and cyclophosphamide. The role of other drugs such as mycophenolate and rituximab has not been proven.

KEY POINTS TO REMEMBER

1. Pulmonary hypertension (PH) occurs when the blood pressure in the lungs' arteries is high.

2. Echocardiogram, PFTs, and right-sided cardiac catheterization can diagnose PH. Cardiac cath is the most accurate test.

3. Mild PH may not cause symptoms and not need treatment. It may be monitored using an echocardiogram, six-minute walk testing, and PFTs at regular intervals.

4. Moderate to severe PH can cause shortness of breath and chest pain, and over time, it may cause heart failure.

5. PH is treated with medicines that relax the lungs' arteries and patients live much longer than in the past.

Bronchiectasis

Bronchiectasis occurs when the lungs' airways (bronchi) are abnormally enlarged. In addition, the bronchus walls become soft, limp, and easily collapsible. Normal working bronchi are essential for moving lung secretions and bacteria out of the lungs. If they do not work correctly and collapse, phlegm accumulates in the lungs, increasing infection risks. Patients with bronchiectasis often have frequent cough, sputum production, and increased lung infections. The diagnosis is made by chest CT scan. Unfortunately, bronchiectasis damage is permanent, and no treatments reverse it.

Chest HRCT scans show bronchiectasis in 12% to 30% of SLE patients (depending on the study). The most likely cause of bronchiectasis is bronchial wall damage due to recurrent infections. This can happen because of immunosuppressant use, the abnormal SLE immune system, and IgG2 subclass deficiency (chapter 22). Patients with SLE-related systemic autoimmune diseases (such as rheumatoid arthritis [RA] and Sjögren's) also tend to have higher rates of bronchiectasis. Although not well defined yet, underlying genetic mutations also probably play a role in its development.

The primary goals of bronchiectasis management are to clear the airways of excess phlegm and prevent lung infections. Lung infections are typically treated with antibiotics. For patients with frequent infections, regular prophylactic (preventative) antibiotics, especially the macrolide group (including azithromycin), are recommended.

A treatment strategy called bronchial hygiene, or airway clearance is also recommended. This includes regular exercise (such as aerobic exercise) and breathing exercises that include forceful coughing and exhalation. Breathing through a flutter valve or acapella valve device can vibrate and break up mucous. Chest physical therapy (clapping the hands on the chest) and using mechanical devices such as chest percussion cups can help dislodge phlegm.

Some patients with bronchiectasis have reactive airway disease (similar to asthma). This can be diagnosed by PFTs, which would show improvement after the patient has inhaled a bronchodilator medicine (such as albuterol). In these individuals, using bronchodilator inhalers can be valuable.

Pulmonary rehabilitation, controlling GERD, and getting vaccinations are also important.

In rare, severe cases, surgical removal of the involved part of the lung or lung transplantation are also options.

Shrinking Lung Syndrome

Shrinking lung syndrome is a rare complication in SLE, occurring in around 1% of patients (but in 6% of patients with severe SLE). People with this syndrome have shortness of breath and pleuritic chest pain (pain worsened when they breathe). Chest x-rays can show that the diaphragm (the muscle at the bases of the lungs) is higher up in the chest than usual. However, up to 40% of chest x-rays can be normal. PFTs demonstrate reduced lung volumes, and often the DLCO is reduced. The cause of this disorder is unknown. Immunosuppressants can stabilize or improve lung function over time.

KEY POINTS TO REMEMBER

1. Shrinking lung syndrome causes shortness of breath and pleuritic chest pain. It is rare.

2. It is diagnosed with chest x-rays and PFTs and treated with immunosuppressants.

Upper Airway Involvement

Every condition mentioned so far involves the lower airways, including the bronchi (small breathing tubes), to the lungs. The upper airway is from the mouth and nose down to the trachea (the largest breathing tube). The back of the mouth is called the pharynx, and below that are two different passageways. One is the esophagus, which is a flattened, muscular tube leading to the stomach (part of the digestive system, chapter 15). The other passage is covered by a flap of tissue called the epiglottis. The epiglottis is part of the upper airway, and its purpose is to prevent food from going down into the lungs. Below the epiglottis is the larynx, which contains your vocal cords. Below the larynx is an open tube surrounded by a thick cartilage wall (trachea) leading down to the smaller bronchi.

Since the mouth and nose are part of the upper airway system, mouth and nose sores (ulcers, chapter 8) due to lupus are the most common upper airway problems. Dryness also occurs, primarily in people with Sjögren's disease (chapter 14). Dryness inside the nose can cause itching, soreness, congestion, crusting, and bleeding, while dryness of the mouth can cause a sore tongue and increased thirst. The combination of dry mouth and dry nose can cause a decreased ability to taste food.

Compared to healthy individuals, SLE patients are twice as likely to have a decreased ability to smell (hyposmia) or a total loss of smell (anosmia). Dry nasal mucosa from Sjögren's overlap syndrome is a possible cause. This can be treated by regularly using nasal saline sprays and ointments to keep the inside of the nose moisturized.

Inflammation of other parts of the upper airway is unusual. Inflammation of the epiglottis (epiglottitis), larynx (laryngitis), trachea (tracheitis), and the cricoarytenoid cartilage (cricoarytenoiditis) have been described in individual case reports in the medical literature. These different areas of inflammation can cause similar symptoms, such as sore throat, hoarseness, dry cough, shortness of breath, and stridor (a high-pitched wheezing sound when breathing). They usually respond to immunosuppressants. In rare cases, the inflammation can be severe enough to cause airway narrowing, leading to death.

If the soft tissues of the neck compress the upper breathing passages, this can potentially lead to obstructive sleep apnea, causing fatigue, memory problems, and heart problems if not diagnosed and treated. It is discussed in chapter 6.

Xerotrachea

Around 30% of SLE patients have dry mouth due to an overlap syndrome with Sjögren's disease (chapter 14). One of the potential complications of Sjögren's is a persistent dry cough from dryness of the trachea (main breathing tube). This problem is called xerotrachea (*xero-* comes from the Greek word for "dry"). When the trachea is dry, it can be irritated and cause persistent cough (just as dry skin can feel itchy).

Other than xerotrachea, the most common causes of a persistent dry cough in SLE are postnasal drip (PND), GERD (chapter 28), asthma, or other lung problems such as ILD. The doctor needs to do tests for these. Sometimes, treatments are given for each potential cause (fluticasone nasal spray for PND, antacids for GERD, and inhalers for asthma) to see if these resolve the cough. A response to therapy can confirm that problem as the cause of the cough. If these possible causes are ruled out by the tests and treatments, then xerotrachea may be the reason.

The treatment for cough due to xerotrachea is to moisten the mouth and increase saliva flow (see chapter 14). These interventions include using a humidifier in the home (especially the bedroom), using xylitol-based mouth moisturizers, and medications such as pilocarpine (Salagen) or cevimeline (Evoxac). Daily guaifenesin (Mucinex) use helps thin out pulmonary mucus, resulting in less cough.

Do not discount xerotrachea if you don't notice dry mouth. It takes a significant decrease in saliva production (often more than a 50% reduction) before people realize that their mouth is dry. The doctor can check the physical exam for saliva under the tongue. The absence of a small amount of saliva pooled under the tongue with tiny bubbles (salivary pooling), which is a normal condition, can be a subtle sign of dry mouth. The doctor can also measure the volume of saliva you can produce to figure out if you have decreased saliva flow. If decreased saliva is detected by these methods, then the treatments mentioned in the previous should be implemented.

KEY POINTS TO REMEMBER

1. Xerotrachea is an underrecognized cause of unexplained dry cough.

2. It is especially common in Sjögren's overlap syndrome.

3. Diagnosis is based on improvement after treatments that moisturize the upper airways (humidifiers, pilocarpine, cevimeline, and guaifenesin).

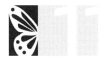

The Heart and Blood Vessels

Rachel C. Robbins, MD, FACP, *Contributing Editor*

The heart (figure 11.1A) consists of four chambers (two large ventricles and two smaller atria) that fill with blood and two sides—a right and a left side. The illustration's right and left sides are oriented as if you were looking directly at the heart through the front of the chest. Each atrium (the singular form of atria) allows blood to flow into its corresponding ventricle through a small hole. Each connecting hole is covered by a valve that can open and close. The heart's valves are like one-way doors (when working correctly) that allow blood to flow in only one direction (from the atria to the ventricles).

Blood arrives at the heart through large veins (the superior vena cava from the upper body and the inferior vena cava from the lower body). These veins empty blood (from which the body has removed most oxygen) into the right atrium. The right and left atria squeeze simultaneously, which causes the blood in the right atrium to travel through an opening covered by a valve (the tricuspid valve) into the right ventricle. Then the two ventricles (left and right) squeeze. This causes the tricuspid valve to close and push blood through the pulmonary valve. The pulmonary valve directs the blood into the pulmonary (meaning lung) artery. This large blood vessel carries this oxygen-depleted blood into the lungs. The blood entering the pulmonary artery travels to smaller pulmonary arteries and subsequently smaller arterioles until it reaches the tiniest blood vessels (capillaries). The capillaries are in the walls of the lungs' tiny air sacs, called alveoli (figure 10.1). Oxygen from the lungs is absorbed into the blood; gases not needed by the body (such as carbon dioxide) are released into the lungs so they can be breathed out.

The oxygen-rich blood in the tiny capillaries of the lungs travels to larger and larger blood vessels called pulmonary veins, the largest of which empties into the left atrium. Again, the left and right atria squeeze simultaneously, causing blood to flow from the left atrium through the mitral valve and into the left ventricle. When the right and left ventricles squeeze, the mitral valve closes. The blood in the left ventricle flows out of the heart through the aortic valve into the body's largest artery (the aorta).

The aorta divides into smaller blood vessels (arteries). The arteries divide into even smaller arterioles and finally into the tiniest blood vessels (capillaries). The body's cells absorb the oxygen and nutrients from this capillary blood. The body's cells also release

Dr. Rachel Robbins contributed to this article in her personal capacity. The views expressed are her own and do not necessarily represent the views of the Walter Reed National Military Medical Center, the Uniformed Services University, or the United States Government.

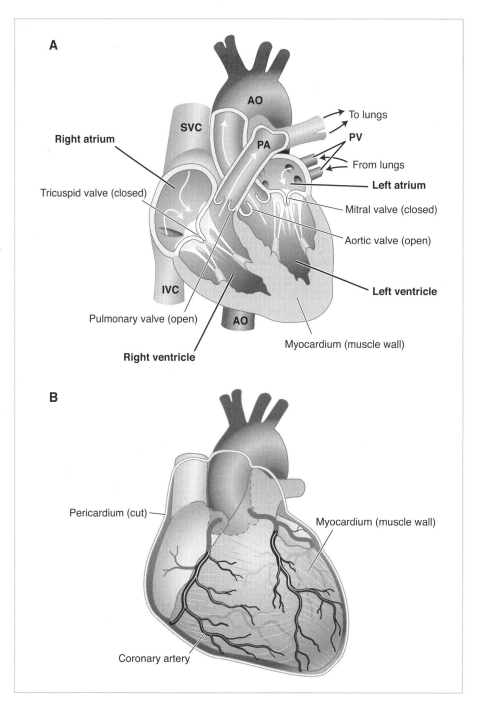

Figure 11.1 Inside the heart (A) and outside of the heart (B); abbreviations: IVC, inferior vena cava; SVC, superior vena cava; AO, aorta; PA, pulmonary artery; PV, pulmonary veins

waste products into the capillaries, and the blood carries them away for proper disposal. From the capillaries, blood flows into slightly larger blood vessels (venules) and then into larger blood vessels (veins).

The veins contain blood from which most of the oxygen has been absorbed by the body's cells. This oxygen-depleted blood appears bluish in color under the skin. The blood in arteries, rich in oxygen, is a deep red.

All the above make up the cardiovascular (CV) system. This chapter discusses the ways that SLE can affect the CV system with inflammation. Note, though, that the CV system is a major cause of problems in SLE patients for other reasons as well (chapter 21).

Pericarditis

The pericardium (figure 11.1B) is the sac of tissue that envelops the heart. Between the heart and the pericardium is a lubricating fluid (pericardial fluid) that allows the atria and ventricles to move effortlessly when they contract. SLE can cause inflammation in the pericardium called pericarditis. *Peri-* comes from the Greek word for "around," *cardio* refers to the heart, and "-itis" means "inflammation." Like pleuritis (chapter 10), it is one of the SLE classification criteria (chapter 1).

Up to 60% of SLE patient autopsies show evidence of pericarditis. However, only around 25% develop pericarditis symptoms, meaning that while most SLE patients get pericarditis, most of those affected do not realize it. Just as pleuritis is the most common lung problem in SLE, pericarditis is the most common heart problem from lupus inflammation.

As with pleuritis, inflammation from lupus pericarditis can cause the pericardium to produce extra fluid. This excessive fluid can accumulate in the pericardial sac (the space between the heart muscle and the pericardium). This fluid usually is slippery and slick, but with lupus inflammation, the number of white blood cells increases. Other inflammation-induced changes cause this fluid to lose its lubricating effects. This combination of events creates the most common pericarditis symptom—pleuritic chest pain (chest pain worsened with breathing).

Pericarditis pain can occur anywhere in the chest. People most commonly describe it as underneath or just to the left of the breastbone (the sternum). Sometimes, this chest pain worsens when the person lies on their back. Leaning forward may reduce the pain. Fever, shortness of breath, and heart palpitations (fluttering sensations) can also occur. The ESR and CRP (measures of inflammation, chapter 4) are usually high.

223

The doctor may identify signs of pericarditis on the physical exam when they listen to the heart and hear a pericardial rub, which sounds like two pieces of sandpaper rubbing against each other with each heartbeat instead of the normal "lub-dub" sound. Pericardial rubs often come and go with pericarditis, so the doctor may not hear anything abnormal.

Doctors typically order an ECG (electrocardiogram) for suspected pericarditis. A technician performs an ECG by placing sticky electrodes on multiple areas of the chest, arms, and legs. These electrodes detect the heart's electrical activity and display it in a graph. An ECG with evidence of pericarditis will show diffuse ST-segment elevations (a highly technical term used by doctors).

Although the ECG is usually enough for diagnosing pericarditis, sometimes an echo, or ultrasound exam of the heart, is performed. Gel is placed on the chest, and a probe (or transducer) is placed on the gel. The probe then sends sound waves into the chest, which bounce back to the probe when they strike solid objects (such as the heart). The ultrasound machine produces pictures of the heart from these sound waves. On an echo, pericarditis can show increased pericardial fluid around the heart.

The usual treatment for pericarditis is non-steroidal anti-inflammatory drugs (NSAIDs, such as naproxen, chapter 36) and colchicine. The anti-malarial hydroxychloroquine (Plaquenil) is usually enough to control the inflammation. However, occasionally more potent immunosuppressants (table 22.1) are used.

When pericarditis is severe, creating a large amount of fluid between the heart muscle and the pericardial sac, it can cause a problem called cardiac tamponade, which prevents the heart from pumping blood properly. When this occurs, the liquid needs to be drained from the pericardial sac (the procedure is called pericardiocentesis). Sometimes, if the doctors are concerned that the fluid might come back, they cut a small hole called a pericardial window, which allows the excess fluid to leak out of the sac so that excessive pressure on the heart muscle is relieved, and it can pump properly.

Constrictive pericarditis is a rare complication. This occurs when the pericardial sac becomes scarred and does not allow the heart to expand and contract normally, causing difficulty pumping blood. To treat constrictive pericarditis, doctors sometimes need to perform a pericardiectomy (-*ectomy* comes from the Greek for "act of cutting out"). The pericardial sac is removed surgically, allowing the heart to pump normally. The heart usually works well without the pericardium.

KEY POINTS TO REMEMBER

1. Pericarditis is the most common heart problem from lupus inflammation.

2. Pleuritic chest pain (pain that worsens with breathing) is the usual symptom. The pain is often worse while lying down and better when leaning forward. Shortness of breath may also occur.

3. Doctors usually diagnose pericarditis with ECG or echo.

4. The treatment is usually colchicine, NSAIDs, and hydroxychloroquine. Occasionally, immunosuppressants are needed.

5. If a large amount of fluid builds up, causing with the heart not to pump properly, then surgery to drain the fluid (pericardiocentesis) or cutting a small hole in the pericardium (pericardial window) or removing the pericardium completely (pericardiectomy) may be required.

Myocarditis and Cardiomyopathy

Myo- is the Greek word for "muscle," and *-carditis* means "inflammation of the heart." The heart muscle is called the myocardium. Its sole function is to pump blood through the body. Lupus myocarditis is due to lupus inflammation of the heart muscle. Over time, the body may heal the inflammation, but it often will leave permanent scar tissue (fibrosis). When there is either active inflammation or fibrosis inside the heart muscle, the heart may not squeeze normally and may have difficulty pumping blood. This can cause breathing problems, chest pain, heart palpitations, lightheadedness, and a rapid heart rate.

If severe, congestive heart failure (CHF) can occur. CHF means that the heart cannot pump blood efficiently and fluid builds up in the lungs and rest of the body. Symptoms of CHF can include shortness of breath, chest pain, fatigue, cough, exercise intolerance, and swelling of the ankles after standing and sitting (called edema). When a person is lying down, fluid can back up into the lungs. Some people instinctively prop themselves up on pillows while they sleep to breathe easier, while some wake up in the middle of the night with breathing difficulties, causing them to have to sit up to catch their breath.

Although only 5% to 10% of SLE patients are diagnosed with myocarditis, autopsy studies show that around one-third of SLE patients have had some degree of myocarditis. This means that, just as with pericarditis, the inflammation may not be severe enough to cause significant problems, or the diagnosis is missed. African ancestry, having a history of myositis (chapter 7) or nephritis (chapter 12), and being positive for anti-RNP or anti-SSA increase the risk for lupus myocarditis. It often occurs during severe lupus flares.

Blood work during myocarditis attacks usually shows inflammation with elevations of CRP and ESR (chapter 4). The inflammation can cause heart muscle enzymes to leak into the blood, causing high CPK and troponin blood levels.

ECG and chest x-ray (CXR) are usually not helpful. However, in severe cases, CXR may show an enlarged heart. The CXR can even show excess fluid built up inside the lungs from CHF.

An echo may show that the heart muscle does not contract or squeeze normally. When the heart muscle is damaged and not squeezing correctly, it is called cardiomyopathy. The ending *-opathy* comes from the Greek word for "suffering" or "disease." "Cardiomyopathy" literally means "a disease of the heart muscle."

There are numerous potential causes. These include lupus myocarditis, blocked coronary arteries (coronary artery disease, chapter 21), high blood pressure (hypertension), medications, viral infections, heart valve problems, and congenital/genetic problems. Hypertension and damage from coronary artery disease are the most common causes. In SLE patients with cardiomyopathy who have no other reasons for the condition (such as uncontrolled hypertension or heart damage from coronary artery disease), one can assume that lupus myocarditis may have occurred at some point.

Cardiomyopathy is diagnosed by echo and/or cardiac catheterization. Cardiac catheterization is performed in most patients with cardiomyopathy to ensure that blocked coronary arteries are not the cause. In this procedure the doctor injects a dye into the blood entering the heart and the blood vessels that feed the heart muscle (the coronary arteries). A special X-ray camera shows the dye, allowing doctors to see how well the heart works and squeezes blood and whether there are blocked arteries.

If the cause of cardiomyopathy is not evident from cardiac catheterization, the doctor can obtain a heart muscle biopsy during the procedure and analyze the biopsy specimen under the microscope. Biopsies are useful to look for lupus myocarditis and hydroxychloroquine-induced cardiomyopathy. It is rare to get heart damage from hydroxychloroquine (Plaquenil). When it does occur, it typically happens in those taking it for more than 20 years.

Cardiac MRI (or cardiovascular magnetic imaging) is a more convenient way of diagnosing lupus myocarditis. It is not invasive and doesn't use radiation. It helps doctors diagnose lupus myocarditis at earlier stages and thus prevent permanent damage in many patients.

Lupus myocarditis is treated with immunosuppressants (table 22.1) or IVIG (chapter 35).

In a case of congestive heart failure (CHF) from heart muscle damage, heart medications may be needed to help the heart muscle squeeze stronger, control blood pressure, and remove excessive fluid (diuretics).

Most patients respond well to lupus myocarditis treatments. However, in those with CHF, up to 25% of patients can die from it.

KEY POINTS TO REMEMBER

1. Cardiomyopathy refers to any damage to the heart muscle.

2. Although lupus myocarditis can cause cardiomyopathy, other possible causes include coronary artery disease, hypertension, diabetes, heart valve problems, and birth defects.

3. Usually, an echo and a cardiac catheterization are necessary to diagnose cardiomyopathy.

4. A cardiac MRI can help diagnose myocarditis.

5. Severe cases of cardiomyopathy and myocarditis may lead to congestive heart failure, causing fluid to accumulate in the lungs and ankles (edema), as well as shortness of breath and chest pain.

6. Lupus myocarditis is treated with immunosuppressants and IVIG.

Valvular Heart Disease (VHD)

The four heart valves function as one-way gates between different sections of the heart and the arteries that carry blood out of the heart (see figure 11.1A). They include the tricuspid valve (between the right atrium and the right ventricle), the pulmonary valve (between the right ventricle and the pulmonary artery), the mitral valve (between the left atrium and the left ventricle), and the aortic valve (between the left ventricle and the aorta). When these valves function normally, they help keep the blood flowing in the right direction. Occasionally there can be problems with the valves. Valve stenosis occurs when the valve opening becomes tighter and smaller than normal, causing the heart muscle to work harder at squeezing blood through the valve. This can cause the heart muscle to enlarge, which causes it to not work as well.

Another potential problem is valvular insufficiency (also called regurgitation). This causes the blood to leak backward (regurgitate) through the valve instead of going in the right direction. This can also cause the heart muscle and heart chambers to become larger than usual and thus not to work properly.

SLE patients have valvular heart disease (VHD) more often than healthy people, but most have mild involvement with no problems. However, chest pain, shortness of breath, heart palpitations, cough, lightheadedness, and even congestive heart failure can occur with more severe VHD. Being positive for antiphospholipid (aPL, chapter 4) antibodies increases the risk for VHD.

A doctor can often detect valvular stenosis and regurgitation (insufficiency) when listening to the heart with a stethoscope. Blood forcefully squeezed through a stenotic valve or flowing backward through a malfunctioning valve can create an abnormal sound called a heart murmur.

An echo and cardiac catheterization (discussed earlier) can show the heart valve problem and severity.

If the VHD is worse than mild, medications to help the heart and blood pressure may be needed. Repeated echo may be necessary to ensure that the condition does not worsen. If severe enough, surgery may be required to replace the valve, but fortunately, this is rare.

Another problem that can occur with the heart's valves is Libman-Sacks endocarditis (also known as verrucous endocarditis and nonbacterial thrombotic endocarditis). *Endo-* is from the Greek term for "inside." The endocardium is the tissue that lines the inside of the heart chambers and valves. Endocarditis means inflammation or infection of the heart valves. In SLE, Libman-Sacks endocarditis is due to inflammation instead of infection and causes wart-like (verrucous) growths on the valves. The growths are composed of cellular debris (pieces of dead cells), a small amount of inflamed tissue, and blood clots. Most patients with Libman-Sacks endocarditis are positive for antiphospholipid (aPL) antibodies and often have antiphospholipid syndrome (chapter 9).

These growths can occasionally break away, travel through the body, and clog blood vessels. If this occurs in the brain, it can cause a stroke. SLE patients with Libman-Sacks are 13 times more likely to have central nervous system lupus (brain involvement, chapter 13) than those without. Kidney damage can occur when clots get stuck in the kidneys' arteries. Rashes that look like vasculitis (blood vessel inflammation, chapter 8) occur with skin involvement. The heart valve may develop valvular regurgitation if the growths are large.

In mild cases of endocarditis, the doctor usually monitors with echocardiograms. If the endocarditis becomes severe, then surgery may be required. Today, we rarely see Libman-Sacks endocarditis, probably due to better treatment of SLE with drugs such as hydroxychloroquine (Plaquenil).

Many cases are treated with blood thinners. A 2020 Chinese study reported that 91% of their patients with Libman-Sacks endocarditis were aPL antibody–positive and that 73% of them had triple positivity (chapter 9). They treated most of these patients with blood thinners, such as warfarin. A patient not on warfarin ended up with a stroke. The authors recommended that all patients with Libman-Sacks and aPL antibodies take a blood thinner (preferentially warfarin).

A rare problem with VHD, especially Libman-Sacks endocarditis, is that the valves are at greater risk for infection. Heart valve infection is called subacute bacterial endocarditis and is very dangerous. This can occur after dental procedures, when bacteria from the mouth enter the bloodstream and infect the heart's valves. Rheumatologists used to give SLE patients antibiotics before dental procedures, hoping to prevent endocarditis. However, the risk for bad side effects from antibiotics is greater than the risk for endocarditis, so this is no longer recommended. The only ones who should be given antibiotics are those who have had surgery on their heart valves or had infectious endocarditis in the past.

KEY POINTS TO REMEMBER

1. SLE can affect any of the four heart valves.

2. Doctors diagnose VHD by echo and cardiac catheterization.

3. Libman-Sacks endocarditis, also called verrucous endocarditis, is usually associated with antiphospholipid antibodies, requiring blood thinners.

4. The medical terms for a leaky valve are "valvular regurgitation" and "valvular insufficiency."

5. "Valvular stenosis" means a damaged valve with a smaller opening than usual.

6. On echo, about one-third of people with SLE have VHD, which is usually mild and doesn't cause problems.

7. Severe cases of VHD may cause shortness of breath, chest pain, and lightheadedness. They require treatment with medicines to help the heart and blood pressure.

8. If someone has a severely damaged valve or has had surgery on one, they may need antibiotics around the time of dental procedures to prevent heart valve infections.

9. Severe heart valve problems may require valve replacement surgery.

Conduction Abnormalities

An electrical system in the heart causes the heart muscle to squeeze and pump blood into the lungs and throughout the body. The medical term for this complex system is the "cardiac electrical conduction system," and problems with it are called conduction abnormalities.

If the electrical activity within the heart muscle is abnormal, it may not squeeze correctly. The atria and ventricles may not squeeze blood in the proper pattern or order, or they may contract too quickly or too slowly. A doctor diagnoses conduction system abnormalities by ECG (discussed earlier). Between 10% and 32% of SLE patients have conduction abnormalities. These may be due to previous episodes of myocarditis. Other possible causes include coronary artery disease or thyroid disease.

Usually, these abnormalities cause only minor changes (such as first- and second-degree heart block, right bundle branch block, and left bundle branch block) that never require treatment. Occasionally, though, someone may develop a severe problem (such as third-degree heart block, atrial fibrillation, or atrial flutter). These can be serious, causing shortness of breath, heart palpitations, chest pain, fainting, or blood clots. Medicines or interventions to help the electrical system work more efficiently may be necessary. Severe cases may require a pacemaker.

The normal heart rate at rest is 60 to 100 beats per minute (bpm). Tachycardia is when the heart beats faster than 100 bpm (*tachy-* from the Greek word for "fast"). There are many types of tachycardia.

The most common is sinus tachycardia, in which the heart produces electrical signals too quickly, making the heart beat faster than usual. Sinus tachycardia is usually a normal response by the heart to pump more blood to the body when the body needs more oxygen, such as during exercise, as well as when someone is dehydrated or has as a fever, low oxygen levels (similar to what can happen in lung disease), or an overactive thyroid (hyperthyroidism, chapter 17). It also occurs when the sympathetic nervous system (chapter 13) is activated (our fight or flight mechanism) in situations that cause pain, fear, or anxiety. Although the heart rate is faster than normal, the rhythm is regular with approximately the same amount of time between each heartbeat. It can also occur from nicotine, caffeine, illegal drugs (like cocaine), and some medications.

Around 15% to 50% of SLE patients (depending on the study) have sinus tachycardia at rest. It occurs most commonly in SLE patients with active lupus (such as during flares), patients with lupus nephritis (kidney inflammation), and patients with a history of myocarditis, pericarditis, and pleurisy. Unexplained sinus tachycardia could indicate undiagnosed myocarditis, pericarditis, or autonomic dysfunction (see POTS below).

Although sinus tachycardia usually does not require any treatment, some patients have heart palpitation episodes that bother them. Blood pressure drugs called beta-blockers (such as metoprolol), calcium channel blockers (such as diltiazem), or a heart medicine called ivabradine (Corlanor) can help slow down the heart rate. A 2018 Polish study showed that calcium channel blockers worked better than beta-blockers for SLE sinus tachycardia.

LUPUS IN FOCUS

Fast heart rate as a sign of active lupus inflammation

Studies show that a heart rate above 90 beats per minute can be an indicator of increased lupus disease activity (flares) in some SLE patients. A high heart rate is more reliable in some patients than blood tests for inflammation.

In atrial fibrillation (Afib) and atrial flutter the conduction system inside the right and left atria works incorrectly. The atria's heart muscles beat and squeeze too quickly and are out of time with the ventricles. The atria cannot squeeze blood into the ventricles as well as they should, and the ventricles may not squeeze enough blood into the lungs and body. This can cause shortness of breath, chest pain, heart palpitations, lightheadedness, and syncope (passing out).

Although around 1% of the US population has Afib, it occurs in approximately 9% of SLE patients. Male SLE patients are four times more likely to have Afib than women. Atrial flutter occurs much less often than Afib.

AFib and atrial flutter are usually treated with medications and electrical cardioversion (where paddles are placed on the chest and electricity is sent into the chest). Surgery or catheter ablation may be needed if drugs don't work. Catheter ablation entails using electrical energy to stop the source of the abnormal Afib and atrial flutter sites in the heart or in the pulmonary veins. Further discussion of ablation therapy is beyond the scope of this book.

In Afib, blood clots can develop inside the atria due to the decreased strength of the muscle contractions (clots can form on the muscle wall more easily). These can break off and go to the brain, causing strokes. Many patients with Afib need to take blood thinners to prevent these.

Slow heart rate is called bradycardia (*brady*- comes from the Greek for "slow"). Severe bradycardias cause shortness of breath, palpitations, lightheadedness, and episodes of passing out (syncope). Examples of severe bradycardia include complete atrioventricular block (third-degree AV block) and sick sinus syndrome. Both are due to conduction system abnormalities that cause dangerously slow electrical pulses and are usually treated with a pacemaker.

Severe bradycardias occur in only 1% of SLE patients. They are more common in those patients with coronary artery disease and high blood pressure. A 2018 Canadian study showed that 1 out of every 200 SLE patients had severe bradycardia without coronary artery disease or high blood pressure. Other potential causes included lupus myocarditis and, rarely, long-term hydroxychloroquine (Plaquenil) use.

If lupus affects the conduction system of newborn babies, it is a form of neonatal lupus called congenital heart block. See chapter 18.

KEY POINTS TO REMEMBER

1. Most cardiac conduction abnormalities in SLE are mild, do not cause problems, and are seen on ECG.

2. Severe types (such as third-degree heart block, atrial fibrillation, or atrial flutter) may cause shortness of breath, heart palpitations, lightheadedness, and chest pain.

3. Sinus tachycardia can help identify lupus flares in some patients.

4. In severe cases of conduction abnormalities, medicines, heart interventions, or even a pacemaker may be required.

Postural Orthostatic Tachycardia Syndrome (POTS)

Another potential cause of sinus tachycardia is when lupus affects the autonomic nervous system. Postural Orthostatic Tachycardia Syndrome (POTS for short) is a type of dysfunction of the autonomic nervous system, which involves nerves that we do not have conscious control over. Examples include the nerves that cause your heart to beat or cause the pupil to enlarge in the dark in order to see better.

A 2015 New York study showed that POTS patients are twice as likely to have an autoimmune disease.

When we stand up, gravity usually pulls blood downward, away from the brain. To ensure that blood remains in critical organs such as the brain, the autonomic nervous system causes the blood vessels in the lower part of the body to squeeze when we stand. The heart does not have to work extra hard to keep blood flowing.

In POTS, this process does not occur properly. When someone with POTS stands, the heart rate increases (tachycardia) to keep the blood flowing and blood pressure stays around normal. This can cause fatigue, weakness, dizziness, blurred vision, heart fluttering, blue fingertips (acrocyanosis), and shakiness. The gastrointestinal autonomic nerves also seem to be affected. Some patients develop bloating, diarrhea or constipation, and stomach cramps. Chronic headaches are common, and some can pass out (called syncope).

The diagnosis of POTS and related disorders can be tricky. It is best to see someone specializing in the autonomic nervous system. A tilt-table test, in which the heart rate and blood pressure are measured while a person is lying down on a table and then measured again when the table is moved upright, can be helpful. The person with POTS will have an exaggerated increase in heart rate in the upright position, while the blood pressure remains about the same or increases.

Patients with POTS should avoid dehydration, alcohol, certain medicines, and a sedentary lifestyle. Regular exercise is essential. POTS usually causes people to become less active due to fatigue, weakness, and dizziness. As a result, their muscles and cardiovascular system become less effective (called deconditioning), which, in turn, makes POTS worse, and so a vicious cycle develops. It is vital to fight it through exercise. Even though it can be hard to exercise when you feel dizzy, weak, and tired, you should force yourself. If you have trouble with upright exercise, swimming is an option. It is crucial to start off slowly. It may take several months before you see the benefits of exercise, but it can make a big difference.

Many people benefit from a high salt diet (greater than 8 grams a day of sodium) along with plenty of water (more than 7 cups daily). If you have high blood pressure, do not increase salt intake without medical advice. You should wear compression stockings or hose daily. This helps squeeze the veins in the legs, forcing fluids up to the brain and heart. Learn how to control stress (chapter 38). Medications such as fludrocortisone (Florinef), midodrine, pyridostigmine, Adderall, droxidopa, ivabradine, and beta-blockers can help.

Whether immunosuppressants helps POTS in SLE is unknown. However, studies at the Mayo Clinic in Minnesota have shown that IVIG and Rituxan (rituximab) help POTS and other dysautonomia problems in Sjögren's, a related autoimmune disease.

Antiphospholipid (aPL) antibodies occur seven times more often in POTS than in healthy people. Antiphospholipid syndrome (APS) experts have noted improvements of POTS in some of their APS patients when treated with blood thinners such as warfarin and aspirin. Two patients with APS responded to IVIG therapy in a 2014 United Kingdom study. The use of blood thinners and IVIG in SLE patients with aPL antibodies and POTS needs more research.

Vasculitis

"Vasculitis" is the medical term for blood vessel wall inflammation. Vasculitis can reduce blood flow and cause fluid to leak out of the blood vessels. As a result, the surrounding tissues can become swollen. Some organs have many blood vessels coming from different directions to provide several blood supply routes to the same tissues. The medical term for this is "collateral circulation." Because of this extra blood flow, if vasculitis occurs in one section of the blood vessels and not the other, the tissues will still get adequate oxygen and nourishment. The vasculitis may not cause significant problems thanks to this additional blood supply. In organs without collateral circulation, the decreased blood flow delivers less oxygen and nourishment, leading to pain, tissue death, and permanent organ damage.

Vasculitis can occur in any organ. However, it is more common in some areas than others. The skin is the most affected area in SLE, and the medical term for this is "cutaneous vasculitis" (chapter 8.) Other commonly affected areas are the eye (retinal vasculitis, chapter 16) and the gastrointestinal tract (mesenteric vasculitis, chapter 15). Vasculitis can occur in the kidneys, liver, and nerves, but only rarely.

A biopsy is sometimes required to diagnose vasculitis. The doctor can also order an angiogram, which is a type of x-ray in which a dye is injected into a vein. The dye travels through the veins and arteries of the body, allowing the doctor to see their shapes and locations. Vasculitis appears as areas of constrictions (narrowing) and dilatations (widening) of the blood vessels, which can look like a string of beads.

People with vasculitis of the internal organs (such as the kidneys, intestines, and liver) and nerves are usually very sick. When there is evidence of internal organ vasculitis, patients require immunosuppressants.

Lupus vasculitis can occasionally be due to abnormal proteins called cryoglobulins (chapters 4 and 8), which can be identified on blood work. If present, a treatment called apheresis (or plasmapheresis, chapter 35) may be necessary.

KEY POINTS TO REMEMBER

1. "Vasculitis" is the term for blood vessel wall inflammation.

2. Skin (cutaneous vasculitis, chapter 8) is the most affected area in SLE.

3. Cryoglobulins are sometimes involved.

4. If severe enough, vasculitis can cause decreased blood flow to the affected organ, leading to pain and tissue death. It can also cause fluid to leak out of the blood vessels, causing swelling of the tissues involved.

5. Mild cases may not require any treatment. More severe cases (especially if they affect the internal organs and nerves) require immunosuppressants.

Aortic Aneurysm

An aneurysm is an area of an artery that is wider than normal in one section, where it bulges or balloons outward. Aneurysms can occur in most arteries. The walls of aneurysms are typically weaker than healthy arteries and are at increased risk of rupture. Depending on the location of the artery, if it ruptures, it can cause severe pain, stroke, severe blood loss, and even death.

Most aneurysms in people with SLE are due to atherosclerotic peripheral vascular disease (ASPVD, hardening of the arteries, chapter 21), but not always. Sometimes aneurysms can be due to artery wall inflammation (vasculitis). Making this distinction is essential. Vasculitis requires immunosuppressant treatment, while ASPVD is treated by controlling blood pressure, cholesterol, and diabetes.

The aorta is the largest artery of the body. It carries blood from the left ventricle through the chest and the abdomen, taking blood to the entire body. An aortic aneurysm inside the chest is called a thoracic aortic aneurysm ("thorax" is the medical term for chest). Aneurysms in the abdomen (the medical term for the belly) are called abdominal aortic aneurysms.

Only 2–3 out of 1,000 SLE patients have aortic aneurysms. Even so, SLE patients are three to five times more likely to develop aortic aneurysms than other people. Patients with SLE are also at higher risk for aneurysm complications.

An aneurysm and artery tear (without rupturing) is called an "aortic dissection." Aortic aneurysm dissections and ruptures are usually accompanied by severe chest or abdominal pain. They are medical emergencies. When identified early, they are treatable with surgery. If not, they are deadly.

Abdominal aortic aneurysms in SLE patients are usually from ASPVD (chapter 21), while thoracic aortic aneurysms are usually from vasculitis (called aortitis or aortic vasculitis). Aortic vasculitis is rare. High fever, shortness of breath, and chest pain are common along with markedly high CRP levels (chapter 4). It is treated with immunosuppressants. Antiphospholipid antibodies are common, so blood thinners (warfarin or heparin) should be considered in these patients.

Complications such as aneurysms, aortic dissections, and recurrences of aortitis a few years after the initial successful treatment are common. An enlarging aortic aneurysm can also damage the aortic valve, which can be dangerous.

Patients with thoracic aortic aneurysms should do everything they can to keep the aneurysm from enlarging, rupturing, or dissecting. Strict blood pressure control should be attempted with the systolic blood pressure (the top number) staying between 105 and 120 (if it doesn't cause dizziness). Blood squeezed out of the heart and into the aorta (as well as the aneurysm) does so with a large amount of force. Blood pressure medicines that reduce this force, especially beta-blockers (medications that end in -olol, such as metoprolol) should be used.

Preventing the formation of ASPVD in the aneurysm is important because ASPVD further increases rupture and dissection risks. Most specialists recommend taking a statin (a cholesterol-lowering medicine). It is also important to prevent diabetes or control it well if present. Regular exercise and a heart-healthy diet (such as the Mediterranean diet, chapter 38) are also recommended.

Surgical repair is usually recommended if the aneurysm diameter is greater than 5.5 cm or if rapid enlargement occurs. Usually, echocardiograms or chest CT scans are performed regularly to monitor the size.

Raynaud's Phenomenon

Raynaud's phenomenon (Raynaud's for short) is the most common SLE cardiovascular problem. It affects around 25% to 60% of SLE patients (depending on the study). Raynaud's causes the fingers and/or toes (rarely the ears, nose, tongue, or nipples) to become pale or dark purple with cold or stress (figure 11.2). This is sometimes followed by reddish coloration when the affected areas are rewarmed. Sometimes the fingers may become painful or have a tingling sensation. Reactions can even occur while shopping in the frozen food section of the grocery store or holding a cold drink.

When someone is exposed to cold temperatures, the brain sends chemical messages along the nervous system to the arteries of the skin, hands, and feet, telling them to

---

LUPUS IN FOCUS

Add fluoroquinolones to your allergy list if you have an aortic aneurysm

Fluoroquinolones are some of the most prescribed antibiotics. They include Levaquin (levofloxacin), Cipro (ciprofloxacin), and others that end in -oxacin. The FDA recommends that people with aortic aneurysms avoid these because they increase the risk for rupture and dissection.

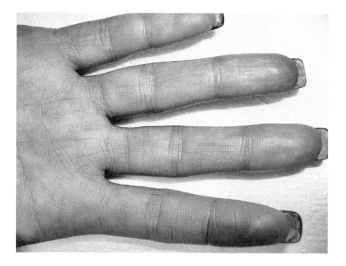

Figure II.2 Dark coloration at the ends of the fingers due to decreased blood flow from Raynaud's phenomenon. It can be more pronounced in one finger, such as in this woman's pinkie.

LUPUS IN FOCUS

Raynaud's phenomenon in the feet

Raynaud's is much more common in the fingers than in the toes. If there is significant RP in the toes, or if the toes tend to stay a purplish color, hardening of the arteries of the legs and feet (atherosclerotic peripheral vascular disease, chapter 21) needs to be strongly considered. A correct diagnosis is essential. Get the proper diagnostic tests, usually done by a heart doctor (cardiologist) or a vascular doctor.

---

constrict (get smaller). This keeps as much warm blood as possible away from the skin, fingers, and toes, preventing the body from losing vital warmth through the skin. The warmer blood is reserved for essential organs (such as the brain, kidneys, and heart). In most people, this chain of events just causes the skin to feel colder than usual.

In Raynaud's, cold makes the blood vessels spasm, restricting blood flow so much that there is too little blood flow to the fingers and toes. Since there is less blood, the fingers and toes (and sometimes the ears and nose) become pale and colder. Then, as the tissues and cells use up the oxygen and release carbon dioxide into the blood, the fingers or toes become blue or purple. After the attack, when the small arteries open, and more blood flows to the digits, the fingers can become reddish in some people.

After repetitive, severe episodes, the tissues of the fingertips may not receive enough nutrients and oxygen. Over time, the fleshy parts of the fingertips (on the palm side) may lose tissue and become tapered and thin instead of staying plump. In more severe cases, blood flow may be so restricted that fingertip tissue may die. This can cause open sores (ulcers). These can be very painful and are prone to infection. Trauma to the fingertips, even minimal trauma, increases the possibility of ulcers occurring.

235

Thickened blood vessels can increase the risk of Raynaud's. The thickened blood vessel walls are usually a result of previous inflammation that formed scar tissue. These thickened walls are permanent and not reversible.

Raynaud's is not as common in the toes. When the toes develop Raynaud's-like episodes, it is important to have the arteries of the legs evaluated to ensure that blood flow is not reduced from arteriosclerosis (hardening of the arteries, chapter 21).

Raynaud's usually does not improve over time and or with anti-inflammatory medicines or immunosuppressants. Raynaud's also usually does not vary between lupus flares and remissions.

It is essential for people with Raynaud's to keep their core body temperature warm (table 11.1) and avoid drugs that can worsen Raynaud's (table 11.2).

Table 11.1 Non-Drug Ways to Address Raynaud's Phenomenon

- Avoid cold places.
- Wear layers of clothing in cool temperatures.
- Wear insulated mittens or gloves (mittens are better).
- Wear battery-heated gloves.
- Wear heavy wool stockings or layers of socks.
- Wear a hat. Always carry a hat, mittens, and jacket with you.
- Wear a scarf to cover your face and ears.
- Keep hand warmers in your pockets.
- Wear long-sleeved shirts when possible.
- When fingers/toes feel cold, immediately start to wiggle them, and run warm water over them.
- Keep your house temperature warm, over 70°F. Keep a space heater or heated humidifier near you.
- Let the water warm up before getting into the shower or bath; close the door.
- Warm up the car before getting in for travel. Having someone do this for you is optimal.
- If possible, have someone else grab things for you from the freezer at home and in stores.
- Use insulated containers around cold beverages or food.
- Rinse food with warm water, not cold water.
- Avoid vibrating tools, which worsen Raynaud's.
- Avoid decongestants, amphetamine-like diet pills, caffeine, and cigarettes (which constrict blood vessels).
- Wear protective gloves when washing dishes (to protect your fingers and fingertips).
- Prevent dry skin; prevents fingertip skin cracking and tenderness (table 14.7).
- Protect your fingertips to prevent sores.
- Avoid all substances in table 11.2.
- *To stop a Raynaud's attack, wiggle your fingers, rub your hands together, run them under warm water, put them under your armpits, or whirl your arms around like a windmill to increase blood flow.*

Table II.2 Substances That Can Worsen Raynaud's Phenomenon

beta-blockers (such as metoprolol, labetalol, and atenolol)

bleomycin

bromocriptine

cabergoline

caffeine

cisplatin

clonidine

cocaine

cyclosporin

dextroamphetamine

dihydroergotamine (Migranal)

erlotinib (Tarceva)

interferon therapy

methylphenidate

nilotinib (Tasigna)

phentermine

pseudoephedrine (Sudafed, Chlor-Tremeton)

vinyl chloride

Allowing mild Raynaud's attacks to occur is acceptable if they are not painful, easy to control, and do not cause tissue loss or fingertip sores. But if the attacks are moderate to severe, medications may be necessary. Medicines help relax the artery walls and allow more blood to flow to the fingers and toes. A group of drugs used to treat high blood pressure called calcium channel blockers, especially nifedipine (Procardia), are helpful in most people. Other channel blockers, such as amlodipine (Norvasc) and diltiazem (Cardizem), and other blood pressure medicines, including reserpine, prazosin, hydralazine, minoxidil, and losartan, can also be helpful.

Nitroglycerin can also help. It comes in pills, cream/gel, and patches. Bosentan (Tracleer) is FDA-approved to treat pulmonary hypertension, and it also helps Raynaud's. So do Prozac and Viagra. Some people may benefit from taking a low dose of aspirin daily (81 mg). This can help thin out the blood and decrease the severity of attacks.

More drastic measures may be necessary for particularly severe, resistant cases. One is a sympathectomy, a surgical procedure in which a surgeon cuts the sympathetic nerves to the hands. A doctor can also inject an anesthetic around the nerves (called a sympathetic nerve block) to keep them from causing blood vessel constriction.

KEY POINTS TO REMEMBER

1. Raynaud's phenomenon is common in SLE, causing the fingers and toes to become cold, pale, and/or purple-colored.

2. Raynaud's is due to artery spasms during cold or stress. It usually does not fluctuate with lupus disease activity or improve when SLE is under reasonable control.

3. It is essential to follow the suggestions in table 11.1 to keep the core body temperature warm and the body's blood vessels relaxed.

4. Medicines may be required to relax the blood vessels.

5. Significant Raynaud's of the toes is not common. Patients with this problem should have studies done to eliminate the possibility of hardening the arteries (arteriosclerosis).

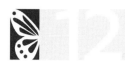

The Urinary System

Fotios Koumpouras, MD, *Contributing Editor*

Monitoring the urinary system, particularly the kidneys, is important in SLE. This is because the start of nephritis (kidney inflammation) is usually asymptomatic (you feel fine even though there is active inflammation). Nephritis varies by ethnicity. It occurs in 25% to 40% of Caucasian SLE patients and in around 50% of African American, Asian, Pacific Islander, and Hispanic SLE patients. Afro-Caribbean SLE patients develop nephritis close to 80% of the time. Other factors also increase the risk of this serious complication (table 12.1). This chapter goes into much more detail about this important body system.

The urinary system (figure 12.1) begins with the kidneys, which are bean-shaped organs in the back of the abdomen around the lower ribcage level. One of their functions is to filter out waste products from blood (creating urine) and to normalize electrolytes (such as potassium, calcium, and sodium) in the blood. The kidney also plays a role in regulating your blood pressure and producing a hormone to help make red blood cells, called erythropoietin.

When blood arrives at the kidneys through the renal arteries ("renal" is the medical term for "kidneys"), it is diverted into a branching system that becomes smaller and smaller until it is microscopic. This microscopic area is comprised of the kidneys' filtering units, which are called nephrons (figure 12.2). There are more than a million nephrons in each kidney.

The nephron contains a glomerulus (a tight collection of blood vessels and other specialized cells, like podocytes, mentioned later in the chapter) that filters waste products from the blood. Note a light-colored, C-shaped area to the right of the glomerulus in figure 12.1. This is Bowman's capsule (not labeled in the figure) into which the filtered waste products are deposited from the blood vessels of the glomerulus, creating newly formed urine. This urine flows into the light-colored tube (a microscopic renal tubule, also not labeled) to the right of Bowman's capsule.

Note the tiny blood vessels (capillaries) that wind around the tubules. The tubules hold on to the urinary waste products but put important fluids and minerals that are in this newly formed urine back into the blood through the walls of these capillaries. The renal tubules then dump the urine into a larger tube, the collecting duct, which connects to a larger collecting tube (the ureter) that carries the urine to the urinary bladder (figure 12.1). The bladder is a muscular organ and is sensitive to filling. When the bladder fills with urine, the muscular walls expand, letting the person know it is time

Table 12.1 Factors That Increase the Risk of Lupus Nephritis

Ethnicity	African
	Hispanic
	Asian
	Mestizo
	Pacific Islander
Age	Younger age of lupus onset (especially teenagers and children)
Weight	Obesity
Gender	Men
Labs	High anti-ds DNA
	Positive anti-C1q antibody
	Low C3, C4, or CH50
	High anti-chromatin
	Many autoantibodies at SLE diagnosis
	Low lymphocyte count at SLE diagnosis
Psychosis	Hallucinations
	Delusions
	Lupus cerebritis

to urinate. The urinary bladder's muscular wall squeezes the urine into one large tube (called the urethra) that empties the urine from the body.

Although the urinary system includes four organ structures—the kidneys, ureters, urinary bladder, and the urethra—SLE affects the kidneys most, especially at the nephron filters. The urinary bladder is rarely involved—when it is, the medical term is "lupus cystitis." The ureters and urethra are not involved.

Kidney Function and Lupus Nephritis

Significant kidney inflammation occurs in 40% to 50% of SLE patients, most often in the first five years. Inflammation and damage of the glomerulus from lupus are the most common SLE kidney complication, causing problems with proper filtering of blood waste products. This is often accompanied by inflammation and damage to the renal tubules, which causes problems with the balance of fluid and electrolytes in the blood. The medical term for this is "lupus glomerulonephritis" ("lupus nephritis" for short). In countries where modern health care is not as accessible, lupus nephritis is the primary cause of death in SLE patients. Treatments typically have excellent results when doctors can identify nephritis early (with regular urine and blood tests).

Although 50% to 60% of those with systemic lupus will never develop any significant kidney problems (on urine and blood testing), lupus nephritis is more common microscopically. A 2012 research study performed renal biopsies on SLE patients with no evidence of kidney involvement on urine and blood tests. Close to 60% showed some

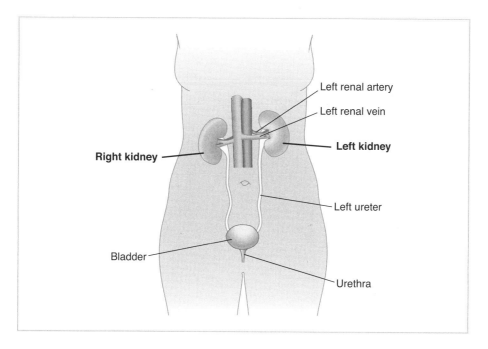

Figure 12.1 The urinary system

LUPUS IN FOCUS

Lupus podocytopathy is a form of SLE kidney disease

Between the glomerulus capillaries (containing blood) and Bowman's space (containing the earliest form of urine) is a network of cells called podocytes. Podocytes make up the primary filtering system of the glomerulus. Podocytes can be damaged by lupus (lupus podocytopathy) and are an area of the kidney that some drugs (especially calcineurin inhibitors) can act on to help lupus nephritis patients. Although lupus podocytopathy is a form of SLE kidney disease, it is not included in the classification system described in this chapter.

lupus kidney inflammation. Therefore, even though the blood and urine tests suggested they were doing well, they still had evidence of mild lupus nephritis. This is called silent lupus nephritis. That it occurs highlights the importance of checking urine and blood tests frequently on patients (every three months in our clinics) even if all their labs are perfect.

It may be difficult to have regular lab work when you feel well. But even if you feel fine, you can still have lupus nephritis. Treating it early increases the chances of good responses. Lupus nephritis experts in Hong Kong showed that even a three-month delay in diagnosing and treating lupus nephritis increases the chances for kidney failure (and even death).

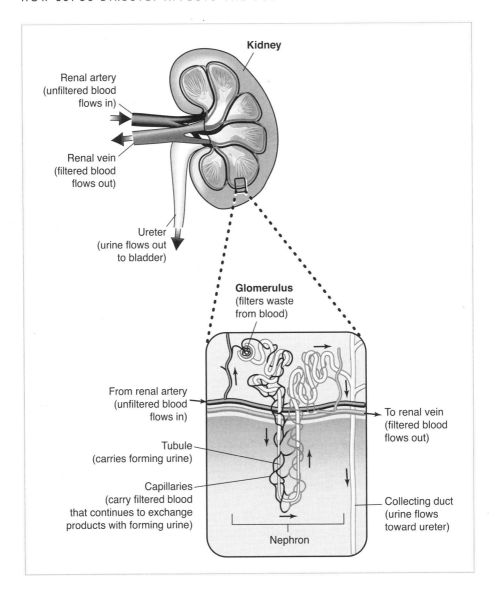

Figure 12.2 Parts of the nephron

SLE affects the kidneys primarily by depositing immune complexes in the filtering glomeruli. Immune complexes are formed by immune molecules binding together during inflammation. In SLE, autoantibodies (especially anti-dsDNA) produce large amounts of abnormal immune complexes and deposit in body organs, leading to organ inflammation and damage. These abnormal immune complexes get trapped (deposited) in the kidneys' glomerulus filters. This leads to kidney inflammation, injury, and abnormal kidney function. The immune complexes use up complement proteins, such as C3 and C4 (chapter 4). Another part of the immune complement system, C1q, is absorbed into these kidney-trapped immune complexes, attracting the formation of anti-C1q antibodies.

Elevated anti-dsDNA, low C3, low C4, elevated EC4d, and high anti-C1q levels (chapter 4) often occur in the blood during periods of increasing kidney inflammation. Rheumatologists regularly order these blood tests, even when SLE patients seem to be doing well, to look for possible early signs of lupus nephritis. Early recognition is key to the best treatment outcome.

Increased protein (including albumin) usually leaks into the urine during lupus nephritis. A simple urine test can detect urinary cells and protein (chapter 4). Almost everyone with significant lupus nephritis has increased urinary protein (proteinuria). In addition to protein, red and white blood cells can also leak into the urine because of the damaged glomeruli filters. Finding more of these blood cells in the urine can also suggest possible lupus nephritis.

When cellular products and proteins clump inside the microscopic urinary tubules, they form urinary casts. Casts are visible in urine only under a microscope. They are cylindrical or cigar-shaped as they compress together and adopt the shape of the tubules. Some casts (such as hyaline casts and granular casts) are common in healthy people. However, other casts (such as white blood cell casts and red blood cell casts) can be seen in lupus nephritis (see chapter 4).

Low kidney function refers to the kidneys' inability to properly filter waste products from the blood. Doctors determine how well the kidneys are functioning by using blood tests that look for blood urea nitrogen (BUN for short), serum creatinine (sCr), and the estimated glomerular filtration rate (eGFR) (see chapter 4). The lower the eGFR, the worse the kidney function. However, kidney function depends on other variables, such as age, sex, and genetics. The eGFR is more accurate than the sCr for assessing kidney function. Sometimes doctors will order a 24 -hour urine collection to measure kidney function and the amount of protein loss.

In addition to filtering, the kidneys secrete a hormone called erythropoietin, which travels through the blood and then to the bone marrow to stimulate red blood cell production. When damaged, the kidneys produce less erythropoietin, which, in turn, causes anemia (chapter 9). The severity of anemia usually parallels the amount of kidney function loss. Worse anemia usually accompanies worse kidney function (lower eGFRs).

The kidneys also play an essential part in helping to maintain normal blood pressure. If enough inflammation or damage occurs, the person's blood pressure can rise. High blood pressure can, in turn, cause additional kidney damage. This creates a dangerous cycle of high blood pressure and kidney damage worsening each other. Therefore, blood pressure must be kept normal in people with kidney problems. This should be a constant goal for people with lupus and kidney disease. Normalizing blood pressure reduces the risk for permanent kidney damage.

The kidneys play an important role in regulating minerals and electrolytes, such as potassium and calcium. The doctor usually monitors these levels closely.

The kidneys are essential for vitamin D production. Although we naturally produce vitamin D in the skin (chapter 3 and 38), and a small amount comes from food, these forms of vitamin D are inactive. Normal working kidneys convert inactive vitamin D into its active form. This active vitamin D is necessary for proper calcium absorption from food in the intestines, regulation of blood calcium and phosphorus levels, and keeping bones strong by promoting proper bone use of calcium and phosphorus. When vitamin D cannot be activated because of kidney damage, the parathyroid glands (located in the neck behind the thyroid gland) make more parathyroid hormone (PTH for short) to help regulate calcium blood levels. These increased PTH levels cause the bones to lose additional calcium, which can make them fragile and more likely to fracture.

In short, the kidney is an important regulator of many vital bodily functions.

Most lupus nephritis symptoms occur when the inflammation and damage are severe. However, it takes a considerable decrease in kidney function before most people feel ill, and the symptoms are nonspecific. Common symptoms include a vague sense of not feeling well (malaise), fatigue, headaches, nausea, and upset stomach. When lupus nephritis is more severe, it can cause shortness of breath, chest pain, ankle swelling, and itchy dry skin.

One typical symptom in lupus nephritis is edema, in which extra fluid accumulates in the body's soft tissues. The effects of gravity then cause this fluid to collect into the body parts closest to the ground—namely, the legs and ankles. Edema typically gets worse throughout the day as people walk and sit. When affected people lie down, the fluid redistributes to the rest of the body. There tends to be a need to urinate more frequently when trying to sleep.

Edema can occur for two main reasons. First, proteins (mainly albumin) are needed to hold the liquid part of the blood inside the blood vessels. If too much albumin leaks into the urine, causing low blood albumin levels, fluid leaks from blood vessels into the soft tissues. Second, when kidney function worsens, the kidneys' ability to regulate the amount of salt (sodium) and water retained in the body worsens, too. The body's retention of too much water and sodium causes fluid retention and edema.

Lupus nephritis rarely causes lower back pain, which usually occurs for other reasons such as being overweight, having back osteoarthritis and degenerative disc disease, or straining the back while lifting. Other kidney problems may cause pain in this area, including kidney infection (often with high fever, chills, and increased urinary frequency) and kidney stones (usually incredibly painful, requiring emergency room treatment). The most dangerous (but least common) cause is kidney cancer. Kidney cancer usually also causes blood in the urine (identified in a urine sample) and requires an ultrasound or CT scan to diagnose.

A physical examination usually does not show any abnormalities in the early stages. However, the blood pressure may be elevated in more severe cases, and ankle edema (swelling) may be present. If there is a severe loss of blood albumin (as in nephrotic syndrome discussed below), edema can occur in the upper legs, abdomen, and face (typically around the eyes).

When the doctor notes abnormal urine test results, they try to determine the exact cause, which may not be related to SLE. For example, it is common for menstruating women to have increased blood and protein in the urine.

Urinary tract infections also can increase urine protein, red blood cells, and white blood cells. Some substances, like non-steroidal anti-inflammatory drugs (NSAIDs, chapter 36) and Chinese herbs, can damage kidneys or cause reduced kidney blood flow, causing increased protein in the urine and decreased kidney function. These effects are potentially reversible when caught early and the drug is stopped. The doctor may also order an ultrasound of the kidneys to ensure that there are no kidney stones or other problems, such as a tumor.

A kidney biopsy is needed to accurately understand what is wrong. The 2019 European League Against Rheumatism guidelines recommend obtaining a biopsy if there is more than 500 mg of protein in the urine per day or if there is an unexplained decrease in kidney function. We also repeat biopsies when the results are important for management decisions, such as if treatment needs to be changed, or to see if we can reduce treatments in patients who have been in remission for a few years.

The kidney biopsy is usually an outpatient procedure. An interventional radiologist (an x-ray doctor specializing in biopsies under x-ray) or a nephrologist (kidney specialist) usually performs the biopsy. They typically use a CT scan or ultrasound to determine the best spot for the biopsy. Before the biopsy, numbing medication is injected into the back tissues to reduce discomfort from the procedure.

A kidney biopsy is typically very safe, and the patient goes home shortly afterward. However, bleeding from the biopsy is a possible complication. This can cause abdominal pain or blood in the urine. In this case, the doctor may admit the person to the hospital for observation after finishing the biopsy. Before the procedure, it is essential to stop all medicines that can cause bleeding (such as aspirin, NSAIDs, warfarin, and Plavix). Infection is also a possible complication and can cause pain and fevers. Fortunately, these complications are very uncommon.

The biopsy doctor sends the specimen to a lab that specializes in kidney biopsies. The kidney specimen is prepared and studied using various techniques, including electron microscopy and immunofluorescence, which looks for deposits of immune system molecules in the kidneys.

If the biopsy shows lupus nephritis, it is classified according to the severity and distribution of the inflammation. There are two different methods of reporting these results. The first method, developed in 1982, is from the World Health Organization (WHO) and is called the WHO classification. The International Society of Nephrology (ISN) and the Renal Pathology Society (RPS) designed the more modern method (abbreviated as the ISN/RPS classification). Although the ISN/RPS is more detailed, the two classification systems have similarities (table 12.2).

Each classification method includes six possibilities, and each uses a roman numeral (I–VI) for identification. Today, most biopsies use the ISN/RPS system. If you have had a

---

LUPUS IN FOCUS

Kidney biopsy complications

Bleeding is a serious potential side effect of a kidney biopsy. Fortunately, using ultrasound to visualize the needle and kidney simultaneously during the biopsy has greatly decreased this complication. When bleeding does occur (10%– 30% of biopsies), it is usually minor. Patients at the highest risk for bleeding are those with low platelet counts, anemia (low red blood cell counts), and low kidney function, especially those with platelets fewer than 150,000 platelets/mm^3, hemoglobin < 10 g/dl, or eGFR < 30 ml/min per 1.73 m^2.

Table 12.2 Lupus Nephritis Biopsy Classifications

WHO Class	WHO Name	ISN/RPS Class	ISN/RPS Name	Treatment
I	Minimal mesangial nephritis	I	Minimal mesangial lupus nephritis	None
II	Mesangial, or purely mesangial disease	II	Mesangial proliferative lupus nephritis	None, unless it worsens
III	Focal segmental proliferative glomerulonephritis	III	Focal lupus nephritis	Steroids and immunosuppressants
IV	Diffuse segmental proliferative glomerulonephritis	IV	Diffuse lupus nephritis	Steroids and immunosuppressants
V	Membranous glomerulonephritis	V	Membranous lupus nephritis	Steroids and immunosuppressants
VI	Advanced sclerosing glomerulonephritis	VI	Advanced sclerosing lupus nephritis	None; possibly prepare for dialysis

kidney biopsy for lupus nephritis, you should find out what your actual result showed. You can use the following section to understand your results. Keep your kidney biopsy result in your personal health records at home for possible future need by other doctors.

Classification of Lupus Nephritis

ISN/RPS Class I. This is minimal mesangial lupus nephritis. This result shows some deposits of immune complexes in the kidneys but without any significant inflammation. There is usually little to no proteinuria and normal kidney function (eGFR). Class I lupus nephritis usually does not progress nor needs treatment.

ISN/RPS Class II. This is mesangial proliferative lupus nephritis. The mesangium is the thin layer of tissue that supports the glomerular blood vessels. Lupus inflammation in this area is referred to as mesangial lupus nephritis. Most patients require no treatment, and usually it does not worsen. Sometimes Class II nephritis can progress to a more severe type of lupus nephritis over time, usually requiring another biopsy and treatment based on the results.

ISN/RPS Class III. This is focal lupus nephritis. Focal means that less than half of the glomeruli are involved with lupus inflammation. It is basically a milder version of Class IV lupus nephritis. Sometimes, Class III lupus nephritis can be mild with absolutely no symptoms at all. It can be severe on the other end of the spectrum, causing fatigue, anemia, edema, high blood pressure, lots of protein in the urine, and decreased kidney function. Nephrotic syndrome (see Class V below) can occasionally occur. Biopsy features that indicate more aggressive and dangerous inflammation are fibrinoid necrosis, karyorrhexis, and crescents. Explaining these is beyond the scope of this book.

Class III nephritis is serious and, left untreated, will progress and lead to kidney failure. Treatment usually consists of steroids and an immunosuppressant such as mycophenolate mofetil (CellCept), azathioprine (Imuran), or occasionally cyclophosphamide. Adding belimumab (Benlysta) or voclosporin (Lupkynis) to these treatments increases the chances of controlling lupus nephritis. Rituxan (rituximab), tacrolimus, and cyclosporine are other potential options.

ISN/RPS Class IV. This is diffuse lupus nephritis. Diffuse means that more than half of the glomeruli are involved. This is the most aggressive form of nephritis, and most patients develop kidney failure if not treated promptly and aggressively. It is more likely to cause fatigue, anemia, edema, high blood pressure, lots of protein in the urine, decreased kidney function, and nephrotic syndrome than Class III. Biopsy features that indicate more aggressive and dangerous inflammation are fibrinoid necrosis, karyorrhexis, and crescents.

The treatment for Class IV lupus nephritis is like the treatment for Class III. Since severe Class IV nephritis has a high risk of rapidly going into kidney failure, some doctors choose more rapidly acting therapies such as cyclophosphamide. Findings that would suggest more severe disease include uncontrollable high blood pressure, worsening kidney function or if the biopsy shows significant amounts of fibrinoid necrosis or crescents. Temporary dialysis for very severe sudden cases is sometimes needed.

ISN/RPS Class V. This is membranous lupus nephritis. Class V lupus nephritis is not more severe than Class IV. Membranous nephritis (Class V) inflammation occurs in a different section of the glomerulus than the previous classes. It is less likely to worsen to the point of complete kidney failure compared to Classes III and IV. Even so, about 30% of patients need dialysis over the long term if not treated.

Membranous nephritis can cause many problems. The reason is that typically Class V nephritis can cause the kidneys to lose a lot of protein. Sometimes the amount of protein lost can be massive, creating a condition called nephrotic syndrome. In nephrotic

LUPUS IN FOCUS

The number of crescents on biopsy is important

The percentage of the glomeruli (plural of glomerulus) containing crescents is significant. If the glomeruli on biopsy have fewer than 50% crescents, the patient has a better chance of responding to treatment. If the biopsy is greater than 80%, patients tend to have kidney failure and may not respond well.

More than 10% of glomeruli with crescents and worsening kidney function over a short time is called rapidly progressive glomerulonephritis. This often requires IV cyclophosphamide and other aggressive treatments.

syndrome, the protein loss is so substantial that the blood albumin level is low, edema occurs, and cholesterol levels rise. A primary role of albumin is to hold onto water molecules and keep them inside blood vessels. When there is reduced blood albumin, fluid leaks into the soft tissues. This can result in severe edema throughout the body (anasarca), even around the eyes. Treatment can sometimes be challenging and usually requires large doses of diuretics (fluid/water pills). Class V nephritis is much more likely to cause nephrotic syndrome than Classes III and IV.

Blood clots are another complication. They develop when the nephrotic syndrome causes the loss of proteins of the clotting system (particularly those that decrease clotting), which makes the blood to clot more easily. A blood clot will often occur in the large veins leading out of the kidneys (the renal veins), causing back or flank pain and reduced kidney function. This is called renal vein thrombosis. Blood clots can also occur in other areas such as the legs (deep venous thrombosis) and the lungs (pulmonary embolism). They are treated with blood thinners.

Recently, treatments for Class V lupus nephritis have improved. Studies suggest that adding voclosporin (Lupkynis) on top of other therapies (such as hydroxychloroquine, mycophenolate, cyclosporine, and steroids) may improve outcomes, especially in those with the largest amounts of urinary protein loss (more than 3 grams per day).

ISN/RPS Class VI. This is advanced sclerosing lupus nephritis. The biopsy findings are often termed as "glomerulosclerosis." In Class VI, permanent scar tissue (sclerosis) is the predominant finding. Class III, IV, and V lupus nephritis can all have small amounts of scar tissue on biopsy and can be reported as a chronicity index measurement. The higher the chronicity index, the more scarring there is. Immunosuppressants are less effective when there is a predominance of scar tissue. The main treatments for Class VI are blood pressure medicines and diet, as well as dialysis and a kidney transplant.

Other Lupus Nephritis Biopsy Results

Other abnormalities can be seen on kidney biopsies. These are usually noted under "impressions" or "comments" in a biopsy report. Check whether any of the following appear on yours.

Lupus Podocytopathy. Podocytopathy is a kidney problem that has been identified more often in lupus patients since 2005. *Podo-* comes from the Greek for "foot" (as in podiatrist, foot doctor), and *-cyte* means "cell." Podocytes are essential cells inside the filters (glomeruli) of the kidneys. The podocytes wrap around the glomerular capillaries forming an essential part of the glomerulus filter. Each podocyte has projections like feet and fingers that wrap around the outside of the capillary walls, intertwining each other. Waste from inside the capillary filters through the tiny slits between the podocytes' intertwining projections.

Podocytopathy is when the podocytes are damaged. *-Opathy* comes from the Greek for "suffering" and is often used to denote a body structure that is abnormal or damaged. When the podocytes are damaged, the filtering slits are not as tight, and larger-sized blood molecules (primarily proteins) leak into the urine. This results in high levels of urinary protein (proteinuria).

> **LUPUS IN FOCUS**
>
> **Think of podocytes as being like a pasta colander**
>
> Think of the feet of podocytes being like the interlocking parts of a sieve, strainer, or colander used to drain pasta. The colander's small holes are the tiny filtering spaces in the slits of the podocytes' feet. When the podocytes' feet are damaged (podocytopathy), the slits between the feet are more prominent. This allows much of the essential blood proteins that we don't want to lose to pass through. Think of a damaged colander with large holes in it, allowing pasta to pass through.

People with lupus podocytopathy have a lot of protein in the urine (proteinuria). Fortunately, it usually responds well to steroids. It is common for patients with lupus podocytopathy to go into remission after just one or two months of treatment.

Calcineurin inhibitors (voclosporin, tacrolimus, and cyclosporin) can help patients who do not adequately respond to steroids. The calcineurin inhibitors improve podocyte function and can help treat podocytopathies such as lupus podocytopathy and collapsing glomerulopathy (discussed next). Calcineurin inhibitors also improve the filtering capabilities of the glomeruli in lupus nephritis, helping to decrease the amount of protein loss. Mycophenolate, azathioprine, leflunomide, and cyclophosphamide can also be used for lupus podocytopathy.

Over 90% of lupus podocytopathy patients respond well to therapy, with three out of four going into complete remission. Kidney failure is uncommon.

Collapsing Glomerulopathy. This is rare and is classified as a severe form of podocytopathy. It is essential to test all patients with collapsing glomerulopathy for HIV and hepatitis C, since they can also cause it. Recently, this type of kidney disease was also seen in COVID-19 infections. Under the microscope, the glomeruli (microscopic filters) are structurally collapsed. Patients often have significant kidney failure with large amounts of protein in the urine.

The treatment of choice is steroids with a calcineurin inhibitor (cyclosporin, tacrolimus, or voclosporin). However, cyclophosphamide and mycophenolate have also been used.

Tubulointerstitial Nephritis and Damage. The kidneys' microscopic tubules carry freshly created urine away from the glomerulus. The tissue between the tubules is called the interstitium. When inflammation and damage occur in the interstitium, it also usually involves the tubules and is called tubulointerstitial nephritis. Patients with this problem are more prone to issues with their potassium levels (too high and too low). They can also develop problems with blood pH (a measure of acidity) since the tubules are essential for regulating these important functions.

The presence and severity of tubulointerstitial damage can predict worse kidney function. Severe involvement increases the chances of future dialysis and renal transplantation.

Noninflammatory Necrotizing Vasculopathy (NNV). The appearance of the blood vessels on the biopsy can help indicate what kind of inflammation is occurring, predict how the patient may do, and which medicine would treat them best. Blood vessel abnormalities that can be seen on kidney biopsy include NNV, true renal vasculitis, thrombotic micro-angiopathy, arterial sclerosis, and antiphospholipid nephropathy (all discussed below). NNV is a blood vessel problem causing reduced arteriolar blood flow to the kidneys. This is seen in around 5% of lupus nephritis biopsies, usually in severe forms of Class III and IV nephritis, along with other severe nephritis biopsy findings, such as crescents and fibrinoid necrosis (mentioned previously). Most patients have low kidney function, high anti-dsDNA levels, and low C3 or C4 complement levels. This finding suggests the need to use strong immunosuppressants. Fortunately, most patients respond well.

True Renal Vasculitis. As in NNV, there is damage to renal arteriole walls in true renal vasculitis. However, there is also significant blood vessel wall inflammation (hence, vasculitis). Most patients have severe kidney failure. These patients need to be diagnosed quickly and treated aggressively. This problem is rare (3% of biopsies).

Thrombotic Microangiopathy. We discussed thrombotic thrombocytopenic purpura (TTP) in the platelet section of chapter 9. TTP can cause multiple tiny blood clots in the kidneys (termed thrombotic microangiopathy) and rapid, permanent kidney failure. Fortunately, this is a rare complication, but dialysis is often needed. However, it may be temporary if the renal function recovers with aggressive treatment.

Arterial Sclerosis. This is also called arteriosclerosis and atherosclerosis. This is the most common blood vessel abnormality seen on SLE kidney biopsies (approximately 50%). This is like the "hardening of the arteries" that can occur in other body parts, such as peripheral vascular disease and coronary artery disease (chapter 21). Arterial sclerosis is often related to high blood pressure, cholesterol, and glucose levels (diabetes and prediabetes). It is a permanent damage in the kidney blood vessels, causing decreased blood flow. Patients with lupus nephritis, especially those with arterial sclerosis, need strict control of blood pressure, cholesterol, and glucose control, healthy body weight, and exercise to keep it from worsening.

Antiphospholipid Nephropathy. SLE patients with antiphospholipid (aPL) antibodies (chapter 9) may develop multiple tiny blood clots in the kidney's blood vessels. This is a rare finding on kidney biopsies (despite approximately one-third of lupus nephritis patients being positive for aPL antibodies). As in patients with antiphospholipid syndrome (chapter 9), the treatments of choice for antiphospholipid nephropathy are the blood thinners warfarin (Coumadin) and heparin.

Drug-Induced Lupus Nephritis. Drug-induced lupus (DIL) was discussed in chapter 1. Kidney involvement is rare in DIL. Medications that have caused drug-induced lupus nephritis include procainamide, hydralazine, isoniazid, TNF inhibitors, and minocycline. Although most DIL patients are positive for anti-histone antibodies, patients with drug-induced lupus nephritis tend to be positive for ANCA (chapter 4) or anti-dsDNA antibodies. Instead of the Class II–V lupus nephritis described above, it is more common for these patients to have a type of kidney disease typical of patients with vasculitis (called necrotizing glomerulonephritis or pauci-immune-crescentic glomerulonephritis). Steroids and other immunosuppressants are usually needed in addition to stopping the causative drug.

Treatment of Lupus Nephritis

As you can see from the descriptions above, doctors generally treat Class III, IV, and V lupus nephritis with steroids and immunosuppressants. These can help save kidney function. Your doctor may recommend high doses of intravenous (IV) steroids, usually methylprednisolone (Solumedrol), for one to three days. The medical term for this is "IV pulse steroids." This is generally followed by oral steroids, usually prednisone or methylprednisolone. Studies show that using high doses of IV steroids initially improves the chance for remission and allows for less oral steroid use overall.

The current trend is to use lower doses of steroids. As recently as 2021, it was common to give three days of 1000 mg of IV Solumedrol followed by 60 mg a day of prednisone. Research studies using voclosporin (Lupkynis) have changed this habit for most of us. They used only 250 mg to 500 mg of IV Solumedrol for 2 days followed by just 20 mg to 25 mg of daily prednisone. They got most patients down to 5 mg a day by 2 months and more than 80% of patients down to 2.5 mg a day by 4 months. In the past, it was not uncommon to have patients on 20 mg to 40 mg a day for several months, leading to many steroid-induced side effects (see chapter 31).

Which immunosuppressant medicine to use is usually based on the biopsy result and how severe the kidney inflammation is. Doctors sometimes treat the most severe cases with IV cyclophosphamide. This is a strong chemotherapy medication that has been used to treat lupus nephritis for decades.

The most common way of using IV cyclophosphamide is the Euro-Lupus regimen, in which 500 mg is given every 2 weeks for a total of 6 doses. It is then switched over to a different medication (such as azathioprine or mycophenolate).

Several studies have revealed that the lower dose Euro-Lupus regimen has fewer side effects and has better long-term remission than the high-dose National Institutes of Health (NIH) cyclophosphamide regimen. IV cyclophosphamide has many potential side effects (chapter 32).

LUPUS IN FOCUS

Why are pulse IV steroids popular in treating lupus nephritis?

In the 1960s, high doses of IV steroids were used to treat patients with organ transplants. Due to this success, in 1976, doctors at Boston University Hospital gave seven SLE patients with severe class IV nephritis 1 gram of IV methylprednisolone (Solumedrol) three days in a row. Five of the seven had an immediate and marked decrease in urine protein (an excellent result). 3,000 mg of IV methylprednisolone given over 3 days is overall safer than the same amount by mouth over a more extended period (such as 60 mg prednisone pills for 50 days).

When severe kidney disease is controlled, patients enter the phase of maintenance therapy. Many experts prefer using mycophenolate over azathioprine for maintenance therapy. A 2012 study showed that mycophenolate worked better than azathioprine. In Toronto, Canada, a group showed that mycophenolate performed best for maintenance therapy in children with lupus nephritis.

One reason to consider azathioprine over mycophenolate is that azathioprine is cheaper. If someone has no insurance or has a type of insurance that pays a percentage of the cost, then azathioprine may be preferable. Another important reason is that azathioprine could be safe to use during pregnancy, as are tacrolimus and cyclosporin.

Nowadays, mycophenolate (CellCept and Myfortic) is more commonly used than cyclophosphamide. Studies show that it is as effective as cyclophosphamide in leading to remission in Class III and IV lupus nephritis patients. It is also safer than intravenous cyclophosphamide. It does not cause infertility, and hair loss is less common with mycophenolate. Mycophenolate is taken by mouth, which makes it more convenient than cyclophosphamide (chapter 32).

Another medication sometimes used to treat lupus nephritis is cyclosporine (chapter 32). Doctors use it primarily for Class V nephritis. However, the doctor must monitor it (blood pressure and blood tests) more frequently than other medications, and it can increase cholesterol levels. Therefore, doctors do not use it as often as they used to.

In December 2020 and January 2021, the FDA approved the first-ever drugs to treat lupus nephritis: belimumab (Benlysta) and voclosporin (Lupkynis) respectively. In the research studies, when belimumab and voclosporin were used in combination with other lupus nephritis drugs (such as hydroxychloroquine, mycophenolate, cyclophosphamide, and steroids), significantly more patients had faster reductions in proteinuria and higher rates of remission compared to those on older therapies alone. These drugs also appear to slow down the loss of kidney function over time more than older treatment regimens. Because of these impressive findings, many lupus nephritis experts use belimumab and voclosporin in most cases of new-onset lupus nephritis and in patients who are not in remission on other therapies.

LUPUS IN FOCUS

Prescription discount services such as Blink Health and GoodRX

According to UpToDate.com (a continuously updated medical resource for health care professionals), in April 2022, the average retail price of a one-month supply of generic azathioprine at 150 mg a day was $480; the Imuran brand equivalent was $863. Generic mycophenolate mofetil at 3,000 mg a day was $1,431 per month, while the CellCept brand equivalent was $3,886.

Prescription discount services, such as blinkhealth.com and goodrx.com can significantly reduce costs. The monthly costs for these same medicines using GoodRx were $25 for azathioprine and $46 for mycophenolate mofetil. These discount service prices are often cheaper than the copay requirements of medical insurance plans.

Generally, the prescribing physician chooses one of the treatment regimens mentioned above and monitors the patient very carefully, often every two to four weeks at first. If there is an excellent response within the first few months—with decreasing protein in the urine, improving blood pressure, and improving kidney function on blood tests—this is a good sign. Studies suggest that if a patient responds in the first few months, they have a much better chance of having an excellent long-term outcome. A good response to a medication is when the amount of protein in the urine decreases by more than 25% in the first 8–12 weeks or 50% by 12–24 weeks. If a doctor does not see improvement within the first few months, they may change the medication to other drugs. It is not uncommon to repeat the high doses of IV steroids again when the medicine is changed.

The goal in treating lupus nephritis is remission. The only way to know if someone is in remission is to do a kidney biopsy. However, it is impractical to frequently perform kidney biopsies. Therefore, we usually go by blood and urine tests. We hope to see the kidney function (eGFR, chapter 4) and the amount of protein in the urine improve or normalize. After a year of treatment, our goal is to ensure that the urine protein to creatine ratio is less than 0.7 mg/gm. Patients who reach this goal are much less likely to go into kidney failure in the future. A goal of less than 0.5 mg/gm is even better. These patients are often in remission or close to remission.

Everyone with lupus nephritis should also take hydroxychloroquine (HCQ, Plaquenil) unless they cannot tolerate it. A Johns Hopkins Hospital study showed that patients with Class V lupus nephritis who took HCQ with mycophenolate were three times more likely to go into remission than those who took mycophenolate alone. A 2020 Brazilian study showed that lupus nephritis patients who were prescribed HCQ but had low HCQ blood levels did poorly. Of patients who were not taking their medicine regularly, 28% had kidney disease flares over 7 months, while only 5% of the adherent patients flared.

If you have lupus nephritis, be your own best health advocate and pay attention to how you are doing. Do everything in tables 12.5 and 12.6 to make sure you give yourself the best chances of controlling your lupus nephritis. Also, follow your labs and vital signs, as in table 12.3. If your numbers are not going in the right direction, ask your rheumatologist or kidney specialist (nephrologist) what can be done to better control your nephritis. Sometimes a repeat kidney biopsy may be needed to determine the best strategies. If you are having trouble taking or affording your medication, let your doctor

LUPUS IN FOCUS

Combination therapy for lupus nephritis

Using either belimumab or voclosporin along with mycophenolate mofetil (MMF) or cyclophosphamide (CYC) is called combination therapy. Using MMF or CYC alone is called monotherapy. Most patients with lupus nephritis do not go into remission using monotherapy, and achieving remission is our main goal. Remission ensures the highest chances of avoiding kidney failure. The clinical trials using combination therapy showed significantly higher remission rates than did monotherapy and should be considered as standard therapy in most lupus nephritis patients.

Table 12.3 Indicators of Improvements in Lupus Nephritis

- Decreasing proteinuria (random urine protein/creatinine ratio and 24-hour urine protein); this is the most important item
- Good blood pressure control (goal is less than 120/80 at home; less than 125/80 at the doctor)
- Decreasing anti-ds DNA, anti-chromatin, anti-C1q, and EC4d
- Increasing C3, C4, CH50 complements
- Decreasing serum creatinine
- Increasing estimated glomerular filtration rate (eGFR)
- Increasing serum albumin
- Increasing hemoglobin level

know so that appropriate changes can be made. Do not stop taking medicines on your own without getting your doctor involved. If you are a woman and thinking about having children, let your doctor know to optimize timing and medications.

Other Immunosuppressant Treatments

Tacrolimus. Tacrolimus (TAC, chapter 32) is related to cyclosporine and voclosporin (collectively called calcineurin inhibitors). A 2015 study showed that a small TAC dose with mycophenolate resulted in many remissions with few side effects.

Rituxan (rituximab) Treatment with Minimal Steroids. Steroids, such as prednisone, are a lifesaving treatment for severe SLE. However, they also carry a high risk for side effects. Steroids are also a contributor to permanent organ damage in lupus patients when used regularly.

In 2013, a UK research study called the RITUXILUP trial showed that lupus nephritis could successfully be treated with rituximab without using oral (pill form) steroids. Two years after treatment 80% of lupus nephritis patients were in at least partial remission. The possibility of treating SLE with a minimum use of steroids is exciting.

Obinutuzumab (Gazyva). Obinutuzumab is related to rituximab. However, preliminary studies suggest higher rates of remission in lupus nephritis and possibly fewer side effects with obinutuzumab. As of 2023, there are several large phase 3 clinical trials (explained in chapter 37) using obinutuzumab in lupus nephritis to see if these findings can be reproduced. One of these is using it with mycophenolate and no steroids. With our trying to get away from steroids as much as possible, we are anxious to see these results.

Orencia (abatacept). Orencia is given intravenously (IV, chapter 33). It is FDA-approved to treat rheumatoid arthritis and psoriatic arthritis. Preliminary studies suggested that it may be beneficial for lupus nephritis. However, it failed to show benefit in phase 3 clinical trials. Even so, those patients who received Orencia improved significantly faster than those on placebo. More of them were also in complete remission one year into the study. Orencia can be considered by some lupus experts for patients who do not respond to other medicines.

Additional Treatments

The treatment of lupus nephritis is complex and includes controlling proteinuria (protein in the urine), anemia, abnormal electrolytes, low vitamin D levels, and edema. These require a balance of medical therapies.

Lupus nephritis patients with proteinuria should take either an angiotensin-converting enzyme inhibitor (ACE inhibitors for short) or an angiotensin receptor blocker (ARB for short). The commonly used medicines are listed in table 12.4. These medicines are used to lessen the leakage of protein and prevent a decrease in kidney function. ACE inhibitors and ARBs can also decrease kidney scar tissue formation and keep the kidneys functioning better. With treatment, it can take almost 12 months for protein levels to fully respond in some cases.

ACE inhibitors can sometimes cause a nagging, dry cough. Other side effects include light-headedness and allergic reactions. If any of these side effects occur, you should let your doctor know. Your doctor will also monitor your blood because the ARBs and ACE inhibitors can increase blood potassium, sCr, and reduce eGFR. These side effects are reversible by reducing the drug dose.

Other blood pressure medicines that can also reduce the amount of protein in the urine include diltiazem and verapamil, used alone, or combined with an ACE inhibitor or an ARB. The diuretic (fluid pill) called spironolactone can also lower proteinuria when added to an ACE inhibitor.

Empagliflozin (Jardiance) and dapagliflozin (Farxiga) are diabetes drugs that are helpful in diabetic kidney disease. However, large studies show they are also effective

Table 12.4 ACE Inhibitors and ARBs for Lupus Nephritis

ACE Inhibitors	ARBs
benazepril (Lotensin)	azilsartan (Edarbi)
	candesartan (Atacand)
captopril (Capoten)	eprosartan
	irbesartan (Avapro)
enalapril (Vasotec)	losartan (Cozaar)
fosinopril (Monopril)	olmesartan (Benicar)
	telmisartan (Micardis)
lisinopril (Prinivil, Zestril)	valsartan (Diovan)
moexipril (Univasc)	
perindopril (Aceon)	
quinapril (Accupril)	
ramipril (Altace)	
trandolapril (Mavik)	

in patients with proteinuria due to kidney disease from non-diabetic causes, reducing kidney function loss and the need for dialysis and kidney transplants. They may also reduce death rates. They should be considered in lupus nephritis patients who have proteinuria as well.

It is vital to control blood pressure in lupus nephritis. Elevated blood pressure can cause increased kidney damage and lead to heart attacks and strokes. Doctors recommend keeping the blood pressure less than 125/80 (less than 120/80 on home blood pressure readings) in lupus nephritis. Home blood pressure readings are useful. Regular exercise can help regulate your blood pressure, especially if it remains elevated despite medications.

In addition to treating high blood pressure, high cholesterol must be addressed. People with lupus nephritis and high cholesterol should generally take a cholesterol-lowering medication (especially a statin). Statins appear to have anti-inflammatory effects in addition to their cholesterol-lowering results. These anti-inflammatory effects may provide additional benefits in SLE.

Lupus nephritis–associated anemia is due to decreased kidney production of the hormone erythropoietin. Anemia can cause fatigue and, if severe, heart problems and difficulties with memory and thinking. If fatigue or memory problems occur or the hemoglobin drops below 10 g/dL, erythropoietin injections may help. It is important to take iron supplements before starting these drugs. If your hemoglobin rises to 13 g/dL on erythropoietin, then it should be stopped.

Sometimes, patients with lupus nephritis need to take extra potassium and calcium, depending on their blood test results. Diuretics (fluid pills) such as furosemide (Lasix) commonly decrease potassium levels, often requiring a potassium supplement.

Diet can be beneficial, depending on the circumstances. Diet recommendations can vary according to the degree of kidney damage, proteinuria, and edema. A proper diet is best prescribed by a kidney doctor (called a nephrologist) with a dietician's help. An essential part of the diet is decreasing salt intake (specifically, sodium). High sodium salt intake counteracts the effects of blood pressure medicines such as ACE inhibitors and ARBs.

If significant edema occurs, you can treat it by elevating your feet and legs when you sit and lie down. Compression stockings, which are tight stockings you can buy from medical supply stores, can decrease leg swelling, especially if you put them on soon after getting up after sleeping. Sometimes people need medications (diuretics or fluid pills) to reduce edema. Note, though, that diuretics can sometimes cause problems with kidney function. They can also cause electrolyte (like potassium, sodium, and calcium) imbalances. Doctors usually follow blood tests closely.

In patients taking steroids (such as prednisone), it is essential to prevent osteoporosis, which can lead to broken bones (chapters 24 and 31).

End-Stage Renal Disease, Dialysis, and Kidney Transplants

A variety of factors can increase the risk of the kidneys doing poorly over time. Some of these factors you have no control over (such as your genetics), but you do have control over others, such as taking your medications regularly, working on your blood pressure, and not smoking (table 12.5).

Lupus nephritis remission

Our goal in treating lupus nephritis is to reach remission, or near-remission, as quickly as possible. This includes using the most effective drugs in the safest ways, especially using the lowest doses of steroids needed. The European League Against Rheumatism published new treatment recommendations in 2019 recommending remission within one year of the initial diagnosis of kidney inflammation. Their remission definition is normal to near-normal kidney function (the eGFR result on blood work) and less than 500 to 700 grams of protein in the urine during a 24-hour urine collection.

If the kidneys completely stop working, the medical term is "end-stage renal disease" (ESRD). This occurs when the eGFR on blood testing or the creatinine clearance on the 24-hour urine test stays below 15 ml/min. At this point, the kidneys can no longer filter harmful substances (toxins) out of the blood and secrete them into the urine adequately. When this occurs, dialysis or a kidney transplant is eventually necessary.

Dialysis filters toxic substances out of the blood, doing the work that the kidneys should do. There are two forms. For hemodialysis, the person goes to a dialysis unit. A needle connected to tubing is inserted into the person's arm so that a dialysis machine can filter the blood. This is typically done three times weekly. Patients on hemodialysis seem to have better control of their SLE, most likely due to the hemodialysis removing harmful autoantibodies. Some people with lupus can get off steroids when they are on hemodialysis.

For peritoneal dialysis, a machine connected to tubing goes into the person's peritoneal cavity (which surrounds the abdomen) to filter the blood. This can be done at home. However, it is usually done nightly.

Although people with ESRD can live long using dialysis, the risk of dying is substantial. SLE patients with ESRD who undergo kidney transplants have a 70% lower death rate than those who stay on dialysis because they have fewer infections, heart attacks, strokes, and blood clots. Therefore, it is important to consider a kidney transplant as early as possible. Waiting lists can be long, and preparation for kidney transplantation can take a long time. You should follow up closely with your kidney doctor and rheumatologist during the transplant evaluation period.

A big concern in kidney transplant patients is the possibility of losing the kidney through organ rejection or other causes. Organ rejection occurs when the patient's immune system attacks the new kidney. SLE patients have similar organ rejection rates as patients without SLE. How often the transplanted kidney fails varies between different transplant centers and countries, and this should be discussed with your transplant team.

A critical factor predicting success after kidney transplantation is treatment adherence. This is a real problem in SLE. A 2019 UK study of lupus kidney transplant patients showed that 42% were not taking their medications regularly. Nonadherent patients are four times more likely to lose their kidneys.

Table 12.5 Factors Associated with Worse Lupus Nephritis Outcomes

Factors you have little or no control over

Factors present at nephritis onset	African or Hispanic ancestry
	Biopsy showing Class III or IV nephritis, scarring, crescents, fibrinoid necrosis, tubulointerstitial damage, arterial sclerosis, vasculopathy, vasculitis
	Negative for anti-SSA and anti-SSB
	Positive anti-phospholipid antibodies
	Lower kidney function
	High blood pressure
	Delay in diagnosis and treatment by the doctor
	Not being prescribed an anti-malarial such as hydroxychloroquine
Factors present after 8–24 weeks of treatment	Urine protein not lowered more than 25% in 8–12 weeks or 50% in 12–24 weeks
	Unable to reduce anti-ds DNA by 8 weeks
Factors present after 1 year of treatment	A urine protein level > 700 mg/day

Factors you have some control over

Delay in starting treatment (if you procrastinate in accepting treatment)

Smoking

Obesity

Not exercising regularly

Not taking medications regularly

Not taking hydroxychloroquine regularly, if prescribed

Blood pressure > 125/80

Having untreated high cholesterol, prediabetes, and diabetes

The best type of kidney to transplant is one from a family member with the same blood type. Otherwise, a properly matched kidney from a non-live (cadaveric) or a live nonrelated donor can also work.

Immunosuppressants used to prevent organ rejection help keep lupus nephritis in remission. However, lupus nephritis recurs within the first three years in around 10% of patients. When this happens, the chances of losing the kidney or dying are three times higher than they are for patients who do not develop lupus nephritis in a new kidney.

In the long run, people with SLE who have a kidney transplant appear to do as well as those who get transplants for other reasons. Ten years after kidney transplantation, over 70% of patients are still alive in both groups. In those SLE patients who die, heart-related conditions, such as heart attacks, are the cause two thirds of the time. It is important to work on preventing heart disease (see chapter 21).

Some Good News

Lupus nephritis used to be the number 1 cause of death in people with SLE. Better treatments and diagnostic accuracy have markedly improved over the years. Today, in countries with good health care, heart attacks, strokes, and infections are more common causes of death. Many of these other problems can be prevented (chapters 21 and 22) by being proactive in your health care.

Between 2018 and 2020, three studies looked at how we are doing with nephritis. One was done at Massachusetts General Hospital, and two in Europe. They showed that compared to earlier times (such as the 1990s), today we are diagnosing patients faster with kidney biopsies. Kidney disease is not as severe at the onset, and there are many more patients with mild proteinuria and minimal kidney inflammation. Patients are 45% less likely to go on dialysis, deaths decreased by 50%, and as few as 1% of lupus nephritis patients develop ESRD by 10 years. These improvements have been attributed to better SLE and lupus nephritis treatments, the use of HCQ in almost all patients, kidney biopsies being done sooner and resulting in faster diagnoses at earlier stages, and therapies such as ACE inhibitors, ARBs, and statins being used more often. However, some patients are still going into kidney failure, needing dialysis and kidney transplants, and dying prematurely. Don't let this happen to you. Do everything in tables 12.5 and 12.6 and in the Lupus Secrets (chapter 44) so that you can be as healthy as possible.

How Can I Do My Best to Do Well with Lupus Nephritis?

Many factors that increase the chances for complications in lupus nephritis have been identified and listed in table 12.5. These complications include lupus nephritis flares (episodes of kidney inflammation, lower kidney function, and increased proteinuria), worsening kidney function over time (chronic kidney disease), increased risk of needing dialysis, kidney transplantation, and even death. Your risk for these complications increases with the more factors you have. While you have no control over some (for example, race), you do have control over others, such as taking your medications regularly. To preserve your kidneys and do well after a diagnosis of lupus nephritis, follow the recommendations in tables 12.5 and 12.6.

Lupus Cystitis

In addition to the kidneys, SLE can occasionally affect the bladder, though this is rare. Lupus cystitis affects only 1% (or less) of SLE patients and is more common in Asians. The term "interstitial cystitis" was used in the past for lupus cystitis. Today, however, "interstitial cystitis" refers to "bladder pain syndrome," which often accompanies fibromyalgia and irritable bowel syndrome.

Common lupus cystitis symptoms include increased frequency in urination and a feeling of urgency to urinate (like those caused by a bladder infection). Most patients

Table 12.6 Preserving Kidney Function after a Lupus Nephritis Diagnosis

- Take your medicines, including hydroxychloroquine and vitamin D, regularly.
- Keep your blood pressure less than 125/80 at the doctor's and less than 120/80 at home.
- Ask your doctors if you can take a statin.
- Work on normalizing cholesterol levels.
- Do moderate aerobic exercise 150 minutes weekly and strengthening exercises 2–3 days weekly.
- Eat a low-salt diet if you have high blood pressure or decreased kidney function.
- Eat a heart-healthy diet (like the Mediterranean diet, chapter 38).
- Avoid drugs that can worsen kidney function, such as NSAIDs (table 36.1) and Chinese herbs.
- Do everything listed in "The Lupus Secrets" checklist (chapter 44).

also have inflammation of the intestines (called enteritis), causing abdominal pain, diarrhea, nausea, and vomiting. These abdominal symptoms often occur before the urinary symptoms. Enteritis can be identified with a CT of the abdomen showing intestinal bowel wall thickening. The doctor should search for lupus cystitis in SLE patients diagnosed with lupus enteritis. Lupus cystitis patients also have an increased risk for mesenteric vasculitis (chapter 15), a potentially lethal complication. A high suspicion of and appropriate workup for vasculitis are important.

A cystoscopy can help diagnose lupus cystitis. In this procedure a urinary tract surgical specialist (a urologist) inserts a tiny fiber optic scope into the urethra, enabling them to look inside the bladder and get a small biopsy. Biopsies typically show tiny blood vessel inflammation (vasculitis) within the bladder wall. It is treated with immunosuppressants.

If lupus cystitis is not identified early and treated quickly, it can cause significant problems. The bladder wall can become permanently scarred, causing difficulties such as needing to urinate more frequently and with just a small quantity at a time. Also, urinary retention can cause the kidneys to become swollen and congested, resulting in reduced kidney function.

KEY POINTS TO REMEMBER

1. African Americans, Asians, and Hispanics are at especially high risk for lupus nephritis.

2. Lupus nephritis can be silent and causes symptoms only when significant damage has already occurred.

3. It is important to have blood and urine tests regularly to look for the possibility of lupus nephritis even when feeling well. We want to identify lupus nephritis at its earliest stages so that treatments are more successful.

4. If you get a kidney biopsy, make sure to keep a permanent copy for your personal records. You will need it for future doctors.

5. If you have lupus nephritis, ensure that your blood pressure remains below 125/80 (or less than 120/80 on home blood pressure readings). If it is higher, see your doctor to lower it (usually using medicines) to protect your kidneys. Exercise helps!

6. If you have increased protein in your urine, make sure your doctor treats you with an ACE inhibitor, ARB (table 12.3), empagliflozin (Jardiance) or dapagliflozin (Farxiga).

7. Lupus nephritis treatment requires multiple medications to control the immune system, treat electrolyte disorders, high blood pressure, proteinuria, edema, high cholesterol, anemia, and to prevent drug side effects (such as using drugs to prevent osteoporosis from steroids).

8. With early targeted treatment, most patients with lupus nephritis do well and do not develop end-stage renal disease, which requires dialysis treatment.

9. Patients with kidney problems should avoid NSAIDs (such as ibuprofen and naproxen) and Chinese herbs as these can worsen kidney function.

10. Do everything that you can have control over (tables 12.5 and 12.6) to do the very best if you have lupus nephritis.

11. Lupus inflammation of the urinary bladder (lupus cystitis) is rare. It occurs primarily in Asians and is treated with immunosuppressants.

The Nervous System

David Hunt, MB, BChir, PhD, *Contributing Editor*

The nervous system handles how you think, love, and hate, and it affects your personality. It regulates your ability to move your muscles, your senses of touch, pain, smell, taste, hearing, and seeing, and your blood pressure and heartbeats. Nerve cells communicate via chemical messengers called neurotransmitters and electrical activity traveling up and down the nerves.

The nervous system is divided into the central nervous system (CNS) and the peripheral nervous system (PNS). The CNS is made up of the brain and spinal cord. The PNS includes the nerves that lead to and from the CNS to the rest of the body (figure 13.1). In 1999 the American College of Rheumatology (ACR) created a list of neuropsychiatric syndromes (*neuro-* referring to the nerves and "psychiatric" referring to psychiatric conditions) in order to help doctors describe their patients similarly to standardize treatments and research. When SLE patients have any of these problems defined by the ACR, they arè said to have neuropsychiatric systemic lupus erythematosus (NPSLE). The different types of NPSLE defined by the ACR are separated into those that affect the CNS and those that affect the PNS. Psychiatric conditions (such as depression and anxiety disorder) are included because they are disorders related to abnormalities in brain nerves.

We use this system to organize this chapter because the ACR and many lupus experts use it. We previously mentioned that we would list lupus problems directly due to lupus inflammation in part II. Complications of lupus due to other issues are in part III. The ACR includes both types in this system; we do so in this chapter as well because they would be difficult to separate. Some neuropsychiatric syndromes due to problems other than the direct influence of immune system inflammation include headaches, anxiety, and mood disorders.

This chapter discusses the neurologic complications and controversies of SLE.

Neuropsychiatric Systemic Lupus Erythematosus (NPSLE)

We don't know exactly how many people develop NPSLE. Neurological conditions such as migraine, anxiety, and mood disorders are common in the general population and in SLE. Some studies have suggested that NPSLE can occur in up to 25% of SLE patients during their lifetime. It often develops at SLE diagnosis or soon after.

The abnormal SLE immune system causes these neurologic problems around 30% of the time. The rest of the time (70%) it is due to non-lupus causes. It is crucial to look

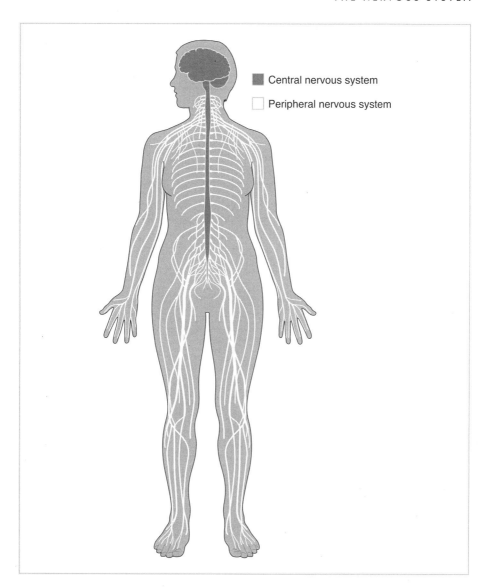

Central nervous system

Peripheral nervous system

Figure 13.1 The central nervous system and the peripheral nervous system

for these other causes (table 13.1) to treat them correctly. Even some of the drugs used to treat lupus can cause these problems. In those cases, the right move is usually to stop the medicine or reduce its dose. This is the opposite of when the problem is due to lupus inflammation, where the correct treatment may be to increase the dosage. It is best to have the help of a nerve expert (neurologist) experienced in treating SLE patients.

Lupus inflammation, which can affect the nerves or surrounding structures (such as the blood vessels in vasculitis), is treated with drugs that calm down the immune system and reduce inflammation.

Table 13.1 Non-Lupus Problems That Mimic NPSLE

Other neurologic and psychiatric diseases

Infections

Depression

Medication side effects

High blood pressure damage

Kidney failure

Electrolyte problems (such as low or high sodium levels)

Obstructive sleep apnea

Fever

Thyroid disease

Aneurysms

Cancer

LUPUS IN FOCUS

Anti-ribosomal P antibodies (Anti-P)

Anti-P (chapter 4) attaches to brain cells, including those involved with emotions and memory. When anti-P is injected into mice, they develop memory problems and depression. Anti-P antibodies can be present in SLE patients with psychosis, memory problems, and depression.

Antiphospholipid syndrome (APS, chapter 9) due to SLE causes blood clots, which can, in turn, cause a loss of blood flow to nerves. If APS is the cause, blood thinners such as warfarin and heparin are used (chapter 9). Overall, treatment of NPSLE events from blood flow loss (ischemia) is not as effective as those from inflammation. Lupus inflammation is potentially reversible, while ischemic (loss of blood flow) events are often irreversible. A 2017 study from the Netherlands showed that while only 16% of their ischemic NPSLE patients improved with treatment, over half of their inflammatory patients did. However, those who received blood thinners, such as warfarin (Coumadin), had reductions in death rates, showing how essential blood thinners are in APS.

A big problem with treating NPSLE is the lack of any large, well-done research studies proving what therapies work best. This is in stark contrast to lupus nephritis (chapter 12) where there are numerous, large, well-done studies. There are not enough patients with each NPSLE problem to have large studies for each type. Also, while kidney biopsies accurately define exactly what type of nephritis someone has, this is not available for NPSLE. It is challenging to know if a nerve problem is due to active inflammation, permanent damage, or blood clots, or if it is related to lupus at all.

Let's look at one type of NPSLE: seizures. It would not be good enough to do a "seizure" study. There are many different types of seizures, and SLE can cause each type by more than one method—for example, by causing inflammation or by causing blood clots). For each of these two cases, the treatment would be very different. But identifying the cause could also be challenging. That is, it would be extremely difficult to perform a good study of generalized seizures due to inflammation (rather than to blood clots), because a brain biopsy from each patient would be needed, and that would be highly impractical.

Immunosuppressants are usually used for inflammation (table 22.1). For severe CNS problems, prednisone may not always work. Dexamethasone (2–20 mg daily) enters the CNS (crosses the blood-brain barrier) and may work better.

A 2013 Cochrane analysis showed that cyclophosphamide and high dose steroids worked similarly for severe NPSLE.

Many experts use high-dose steroids and mycophenolate mofetil (MMF, CellCept) as drugs of choice. MMF use was supported in a large 2017 Indian study of many different types of NPSLE, of which seizures were the most common. MMF is as effective and safer than cyclophosphamide (a potent chemotherapy agent) to treat another significant organ problem in SLE, lupus nephritis (kidney inflammation).

Rituximab (Rituxan) may help. A 2007 Japanese study used Rituxan in 10 patients with severe NPSLE who did not respond to other therapies. They all went into remission that lasted from 4 to 29 months. Rituximab may especially be useful in aquaporin-4-mediated spinal cord inflammation (myelitis, discussed later) and for vasculitis.

Some of these NPSLE disorders are treated similarly to when they occur in non-lupus patients. For example, we use plasmapheresis and IVIG (chapter 35) for lupus-associated Guillain-Barré syndrome (described later). We use plasma exchange for thrombotic microangiopathies (such as TTP, chapter 9). Plasma exchange can also be used for severe CNS lupus (such as coma from SLE) that does not improve quickly on other treatments.

Stem-cell transplantation (bone marrow transplants) can be also considered in severe cases that do not respond to other treatments. A 2000 US study did bone marrow transplants on seven NPSLE patients who did not respond to cyclophosphamide. All seven survived and were in remission two years later.

One possible way that SLE can cause some of these NPSLE syndromes (strokes and seizures, for example) is thrombotic microangiopathy (such as TTP, chapter 9). In this condition, blood clots develop in numerous small blood vessels and affect the nervous system and other organs such as the kidneys. Low platelet counts and fever are usually present. Appropriate therapies include plasma exchange, rituximab (Rituxan), and eculizumab (Soliris). If antiphospholipid antibodies are present, blood thinners such as heparin are usually used.

If catastrophic antiphospholipid syndrome (chapter 9) causes NPSLE, then triple therapy, consisting of plasma exchange, intravenous heparin, and high dose steroids, is recommended. IVIG, rituximab (Rituxan), or eculizumab (Soliris) are also sometimes used.

The following sections are divided up into each type of NPSLE syndrome, as defined by the ACR. Those that affect the central nervous system are described first, followed by those that affect the peripheral nervous system.

Central Nervous System Disorders

The brain and spinal cord make up the central nervous system (CNS). When SLE affects most of the brain (the cerebrum), some doctors call it "lupus cerebritis," but this term is outdated and should not be used. "CNS vasculitis" is often used if the inflammation mainly affects blood vessels. However, this term is overused, and actual blood vessel inflammation in the brain is rare.

Aseptic Meningitis

The meninges are the tissues and membranes surrounding the brain and spinal cord. Inflammation of the meninges is called meningitis (-*itis* means "inflammation of"). Meningitis typically causes headaches, trouble thinking, fever, neck stiffness, and intolerance of light shining in the eyes. It may be hard to keep the hips and knees straightened out while laying down. Physical exam may show nuchal rigidity ("nuchal" refers to the neck). The doctor pushes the person's head down toward the chest, causing neck muscle spasms and pain.

The most important thing with meningitis is to make sure it is not due to infection. Meningitis infection can be deadly if not treated immediately. Therefore, someone with suspected meningitis is treated quickly with antibiotics (just in case there is infection), and a lumbar puncture, described next) is performed.

During a lumbar puncture (commonly called a spinal tap) the lower back is numbed up with an anesthetic (usually lidocaine) using a thin needle. A larger needle is inserted through the numbed-up area until it reaches the spinal canal to collect some cerebrospinal fluid (CSF) for examination. Cerebrospinal fluid (*cerebro-* comes from the Latin word for "brain") is the nourishing fluid around the brain and spinal cord.

Major lumbar puncture complications are rare. The most common side effect is a headache (occurs around half the time), which lasts for a few days and is typically worse when standing up. Bleeding and infection are possible but rare. Special considerations are needed for lumbar puncture if you take blood thinners. Your doctor will advise on this. The spinal cord ends a few levels up from where the lumbar puncture is performed, so spinal cord injury should not be possible.

The CSF is sent to the lab to help differentiate different types of brain and spinal cord problems. The fluid is examined under a microscope to look for bacteria. Tests, including cultures, are done to exclude infections from Lyme, bacteria, viruses, fungi, and other microorganisms. A culture is performed by placing fluid in various containers containing food (agar) that different bacteria and microorganisms can grow on. It

---

LUPUS IN FOCUS

Meningitis and Kikuchi disease

It can be difficult to tell if someone has SLE or Kikuchi disease (chapter 9), since they have many similarities. For example, meningitis can occur in both. KD and SLE should be considered in someone with meningitis, swollen lymph glands, fever, and other lupus-like symptoms.

is often vital to keep the person on antibiotics "just in case" until the final results. While infections can sometimes be diagnosed quickly, culture results take several days.

Elevated white blood cells in the CSF indicate inflammation around the brain and spinal cord. This confirms a meningitis diagnosis.

If no bacteria or other microorganisms are found, the meningitis is called aseptic meningitis (*a-* means "not," and "septic" means "infectious"). Virus infections are a common cause of aseptic meningitis and usually resolve over time.

Various drugs, including non-steroidal anti-inflammatory drugs (NSAIDs, such as naproxen and ibuprofen) and, more rarely, azathioprine (Imuran) and intravenous immunoglobulin (IVIG), can cause aseptic meningitis. It usually resolves after stopping the drug. Blood vessel bleeding and even cancer can also cause aseptic meningitis.

If the above causes are excluded (drugs, infection, and so on), it is presumed that the aseptic meningitis is due to SLE and is treated with immunosuppressants. Less than 5% of SLE patients develop aseptic meningitis from NPSLE.

Hypertrophic Pachymeningitis

This condition is also called pachymeningitis (*pachy-* from the Greek word for "thick"), for short. It is very rare. It occurs when the outermost layer of tissue surrounding the brain and spinal cord (called the dura) becomes thicker due to chronic (going on for a long time) inflammation. Most patients have headaches, but confusion and cranial neuropathies (discussed later in this chapter) can also occur. Brain MRI reveals the thickening. Since infections, cancer, sarcoidosis, and IgG4-related disorder (chapter 4) can also cause pachymeningitis, a biopsy is recommended to exclude these.

SLE pachymeningitis usually responds well to immunosuppressants such as high-dose steroids, cyclophosphamide, IVIG, rituximab (Rituxan), and mycophenolate (CellCept).

KEY POINTS TO REMEMBER

1. Headache, fever, difficulty tolerating light in the eyes, and a stiff neck are common in meningitis.

2. Bacterial meningitis is potentially deadly and requires immediate antibiotics. A lumbar puncture is performed to send the CSF to the lab for cultures and other tests.

3. NSAIDs such as ibuprofen and naproxen can cause aseptic meningitis. It resolves when the NSAID is stopped.

4. Lupus aseptic meningitis is treated with immunosuppressants.

5. Lupus pachymeningitis is due to inflammation and thickening of the lining around the brain and is usually diagnosed by MRI and a biopsy.

6. Pachymeningitis usually causes headaches and is treated with immunosuppressants.

Cerebrovascular Disease

Cerebrovascular disease refers to brain blood vessel problems (*cerebro-* meaning "brain" and -*vascular* referring to blood vessels). There are many ways that the brain's blood vessels can become damaged, and many types of cerebrovascular disease can develop in SLE. These specific problems (such as stroke, seizures, memory loss, and so on) are discussed below. Many of them (such as headaches, seizures, and cognitive dysfunction) are ACR-listed NPSLE syndromes.

Cerebrovascular Accidents (Strokes)

A cerebrovascular accident (CVA, also called a stroke) can be thought of as a heart attack of the brain. CVAs are twice as common in people with SLE than in the general population. They are due to blood supply loss to an area of the brain. The blood-flow loss damages that part of the brain, and that area can die. Which problems occur depends on what part of the brain is affected. For example, if the CVA involves the part of the brain responsible for right leg and arm movement, the person may develop sudden onset of weakness on the body's right side. Other common symptoms of stroke include headaches, numbness, difficulty speaking, and incoordination. Stroke-induced vision loss that comes and goes in one or both eyes is called amaurosis fugax (*amaurosis* is from the Greek for "dark," and *fugax* is from the Latin word for "fleeting").

Stroke causes permanent brain nerve damage, but with varying degrees of severity, ranging from being so mild that they don't bother the person to so devastating that the person requires continuous nursing help. One out of five people die from a stroke. The faster someone gets medical attention, the sooner treatment can be given, and the less likelihood for severe problems.

A transient ischemic attack (TIA, often called mini-stroke) is when stroke symptoms occur but then resolve. If someone has a TIA, they are at high risk of a full-blown CVA in the future. Immediate medical attention is needed, as with a CVA.

People with SLE are at least twice as likely to develop CVAs and TIAs. Strokes and heart attacks are among the most common causes of death in SLE and occur earlier than in those without SLE (chapter 21). Therefore, SLE patients should do everything possible to decrease their chances for these. This includes keeping proper body weight, exercising regularly, not smoking, eating healthy, and ensuring that blood pressure, sugar levels, and cholesterol levels are kept under control.

CVAs and TIAs occur from many different causes. Many medical tests are needed to figure out the cause so proper therapies can be given.

For example, if a CVA is due to a blocked blood vessel from a blood clot, doctors can administer a blood thinner (called thrombolytic therapy). If given quickly enough, this therapy can reverse the stroke, preventing permanent damage. As they say in the emergency room, "Time is Brain." The faster someone gets treatment, the more brain that can be saved. The person who waits at home, hoping things will get better, risks permanent brain damage. The best results occur when treatment is given within 90 minutes of symptom onset. However, it can still be effective up to four and a half hours later. Before the medicine is given, a brain CT is important to ensure that there is no bleeding. Thrombolytic therapy can be lifesaving, and more than one-third of people fully recover.

After this acute stage, one of the most important things is figuring out what caused the stroke so proper treatment can be given.

Between one-third and one-half of SLE patients have antiphospholipid (aPL) antibodies, which cause strokes or heart attacks in around half of them. When aPL antibodies cause strokes or heart attacks, it is called antiphospholipid syndrome (APS). APS causes

TIAs and CVAs by causing brain artery blood clots. One APS-induced TIA or CVA greatly increases the risk of future CVAs. If a stroke (CVA) occurs in someone with aPL antibodies and livedo reticularis (chapter 8), it is called Sneddon's syndrome. APS is treated with lifelong blood thinners such as warfarin, heparin, and aspirin.

Lifelong warfarin use applies primarily to APS patients with persistently high-positive aPL antibodies. Treatment for those with intermittent or low positive antibodies is not straightforward, since it is not known if the aPL antibodies caused the stroke or not. In this case, low-dose aspirin may be sufficient.

SLE vasculitis (blood vessel inflammation, chapter 11) can also cause strokes. Artery inflammation from vasculitis causes reduced brain blood flow and brain blood leakage. This typically occurs in extremely sick patients. They often have fever, headache, confusion, seizures, and even coma. However, "CNS vasculitis" is used too loosely. NPSLE patient autopsies rarely show vasculitis.

An angiogram x-ray visualizes the brain's arteries. A magnetic resonance angiogram (MRA), using an MRI machine, is an alternative test. These studies may show narrowing and dilatations (called "beading") in the brain's arteries from vasculitis. They could also show an abnormal artery bulge (aneurysm, chapter 11).

Cerebrospinal fluid (CSF) from a spinal tap may show elevated white blood cells and protein from vasculitis inflammation. Vasculitis can be diagnosed with certainty only with a brain biopsy. This is an operation that removes a small piece of brain to look at it under the microscope. This operation can be risky and is not always used.

If vasculitis is suspected, it is treated with immunosuppressants.

Bleeding can also cause CVAs and TIAs, especially in those with very low platelet counts (thrombocytopenia). SLE-induced thrombocytopenia is treated with immunosuppressants and platelet transfusions.

Blood thinners such as aspirin, warfarin (Coumadin), or clopidogrel (Plavix) can also cause bleeding. Stopping the medication is the treatment of choice. In the case of warfarin, vitamin K and transfusions containing clotting factors can help.

Thrombotic thrombocytopenic purpura (TTP) can also cause CVAs and TIAs by causing many blood clots in the brain's smaller arteries. See chapter 9.

Hardening of the arteries, also known as atherosclerosis or arteriosclerosis, is the main cause of heart attacks and strokes in older people. SLE patients develop hardening of the arteries at a younger age and at a faster pace than others. Read chapter 21 for more information, including treatments.

LUPUS IN FOCUS

NPSLE-like problems from steroids

Of people who take steroids, 20% develop NPSLE-like problems (moodiness, depression, anxiety, aggressiveness, tremors, muscle weakness, behavioral changes, memory problems, psychosis, headaches, difficulty concentrating, and trouble sleeping). The higher the dose, the more likely the side effect. But whether it is caused by NPSLE or steroids can be difficult to figure out. If due to steroids, the treatment is to lower the steroid dose.

Another potential cause of stroke is an embolus, which is a blood clot that travels through the bloodstream. There are several common origins for stroke-causing emboli (plural of embolus), including the carotid arteries, the aorta, and the heart. Vascular studies such as ultrasound, MRA, and echocardiogram can search for embolic sources. If one is found, treatment is directed at whatever caused the embolus. If it is due to arteriosclerosis, a substance called plaque may be found inside the arteries (chapter 21). Plaque is a buildup of cholesterol mixed with inflammation and clotted blood that can loosen and travel to the brain. If there is severe carotid artery narrowing, surgery may be needed to open the affected arteries.

Libman-Sacks endocarditis (chapter 11) can produce emboli-causing strokes. Often, aPL antibodies are present, requiring lifelong warfarin.

Birth control pills can cause strokes; aPL-positive SLE patients should not take birth control pills.

Cerebral Venous Thrombosis

The cerebral (brain) veins drain blood from the brain. When blood clots occur, it is called cerebral venous thrombosis, and it is rare in SLE. The cavernous and dural sinuses are types of cerebral veins, and they can also develop blood clots: cavernous sinus thrombosis and dural sinus thrombosis. Headaches and nausea that do not respond to therapy are the most common symptoms. Seizures can also occur. Brain MRI usually diagnoses it. Sometimes a venous angiogram, which is done by injecting a dye while performing an MRI or CT, is needed.

Treatment is usually blood thinners and immunosuppressants (table 22.1). Antiphospholipid syndrome causes 10% to 15% of cases and should be treated with lifelong warfarin.

Reversible Cerebral Vasoconstriction Syndrome

This is another rare problem with multiple areas of brain artery (*vaso-*) spasms (*-constriction*). It causes a "thunderclap headache," which is a severe headache that comes on abruptly, with the maximum intensity occurring within seconds. Some patients develop a TIA or stroke, and a few have seizures. Brain MRA shows multiple areas of arterial narrowing (the condition can look like vasculitis). However, brain MRI can distinguish between vasculitis and reversible cerebral vasoconstriction. These findings along with the thunderclap headache, are diagnostic.

Immunosuppressants are not useful. Instead, blood pressure medicines are used to relax the arteries. The symptoms resolve over days to weeks. Fewer than 15% of patients are left with residual stroke problems (such as weakness, numbness, difficulty talking).

Small Vessel Cerebrovascular Disease (Cerebral Microangiopathy)

This refers to brain small blood vessel damage. It is the most common finding on SLE brain MRIs. Radiologists often describe these as "white matter hyperintensities" (WMHIs) or nonspecific white matter changes. They are especially common after strokes, severe SLE inflammation, and in those with aPL antibodies. These MRI findings are sometimes mistaken for multiple sclerosis. However, the location and pattern of changes should lead to a correct diagnosis. Small vessel disease is expected in the general population as they age. However, SLE patients tend to get these changes at a much younger age due to inflammation (due to cytokines, chapter 3) and accelerated

Brain MRIs and NPSLE

Brain MRIs are not usually helpful in diagnosing NPSLE (except in some cases such as stroke). They are most beneficial in excluding non-lupus problems (such as cancer and infections). A 2020 Italian study recommended that all SLE patients get brain MRIs at their lupus diagnosis. A repeat MRI could be done if a suspected NPSLE event occurs. The study showed that new NPSLE events were often associated with new MRI findings (such as non-specific white matter changes) and supported NPSLE diagnoses. However, MRIs are expensive, so this approach of getting baseline MRIs needs further study.

atherosclerosis (chapter 21). Most people with mild, early small vessel disease do not have any problems related to it.

KEY POINTS TO REMEMBER

1. A cerebrovascular accident (CVA, also called a stroke) occurs when blood flow decreases to part of the brain, causing permanent damage.

2. Common symptoms of a CVA include weakness, numbness, difficulty walking or speaking, and vision loss.

3. If a person develops CVA symptoms that resolve, it is called a transient ischemic attack or a mini-stroke.

4. If CVA symptoms occur, it is vital to immediately seek medical attention to minimize permanent brain damage.

5. CVAs and heart attacks are among the top causes of death in SLE. It is crucial to control weight, blood pressure, diabetes, and cholesterol levels, exercise regularly, and not smoke.

6. Sometimes, CVA and TIA can be due to APS where lifetime warfarin treatment is needed.

7. Low platelet-induced brain bleeding can potentially cause a CVA. If the low platelets are due to SLE, it is treated with platelet transfusions and immunosuppressants. If the bleeding is due to blood-thinning drugs such as aspirin, Plavix, or warfarin (Coumadin), the medication needs to be stopped.

8. Small vessel cerebrovascular disease is the most common SLE brain MRI abnormality. It is most commonly due to hardening of the arteries.

Demyelinating Syndrome

Many nerves are covered with a thin layer of tissue called myelin, which increases the speed of electrical impulses up and down the nerve. Myelin is similar to the rubber coating around electrical cords.

Myelin loss is called "demyelination." Demyelination can happen in the brain, spinal cord nerves, and the peripheral nerves (discussed later in this chapter). The main demyelinating disorders in SLE are multiple sclerosis, neuromyelitis optica spectrum disorders (NMOSD), aquaporin-4-mediated inflammation, Guillain-Barré syndrome, and chronic inflammatory demyelinating polyradiculoneuropathy. The first three affect the CNS, while the last two affect the peripheral nervous system. The latter four are discussed later in this chapter.

MS is an autoimmune disease and is the most common cause of CNS demyelination. NPSLE can cause CNS demyelination that looks like MS. In the past, these cases were often called lupoid sclerosis when older MRI machines had difficulty discriminating between MS in SLE patients and lupus CNS demyelination. Today, diagnostic methods are better, and this term is rarely used.

Headache (Including Migraine and Pseudotumor Cerebri)

Like the general public, around 70% of SLE patients have headaches. Similarly, the most common are migraine, tension, and fibromyalgia headaches (chapter 27). These headaches can occur during stressful events (such as lupus flares). These are not due to lupus inflammation and are treated similarly to those in people without SLE.

True lupus headaches from lupus inflammation are rare. They typically improve or resolve promptly with steroids. However, headaches such as migraines can also improve with steroids. Other NPSLE disorders can also cause headaches (table 13.2), and treatment is directed at these. In such cases, the headache-producing disorder (for example, meningitis) should be the diagnosis, not "lupus headache."

Migraines are usually located on one side of the head, pulsate, can be moderate to severe, and are worsened by body movement. Nausea or intolerance of noise or light often occur. Some migraines occur with or after what is called an aura. The aura can be visual (such as seeing zig-zag lines) or sensory (such as tingling sensations over an arm or leg), which develops over minutes. Sometimes auras can cause difficulty speaking or seeing.

Migraines probably occur more often in patients with antiphospholipid (aPL) antibodies, and having Raynaud's may increase this risk. Some APS experts treat SLE pa-

Table 13.2 NPSLE Disorders That Can Cause Headache

Lupus meningitis and pachymeningitis

Stroke or transient ischemic attack

Vasculitis

Antiphospholipid syndrome

Thrombotic microangiopathy and thrombotic thrombocytopenic purpura (chapter 9)

Central venous thrombosis

Reversible cerebral vasoconstriction syndrome

Reversible posterior leukoencephalopathy syndrome

Benign intracranial hypertension (pseudotumor cerebri)

LUPUS IN FOCUS

Lupus headache

Less than 10% of headaches occurring in SLE patients are due to lupus inflammation (also called lupus headache). Even NPSLE experts are unsure how to accurately define "lupus headache." The SLEDAI (chapter 29) measures disease activity for research. More severe SLE gets more SLEDAI points. Having a lupus headache gives someone the maximum allowed number of SLEDAI points. Because some research patients may be earning points for headaches that may not be due to lupus, some experts recommend removing lupus headache from the SLEDAI.

tients with migraines and aPL antibodies with blood thinners. But this approach is controversial and has no good studies to support its use.

Migraines may increase the risk of strokes and heart attacks. A large 2020 study of 27,858 women (non-lupus patients) showed that those with migraine headaches with an aura had a 50% higher chance of heart attacks and strokes. SLE patients with migraines and aura should exercise regularly, eat well, and control weight, blood pressure, cholesterol, and sugar levels.

Pseudotumor cerebri (also called idiopathic intracranial hypertension, IIH) is another headache-causing condition. It is due to increased fluid pressure around the brain and spinal cord. The headaches can be severe, and they can cause blurred and double vision. On physical exam, the doctor will note swelling around the optic nerve in the back of the eye (papilledema). Papilledema can also be caused by a tumor in the brain, so an MRI or CT scan is performed to ensure that there is no cancer. When there is no tumor or cancer, the condition is called pseudotumor cerebri. *Pseudo-* means "false," and *-cerebri* means "of the brain." So "pseudotumor cerebri" means "false brain tumor"—a condition that looks like it could be a brain tumor, but it is not.

A lumbar puncture (spinal tap) can find elevated cerebrospinal fluid (CSF), which is what causes the symptoms. Draining some CSF from the spinal canal decreases the pressure and symptoms. This elevated pressure is the source of the other name for the disorder—"benign intracranial hypertension," where "benign" means "not due to cancer." "Intracranial" means "inside the brain," and "hypertension" means the pressure is increased. "Idiopathic intracranial hypertension" (IIH) is preferred by many neurologists, where "idiopathic" means "we don't know the cause."

Other therapies include immunosuppressants. Steroids can worsen IIH, so they are used sparingly. Acetazolamide (a fluid pill or diuretic) reduces CSF pressure. In resistant cases, eye surgery to reduce high pressure around the brain can be a permanent solution.

In some SLE patients with IIH, it is important to consider the possibility of blood clots, such as dural venous sinus thrombosis, which form in a collection of veins around the brain (dural venous sinus) These can occur in patients with or without aPL antibodies and are treated with blood thinners such as heparin and warfarin (chapter 9).

Other potential causes of headaches include infections, medications (which cause analgesic rebound headache), cancer, and high blood pressure. The doctor needs to consider these, and treatments vary among these causes.

1. Headaches (especially migraines, fibromyalgia, and tension headaches) are common in the general population and in SLE patients.

2. SLE patients are predisposed to other causes of headaches. Therefore, headaches, especially new ones, should always be taken seriously with a full clinical assessment.

Movement Disorders

There are several NPSLE movement disorders. These most commonly occur from lupus inflammation or blood clots in the cerebellum or basal ganglia of the brain. The cerebellum lies inside the back of the skull and manages balance and coordination. The basal ganglia are deep in the brain and help purposeful muscle movement.

Tremors are the most common movement disorders in people with and without SLE. The hands or head can shake with tremors, either when resting or moving. Tremors can occur for many reasons, including drugs such as mycophenolate (CellCept), tacrolimus, voclosporin (Lupkynis), and antidepressants. If these occur, your doctor may decrease the drug dose or change to a different drug. Caffeine and smoking are common causes and should be stopped for a few days to see if the tremors improve.

The most common movement disorder from NPSLE is chorea (from *choros*, the Greek word for "dance"). It occurs in around 4% of pediatric SLE patients but is rare in adults. It causes sudden, uncontrollable, brief movements of the arms, legs, or head, and typically occur during the first few years of SLE. Brain MRI and CT are usually normal. These episodes may last several weeks and often resolve with no treatment. However, sometimes steroids and neurologic medicines are needed. There are other movement disorders, but they are so rare that we omit them.

APS rarely causes movement disorders, but if it does, they are treated with blood thinners (chapter 9).

1. Tremors in people with SLE are most commonly due to other causes, such as medications, smoking, or caffeine.

2. The most common NPSLE movement disorder is chorea, which causes uncontrollable, sudden movements of the arms, legs, or head and is treated with steroids. However, it often resolves without treatment.

3. Antiphospholipid antibodies can be associated with NPSLE movement disorders.

Myelitis and Myelopathy

Myelo- comes from the Greek word for both "spinal cord" and "bone marrow." *-Pathy* comes from the Greek word for "disease" or "suffering." "Myelopathy" refers to abnormalities of the spinal cord. Other terms for lupus myelopathy include "lupus myelitis," "longitudinal myelitis," and "transverse myelitis." Although myelitis and myelopathy are commonly used interchangeably, "myelitis" refers specifically to spinal cord disease arising from inflammation. It is the preferred term in SLE.

Lupus myelitis, though rare and often severe, is potentially reversible with treatment. Myelitis is included as one of the classification criteria for SLE (chapter 1).

Vertebrae (plural of vertebra) are the bones that make up the spine. The thoracic vertebrae are those attached to the ribs and are numbered 1 to 12 (abbreviated T1 to T12), starting at the top. The peripheral nerves originate from the spine and exit below their corresponding vertebra. These are called spinal nerves. For example, the nerves that leave the spinal cord from underneath the T12 vertebra are labeled the left and right T12 spinal nerves. These spinal nerves originate from a segment of the spinal cord located higher than the vertebra. These spinal cord segments (T1 to T12) can be identified on MRI.

Short segment transverse myelitis involves one or two spinal cord areas (such as thoracic levels 8 and 9, T8–T9). Longitudinally extensive transverse myelitis is used if the injury involves at least three spinal nerve areas (for example, T8–T10). Around 30% of lupus spinal cord myelitis are short, while 70% of cases are long. Those with the long type tend to have more severe nerve problems.

Myelitis disrupts communication between the brain and anything below the damaged area, causing paralysis and numbness below this level. Loss of bowel and bladder control may occur. For example, in longitudinal myelitis T8–T10, the spinal nerves below T10 cannot function (can't relay messages to the brain and vice versa). The T8 to T10 spinal nerves may or may not function well (depends on the damage severity). Since the T10 spinal nerves convey sensation from the belly button to around the back, the result would be leg weakness and decreased feeling below the belly button, or, if severe, complete loss of feeling below the belly button and leg paralysis (paraplegia). If myelitis developed in the neck (cervical area), paralysis of the arms and legs (quadriplegia or tetraplegia) could be the result.

Lupus myelitis is a medical emergency requiring quick diagnosis and treatment to prevent bladder and bowel function loss with permanent limb paralysis. The symptoms are profound, and it would be unusual for someone not to seek medical attention at once.

Brain and spine MRI is needed to show the damaged area. The MRI can look for other potential causes such as cancer, infection, bulging discs, and spinal cord bleeding. A spinal tap can ensure that there is no infection, cancer, or multiple sclerosis (MS). Telling the difference between lupus myelitis and MS can be challenging, since both SLE and MS both can have similar MRI and CSF results. But SLE patients with myelitis usually also have severe, active lupus involvement in other areas. Testing for aquaporin-4 (AQP4) antibodies should also be done (discussed below).

Lupus myelitis (not due to NMOSD) is often treated immediately with IV high-dose steroids plus cyclophosphamide. Early use of plasma exchange may help some patients, especially if NMO-IgG positive.

After initial treatment, maintenance therapy is continued using an immunosuppressant medicine to prevent a recurrence. How long the immunosuppressant should be continued is unknown. Some experts recommend at least five years for NMO spectrum disorder (discussed below) because most patients have recurrent attacks without

Cyclophosphamide and bladder problems

Cyclophosphamide (CYC) can become concentrated inside the bladder causing bleeding (hemorrhagic cystitis) and increase the risk of bladder cancer. Therefore, in people who must self-catheterize their urinary bladder, it is important to empty the bladder with a catheter more often than usual if receiving CYC.

treatment. In particular, the presence of AQP4 antibodies is associated with an elevated risk of further attacks.

Between 50% and 75% of patients have full recovery (depending upon the treatment center). The rest are left with various degrees of paralysis, numbness, and bladder control problems. Some are left with complete paralysis. Patients who become bedridden are at high risk of blood clots, bedsores, and infections. Before permanent spinal cord damage occurs, patients treated most quickly do best. Younger patients, those with a high fever, or more spinal cord involvement, tend to do worse.

If APS is playing a role, MRI would show an area of dead spinal cord tissue (spinal cord infarction), and the patient would be aPL antibody–positive. In addition to the immunosuppressant therapies described above, blood thinners, such as heparin and warfarin, may be needed.

Neuromyelitis Optica Spectrum Disorders (NMOSD)

NMOSD used to be called Devic disease, named after the doctor who described it. It involves myelitis and optic nerve (the main eye nerves) inflammation (called optic neuritis). Myelitis and optic neuritis can also be seen in MS. So, NMOSD can sometimes be mistaken for MS. It is caused by an autoantibody that attacks a critical protein called aquaporin-4 (AQP4). AQP4 is found on central nervous system cell surfaces, particularly on cells called astrocytes that supply structural support to electrical nerve cells. AQP4 regulates water flow in and out of astrocytes, and this water flow is needed for proper nerve function. Most NMOSD patients have autoantibodies called AQP4-IgG antibodies (also called neuromyelitis optica-IgG or NMO-IgG antibodies). When these antibodies attack AQP4 on nerve cells, cellular water flow is disrupted, causing nerve damage.

All SLE patients with spinal cord problems should be checked for NMO-IgG antibodies. They can be negative initially, so they should be repeated. Patients who are persistently negative for NMO-IgG antibodies are labeled as having seronegative NMOSD.

When optic neuritis occurs, patients can experience eye pain that worsens with eye movement, as well as blurred vision, sometimes described as "looking through frosted glass." This most commonly occurs in one eye at a time but can progress to both eyes. Permanent vision loss can occur without prompt treatment. Although the optic nerve is the brain's primary target, the autoantibodies can attack other areas, causing nausea, vomiting, hiccups, confusion, incoordination, and breathing problems.

NMOSD myelitis usually affects three or more spinal levels (longitudinally extensive transverse myelitis). This can occur over hours to days, causing leg paralysis, lower body numbness, bladder problems, and painful muscle spasms.

NMOSD myelitis appears to be a distinct autoimmune disease. Most NMOSD patients do not have SLE, and the autoantibody anti-IgG-NMO is unique for NMOSD. SLE patients with this antibody usually have an overlap syndrome (chapter 2) with NMOSD. This is different from the other myelopathies discussed, which are most likely due to SLE attacking the spinal cord.

Plasma exchange (plasmapheresis) can remove NMO-IgG antibodies and is considered an important treatment that should be given immediately along with high-dose IV corticosteroids, which is followed by rituximab (Rituxan), or an FDA-approved NMOSD drug, such as eculizumab (Soliris), inebilizumab (Uplizna) or satralizumab (Enspryng). Eculizumab, inebilizumab, satralizumab are not discussed in this book as they are rarely used in SLE (as of 2023).

Tocilizumab (Xeljanz) proved to be superior to azathioprine in patients who failed standard therapies (such as rituximab).

Other immunosuppressants that may be useful in patients who fail these treatments include azathioprine (Imuran), cyclophosphamide, and mycophenolate mofetil (CellCept).

In a 2019 Mexican study at a center specializing in myelitis, over 90% of their patients achieved partial remission, and over 50% complete remission. If attacks are severe or treatment is delayed, paralysis, numbness, or decreased vision (even blindness) can be permanent. NMOSD can also be deadly if it affects breathing.

KEY POINTS TO REMEMBER

1. Spinal cord inflammation from SLE is called lupus myelitis. A particular overlap syndrome with an autoimmune disease called NMOSD causes severe spinal cord inflammation.

2. Lupus myelitis is rare and can be devastating.

3. Myelitis can cause numbness in the lower part of the body on both sides, urination problems, and leg paralysis on both sides (paraplegia) or all four limbs (quadriplegia).

4. Lupus myelitis treatment depends on accurately identifying the underlying cause. Inflammatory spinal cord disease is treated with long-term immunosuppressants.

5. NMOSD is treated with plasma exchange with high-dose IV steroids followed by rituximab, eculizumab, inebilizumab, or satralizumab. Tocilizumab is another choice.

6. Spinal cord infarction due to APS is treated with blood thinners.

7. Unfortunately, many patients do not return to their usual selves.

8. If NMOSD is not identified and treated rapidly, it can result in blindness, permanent paralysis, and numbness.

Seizure Disorders

Seizures (also called epilepsy) are due to repeated episodes of abnormal electrical brain activity. The symptoms depend on which part of the brain is affected. It is one of the most common NPSLE problems, occurring in approximately 10% of SLE patients. They occur more often in SLE patients of African descent. Seizures are one of the SLE classification criteria (chapter 1).

Many people think that seizures cause a person's body to shake uncontrollably, bite their tongue, and become unconscious. This certainly can happen and is called a generalized tonic-clonic seizure. However, there are numerous other types, and many do not cause loss of consciousness. Sometimes only one part of the body will shake. Some seizures do not cause abnormal movements but may cause the person to experience hallucinations—see, hear, or even smell things that are not actually present.

Infections, stroke, drugs, cancer, high blood pressure, and metabolic problems (such as diabetes, low sodium, or low calcium) can cause seizures. Blood tests, lumbar puncture (spinal tap), and brain MRI are needed to determine the cause. An EEG (electroencephalogram) is also done. This is a special test, usually done by a neurologist (a nerve specialist), in which electrodes are attached to various parts of the head to monitor the brain's electrical activity, including seizure activity.

Accurately diagnosing a seizure is essential. Medical conditions, such as heart conditions, can mimic seizures and vice versa. Involving a neurologist in the evaluation is critical.

Lupus can cause seizures in many ways. If a neurologist thinks that seizures might recur, then treatment with anti-seizure drugs may be needed. Examples of such drugs are lamotrigine (Lamictal), carbamazepine (Tegretol), levetiracetam (Keppra), phenytoin (Dilantin), clonazepam (Klonopin), gabapentin (Neurontin), topiramate (Topamax), and pregabalin (Lyrica).

Neurologists base treatment on factors such as drug interactions, MRI and EEG findings, pregnancy safety, and whether the seizures start in a single place in the brain or arise spontaneously all over.

In rare cases, some anti-seizure medicines can cause drug-induced lupus in people without SLE. They do not appear to worsen lupus in those who already have SLE.

Seizures can be due to lupus inflammation. When this occurs, SLE is usually active elsewhere (such as arthritis, pleurisy, rash). Seizures due to inflammation are treated with immunosuppressants.

In some cases, a tiny area of permanent brain damage, such as scarring from earlier lupus inflammation or an earlier CVA (stroke), can create a seizure focus or an epileptic nidus (*nidus* comes from the Latin word for "nest" and refers to a place where something originates). This nidus can cause recurrent brain nerve irritation, resulting in seizures. Focal seizures usually do not cause loss of consciousness (as do generalized seizures). However, the person may not respond to others and may stare into space. Special brain scans and electrical recordings are sometimes done to identify where this nidus is located.

In APS, brain blood clots can cause seizures, and blood thinners are used.

Hydroxychloroquine reduces the risk for seizures. This may be due to its ability to reduce SLE inflammation, as well as to lower the risk of blood clots.

Thrombotic microangiopathy (such as TTP; chapter 9) and PRES (discussed below) can also cause seizures.

After treatment, some SLE patients can stop anti-seizure medications, while others need to stay on them for a long time. Seizure patients should not drive unless they have been free of seizures for at least several months.

KEY POINTS TO REMEMBER

1. Seizures (epilepsy) are due to uncontrollable, repetitive electrical activity in the brain. They can cause many problems such as loss of consciousness, jerking movements, twitching, and hallucinations.

2. Seizures are one of the classification criteria for SLE.

3. Seizures caused by lupus inflammation are treated with immunosuppressants.

4. Hydroxychloroquine can reduce seizure risk.

5. If the seizures are due to blood clots, they are treated with blood thinners, such as heparin and warfarin (Coumadin).

6. Seizures can be difficult to diagnose and treat. A neurologist should be consulted.

Acute Confusional State

Acute confusional state is also called delirium or acute encephalopathy (*encephalo-* from the Greek word for "brain," *-pathy* for "suffering"). It often occurs suddenly, and it can vary from mild drowsiness at one end of the spectrum or complete coma (unable to be awakened) on the other. If awake, the person has difficulty focusing and has problems answering questions appropriately. They do not respond appropriately to the environment and other people. It is included as one of the classification criteria for SLE (chapter 1).

It is usually seen in someone with a severe lupus flare and significant brain inflammation. Doctors usually need to order many tests to ensure there are no other causes,

---

LUPUS IN FOCUS

One treatment approach for severe, refractory NPSLE

Dr. Sterling West, a well-regarded rheumatologist and author of *Rheumatology Secrets*, suggests the following regimen for severe NPSLE:

- IV pulse methylprednisolone (SOLU-Medrol) 1,000 mg daily × 3 days
- Then the Euro-Lupus cyclophosphamide regimen (chapter 12)
- Then IV rituximab (Rituxan) 1,000 mg the day after the first and second doses of cyclophosphamide
- Mycophenolate (CellCept) maintenance therapy 2 weeks after the last cyclophosphamide dose, gradually increasing the amount to 1.5 gm bid over 2–4 weeks

such as infection, medicines, metabolic issues, or TTP (chapter 9). Antibodies against brain proteins such as NMDA-receptors can also cause similar symptoms. For these reasons, thorough testing, including MRI of the brain, blood tests, and a lumbar puncture, is usually needed.

There is very little evidence to guide treatment, and sometimes it resolves on its own. Many doctors use immunosuppressants, IVIG, or plasma exchange (chapter 35).

KEY POINTS TO REMEMBER

1. Acute confusional state (delirium, acute encephalopathy) in SLE can have many potential causes. Its effects include difficulty thinking and responding appropriately to the environment.

2. It is essential to rule out other causes, such as brain infection.

3. Acute confusional state is one of the SLE classification criteria.

4. Acute confusional states require detailed neurological investigation. Treatment is targeted at the underlying cause.

5. Acute confusional state due to lupus inflammation is treated with immunosuppressants, IVIG, and plasma exchange.

Posterior Reversible Encephalopathy Syndrome (PRES)

The name of this condition comes from brain MRI findings. The brain MRI in PRES most commonly shows brain tissue swelling (edema) in the posterior (back) brain. It is reversible (goes away with treatment) most of the time, but not always. "Encephalopathy" refers to the brain not working correctly. The name "posterior *reversible* encephalopathy syndrome" can be misleading because it does not always go away (it can occasionally be irreversible). It can also occur in other areas of the brain (not always in the back).

PRES goes by many other names, including "reversible posterior leukoencephalopathy syndrome" (*leuko-* comes from the Greek for "white"; it tends to affect the white colored parts of the brain), "brain capillary leak syndrome," "posterior leukoencephalopathy syndrome," "posterior reversible encephalopathy syndrome," and "reversible posterior cerebral edema syndrome." Uncontrolled high blood pressure is the leading cause, in which case, some doctors call it "hypertensive encephalopathy."

PRES is not included in the ACR list of NPSLE syndromes. However, it is important to mention since it can occur in SLE. It can cause many earlier mentioned problems, including seizures (75% of patients), headaches, and delirium. It occurs in SLE and other autoimmune diseases, kidney disease, cancer, infections, during pregnancy, and from medications. Anything that can cause an abnormal fluid leakage within the brain can cause it.

Around 90% of PRES patients have uncontrolled high blood pressure. Blood pressure control is one of the essential treatments.

Some of the lupus drugs that may cause PRES include tacrolimus, IVIG, methotrexate, and rituximab. In 80% of patients with drug-induced PRES, symptoms begin within two weeks of starting the drug. However, 20% of the time, PRES starts weeks to months afterward. When a medication causes PRES, the treatment of choice is to stop the medicine.

If lupus brain inflammation (cerebritis or vasculitis) causes PRES, immunosuppressants are needed. Since PRES can resolve relatively rapidly, it is recommended not to increase immunosuppressant therapy during the first few days. Instead, we monitor the patient, treat high blood pressure, and treat any seizures if they occur. PRES usually resolves with these interventions.

When a brain MRI is repeated after treatment, it usually shows partial to complete swelling (edema) resolution. However, occasionally there can be permanent brain damage.

PRES is often described as benign, meaning that it is not a harmful medical condition, but this is misleading. Several studies have shown high death rates of around 30% in SLE patients who develop PRES. Up to half of these occur within the first three months of the event, especially in those with severe SLE and uncontrolled high blood pressure.

Anxiety Disorder

Excessive worrying is the predominant symptom of anxiety. It is often accompanied by feeling nervous or "on edge," decreased appetite, difficulty relaxing or sitting still, and being easily annoyed, irritable, or moody. The person with anxiety disorder may have trouble sleeping, with their mind racing, recalling troubling things from the past and worrying about the future. Untreated anxiety can cause chronic pain. It is not uncommon to have anxiety disorder and depression; many of their treatments are similar.

Around one-third of SLE patients will have anxiety, which is common in chronic illnesses (disorders that last a long time). If symptoms are moderate to severe, affect the person's quality of life, impact relationships, or cause other significant problems—such as insomnia, fatigue, memory problems, and pain—the anxiety is a health problem. At the extreme, panic attacks, with sudden chest pain episodes, shortness of breath, heart palpitations, sweating, dizziness, and a general sense of doom, may occur. Some people develop phobias, such as a fear of being in public.

Anxiety often worsens when lupus gets worse and improves when lupus gets better. Patients who do not understand SLE and its treatment tend to have worse anxiety than those who educate themselves. By reading this book and learning about what aspects of lupus management are in your control, you are taking one step in the right direction in reducing anxiety.

Lupus experts do not believe that lupus inflammation causes anxiety.

Some drugs can cause anxiety. The anxiety feelings typically begin soon after starting the medicine. Some anxiety-causing substances include thyroid medications, steroids (such as prednisone), ADHD drugs, albuterol (used for asthma and COPD), phenytoin (Dilantin, used for seizures), alcohol, caffeine, and illicit drugs. The offending drug is usually stopped, or the dosage is lowered.

To see whether you have an anxiety disorder, take a self-survey, such as the GAD-7 (Generalized Anxiety Disorder-7) questionnaire (table 13.3). If you score five or higher, you may have an anxiety disorder, and you should show the results to your doctor.

Table 13.3 GAD-7 (Anxiety Screening Test)

Circle the appropriate number to the right of each list of problems.
Add up each column of numbers; then add the column totals to get your total score.
If you score 5 points or higher, you may have an anxiety disorder.

Over the last two weeks, how often have you had the following problems?	Not at All	Several Days	More than Half the Days	Nearly Every Day
Feeling nervous, anxious, or on edge	0	1	2	3
Not being able to stop or control worrying	0	1	2	3
Worrying too much about different things	0	1	2	3
Having trouble relaxing	0	1	2	3
Being so restless that it is hard to sit still	0	1	2	3
Becoming easily annoyed or irritable	0	1	2	3
Feeling afraid as if something awful might happen	0	1	2	3
Column totals Total score = _____	_____	+ _____	+ _____	+ _____

LUPUS IN FOCUS

Attention deficit and hyperactivity disorder (ADHD)

A 2013 State University of New York study found elevated rates of ADHD in their SLE patients compared to the general population. ADHD can negatively impact the quality of life, so this subject should be investigated further.

Psychological counseling can help. Counselors include sociologists, psychologists, and psychiatrists. A counselor can help people learn new coping skills for SLE, interacting more appropriately with others, and handling stress (chapter 38). These coping strategies are also called cognitive behavioral therapy, or CBT. People who learn and practice good disease coping techniques (chapter 44) do better in the long term.

Regularly practicing mindfulness helps (see chapter 39).

Regular aerobic exercise may be as helpful as medications, so it is essential to exercise regularly (chapters 7 and 38).

Many people improve significantly using medications that adjust the brain's chemical imbalances. Most of these medications are also listed as antidepressants. Selective serotonin reuptake inhibitors (SSRIs) such as sertraline, paroxetine, and fluoxetine are considered the first-line therapies.

KEY POINTS TO REMEMBER

1. Anxiety disorder causes excessive worrying and racing thoughts, often accompanied by a feeling of being on edge, moodiness, insomnia, and fatigue.

2. Anxiety disorder can sometimes be accompanied by panic attacks, with shortness of breath, chest pain, palpitations, sweating, and a general sense of doom.

3. Take the GAD-7 self-survey (table 13.3). If you score 5 points or higher, you may have an anxiety disorder, and you should show your doctor the results.

4. Treatment options include counseling, mindfulness, regular aerobic exercise, and SSRIs.

Cognitive Dysfunction

"Cognitive dysfunction" refers to having problems with memory, paying attention, problem-solving, understanding language, planning, and self-control. It can also be accompanied by problems with judgment, abstract thinking, and personality changes. Its mildest form is commonly called mild cognitive impairment. Patients often call this "lupus fog," and it can fluctuate over time. In severe form, serious memory impairment, including dementia, may occur. Formal neuropsychiatric testing shows that up to half of SLE patients have cognitive dysfunction. Memory problems can be devastating, causing difficulties with jobs, social interactions, and family, while also significantly affecting quality of life.

In people with CNS neuropsychiatric lupus (such as stroke, meningitis, seizures, or acute confusional state), residual cognitive dysfunction from an earlier brain injury is common.

Problems that can cause cognitive dysfunction in SLE include thyroid disease, low vitamin B12, depression, anxiety disorder, fibromyalgia, steroids, and lack of sleep. The doctor attempts to figure out any potentially treatable causes for cognitive dysfunction, such as depression.

Suppose you have significant memory problems, and your lupus is not particularly active. In that case, your doctor may test for treatable causes such as thyroid disease and low vitamin B12.

If those are not found, depression, anxiety disorder, and fibromyalgia are common causes. You can take self-surveys for fibromyalgia (chapter 27), anxiety (table 13.3), sleep apnea (table 6.4), or depression (table 13.5). One study showed that close to one-third of patients with recently diagnosed SLE and cognitive dysfunction also had depression. If any of these causes are found, it should be treated.

Table 13.4 Coping with Memory Problems

- Exercise regularly. This is your most important tool.
- Do not multitask. Concentrate on one activity.
- Eliminate clutter. Throw away or give away excessive objects and papers.
- Keep organized.
- Carry a small notepad. Take notes frequently and review later.
- Use sticky notes; put them in places to help you remember.
- Keep a calendar, addresses, and phone numbers with you (use your smartphone contacts)
- Ask that only one person speaks during conversations.
- During a conversation, concentrate on listening. Do nothing else (such as eating, looking at your cell phone, newspaper). Do not think about what to say back to the person.
- Do not be afraid to ask people to repeat themselves.
- Repeat things out loud or in your head. When you meet someone, say the person's name in your mind repeatedly; repeat their name in the conversation.
- "Train the brain": do mental exercises such as crosswords, Solitaire, Scrabble, or Sudoku daily.
- Read memory improvement books such as *The Memory Book* by Harry Lorayne.
- Keep your mind active: volunteer, don't retire.
- Challenge your brain by learning new skills, hobbies.
- Increase interactions to stimulate your mind by making new friendships and relationships.
- Get treatment for memory problem disorders. Take the self-surveys for anxiety disorder (table 13.3), depression (table 13.5), and obstructive sleep apnea (table 6.4).
- Decrease stress. Learn to say "no" when asked to do favors if you are a "yes" person.
- Be open about your memory problems with others so they can understand and help.
- Get plenty of sleep. Practice sleep hygiene techniques (chapter 6).
- Get professional help (neuropsychologist, vocational counselor, cognitive therapist, or occupational therapist) specializing in cognitive rehabilitation.
- If it is causing problems at work, contact the Job Accommodation Network (www.askjan.org) to understand your rights (under the Americans with Disabilities Act).

A 2016 Taiwanese study showed that SLE patients were twice as likely to develop dementia as the general Taiwanese population. Many SLE patients develop peripheral vascular disease (PVD, hardening of the arteries, chapter 21) at a younger age than people without SLE. This can sometimes lead to "vascular dementia" from decreased brain blood supply. The Taiwanese researchers thought this could be a reason for increased dementia in SLE.

The researchers also pointed out that other studies have shown that parts of SLE patients' brains tend to shrink in size faster than they should. In particular, the hippocampus and amygdala, parts of the brain that are important for memory, become smaller. Therefore, this could also explain memory problems.

Two 2012 studies from the University of California, San Francisco, found that 15% of their SLE patients had memory problems. High blood pressure, obesity, history of stroke, not exercising, and being aPL antibody–positive were more common in these patients. These findings support the Taiwanese study regarding peripheral vascular disease (PVD, hardening of the arteries, chapter 21) playing a role.

To reduce memory problems, SLE patients should reduce PVD risks by eating a healthy diet, exercising, reducing cholesterol, maintaining a healthy body weight, and not smoking (chapter 21).

Another possible cause is that an anti-dsDNA antibody called an anti-NMDA receptor antibody can cause brain cell death. A mouse study showed that these antibodies caused damage to mice hippocampus, resulting in memory problems.

Antiphospholipid (aPL) antibodies may be responsible for cognitive dysfunction in some people. APL antibodies may damage brain cells directly, and they can cause brain blood clots. A 2005 NIH study showed that SLE patients who took low-dose aspirin had some improvements in memory. However, more extensive studies are needed regarding aPL antibodies and cognitive dysfunction.

Anti-ribosomal-P has also been suggested as a possible brain cell damaging antibody. However, further studies are needed.

One interesting approach is the blood pressure-lowering drug captopril, an angiotensin-converting enzyme inhibitor. An angiotensin II molecule produced in our bodies can interact with brain cells called microglia, causing inflammation and leading to a loss of nerve cells and memory problems. Captopril can cross the blood-brain barrier, enter the brain, and stop this action.

LUPUS IN FOCUS

Drugs can cause memory loss and other cognitive problems

Drugs that can cause cognitive problems include pain medications, anti-seizure medicines (especially Topamax), beta-blockers (for blood pressure), antihistamines, antidepressants (especially tricyclic antidepressants such as amitriptyline), benzodiazepines (such as Valium), incontinence drugs (such as Ditropan, Oxytrol, and Detrol), statins (primarily simvastatin and atorvastatin), and sleeping aids. Ask your doctor about temporarily stopping any of these to see if memory improves.

Researchers at the Feinstein Institute for Medical Research in New York studied mice with lupus autoantibodies, called anti-DNRAbs, which attack brain cells and cause memory problems. Mice treated with captopril showed decreased brain nerve cell loss. They also did better than mice treated with enalapril, an ACEi unable to cross the blood-brain barrier. Other studies suggest that ACEi drugs may slow memory loss in Alzheimer's disease (a severe dementia). Note that captopril is not a proven remedy. However, this research is intriguing.

Alzheimer's has not been shown to occur more often in SLE patients than in others.

Drugs for memory problems in dementia have not been proven helpful in SLE cognitive dysfunction. A Johns Hopkins Hospital (Baltimore, Maryland) study found no benefit for memory in SLE patients using the Alzheimer's drug memantine (Namenda).

A memory specialist can help you learn how to cope with forgetfulness by using special techniques. You can also do things on your own to improve your memory (table 13.4).

One key recommendation is regular exercise. Studies consistently show the importance of exercise and its role in cognitive dysfunction, especially preventing dementias like Alzheimer's. Lupus experts do not know why exercise is essential for good memory and thinking abilities. It may very well play a role in the maintenance of adequate brain blood supply. Read chapters 7 and 38 about exercise.

Illustrating the importance of exercise, a 2012 study evaluated 138 women with SLE and found that only 5% of physically active women had cognitive dysfunction. In contrast, 23% of sedentary (non-exercising) women had significant memory problems. The women with cognitive dysfunction were also more likely to be obese.

Some studies suggest that healthy dietary habits, such as eating a Mediterranean-style diet (chapter 38), may help slow down memory loss and cognitive decline. A 2020 research report evaluated close to 10,000 people aged 50 to 85 and showed that those who closely followed a Mediterranean diet (especially fish consumption), had the highest cognition scores.

No vitamins or supplements have been shown to improve memory. Be skeptical of the memory improvement claims made by supplement manufacturers.

Brain games (such as lumosity.com) that are touted to exercise the brain have been popular. Although they promote themselves as helping with memory and quote small, uncontrolled studies, these games have not yet been proven to help with memory.

Fortunately, SLE cognitive dysfunction can improve. A 2018 Italian study showed that 21% of their SLE patients had cognitive dysfunction. Over a ten-year period, 50% improved, while 10% worsened. Only 13% were affected at ten years. An earlier Canadian study that followed SLE patients for five years showed similar numbers.

LUPUS IN FOCUS

Exercise directly improves brain activity and test scores

Professor Charles Hill at the University of Illinois showed that children who walked on a treadmill for 20 minutes performed better on memory and attention span tests (done right after exercise) than those who did not exercise.

1. Cognitive dysfunction involves difficulties with memory, attention, problem-solving, understanding language, planning, self-control, judgment, and abstract thinking.

2. Cognitive dysfunction is a common problem in SLE.

3. Cognitive dysfunction can be caused by depression, anxiety, fibromyalgia, medications, sleep disorders, or thyroid problems.

4. Take the self-surveys for fibromyalgia (chapter 27), anxiety (table 13.3), sleep apnea (table 6.4), and depression (table 13.5) if you have cognitive dysfunction.

5. Treatment is aimed at the cause of the memory problem (such as treating depression).

6. Seeing someone experienced in memory problems (like psychologists and neurologists) and attending clinics specializing in dementia or closed brain injuries can help.

7. Do everything in table 13.4. It is especially crucial to exercise regularly.

8. Cognitive dysfunction tends to improve in many SLE patients over time.

Mood Disorders (Depression, Mania, and Bipolar Disorder)

Mood disorders include depression, mania, and bipolar disorder and are some of the most common neuropsychiatric problems in SLE. This includes children with SLE, who tend to have depression more frequently than young adults.

Discoid lupus patients (chapter 8) are five times more likely to have moderate to severe depression than people without lupus. SLE patients with Sjögren's disease overlap (chapter 14) are three times more likely to have depression than SLE patients who do not.

Research suggests that depression in SLE is most often related to dealing with a chronic disease, taking multiple medications, and avoiding sunlight.

Low body image appears to be a major contributor. A 2019 US study followed 135 SLE patients over 17 years. One-quarter of them had had problems with depression, and half of those depression events could be attributed to low self-body image. It is common for lupus patients not to like the way they look due to weight gain from prednisone, hair loss, permanent pigment changes, skin scarring, and finger joint deformities from lupus arthritis.

There is much ongoing research to understand if inflammatory molecules contribute to depression. These include the study of cytokines such as interferon-alpha, IL-6, and antibodies (such as anti-ribosomal-P) binding to brain cells. If specific causes such as these are identified, this research could help us figure out treatments for SLE-associated depression.

Depression is the most common psychological problem in lupus. People with depression may feel "down in the dumps" or "have the blues." They often have insomnia and may have increased or decreased appetite, causing weight changes. They often

LUPUS IN FOCUS

Depression may trigger SLE (or vice versa)

The Nurses' Healthy Studies I and II tracked close to 200,000 nurses over 20 years and showed that depressed nurses developed SLE 3 times more often than non-depressed nurses. Just as stress appears to be a trigger for SLE, depression may be as well. Another possibility is that the depression could have been an early warning sign of SLE. In other words, the depression may be caused by SLE.

withdraw from social situations. People with depression may have memory problems and become afraid of developing dementia or Alzheimer's disease. Many depressed people will stop doing activities that they find enjoyable (called anhedonia) and often lose interest in sex (reduced libido). Many people with depression also have feelings of guilt above and beyond what is rational.

Depression can cause problems that the person may not even realize are due to depression, such as body pain, severe fatigue, and stomach upset. Extremely depressed people may feel like it is not worth living and feel like they cannot go on. They may even consider suicide.

Depressed people are more apt to be nonadherent in their lupus treatment. SLE patients with severe depression are four times more likely not to take their drugs than those with mild depression. This leads to a higher rate of severe lupus complications.

Identifying and treating depression in SLE patients are essential. It does not always correlate with lupus severity and can be more disabling than lupus itself. It can be a significant cause of memory problems, insomnia, pain, and reduced life quality.

It is common for people with depression to resist diagnosis and treatment. It is easier to blame their lupus, stress, or pain as the cause of their depression than to realize that it may be the depression causing their pain, fatigue, and insomnia.

A 2011 study in the journal *Lupus*, which evaluated 125 SLE patients, reported that they were more apt to have a poor quality of life from depression rather than from lupus. In this situation, getting their lupus under better control would not necessarily help them feel better, so treating the depression would be a priority.

Depression is underdiagnosed and undertreated in SLE. If you have memory problems, we encourage you to take the depression screening test called the PHQ-9 (Patient Health Questionnaire-9) depression questionnaire (table 13.5). A score of 5 or higher suggests you may have depression; 10 or above suggests major depression. If you score 5 or higher, you should show your doctor the results.

If you have any thoughts of hurting yourself or others, please immediately contact your doctor. In the United States, call the Suicide Hotline at 800-273-8255. Suicide and injuring others are two of the most dangerous complications of severe depression and are avoidable with treatment.

If the self-survey test indicates that you may have depression, first consider exercising for treatment. Regular aerobic exercise (chapters 7 and 38) can be as effective as antidepressants.

Table 13.5 PHQ-9 Depression Questionnaire

Circle the corresponding number score to the right of each list of columns.
Add up the circled numbers in each column, then total these results.
A score of 5–9 suggests mild depression; a score of ≥ 10 suggests major depression.

Over the last two weeks, how often have you had the following problems?	Not at All	Several Days	More than Half the Days	Nearly Every Day
Little interest or pleasure in doing things	0	1	2	3
Feeling down, depressed, or hopeless	0	1	2	3
Trouble falling or staying asleep or sleeping too much	0	1	2	3
Feeling tired or having little energy	0	1	2	3
Poor appetite or overeating	0	1	2	3
Feeling bad about yourself or that you are a failure or have let yourself or your family down	0	1	2	3
Trouble concentrating on reading the newspaper, watching television, or the like	0	1	2	3
Moving or speaking so slowly that other people could have noticed; or the opposite, being unusually fidgety or restless	0	1	2	3
Having thoughts that you would be better off dead or of hurting yourself in some way	0	1	2	3
Column totals Total score = _____	_____	+_____	+_____	+_____

As with anxiety disorder, psychotherapy and cognitive behavioral therapy (CBT) can help. Psychotherapy and CBT are as beneficial as taking antidepressants. Around 41% of patients go into remission with CBT. A significant advantage over medicine is that the positive effects last much longer after stopping CBT.

If depression significantly affects your quality of life, there are numerous antidepressants available (too many to discuss). If you are affected by depression, consult your rheumatologist or primary care provider for help.

In cases where the depression is caused by or worsened by steroids (such as prednisone), it is important to try to lower the dosage. This should always be done under the direct supervision of your doctor. Too rapid a taper could cause a lupus flare or adrenal insufficiency (chapter 26).

Mania and hypomania (a milder version of mania) are the opposite of depression. These mood disorders cause excessive happiness, or euphoria, and make people feel like they are on top of the world. They may need little sleep and have lots of energy. Other signs are moodiness, unusually increased sexual desire, aggressive behavior, and religiosity (excessive religious thoughts). The most common cause of mania and hypomania in SLE patients is steroids. Just as with steroid-induced depression, steroid-induced mania gets better on lower doses.

Even without steroids, mania and hypomania occur more commonly in SLE patients than in those without SLE. Mania more commonly occurs as part of bipolar disorder (rather than occurring alone). In bipolar disorder, there are alternating episodes of depression and mania or hypomania. Bipolar disorder is not nearly as common in SLE as depression. It is essential for bipolar disorder patients to take medications regularly, although unlike depression and anxiety disorder, non-drug treatments are rarely sufficient, and psychiatric care is often needed.

KEY POINTS TO REMEMBER

1. Mood disorders include depression on one end of the spectrum and elevated mood (mania and hypomania as a part of bipolar disorder) on the other.

2. Mood disorders are brain chemical imbalance disorders. They are probably not due to lupus inflammation.

3. Depression is a common cause of fatigue, memory problems, and pain. The depression needs to be treated to help with those symptoms.

4. Take a self-survey (table 13.5) to see if you may be depressed.

5. If you have suicidal thoughts or think about injuring others, contact your doctor right away, go to an urgent care center, or call the Suicide Hotline at 800-273-8255

6. Perform regular aerobic exercise or consider seeing a counselor specializing in depression. Antidepressants may be needed.

7. Many people with mood disorders do not realize they have it.

8. People with bipolar disorder need to take medications regularly.

Psychosis

Psychosis is characterized by disordered and bizarre thinking, including delusions and hallucinations. Delusion refers to believing that something is occurring when reality shows otherwise. Classic examples include thinking that people, such as CIA agents, are out to get you or that you are someone else, such as Napoleon or Albert Einstein. Hallucinations are when a person senses things that are not actually present. These can occur with any of the senses. For example, you may hear voices that are not there, see things that are not there, smell unusual smells that are not present, or believe that snakes are crawling under your skin. Psychosis can present along with an acute confusional state (discussed earlier). Psychosis is one of the SLE classification criteria (chapter 1).

Around 2% of SLE patients have psychosis, most commonly within the first three years, especially the first year. It occurs more often in men, those of African ancestry, and younger patients.

NMDA-R antibodies and other antibodies, such as anti-ribosomal-P, can bind to brain cells and alter behavior. If psychosis occurs with other neurological features, such as movement disorders and seizures, NMDA-R antibodies should be evaluated in the blood and cerebrospinal fluid (from a spinal tap).

Lupus psychosis is treated with immunosuppressants. Psychiatric medications used to treat psychotic conditions, such as schizophrenia (a psychiatric disease), are often needed.

Illicit drugs (cocaine, Ecstasy, methamphetamines, and the like) can cause psychosis.

So can steroids (such as prednisone), especially in high doses. Reducing the dose helps, but this can be challenging because most people with SLE psychosis have lupus affecting other areas (such as rash, arthritis, or pleurisy) and so they may need the steroids. In this case, antipsychotic drugs (such as those used in schizophrenia) may be prescribed.

Fortunately, most patients do well in the long run, and most patients have only one episode.

KEY POINTS TO REMEMBER

1. Psychosis is characterized by disordered, bizarre thinking and includes problems with hallucinations and delusions.

2. Other causes of psychosis should be excluded, including medications like steroids and using illicit drugs such as cocaine.

3. If psychosis is due to SLE, immunosuppressants are needed.

4. Therapies used to treat other psychotic disorders (like schizophrenia) may be needed.

Peripheral Nervous System Disorders

While the previously discussed syndromes involve the CNS, the rest of the chapter is about the peripheral nervous system (PNS). The PNS involves all the nerves that travel between the brain and spinal cord to and from the rest of the body. It can further be divided into the somatic and autonomic nervous systems. The somatic nerves are used for purposeful movements (such as the nerves telling your muscles to move when you lift a cup of coffee). The autonomic nerves deal with involuntary activities (think of "automatic"). These include, for instance, the nerves responsible for your pupils enlarging in the dark.

Lupus can affect the PNS in many ways, but so can many non-lupus factors. These include diabetes, toxins, medications, metabolic problems, and infections such as Lyme disease. Therefore, multiple tests are often necessary. These may include blood tests, EMG with nerve conduction velocity testing (discussed under myositis in chapter 7), and sometimes a lumbar puncture.

Somatic Nervous System Disorders

Acute Inflammatory Demyelinating Polyradiculoneuropathy (Guillain-Barré Syndrome)

Acute inflammatory demyelinating polyradiculoneuropathy is a rare lupus complication. It is also called Guillain-Barré syndrome (GBS; pronounced GHEE-ahn bah-RAY). Very few cases have been reported. It occurs when there is damage to the myelin sheaths around the nerves of the peripheral nervous system. The myelin sheath is the coating surrounding nerves (like the rubber coating around an electrical cord). It allows nerves to send electrical signals faster. GBS causes weakness of the legs, arms, and sometimes the face. The autonomic nervous system, which controls blood pressure, heart rate, and gut movement, can also be affected. Physical exam shows loss of reflexes. A lumbar puncture and EMG with nerve conduction velocity testing confirm the diagnosis, and a spinal cord MRI may be needed. GBS is an autoimmune disease itself. It is unknown whether GBS is due to SLE or whether its occurrence in an SLE patient is an overlap syndrome (the presence of two autoimmune diseases in the same person).

Plasmapheresis or IVIG are the treatments of choice (chapter 35). Plasmapheresis is a highly specialized treatment usually performed at large hospitals and major medical centers. Although high-dose steroids are typically used for severe SLE nerve involvement, they should probably be avoided in GBS unless other organs are affected. Plasma exchange and IVIG are usually better than steroids. Most people recover, but it is essential to diagnose promptly since breathing, swallowing, and heart problems can occur without prompt treatment. Although GBS typically happens once and then improves, it can relapse and sometimes requires prolonged treatment.

A more chronic version of GBS called chronic inflammatory demyelinating polyradiculoneuropathy (CIDP), develops over months rather than days and requires long-term treatment. CIDP can cause permanent problems with leg and arm weakness and tingling. Lupus-associated CIDP is treated like GBS, usually with IVIG or plasmapheresis. However, cyclophosphamide and rituximab are other options.

KEY POINTS TO REMEMBER

1. Acute inflammatory demyelinating polyradiculoneuropathy is commonly known as Guillain-Barré syndrome. CIDP is a chronic, long-lasting form.

2. These are rare in SLE, causing progressive arm and leg weakness with loss of normal reflexes on physical examination.

3. They are usually treated in the hospital with IVIG or plasmapheresis.

Mononeuropathy and Mononeuritis Multiplex

When SLE attacks one large peripheral nervous system nerve, it is called mononeuropathy (*mono-* means "one"). Mononeuropathy can cause weakness and/or numbness in one body part.

One of the most common SLE mononeuropathies is carpal tunnel syndrome (CTS), which accounts for 5% to 10% of SLE peripheral neuropathies. CTS is an entrapment neuropathy, meaning that the nerve gets compressed or squeezed by a surrounding structure.

The carpal tunnel is a tight tunnel that leads from the underside of the forearm into the palm side of the wrist. The tunnel has tendons, muscles, blood vessels, and nerves. CTS is also called "median neuropathy" and "median nerve mononeuropathy," because increased pressure inside the tunnel (such as from lupus wrist arthritis or tenosynovitis, chapter 7) squeezes a nerve called the median nerve.

The median nerve is essential for feeling in the thumb, index finger, middle finger, and ring finger. CTS can cause tingling, numbness, or burning pain in these areas. This nerve is also needed for muscle strength, so hand weakness and clumsiness can occur. People sometimes feel only vague hand or wrist pain. It is diagnosed by EMG or ultrasound (chapter 7).

Treatment is similar to its treatment in non-lupus patients, including wearing carpal tunnel braces, performing hand exercises, and improving ergonomics (such as using wrists rests with the keyboard and computer mouse). Carpal tunnel cortisone injections can help, but sometimes surgery is needed.

If a large nerve coming directly from the spinal cord (called a radicular nerve) is affected, it is called a radiculopathy. It is also a type of mononeuropathy.

If SLE attacks more than one large separate nerve (occurring in different areas), it is called mononeuritis multiplex. Multiplex (*multi-* means many, and -plex comes from the Greek for "to strike") refers to more than one large nerve being affected.

"Foot drop" in one foot (not being able to raise the foot upward) while the other muscles of the legs work fine is an example. If someone has a right foot drop and inability to move the left wrist, they could have mononeuritis multiplex.

Mononeuritis multiplex is usually due to vasculitis (blood vessel inflammation) affecting the nerve blood supply, causing the nerves to not function properly and resulting in weakness and numbness. Sometimes, a nerve biopsy is needed to confirm a diagnosis of vasculitis.

It is treated with immunosuppressants or IVIG. It may take a long time to recover—up to a year before maximum improvement. Nerve damage severity and the length of time that lapses before treatment predict recovery chances. If a long time passes before treatment, or if involvement is severe, there may be permanent weakness and numbness.

Mononeuropathy and mononeuritis multiplex are SLE classification criteria (chapter 1).

KEY POINTS TO REMEMBER

1. In mononeuropathy, one large peripheral nerve is affected. One of the most common forms is foot drop with difficulty lifting the foot and walking.

2. In mononeuritis multiplex, two or more large nerves are affected.

3. Vasculitis is the most common cause of mononeuritis multiplex and is usually treated with immunosuppressants.

4. CTS is one of the most common mononeuropathies. It is treated the same way as in people who do not have lupus.

Myasthenia Gravis

Myasthenia gravis (MG) is an autoimmune disease that causes muscle weakness. It is separate from SLE. However, 1% of SLE patients have MG, while 5% of MG patients also have SLE. People with MG and SLE tend to have milder cases of SLE. For example, they are less likely to have nephritis (kidney inflammation).

In MG, the immune system usually produces acetylcholine receptor antibodies that attach to muscle cells acetylcholine receptors. This prevents much-needed acetylcholine neurotransmitters from causing muscles to contract and squeeze. These antibodies also destroy the receptors. The person with MG will have muscle weakness that worsens with each attempt to use a muscle. MG's typical symptoms include having a droopy eyelid (ptosis), double vision, and difficulty chewing and talking. For example, if the chewing muscles (masseters) are affected, eating gets harder and harder as the muscles tire.

MG is diagnosed by EMG and nerve conduction velocity tests. Acetylcholine receptor antibodies (AChR-Ab) are present in 85% of patients. In AChR-Ab-negative patients, another antibody, called the MuSK antibody, may be positive.

Some MG patients have a large thymus (an important immune system gland in the upper chest). Thymectomy (surgical thyroid gland removal) improves MG symptoms in some of these patients. However, thymectomy can sometimes worsen SLE, so close rheumatologic follow-up is important. Around 10% of MG patients have a thymoma (a thymus gland tumor), in which case, thymectomy is the treatment of choice.

KEY POINTS TO REMEMBER

1. Myasthenic gravis, an organ-specific autoimmune disease (chapter 2) that affects muscles, occurs in 1% of SLE patients.

2. It causes weakness of muscles that gets worse as the affected muscles are used.

3. If the thymus gland is enlarged, thymectomy can help. However, this can sometimes worsen SLE, so close rheumatologic follow-up is important.

LUPUS IN FOCUS

Is hydroxychloroquine safe in myasthenia gravis patients with SLE?

Myasthenia gravis (MG) has rarely occurred after starting hydroxychloroquine (HCQ, Plaquenil). While some MG experts recommend avoiding HCQ in MG patients, a 2012 French study showed that HCQ was safe to use in SLE patients with MG.

Cranial Neuropathy

The cranial nerves (arising within the skull, or cranium) are peripheral nerves that come directly from the brain. They manage blinking, smiling, tongue movement, eye movement, seeing, hearing, and similar functions. Cranial neuropathies (inflammation or damage to cranial nerves) in SLE can cause problems such as double vision, drooping of the eyes or mouth, face numbness, vision loss, vertigo (a type of dizziness), ringing in the ears, or hearing loss.

Bell's palsy is a cranial neuropathy. When it occurs in SLE, it is more appropriately called seventh cranial nerve palsy or facial nerve palsy. Facial nerve palsy causes the muscles on one side of the face to weaken and makes smiling and closing the eye difficult. Cranial neuropathy is an SLE classification criteria (chapter 1).

Other causes of cranial neuropathies (such as sarcoid, Lyme, and myasthenia gravis) must be excluded through blood work and imaging studies (such as brain MRI and chest x-ray).

SLE cranial neuropathy is usually due to nerve inflammation, which can be caused by meningitis or vasculitis of the blood vessels that nourish the nerve. It is treated with immunosuppressants.

Sometimes, cranial neuropathy is due to blood clots from antiphospholipid antibodies. In this case, blood thinners are used (see antiphospholipid syndrome, chapter 9). In some people with antiphospholipid antibodies, the exact cause may not be easy to determine. Both immunosuppressants and blood thinners may be used.

If the second cranial nerve (optic nerve) is affected, it is important to test for NMO-IgG antibodies to exclude NMO spectrum disorder.

Four of the five senses are controlled by cranial nerves. These include smell (first cranial nerve or olfactory nerve), sight (second cranial nerve or optic nerve), and sound (eighth cranial nerve or vestibulocochlear nerve). Taste involves the seventh cranial nerve (facial nerve) and the ninth cranial nerve (glossopharyngeal nerve).

Touch is more complicated. Nerves from the CNS (including the brain's cranial nerves) and the peripheral nervous system control this sense. Difficulties in feeling and touch can be due to many problems discussed in this chapter (such as stroke, cranial neuropathy, and polyneuropathy).

SLE patients can have decreased ability to smell (hyposmia) or complete loss of smell (anosmia); these occur twice as often as in non-SLE people. Loss of the sense of smell occurs more often in those with higher lupus disease activity and in CNS lupus. Anti-ribosomal P antibody (chapter 4) increases this risk.

Non-neurologic problems such as SLE nose ulcers, Sjögren's dryness, nose fungal infections, COVID infection, and drug side effects can also cause loss of smell.

Hearing loss occurs up to seven times more often in those who have SLE than in those who do not. It can be caused by inflammation and damage to the eighth cranial nerve (eighth cranial neuropathy). This nerve is also responsible for balancing. When affected, people often have vertigo (feeling like the room is moving). Tinnitus (ringing in the ears) is also common. One or both ears can be affected. Inner-ear biopsies (in research studies) from SLE patients with eighth cranial neuropathy usually show inflammation and vasculitis (blood vessel inflammation). It is also important to exclude non-neurologic problems such as excessive ear wax, ear infections, and aging, among others.

Although SLE patients often get hearing loss from other causes (such as aging), when it occurs suddenly, inflammation should be suspected, and immunosuppressants should be considered. It is essential to involve an otorhinolaryngologist (ear, nose, and throat specialist).

The sense of taste involves two cranial nerves. Decreased taste (hypogeusia) and abnormal taste (dysgeusia) are often caused by fungal tongue infection (thrush, chapters 14 and 22), tongue inflammation (glossitis) due to drugs such as methotrexate, or dryness. Sjögren's disease (chapter 14), which causes mouth and nose dryness, occurs in 30% of SLE patients. The glands that taste and smell (our ability to smell is essential for taste) rely on mouth and nose moisture to work properly.

KEY POINTS TO REMEMBER

1. The cranial nerves are peripheral nerves coming directly from the brain.

2. SLE cranial neuropathies can cause problems like double vision, face numbness or drooping, vision loss, vertigo, ringing in the ears, or hearing loss.

3. They are usually treated with immunosuppressants. However, blood thinners may be needed if antiphospholipid antibodies are present.

4. Loss of taste and smell occur more commonly in SLE patients than in the general population.

Plexopathy

The peripheral nerves from the spinal cord are called radicular or spinal nerves. One pair of nerves (one each for the left and right sides of the body) exit each spine's vertebral segment. There are usually five lumbar vertebrae in the lower back. Each vertebra has its own pair of radicular nerves leaving the spinal cord. They are numbered L1–L5 ("L" for "lumbar"). These radicular nerves intertwine into a plexus (from the Latin word for "braid"). Plexopathy occurs when lupus causes damage or inflammation to this collection of nerves. Its symptoms include numbness, weakness, and nerve pain in one arm or leg. Nerve pain is often described as burning, tingling, or like an electrical shock. It is diagnosed with an EMG with nerve conduction velocity testing (discussed earlier). MRI of the nerves can help. Plexopathy is rare in SLE. Treatment can include immunosuppressants or IVIG and should involve a neurologist. Plexopathy is one of the SLE classification criteria (chapter 1).

Polyneuropathy

Polyneuropathy involves multiple peripheral nerves. Although all the nerve problems discussed in this section on the peripheral nervous system are technically "peripheral neuropathies," doctors more commonly use the term "peripheral neuropathy" in place of "polyneuropathy." The other peripheral neuropathy types are usually given their specific names, such as "cranial neuropathy" and "plexopathy."

Peripheral neuropathy (meaning polyneuropathy) typically affects the nerves for sensation and feeling things more often than those related to muscle function. Typical symptoms are burning pain, numbness, and tingling. Often the pain is worse when the person is in bed, where the feet become colder, and the nerves become more sensitive and more susceptible to damage.

Peripheral neuropathy usually first affects the feet. The length of nerves from the spinal cord (where they begin) until they reach the feet are the longest in the body and are more easily damaged. Numbness (decreased sensation to feel things) affects the toes first, followed by the foot and ankle. When it occurs in the upper limbs (indicating more severe peripheral neuropathy), it affects the fingers and hands before affecting the arms. This pattern of numbness is called a stocking-glove distribution. Foot sensation loss can cause balance problems, falls, and unnoticed foot ulcers. There may be weakness lifting the toe or walking on the heels if severe. The reflex action caused by tapping a reflex hammer behind the ankle may be decreased.

Around 10% of patients with lupus peripheral neuropathy will also have autonomic neuropathy (described below). These patients often have lightheadedness while standing, but urine incontinence can also occur.

Peripheral neuropathy occurs in 10% to 25% of SLE patients, and around 60% of these are directly due to lupus. The other 40% is due to other causes such as diabetes, aging, obesity, and alcohol. Therefore, the range for SLE-induced peripheral neuropathy is around 6%–15%. EMG and nerve conduction velocity (NCV) testing diagnose peripheral neuropathy. Peripheral neuropathy is an SLE classification criterion (chapter 1).

Other causes for peripheral neuropathy must be checked. These include diabetes (and prediabetes), vitamin B12 deficiency, monoclonal gammopathy (chapter 9), alcohol use, thyroid disease, and Lyme disease. Some drugs used to treat SLE can cause neuropathy (such as leflunomide, dapsone, thalidomide, colchicine, phenytoin, and statins). In this case, the correct treatment is to stop the medicine.

We do not know how SLE causes peripheral neuropathy. Therefore, we do not know the best treatment. EMG with NCV testing often shows the same type of neuropathy that we see with aging and obesity (axonal neuropathy). It is thought that axonal neuropathy is due to hardening of the arteries (with decreased blood flow), high cholesterol, and high glucose (diabetes and prediabetes). Since hardening of the arteries occurs at a much younger age in SLE (accelerated atherosclerosis, chapter 21), this could cause lupus peripheral neuropathy. A 2013 study from Johns Hopkins University in Baltimore, Maryland, supports this view. In it, SLE patients with peripheral neuropathy had nerve damage but not much active inflammation. Steroids and immunosuppressants would not help these SLE patients.

If peripheral neuropathy comes on abruptly and is severe, inflammation may be the cause. In these cases, some experts recommend high-dose steroids and other immunosuppressants.

In 2017, an Italian group published their results of treating most of their lupus peripheral neuropathy patients with high-dose steroids, cyclophosphamide, or mycophenolate over a 14-year period. Around 64% of their patients improved with treatment, while only 20% got worse.

If there is a strong suspicion for inflammation, a nerve biopsy (especially on the foot's sural nerve) can be useful. A sural nerve biopsy can, however, be risky in people on immunosuppressants. It can also leave a permanently numb area of the skin.

Many different medications can decrease nerve pain. These include opioids such as tramadol, antidepressants such as nortriptyline and duloxetine (Cymbalta), and antiepileptic medicines such as pregabalin (Lyrica) and gabapentin (chapter 36). Note, though, that these drugs can cause side effects, such as dizziness and drowsiness, so if nerve pain symptoms are mild, it is usually best to cope with them without medication. Over-the-counter lidocaine patches and capsaicin can help and are usually well tolerated.

Wearing comfortable shoes and soft socks, soaking the feet in cold water, exercising regularly, maintaining normal body weight, cognitive-behavioral therapy, and biofeedback are non-drug ways to help (chapters 11 and 39).

Diabetes and prediabetes (borderline diabetes) can worsen neuropathy. It is important to be exceptionally good with diet, exercise, and taking glucose-lowering (sugar-lowering) medications to keep it under control. Hydroxychloroquine (Plaquenil) can help glucose control.

When there is foot numbness, it is possible to develop sores on the bottom of the feet and not notice them. This increases the chances of dangerous foot ulcers and infections. It is crucial to examine the bottom of the feet daily. If any sores occur, see your doctor right away. Seeing a foot specialist (podiatrist) regularly for proper foot and nail care helps. It is essential to wear proper shoes (good cushions, wide toe box in the front, and avoiding heels).

Seeing a physical therapist to learn balance (proprioception) exercises and fall-prevention strategies should also be considered.

KEY POINTS TO REMEMBER

1. Peripheral neuropathy is one of the most common nerve problems in SLE.

2. It usually begins in the feet, often with burning pain and tingling, especially when in bed.

3. Non-lupus problems (such as aging, alcohol, diabetes, and obesity) are often the cause.

4. All patients with peripheral neuropathy should work on exercise, diet, and maintaining proper weight to help increase blood flow to the nerves.

5. If inflammation is suspected, immunosuppressants are used.

6. If you have peripheral neuropathy, examine your feet daily for sores, see a podiatrist regularly, and wear good shoes.

Autonomic Nervous System Disorders

The autonomic nervous system is responsible for the electrical activity of all bodily functions over which we do not have conscious control. Some examples of autonomic nerve functions include heart beating, dilation of the pupils in the dark, and sweating in the heat. Autonomic nerves are also responsible for some functions that you can sometimes control, such as breathing and blinking. In other words, you can make yourself breathe and blink whenever you want and as fast as you want. However, we do not consciously think of doing so most of the time. This is when the autonomic nervous system takes over.

It is divided into the sympathetic autonomic nerves and the parasympathetic. These nerves usually cause parts of our bodies to do opposite functions to keep us in balance.

The sympathetic nervous system oversees our "fight or flight" reactions. Its job is to help us survive in dangerous situations.

Let's look at an example. You are alone at night and sleepy. You hear a strange creak. You become nervous—there may be a stranger in the house. Your body goes into protection mode, getting you ready to either "fight" the intruder or run away ("flight"). Your sympathetic nervous system goes into action. Your adrenal glands are activated and secrete adrenaline (epinephrine) that travels throughout your body to get you ready. Your mind becomes more alert (though you were sleepy), and your pupils dilate so you can see better in the dark. Your body needs more oxygen to supply your brain and muscles, so your airway passages expand, and you breathe more quickly. Likewise, your heart pumps harder and faster. Meanwhile some organs, such as your urinary bladder and intestines quiet down, even though your bladder and colon may be full, and you may need to empty them. You may also get goosebumps. All of these occur due to the sympathetic nervous system.

Then, when you realize it was your dog walking on some creaky boards, the sympathetic nervous system quiets down, and you relax. The parasympathetic nervous system becomes active to put all the organs that were affected into balance. You could call it the rest-and-digest system. Those organs that stopped working (such as the stomach, intestines, and bladder) become more active. You now sense that you must go to the bathroom—and feel that you can do so safely.

SLE can affect these nerves. This is called autonomic dysfunction (dysautonomia). Dysautonomia from lupus can cause numerous difficulties depending on the areas involved (table 13.6). For example, less adrenaline causes your heart to pump less vigorously. It may beat faster than normal, trying to keep up (as in POTS, see chapter 11). When you stand up, your blood vessels may not constrict to keep the blood flowing to the brain, and you become lightheaded (or even pass out), feel fatigued, and have difficulty focusing.

When you eat, the muscles from your esophagus to your large colon may not squeeze properly. This can cause difficulty swallowing, feeling full quickly, bloating, feeling nauseated, or having diarrhea or constipation.

Autonomic dysfunction can affect many body parts, as indicated in table 13.6. It can mimic heart and lung disease, eye problems, stomach problems, Sjogren's (chapter 14), and urinary tract infections. However, the cause and treatment are entirely different.

Drugs and other medical issues can cause similar problems, making a proper diagnosis challenging. Since dysautonomia can affect so many different areas, numerous tests may be needed. A neurologist or cardiologist specializing in autonomic disorders would be an excellent resource.

Table 13.6 Lupus Dysautonomia Symptoms Grouped by Organ System

Note: Some of these symptoms can occur due to more than one system.

General

Fatigue and malaise

Trouble concentrating

Blood vessels and heart

Dizziness, especially when standing

Heart palpitations

Shortness of breath

Chest pain

Fainting

Blue fingers or toes

Cold feet and hands

Red, warm feet or hands

Eyes

Blurred vision

Dry eyes

Inner ear

Vertigo (feels like the room is spinning)

Gastrointestinal system

Dry mouth

Nausea and vomiting

Trouble swallowing, heartburn

Diarrhea, constipation

Feeling full quickly or bloated when eating

Belly pain

Bladder

Difficulty emptying bladder

Urinary incontinence

Urinary urgency (a feeling of having to urinate immediately)

Increased urine frequency (daytime or nighttime)

Sweat glands and skin

Increased or decreased sweating

Night sweats without fever

Cold or heat intolerance

Goosebumps

Penis

Erectile dysfunction

KEY POINTS TO REMEMBER

1. The autonomic nervous system is comprised of the peripheral nerves that cause our bodies to do things we usually do not consciously control (such as blinking and breathing).

2. When autonomic nerve problems occur, it is essential to ensure that they are not due to medications.

3. Getting help from a dysautonomia expert (like a neurologist or cardiologist) is important.

Small-Fiber Neuropathy

This occurs when there is the loss of some of the smallest nerves in the skin, causing burning pain in the feet and hands. Some people will have tingling and numbness in unusual areas, such as the chest or the middle of the arms or legs. It is considered a type of peripheral neuropathy and makes up around 17% of lupus peripheral neuropathy cases. It involves nerves in both the somatic and autonomic nervous systems (described above).

EMG and nerve conduction velocity studies evaluate larger nerves, and are often normal in small-fiber neuropathy. However, when a skin biopsy is performed, and special preparations are done on the biopsy, small nerve fiber loss can be seen. If you have unexplained sensations like this, a dermatologist may be able to perform this biopsy. The cause of this problem in SLE is not known. It is treated with nerve pain medicines, as described above. Unfortunately, it tends to worsen over time in two-thirds of patients.

KEY POINTS TO REMEMBER

1. If tingling and numbness occur in unusual places, or if nerve symptoms occur in the feet with normal EMG and nerve conduction velocity testing, a skin biopsy can look for small-fiber neuropathy.

2. Burning pain and tingling from peripheral neuropathies (including small fiber neuropathy) can be treated with nerve pain medicines.

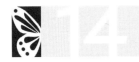

The Exocrine Gland System

Alan N. Baer, MD, *Contributing Editor*

The two large groups of body glands are endocrine glands and exocrine glands. Endocrine glands (*endo-* from the Greek for "inside" and *-crine* is used in medicine meaning "to secrete") produce substances that are secreted into the blood. Examples include the thyroid (secretes thyroid hormones), adrenal glands (secrete cortisol and other substances), and the ovaries (secrete female hormones). Endocrine involvement by SLE is discussed in chapter 17.

The exocrine glands (*exo-* meaning "outside") secrete fluids outside the body (such as outside the skin or into the gastrointestinal tract, which is a tube from the mouth to the anus, and technically outside the body). The main autoimmune problem with exocrine glands is Sjögren's disease, which is the subject of this chapter.

Sjögren's Disease

Sjögren's disease is an autoimmune disease characterized by its targeting of the glands that produce tears and saliva, leading to dry eyes and mouth. It also attacks other moisture-producing glands throughout the body, causing them to not work properly. It can involve many different organs, such as the blood cells, kidneys, nerves, and skin, and is thus a "systemic" disease, like lupus. For many years, it was called "Sjögren's syndrome," but an effort is now underway to change the name to "Sjögren's disease," or simply "Sjögren's." It may occur as a stand-alone condition (so-called primary Sjögren's) or as part of another systemic autoimmune disease (so-called secondary Sjögren's). SLE and Sjögren's share many features, including Raynaud's phenomenon (chapter 9), arthritis, a particular form of sun-sensitive rash (called annular erythema and subacute cutaneous lupus; chapter 8), low white blood cell counts (chapter 9), antinuclear antibodies, anti-SSA (Ro), and low complement levels (chapter 4). Because of these commonalties, it can be difficult to definitively distinguish SLE and Sjögren's. Estimates of the frequency of Sjögren's in SLE patients range from 10% to 30%. Some experts think that this is an underestimate due to Sjögren's being underdiagnosed.

Sjögren's involves not only the parotid, submandibular and sublingual glands that produce saliva and the lacrimal glands that produce tears, but also a myriad of smaller moisture-producing glands that lie just beneath the surface of the membranes that line our eyes (conjunctivae), sinuses, inner mouth, throat, and breathing passages. Thus, the dryness can lead to sinus congestion, dry inner nose, hoarseness, throat pain, cough, and difficulty breathing.

Skin and vaginal dryness are also common but may not be due to inflammation in moisture-producing glands. Involvement of the sweat glands has been thought to cause skin dryness, but this has never been proven. The vagina does not rely on secretory glands for moisture, either at rest or during sexual arousal. Thus, other mechanisms may be at play that impair the passage of fluid across the vaginal wall in women with Sjögren's.

Approximately 1–10 people out of every 10,000 have Sjögren's alone, and 3–18 out of every 10,000 have Sjögren's associated with rheumatoid arthritis or SLE. Thus, in the adult US population, approximately 600,000 people are known to have Sjögren's. However, according to the Sjögren's Foundation, as many as 4,000,000 Americans may have Sjögren's since it is often underdiagnosed. Only 5% of Sjögren's patients are men.

How Sjögren's Is Diagnosed

Just as with SLE (chapter 1), there are classification criteria for Sjögren's. While these classification criteria are used to enroll patients in research studies, they also help with diagnosis. These criteria require anti-SSA (also called anti-Ro, chapter 4) or a positive minor salivary gland lip biopsy. If you run your lower teeth up and down the inside of your lower lip, you can feel tiny lumps under the inner skin (mucosa). Each of these is a minor salivary gland. A lip biopsy is performed in a doctor's office, using local anesthesia of the lower lip. A tiny surgical cut is made, and some minor salivary glands are removed for evaluation under the microscope. Tests that document dryness of the eyes and mouth by measuring tear and saliva flow or assessing dryness damage to the eye's surface are also used in diagnosis.

A lip biopsy is not required for diagnosis. It is used mostly for research purposes. In SLE patients, the finding of eye or mouth dryness assessed by symptoms and one of the tests described below, is often sufficient. However, a lip biopsy may be needed for diagnosis if an individual has dryness symptoms but does not have SLE or another systemic rheumatic disease. It may also be required in someone who does not have anti-SSA (Ro) antibodies (typically seen in 65%–80% of people with Sjögren's and 40%–50% of those with lupus). In addition, a biopsy may be helpful if the antibody tests yield inconsistent results, positive in one lab and negative in another, or are weakly positive (in other words, only slightly higher than normal).

Dry eyes can be diagnosed in several ways. One is the Schirmer test (figure 14.1). In it, a small strip of sterile filter paper is placed under the lower eyelid, with part of it hanging down outside the eye. The person closes their eyes gently for five minutes. Although there is some slight irritation during the test, it is painless. The filter paper absorbs or "wicks" tears from the eyes. When the paper is removed, the amount of paper wetted with tears is measured in millimeters. If less than 10 mm of the paper is moistened, the finding is consistent with decreased tears. Less than 5 mm is required to enroll patients into research (using the Sjögren's classification criteria).

Another test for dry eyes looks for damage to the clear part of the eye (cornea) and the tissue layer (conjunctiva) overlying the white part of the eye (sclera). This is performed by an eye doctor (ophthalmologist or optometrist). A drop of a vegetable dye (fluorescein or lissamine green) is applied to the eyes. Then the eyes are examined with a slit lamp, a type of microscope that allows the eye doctor to inspect the eye surface with magnification and special lighting. Dryness damage to the cornea shows up as pinpoint pits in its otherwise smooth surface. These damaged areas light up with the stain when viewed with a special light in the slip lamp. Damage to the conjunctiva shows up as green dots, generally located in the triangular area next to the cornea, which is not normally covered by the eyelids. These green dots represent dried or dead cells that absorb the dye. This absorption of pigment into the damaged area of the cornea is called "ocular surface staining." The more staining that is present, the more severe the damage and dryness. The coloration resolves in a few hours. Rose Bengal, a red stain that was commonly used in the past, can be irritating and is rarely used today.

Another dry eye test is the tear break-up time test (TBUT). Fluorescein dye is added to the eyes, and the patient is asked to blink once. This spreads the dye evenly over the

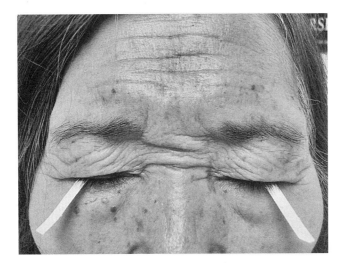

Figure 14.1 Schirmer test to diagnose dry eyes in Sjögren's disease

tear film's outermost layer, which is comprised of oils from the meibomian glands. Then the person is asked not to blink anymore while the eye doctor watches the green coloration of the tear film using a slit lamp. When the colored tear film is first seen breaking apart on the eye's surface, then that is the time entered as the TBUT. It should normally take more than 10 seconds for the tear film to break apart. The TBUT is primarily a measure of tear quality and is typically abnormal in people with meibomian gland dysfunction where tears evaporate too quickly.

Dry mouth can often be diagnosed by physical exam. In some cases, the tongue may develop multiple furrows or cracks on the surface. In others, its surface may become smooth and a brighter red. The wood tongue depressor used to examine the mouth may stick to the tongue or the inside of the cheeks. There may be absence of any accumulation of saliva under the tongue (called salivary pooling) when the tongue is held up for one minute.

Sialometric tests measure saliva flow. The simplest of these is the whole unstimulated saliva flow test. For this test, you sit quietly (no talking or swallowing) and collect the saliva that accumulates over 5 to 15 minutes. The saliva is collected in a pre-weighed tube or cup, either by drooling or spitting into it. At the end of the collection, the cup or tube is weighed, and the volume collected is approximated based on the specific gravity of water (1 gram per milliliter). Normally, you should be able to spit at least 1.5 milliliters within 15 minutes. Amounts less than this indicate poor saliva production. An abnormal result does not by itself indicate Sjögren's. Some people may have low saliva production from drugs such as antihistamines, antidepressants, and blood pressure and pain medicines. Others may be bashful about spitting in front of a stranger and not perform the test optimally.

Another way to detect salivary gland involvement is by ultrasound examination. Many rheumatologists are now using ultrasound in their practices. The parotid salivary glands are the largest and lie below the ears at the angle of the jaw. For a parotid gland ultrasound exam, the doctor has the patient lie on the exam table on their side. The doctor places the ultrasound probe (also called a transducer) covered with gel on the side of the face, just under the ear. The probe assesses the transmission (and back reflection) of sound waves aimed into the parotid gland, allowing an image to be formed. The parotid gland involved by Sjögren's will often contain multiple oval-shaped areas of decreased sound reflection. These areas may represent areas of inflammation in the gland or dilated ducts. The submandibular glands underneath the jaw can also be examined this way.

There are other common causes of dryness that should be excluded before someone is diagnosed with Sjögren's. These include medications, prior radiation therapy to the head and neck, bone marrow transplantation, hepatitis C infection, and other inflammatory diseases, such as IgG4-related disease and sarcoidosis.

Specific Sjögren's Conditions and Treatments

Dry Eyes

When Sjögren's causes inflammation and damage to the tear-secreting glands (lacrimal glands), the result is a decrease in tear production and abnormal tear quality. The symptoms of Sjögren's dry eyes are many (table 14.1).

Table 14.1 Dry Eye Signs and Symptoms

- Dry, gritty eyes
- Foreign object sensation in the eye
- Redness of the white (sclera) of the eyes
- Blurred vision
- Photophobia (intolerance of light)
- Ropey, thick secretions in the eyes, especially when first awakening
- Difficulty opening the eyes after sleeping due to dryness
- Red, tender eyelids (blepharitis)

Eye dryness is a critical problem to identify and treat. Left untreated, it can potentially cause permanent damage to the cornea (clear part of the eye) and lead to vision problems. Usually, the symptoms of dry eyes come on very slowly—over several to many years.

People with Sjögren's can do many things on their own to help with eye dryness as well as dryness elsewhere (tables 14.2 and 14.3). In 2015, the Sjögren's Foundation and the American Academy of Ophthalmology published guidelines for treating dry eyes. These recommendations are included in table 14.3.

Over-the-counter liquid tear supplements (artificial tears) can be used during the day. Try different brands and preparations to see which works best. If you require them four or more times a day, you should use a preservative-free formulation (usually in individual vials) since preservatives can be irritating and aggravate dryness. Because less tear fluid is produced while sleeping, use a gel or ointment at bedtime. Artificial tears that contain lipids (fatty substances) are formulated specifically for people with meibomian gland dysfunction (discussed below). Examples include Oasis Tears Plus, Refresh Optive Advanced, Ocusoft Retaine MGD, Systane Complete, Rohto, and Systane Balance. Over-the-counter liposomal sprays, such as Optrex ActiMist, can help.

Activities that decrease eye blinking aggravate dryness. These include reading, watching TV or movies, doing computer work, and using smartphones. While we typically blink around 20 times a minute, during these activities this drops to around 5 times a minute. A vicious cycle develops in which eye dryness makes it more difficult to see and concentrate, causing you to read more slowly and blink less often, which makes your eyes become dryer, and so on.

Some medical studies suggest that omega-3 fatty acids may be beneficial, while other studies show no benefit. The American Heart Association recommends that people get 1 gram of omega-3 fatty acids daily from food sources such as salmon, flaxseed, chia seed, and walnuts (chapter 38). Six walnut halves contain approximately 1 gram of omega-3 fatty acids.

Many patients with Sjögren's have plugging of the meibomian glands (located inside the eyelids). They secrete an oil called meibum through pores on the eyelid edges. Meibum coats the exposed outer surface of the tear film to decrease its rate of evaporation. Meibum also lubricates, allowing the eyelids to move smoothly over the eyeballs. Less meibum allows the tear film to evaporate too quickly. This is especially problematic

Table 14.2 General Measures to Alleviate Dryness

- Stay hydrated but avoid drinking excess fluids, which results in going to the bathroom frequently at night, contributing to fatigue. It also washes away the mucous salivary lining that keeps your mouth feeling moist.
- Avoid dehydrating fluids, like alcohol and caffeine.
- Avoid smoking (dries out the mouth, eyes, and nose).
- Use a humidifier (at 55%–60% humidity) in each room where you spend significant time.
- A humidifier near the bed is a must (we spend the most time there). Our eyes dry out more when asleep. Turn on at least an hour before bed.
- Clean and dry out humidifiers daily to prevent mold and fungus.
- A centralized humidifier in the furnace is even better.
- Consider a central air UV light plus filter to decrease infections.

in Sjögren's, where there is less tear film being produced already. Less lacrimal gland tear production and faster evaporation of the tear film due to the decreased layer of meibum oil add up to significant problems with lubrication of the eyeballs and overlying eyelids.

If your eye doctor tells you that you have plugged meibomian glands, you can use daily warm compresses (for instance, a washcloth soaked in warm water) followed by gentle eyelid massaging. Do the eyelid massage after applying the warm compress for one minute. Gently close your eyelids. Put your index finger on the outer corner of the eyelid. Pull the eyelid toward your ear so that the upper and lower eyelids are stretched taut. Next, use the index finger of your opposite hand to apply direct pressure to the taut eyelids, starting at the inner aspect of the eyelid near the base of the nose. Sweep with firm but gentle pressure toward your ear. Repeat this maneuver four to five times.

If your meibomian gland blockage is severe, your doctor may recommend other treatments. These may include antibiotics (usually doxycycline or azithromycin) or other newer treatments, such as LipiFlow Thermal Pulsation Therapy. Intense pulsed light (IPL) treatments use pulses of light aimed at the meibomian glands to liquefy the hardened oils that are clogging them. An ophthalmologist can also use a tool to manually open each individual blocked meibomian gland.

Inflammation of the outer edge of the eyelids (blepharitis) may also contribute to eye irritation. When this occurs, the eyelids may become sore and reddish, the eyes can have a gritty sensation, and crusting can develop. These findings are often subtle, requiring examination from an eye doctor.

If you have blepharitis, there are things you can do at home to help. Place a warm, wet cloth on your eyelid for 5 to 10 minutes 4 times daily. This will loosen any crusts. Then gently rub the base of the eyelashes on the eyelid margin with a cotton swab or your clean fingertip. Use a soap that is free of lotion or perfume, such as Neutrogena or baby shampoo (diluted 1:1). Form a lather on your clean fingertips or a cotton swab and apply the soap to the eyelid margins and eyelid base for up to 1 minute. Keep your eyelids gently closed so that soap does not enter your eyes. Then rinse with warm water. You can also purchase cleansing pads (such as OCuSOFT Lid Scrub or Novartis Eye

Table 14.3 Keeping the Eyes Moist

General measures

- Do everything in table 14.2.
- Fish oil, flaxseed oil, or omega-3 fatty acid supplements may help. (Natural sources such as fish, flaxseed, walnuts, and olive oil are even better.) Many eye experts recommend high-quality brands, such as Nordic Naturals Ultimate Omega and PRN's "De 3 Dry Eye Omega Benefits."

Artificial tears and gels

- Use artificial tears a minimum of once daily (even if the eyes do not feel dry). Use regularly; do not wait for your eyes to dry out.
- Use preservative-free brands if you use them more than 4 times a day.
- For severe dry eyes, start using preservative-free artificial tears every 1–2 hours regularly. After 1 week, slowly back off on how often you use it. As soon as your eyes feel any dryness at all, go back to the previous, more frequent application to figure out how often you need them.
- Try different brands and formulations to find the one most suited to you. Some are more viscous and may stay in the eye longer but may also blur vision. Some are for people with coexistent Meibomian gland dysfunction.
- Freshkote and Hylo are preservative-free tears in bottles instead of individual vials.
- If you don't like eye drops, consider aerosolized spray (such as Nature's Tears EyeMist).
- An alternative is the prescription Lacrisert, inserted in the lower eyelids to moisten the eyes all day.
- Use a lubricating eye ointment or gel before bed. At first, apply it just to your eyelids and lashes and blink several times to see if it helps. If not, apply one-eighth inch under your lower eyelids.
- Use artificial tears more often when flying (air is drier in the plane) or when reading or doing computer work (you blink less often).

Eye protection

- Decrease air and wind drying by wearing moisture chamber glasses, moisturizing goggles, or wrap-around sunglasses (Eye Eco, Ziena, and Wiley X brands).
- If light bothers your eyes, wear sunglasses or have the lenses in your eyeglasses tinted with FL-41 (a rose-colored filter).
- Avoid fans, drafts, and air vents; air movement dries out eyes.

Visual attention that decreases blinking

- When reading, watching TV/movies, using a smartphone, or doing computer work, perform "blinking exercises" every 20 minutes. Close your eyes, squeeze hard, hold for a few seconds, open, and repeat a few times.
- Follow the 20:20:20 rule: every 20 minutes, stand and look at something at least 20 feet away for at least 20 seconds.

Workspace modifications

- Have your computer screen about an arm's length away and lower so that your eyes gaze down slightly.

Table 14.3 *(continued)*

- The computer screen should not be brighter than surrounding light, so your eyes do not have to work harder. Use an anti-glare screen filter.
- Use a desktop humidifier.

Blepharitis and Meibomian gland dysfunction treatment

- Use warm moist compresses on your eyes (such as Tranquil Eyes, Eyeseals 4.0, and Bruder wet heat eye compresses).
- Clean sore, irritated eyelids daily with baby shampoo. Use warm, moist cloths on the eyes, and gently massage the eyelids.
- Use products that clean the eyelid edges, such as Cliradex pads, tea tree and coconut oil eye wipes, and Avenova.
- Apply a warm, moist washcloth to the eyes before sleeping and upon awakening for 5 minutes.
- Carry a wet washcloth in a zip-lock bag when you travel; apply to your eyes when needed.
- Keep makeup and lotions away from eyelids.
- For Meibomian gland dysfunction, massage your eyelids after applying a moist warm compress for one minute.

Contact lenses

- If you wear contact lenses, use only special daily replacement lenses (such as Acuvue Oasys and Alcon's Dailies Total-1) designed for dry eyes.
- Therapeutic scleral contact lenses can help severe dry eyes.

Prescription drugs

- Ask your doctor if you would benefit from medicated dry-eye drops, such as Restasis, Cequa, or Xiidra.
- If Restasis or Cequa irritates your eyes when you first start using it, keep it in the refrigerator. Also, apply it 10–15 minutes after using artificial tears first.
- Restasis comes in single-use tiny vials and a large multidose vial. If you want to save money, ask for the small vials. Do not touch the wet edges of the vial while using it; twist the cap back on the vial to reuse. Get two doses out of each vial (a 3-month supply can last 6 months).
- Ask your doctor for Tyrvaya (varenicline) nose drops to help dry eyes (one spray in each nostril twice daily; can take 4 weeks to work).
- Add NSAID eye drops to your drug intolerance list. They can harm dry eyes.

Punctal plugs

- Ask your ophthalmologist to insert tear-duct plugs to decrease tear drainage.

Tear stimulation

- Systemic drugs that stimulate saliva and tear secretion, such as bethanechol, pilocarpine (Salagen), and cevimeline (Evoxac) help.
- Ask your eye doctor about the iTEAR 100 neurostimulator.

Notes: Dry-eye care table reviewed and edited by Dr. Stephen Cohen, OD, an optometrist in Phoenix, Arizona, and previous Chair of the National Board Sjögren's Foundation. Brands mentioned above are included as examples only and are not formal endorsements.

LUPUS IN FOCUS

Moist, warm compresses versus dry heat

Moist, warm compresses can help dry eyes, especially when sleeping. They improve meibomian gland function, decrease dry eye discomfort, and help heal blepharitis. Moist heat works better than dry. Think about putting your hand into a warm oven at 250° Fahrenheit (hotter than boiling water). It takes quite a while before your hand feels hot enough to pull out of the oven. If you put your hand over a boiling pot of water (212° Fahrenheit, cooler than the oven), you must pull it away much faster. This is because moisture transmits heat quicker and more efficiently. Some commercial microwavable "moist" compresses absorb moisture from the air when warmed, allowing them to advertise themselves as "moist." But if you are in a dry climate, this type of compress will not work as well as the ones that have actual moisture added. (Tips from Dr. Stephen Cohen, OD, optometrist in Phoenix, Arizona, and former Chair of the National Board Sjögren's Foundation)

Scrub) instead of using soap or baby shampoo. After the eyelid scrubs, perform the eyelid massage described above to gently squeeze out hardened oils from the meibomian glands located on the eyelid edges.

Another treatment for dry eyes is called the iTEAR100. It is a device that you place on the outside of each side of the nose. It sends gentle electrical waves that stimulate the nerves, causing the tear glands to secrete tears.

Doctors can also prescribe anti-inflammatory drops that contain cyclosporine (Restasis and Cequa). One drop is placed in each eye twice a day. Restasis and Cequa decrease conjunctival lining inflammation, increase eye surface lubrication, and reduce eye dryness. It is essential to use it regularly twice daily for 3 to 12 months for the full effect. If there is no improvement after three or four months, ask your doctor if you can try using it three to four times daily. Many patients find that more frequent usage works better.

Lifitegrast (Xiidra) is another anti-inflammatory drop for dry eyes. Lifitegrast drops are also used twice daily and tends to work faster than cyclosporine.

Sometimes eye doctors will prescribe steroid eye drops for dry eye inflammation. However, they try to limit their use due to potential side effects like glaucoma (high pressure in the eyeballs) and cataracts (clouding of the lenses).

Punctal plugging (punctal occlusion) is another dry eye treatment. The eye doctor inserts tiny plugs into the tear ducts that drain fluid from the eye's surface. These ducts are in the upper and lower eyelids on the sides closest to the nose. After the ophthalmologist plugs the ducts, tears remain longer in the eyes. These ducts can even be permanently closed using heat or laser treatments (cauterization).

Another treatment involves using your own blood to create eye drops called autologous serum tears. These are made in a compounding pharmacy, usually in supplies that each last for three months. The serum contains substances that reduce inflammation and promote dry eye healing.

Custom-made large contact lenses are sometimes used to protect the cornea and keep it moist. These include therapeutic contact lenses, soft bandage contact lenses, and scleral contact lenses (sometimes referred to as prosthetic replacement of the ocular surface ecosystem, or PROSE, lenses). These contact lenses are designed to rest on the sclera (white portion of the eye). A tiny chamber over the central cornea filled with saltwater bathes the cornea while the lens is in place.

If there are eyelid abnormalities making the dry eyes worse, surgical correction can help.

Dry Mouth

When Sjögren's causes inflammation and damage to the glands that secrete saliva (the salivary glands), saliva production decreases. Most people do not notice mouth dryness until there has been a 40% to 50% decrease in saliva formation. Most everyone with Sjögren's will have dry mouth. They may feel like they must drink more water and often get into the habit of carrying a water bottle. They may have difficulty swallowing dry food, such as crackers, without drinking fluids. The dryness can worsen while sleeping and lead to frequent waking. Dryness in the back of the mouth can cause a sore throat. The lips can also become dry, irritated, swollen, and cracked. When a person has dry mouth, deep furrows (figure 14.2) may develop in the tongue caused by the persistent dryness. The papillae (taste bud bumps) of the tongue may be much smaller (atrophied) than usual. The saliva can become thick and frothy.

Like dry eyes, dry mouth causes many problems (table 14.4). Reduced saliva leads to dryness of the throat, trachea (windpipe), and vocal cords. This can result in a dry cough, hoarseness, and difficulty swallowing. This is treated with pilocarpine or cevimeline (see below) and guaifenesin.

The major salivary glands are the parotid, submandibular, and sublingual salivary glands (figure 14.3). The parotid glands are located on both sides of the face just below the ears and cover the jaw angle. The submandibular glands are located underneath the jaw in the soft tissue back toward the throat. The sublingual glands are located underneath the tongue in the floor of the mouth.

Involvement of these glands, especially the parotids, from Sjögren's can cause them to enlarge and lead to a chipmunk-like appearance. If this enlargement persists for three or more months, it should be investigated, since it can sometimes be a sign of lymphoma (though this is uncommon). Most people with Sjögren's who have salivary gland enlargement notice that it comes and goes over days, often associated with mild discomfort. If one gland becomes tender, painful, and swollen in a matter of hours, then medical attention is needed. This can arise in a gland damaged from Sjögren's due to mucus plugs that block ducts in the gland and cause a backup of saliva. An infection may also occur in the gland, particularly in the setting of a blockage. Treatment may include antibiotics, steroids, using hot compresses, sucking on lemon drops, and staying well hydrated.

Saliva is also essential for the sense of taste. It helps dissolve food molecules so that the taste buds can detect flavors accurately. It is common for Sjögren's patients to have a decreased ability to taste and enjoy food. The nose is even more critical for taste. Nose dryness reduces the ability to smell and appreciate food.

Saliva flows down the esophagus to neutralize acidic stomach contents that sometimes reflux up into the esophagus. In Sjögren's, less saliva is available, so gastroesophageal reflux problems (chapter 28) can occur, causing heartburn and even chest pain.

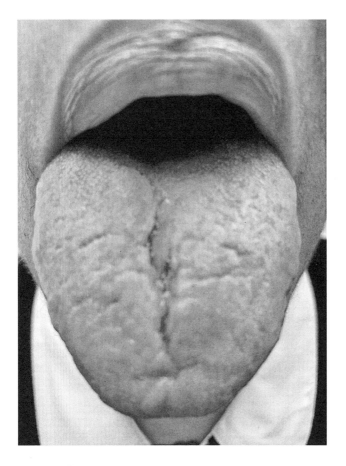

Figure 14.2 Oral candidiasis in a person with SLE and Sjögren's overlap syndrome. She had a tender tongue and loss of taste. The deep furrows are due to chronic dryness. She primarily has chronic erythematous candidiasis (note the darker tint of the center part of the tongue, shows up as red on the color online photo). However, she also has some subtle white coating on the tongue edges (classic for typical thrush).

Saliva is also essential for washing away harmful bacteria and other organisms, which are swallowed and destroyed by stomach acids. When the mouth becomes dry, harmful microorganisms can multiply and cause damage, such as dental caries (cavities) and periodontitis (infection of the tissues that hold your teeth in your mouth). These problems can cause bad breath and tooth loss.

Candidiasis is a fungal infection due to *Candida albicans* and is problematic in Sjögren's. In most people, this fungal infection is characterized by white patches on the tongue, roof of the mouth, and insides of the cheeks. This is called thrush and can develop in healthy people who take steroids or antibiotics.

Table 14.4 Dry Mouth Signs and Symptoms

- Parotid gland swelling (sides of the jaws)
- Parotid gland pain from infections, inflammation (parotitis), or blockages
- Tongue sticking to the roof of the mouth
- Waking up with a dry mouth and having daytime fatigue
- Difficulty swallowing crackers and other dry food without fluids
- Sore throat
- Dry, cracked, swollen, sore lips
- Difficulty tasting food
- Difficulty talking for very long
- Heartburn
- Hoarseness
- Dry cough
- Candidiasis (sore red tongue, sore corners of the lips, sore lining of the mouth)
- Increased dental cavities and tooth loss
- Gingivitis (sore, bleeding gums) and mucosal ulcers (sores inside the mouth)
- Bad breath

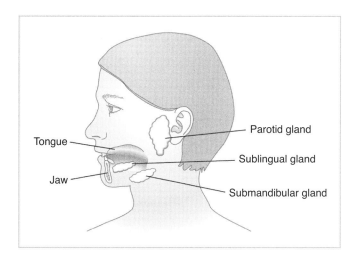

Figure 14.3 Major salivary glands

However, candidiasis is more common in people with dry mouth, and it often has a different appearance, called erythematous candidiasis and atrophic candidiasis. Instead of white patches, the tongue is typically smooth (atrophic), red (erythematous), and tender. The lining inside the cheeks and on the roof of the mouth will have a velvety, red appearance, sometimes with shallow ulcers. This fungal infection leads to

Tips for swallowing drugs (modified with permission from The Sjögren's Foundation)

Difficulty swallowing pills is a common problem in people with dry mouth. To deal with this,

- Ask your doctor and pharmacist for easier-to-swallow forms such as liquids or disintegrating, sublingual (under the tongue), or crushable pills. You can also ask if patches, suppositories, creams, and inhaled versions are available.
- Cut pills in halves, quarters, or crush them (do NOT crush extended-release forms; ask your pharmacist first). Crushed tablets can be placed in applesauce or pudding.
- Moisten your mouth with water beforehand. If you have a significant gag reflex, take a deep breath and hold it before placing the pill on your tongue.
- Place the pill in the center of the tongue lengthwise if oval-shaped. Immediately sip water to wash the pill into the throat while throwing your head back. Some people do better swallowing while placing the chin on the chest.
- Take a larger amount of water into the mouth, allow the pill to float in it, then swallow.
- Chew some moist food beforehand, then place the pill inside the food in your mouth and swallow it together. Or, put a pill in applesauce or pudding and swallow.
- Fill a soda bottle with a narrow opening with water. Place the tablet on the tongue, wrap your lips around the opening, then swallow. Keep sucking in the water. The force of water through the narrow opening pushes the pill back.
- Use a "pill popper" straw specially designed for swallowing pills. Keep sucking water through the straw to distract you from a gag reflex.
- Coat the pill with a flavored swallowing gel (such as Phazix) or swallowing spray to help it go down more easily.
- After swallowing the pill, immediately eat some food to help it go down

Why does my tongue have cracks?

A dry tongue acts similarly to dry skin. Both develop cracks and flaking when dry but it is more exaggerated on the tongue. In the tongue, food particles also tend to get trapped in the cracks, contributing to bad breath. Make sure to brush and scrape your tongue daily (with a scraper available in your drugstore) and frequently rinse your mouth. Using an oral irrigator (Waterpik, Liberex, Akunbem, and many others) on the tongue every day helps.

mouth soreness and burning when eating acidic foods. The corners of the mouth may also become sore and tender. This is called angular cheilitis (also called perlèche).

If you have signs of a *Candida* infection (sore and red tongue, mouth lining, and corners of the mouth), make sure to see your doctor for antifungal medications. Antifungal antibiotic choices include pills that work systemically (such as fluconazole) or topical preparations (such as clotrimazole troches or miconazole tablets). In patients with severe dry mouth, the topicals may work better because if there is not much saliva produced, less fluconazole enters the saliva from the bloodstream. Clotrimazole troches (lozenges) are used five times daily; it may be necessary to sip water while using the lozenge to facilitate its slow dissolution. Another option is miconazole buccal mucoadhesive (Oravig) tablets, which adhere to the lining of the mouth and dissolve slowly. You place one above the bony ridge at the gumline of your upper teeth in the pocket formed by your upper lip and the upper jawbone once daily.

Nystatin is a commonly prescribed antifungal treatment that comes in liquid form as a "swish and swallow" preparation. However, it is not recommended for Sjögren's patients since it has a high sugar (sucrose) content. Clotrimazole and miconazole are preferred.

Saliva production is essential to prevent tooth decay and cavities. The insides of our mouths become more acidic after consuming food and beverages. This acid promotes the loss of minerals from tooth enamel. Saliva contains bicarbonate that neutralizes this acid and promotes remineralization; the tooth enamel becomes stronger and cavity resistant. Enamel remineralization depends on calcium and phosphate minerals in the saliva and is promoted by fluoride in drinking water and supplements. Sjögren's patients are repeatedly in a state of demineralization with low saliva, increased acidity, and reduced fluoride and calcium on their teeth. This promotes the rapid formation of cavities and tooth decay.

Therefore, it is important to do everything possible to increase saliva flow when you have dry mouth. It is also important to use supplemental fluoride daily, either as a mouth rinse or a prescription-strength (1.1%) fluoride toothpaste (table 14.5). Remineralization toothpaste (such as Clinpro 5000 and Prevident 5000 Booster Plus) and chewing gums (Basic Bites) have high concentrations of minerals essential to tooth protection and may also be used.

Just as with dry eyes, many things can help dry mouth (table 14.5). If these measures do not suffice, a doctor can prescribe pilocarpine (Salagen) or cevimeline (Evoxac), both of which stimulate the salivary glands to make more saliva.

Pilocarpine is taken four times a day, and cevimeline three times a day. Both need to be taken regularly and can take up to three months to work. Potential side effects include heart fluttering sensations, stomach upset, increased sweating, flushing, and increased urinary frequency. They can potentially worsen untreated closed-angle glaucoma (a rare form of glaucoma), asthma, and some heart conditions.

Cevimeline may be easier to tolerate than pilocarpine. For both, start with one pill daily after your evening meal. Each week after that, increase by another pill daily (but not at the same time). If you get any bothersome side effects, go back to the previous dose you tolerated well. Another trick to handling these drugs is to take a smaller amount. You can cut the pilocarpine into fourths or halves to find a dose you tolerate.

Table 14.5 Dry Mouth Care

General measures

- Do everything in table 14.2.
- Sip just enough water to keep your mouth moist or let small ice chips melt in your mouth. Avoid drinking too much water: dilutes saliva and increases the chances of getting up at night to urinate.
- To decrease having to get up at night to urinate, don't drink several hours before bed.
- Avoid salty, spicy, carbonated, and acidic foods and drinks (including fruit juices), if they irritate your dry mouth.
- Avoid caffeine and alcohol; they worsen dry mouth.
- Avoid frequent and prolonged exposure of teeth to sugars; they cause dental decay and tooth loss.
- To decrease a metallic or bad taste in your mouth, consider products such as MetaQil.

Stimulation of saliva flow

- Use xylitol-containing gum, mints, and lozenges regularly to stimulate saliva and decrease bacteria. Examples: Ice Chips candies, Spry, Salese lozenges.
- Xylitol gum-chewing tips: saliva production reaches a maximum at 5 minutes, then declines; change gum frequently. Larger pieces are more effective than smaller ones. Chew slowly to decrease the risk for temporomandibular joint (TMJ) pain.
- Place two xylitol adhering discs (like Xylimelts) between cheek and gum before bed to stimulate saliva and reduce bacteria. Use as needed in the daytime.
- Ask your doctor for pilocarpine (Salagen), cevimeline (Evoxac), or bethanechol to stimulate saliva flow.
- To maximize mouth moisture for speaking events, social gatherings: take pilocarpine 1 hour beforehand or cevimeline 2 hours before.

Saliva substitutes

- Use lubricating sprays and saliva substitutes regularly, such as Biotene Moisturizing Spray/Gel/or Rinse, Oasis Moisturizing Mouth Spray, Oral7 gel, BioXtra gel, Lubricity, and Mouth Kote. Keep some on your bedside stand, next to your phone, and when traveling.
- Use artificial saliva before bed and in the middle of the night instead of water, decreasing the need to drink water before bed and get up during the night to urinate.
- Lubricating tips: cover all inner mouth areas (inside lips, under the tongue, front of the tongue, inner cheeks, palate, and so on). The dryness sensation has a lot to do with the mucosal surfaces not sliding easily over each other. You want this lubricating sensation everywhere.
- A saliva substitute alternative is water mixed with olive or coconut oil.
- If you suffer from dysgeusia (metallic or abnormal taste), use MetaQil mouth rinse and brush your tongue at least once daily.

Diet

- Eat soft, moist food if you have trouble swallowing.
- Eat smaller, more frequent meals (stimulates saliva flow more regularly).

Sore lips and mouth

- Use an ointment (better than balm or Chapstick) that contains ceramides or hyaluronic acid (moisturizers) with a sealer (lanolin or petrolatum) on your lips throughout the day; use a lot (you can't use too much; you can use too little). Avoid flavored brands (like menthol and peppermint).

Table 14.5 (*continued*)

- Do not lick your lips.
- Replace your lip balm every 3 months.
- Apply vitamin E oil to sore, dry parts of your mouth. You can squirt out the gel from vitamin E gel capsules.
- If you have a sore tongue, sores on the edges of your lips, or swollen lips, see your doctor for a possible *Candida* infection.

Dental care

- Use fluoride-containing moisturizing toothpaste and mouthwashes (such as Biotene or TheraBreath brands) 2–3 to three times a day.
- Avoid anything with alcohol or witch hazel: they dry out the mouth.
- Avoid whitening toothpaste (irritates teeth and gums).
- Consider an electric toothbrush, especially if you have arthritis and difficulty using a regular one.
- Floss at least daily to decrease plaque, periodontal disease (gum infection), and cavities.
- Daily use of an oral irrigator (Waterpik, Liberex, Akunbem Water Flosser, and so on) removes food particles from crevices unreached by floss and toothbrushes. These do not replace flossing.
- Ask your dental hygienist to teach you how to brush and floss (most people do not do so correctly).
- Rinse with a fluoride mouth rinse twice a day (such as Act, Crest Pro-Health, Closys, Colgate Total Pro-Shield, FluoriGard, and CariFree Maintenance Rinse).
- Use a RX high-fluoride, remineralizing toothpaste (Prevident 5000 Booster Plus or Clinpro 5000). Apply half a pea-sized amount to teeth after brushing twice daily, move around your teeth with your tongue, spit out the excess, do not rinse.
- See your dentist more often than twice a year for fluoride varnish and oral hygiene.
- Ask for fluoride trays if you get cavities.
- If you get cavities, consider crowns instead of fillings.
- Brush and scrape your tongue at least once a day to remove bacteria and fungus. If you have tongue furrows, use an oral irrigator daily to clean out particles.

Candida infections

- If you get recurrent *Candida* infections (thrush), eat yogurt with live cultures (probiotics) daily to decrease *Candida*.
- Ask your doctor for an anti-fungal treatment.
- Disinfect dentures daily (they harbor bacteria and fungus). Ask your doctor for an antifungal powder to use on your dentures.
- Do not sleep with removable dental appliances. Keep them in a container with denture cleaners.

Notes: Dry mouth care table reviewed and edited by Dr. Ava Wu, DDS, Sjögren's Clinic, University of California San Francisco, and member of the National Board Sjögren's Foundation, and by Vidya Sankar, DMD, MHS Division Director of Oral Medicine, Tufts University School of Dental Medicine, Boston, MA, and member of the National Board Sjogren's Foundation. Brands mentioned above are included as examples only and are not formal endorsements.

Cevimeline is a capsule, but you can dissolve the contents in a small glass of water and take only a portion of the liquid, reserving the remaining quantity for a later dose. If you do not tolerate either pilocarpine or cevimeline, or if one or the other does not work, your doctor can prescribe the other one. Sjögren's patients sometimes note that these medications help their dry eyes, nasal congestion, dry skin, chronic cough, and dry vaginal problems. Bethanechol can be prescribed if pilocarpine and cevimeline don't work.

If you continue to have soreness and a sensation of dryness in the mouth despite taking pilocarpine or cevimeline, it may be due to chronic erythematous candidiasis (see above). Treating the infection usually helps.

People with dry mouth should see their dentist more often than twice a year. Sjögren's patients have increased chances of developing gingivitis (gum inflammation), periodontitis, dental cavities, and tooth loss. Your dentist can identify problems early so that proper treatment can be given before things get out of hand, such as the permanent loss of teeth. Make sure to ask your dentist about fluoride applications that can be done in the office (fluoride varnish) or used at home (dental trays with fluoride gel or prescription-strength fluoride toothpaste).

Dry Nose

When dryness occurs inside the nose, it can become itchy and uncomfortable. Sometimes the blood vessels just beneath the mucosal surface can even bleed, causing a bloody nose. Since the sinus passages connect to the inside of the nose, dryness in this area can also cause sinus congestion, sinusitis (sinus infections), and increased allergy problems (itching, sneezing, and nasal congestion). Sjögren's patients are twice as likely to have chronic sinusitis than the general population.

Many Sjögren's patients do not realize that they have nose dryness. A bloody nose, irritation in the nose, nose itchiness, and loss of taste can all be signs of nasal dryness. These problems occur especially during winter, when there is much less air moisture. Measures to help with dry nose are listed in table 14.6.

LUPUS IN FOCUS

Preventing cavities and tooth loss from dry mouth

In 2016, the Sjögren's Foundation published guidelines with the American Dental Association for preventing dental cavities in Sjogren's patients. These guidelines are especially helpful for doctors, such as rheumatologists, who are not trained in tooth and gum care. These guidelines recommend that Sjögren's patients with dry mouth regularly use fluoride, xylitol-based gum and lozenges, and take Salagen or Evoxac. They should also use remineralizing toothpastes (such as Clinpro 5000 and Prevident 5000 Booster Plus). Do not let your pharmacist substitute these with Denta 5000 because it does not have the non-fluoride remineralizing agent called tricalcium phosphate.

Table 14.6 Keeping the Inner Nose Moist

- Do everything in table 14.2.
- Use a moisturizing saline spray followed by saline gel every several hours. Brands include Ayr, Ponaris, Nasogel, Rhinase, and Alkalol. Oil-based products usually work better than water-based.
- Use Vaseline, Neosporin, or Polysporin every few hours if the outer nasal passages are sore and dry.
- Use saline irrigation products (such as Navage Nasal Care, NeilMed Sinus Rinse, Simply Saline, or SinuPulse) regularly to keep the nasal passages moist.
- Avoid systemic antihistamines (Benadryl, Claritin, Alavert, and Zyrtec) that dry out the nose.
- Avoid systemic decongestants (Sudafed and antihistamines that end with a "-D" such as Claritin-D) that dry out the nose.
- A nasal steroid (Flonase, fluticasone) may be better and safer to treat allergies than antihistamines and decongestants. Treat nasal congestion. It contributes to mouth breathing, making dry mouth worse. Try over-the-counter fluticasone nasal spray (Flonase) and guaifenesin (Mucinex) daily for a few weeks.
- For thick mucus, take guaifenesin (e.g., Mucinex).
- Ask your doctor to prescribe pilocarpine (Salagen), cevimeline (Evoxac), or bethanechol.

Note: Brands mentioned above are included as examples only and are not formal endorsements.

Dry Skin

Dry, itchy skin is another common problem in Sjögren's. This is thought to be due to decreased sweat and oil production by the sweat and sebaceous glands of the skin, but this is not known for sure. The dry skin becomes especially apparent in the wintertime when indoor heat makes the winter air even drier. In fact, many of the dryness problems of Sjögren's are often exacerbated in winter. The itchiness can sometimes be quite intense, causing difficulty sleeping. Scratching the skin while trying to alleviate the itching can cause irritation, inflammation, and red patches. Suggestions for caring for dry skin are in table 14.7 and at lupusencyclopedia.com/dry-skin-in-lupus.

Dry Vagina

More than half of women with Sjögren's have vaginal dryness. It can cause a persistent feeling of itchiness and discomfort, pain during intercourse, bleeding, and discharge. It also increases the risk of recurrent yeast infections from *Candida*. Another issue is that estrogen, which is vital for maintaining healthy vaginal tissue and lubrication, decreases with menopause and makes vaginal dryness worse. Helpful recommendations are listed in table 14.8.

Table 14.7 Treating Dry, Itchy Skin

- Do everything listed in table 14.2.
- Do not use soap on most body surfaces. Instead, use a moisturizer (such as CeraVe Cream) as a substitute for soap on face, arms, legs, and trunk. Cream is better than lotion. For underarms, feet, and private areas, use an oil-based soap, like Eucerin Calming Body Wash Daily Shower Oil.
- Shower or bathe in lukewarm water, not hot. Hot water removes natural lubricating oils. Whatever your bath or shower temperature is currently, make it slightly cooler (the cooler, the better).
- Take shorter baths and showers.
- After bathing or showering, pat the skin dry; do not rub (rubbing removes moisturizing oils).
- Apply a moisturizer to dry body areas immediately after bathing.
- Use a heavy-duty moisturizer with urea, glycerin, lactic, or alpha hydroxyl acids (such as CVS Healing Skin Therapy Lotion or AmLactin Cream).
- Consider moisturizers with ceramides: help repair the skin's protective barrier (such as Aveeno Eczema Therapy or CeraVe).
- For areas of very dehydrated skin, use petrolatum (Vaseline) or body oil (such as Neutrogena Body Oil, RoBathol, or Aveeno Skin Relief Shower and Bath Oil). Apply it right after you bathe and while your skin is still moist to trap moisture in the skin.
- Use moisturizers several times a day.
- Avoid fabric softeners, which irritate dry skin.

Note: Brands mentioned above are included as examples only and are not formal endorsements.

Table 14.8 Treating Vaginal Dryness

- Use vaginal moisturizers such as Satisfaite, Replens, Luvena (contains prebiotics), YES VM, Vagisil, Gynatrof, KY Liquibeads, and BeeFriendly Queen Bee (organic) regularly.
- Use only vulva-friendly creams and moisturizers, such as Satisfem, Vulvacare, Vulva Harmony, VMagic, Protégé V-Topia, and NeliDew Organics Vaginal Moisturizer.
- To decrease painful intercourse, use silicone-based or natural oil-based (olive, avocado, coconut, vegetable) lubricants each time. Only use silicone-based with latex condoms. Oil-based destroy condoms.
- See your gynecologist and ask about estrogen cream, rings, or suppositories.

Note: Brands mentioned above are included as examples only and are not formal endorsements.

KEY POINTS TO REMEMBER

1. Sjögren's is an autoimmune disease. It occurs as an overlap syndrome in 30% of SLE patients (sometimes called secondary Sjögren's).

2. Sjögren's causes inflammation and damage to the body's moisture-producing glands, leading particularly to dryness of the mouth, eyes, nose, and airways.

3. Dryness is often present in other body areas, such as the skin, ear canals, and vagina.

4. Decreased saliva production commonly causes gingivitis, periodontitis, dental cavities, and loss of teeth if preventative measures are not taken.

5. Redness and soreness of the tongue, mouth lining, and corners of the lips may indicate an infection due to *Candida albicans* (oral candidiasis) and needs to be treated with antifungal medications and taking steps to improve mouth moisture (table 14.5).

6. Dry eyes can cause problems with vision if not addressed and treated.

7. If you have itchy skin, especially in the winter, you may have dry skin from Sjögren's.

8. Many measures can be taken to help the dryness of Sjögren's. Refer to tables 14.3–14.8.

9. Pilocarpine (Salagen), cevimeline (Evoxac), or bethanechol can increase saliva production.

10. For dry eyes, prescription anti-inflammatory (Restasis, Cequa, and Xiidra) eye drops can help.

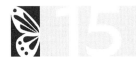

The Digestive System

Darryn Potosky, MD, AGAF, *Contributing Editor*

The digestive system (figure 15.1), also called the gastrointestinal (GI) system, handles what we eat and drink, breaking nutrients down into tiny molecules to be absorbed into the bloodstream. The digestive system starts at the mouth and ends at the anus, where the final waste products are eliminated in the feces. In between are the esophagus, stomach, and intestines. In addition to the gastrointestinal tract, other organs in the digestive system include the liver, gall bladder, and pancreas.

The GI system is the largest organ of the immune system. The walls of the stomach and intestines are lined with important immune system cells, and the intestinal walls contain many types of immune system white blood cells. The GI tract has more of these white blood cells than the entire rest of the body. It should be no surprise that what we eat and the microorganisms (microbiome, chapter 3) in our GI tract regularly interact with our immune system. These interactions play essential roles in autoimmune disorders, such as SLE (chapters 3 and 38).

SLE affects the GI tract in many ways. The main problem from lupus inflammation in the mouth is oral ulcers, discussed in chapter 8. The salivary glands are part of the digestive system and can be affected by Sjögren's disease (chapter 14). This chapter discusses the other areas of the digestive system.

Pharynx

The pharynx is the area behind the mouth and nose. It is involved in the respiratory system (chapter 10) and the gastrointestinal system. Anything that comes into the pharynx from the mouth or nose can go in one of two directions: the gastrointestinal tract if it goes into the esophagus (food and drink) or the trachea (windpipe) with breathing. Just as SLE can cause oral and nasal ulcers, it can also cause inflammation of the pharynx (lupus pharyngitis). Pharyngitis can also result from dryness from Sjögren's. Either way, its effect tends to be a sore throat.

Lupus pharyngitis is treated with immunosuppressants. Sjögren's sore throat is treated with moisturizing measures (chapter 14). However, sometimes a sore throat can be due to an infection that is bacterial (such as strep throat), viral, or fungal (such as *Candida*). In strep throat, the doctor will usually see pus in the back of the throat and large neck lymph glands in someone with fever. It is treated with antibacterial medications (antibiotics). Viral pharyngitis causes redness in the back of the throat, usually

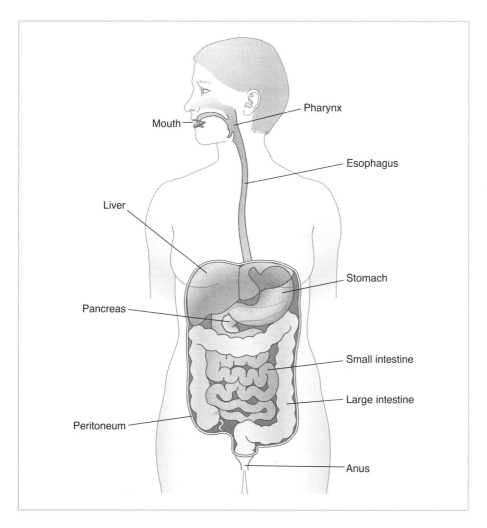

Figure 15.1 The digestive system

Prevent SLE mouth problems

Unfortunately, SLE patients lose teeth more often and at a younger age than others. Dry mouth, sores, and mouth discomfort can make eating difficult and decrease the quality of life. These problems can be caused by Sjögren's disease overlap (chapter 14), lupus inflammation, *Candida* fungal infections, and medications. All SLE patients should be extra vigilant with their dental health care from an early age. Do not smoke and do everything in table 14.5 to lower your chances for tooth loss and other mouth problems.

with no pus. It is due to a virus (such as the common cold virus), and antibiotics do not help. It is treated with medicines that can calm down symptoms (such as throat lozenges). In SLE patients on immunosuppressants (table 22.1) and in those with Sjögren's overlap syndrome, another common cause of pharyngitis is a fungus called *Candida albicans. Candida* infection usually shows white patches in the mouth or back of the throat. In someone with dry mouth, the tongue will be red, tender, and often lack white patches (chapters 14 and 22). It is treated with anti-fungal medications.

Gastroesophageal reflux disease (GERD, chapter 28) due to acidic contents backing up from the stomach can also irritate the pharynx.

KEY POINTS TO REMEMBER

1. Lupus inflammation or Sjögren's dryness can cause pharyngitis, resulting in sore throat.

2. The doctor will consider other possibilities, such as strep throat, *Candida* thrush infection, or irritation from acidic stomach contents due to gastroesophageal reflux. These are all treated differently.

Esophagus

The esophagus is a muscular tube connecting the pharynx to the stomach. Between the esophagus and stomach is a muscular ring, the lower esophageal sphincter (LES). A sphincter is a muscle that squeezes a tube-shaped passageway closed. The role of the esophagus is to push the food and liquid that you swallow down into the stomach. The first part of swallowing is performed consciously by squeezing the muscles of the pharynx and upper part of the esophagus. The muscles lower in the esophagus then continue this downward motion without conscious effort on your part. The LES then automatically relaxes. This allows the food to be pushed into the stomach by the esophagus muscles. After the food enters the stomach, the LES tightens to ensure that swallowed food and liquid remain in the stomach and does not go back up into the esophagus.

Depending on the study, in 10% to 70% of SLE patients the esophagus muscles do not work correctly. This is termed "esophageal dysmotility" (*dys-* means "abnormal," and -*motility* means "motion or movement"), or "hypomotility" (*hypo-* is from the Greek for "under" or "less than"). This condition may be due to SLE inflammation, scarring or decreased blood supply to the esophageal muscles. Esophageal dysmotility is more common in anti-RNP-positive patients (chapter 4) and in those with Raynaud's (chapter 11).

A person with esophageal dysmotility may have difficulty swallowing, pain when swallowing, heartburn, or chest pain. Other problems can cause similar symptoms and need to be excluded. Some drugs used by lupus patients can cause inflammation of the esophagus (table 15.1). Immunosuppressants can increase infections, such as Candidal esophagitis. It is due to the fungus called *Candida albicans* and is treated with anti-fungal medications. Other potential causes of these same symptoms, such as cancer or scarring of the esophagus, also need to be excluded.

Table 15.1 Lupus Drugs That Can Cause Esophagus Irritation

Bisphosphonates for osteoporosis (alendronate, ibandronate, risedronate)

NSAIDs (ibuprofen, naproxen, meloxicam, etodolac, etc.)

Antibiotics (especially doxycycline)

Methotrexate

Blood pressure medicines

Others: aspirin, potassium, vitamin C, iron

If the LES does not work correctly, stomach contents can go into the esophagus. This is called gastroesophageal reflux disease, or GERD (chapter 28). With repeated exposure to acid, problems such as ulcers and scar tissue can form, causing damage to the esophagus. This irritation can even lead to a pre-cancerous condition called Barrett's esophagus. Pre-cancerous means that it is not cancer, but it could turn into cancer over time.

Another harmful complication of esophageal dysmotility occurs when stomach contents travel up the esophagus when someone is lying down. These contents can go into the lungs, causing lung damage or pneumonia. The medical term for this is "aspiration."

It is best to be evaluated by a gastroenterologist (stomach doctor) to help figure out the cause of these esophageal symptoms. They will often perform an esophagogastroduodenoscopy (EGD), also known as an upper endoscopy. While you are sedated (made sleepy with anesthesia), the doctor inserts a thin, flexible camera down into the esophagus, the stomach, and the first part of the small intestine (the duodenum). The doctor can see inflammation (such as esophagitis), scar tissue, ulcers, and cancer. A biopsy is taken of abnormal areas and sent to the lab to look for cancer, celiac disease (gluten intolerance), and infections such as *H. pylori* (chapter 28). However, the EGD cannot diagnose esophageal dysmotility. Its purpose is to exclude conditions that can cause similar symptoms.

Esophageal dysmotility is diagnosed by other tests, such as an upper GI study, esophagram, or barium swallow (the three tests are similar with minor differences). During these tests, the person is asked to swallow a liquid that can be seen on x-rays. The liquid coats the esophagus so that its shape shows up on the x-ray. Sometimes the person is asked to swallow a coated tablet or food. As it is ingested, x-rays show how the esophagus is working.

Another test is esophageal manometry (*mano-* from the Greek for "thin," and *-metry* means "measure"). A thin, flexible tube is inserted into the nose, down the esophagus, and into the stomach. Then the person takes sips of water. The technician measures the pressures exerted by the muscles as the water goes down the esophagus.

If you have esophageal dysmotility, these tests will show where the esophagus muscles are not moving the liquid or food correctly. This can occur at various parts of the esophagus or at the very end where the LES lies.

Sometimes, involving a trained speech therapist helps. A speech therapist, specializing in swallowing, can teach the affected person how to eat and drink appropriately. There are techniques (table 15.2) that can make it easier to eat and decrease complications such as esophageal and lung damage. There are also medications that can help lower stomach content acidity and others that can help the esophageal muscles work better.

Achalasia is a specific type of esophageal dysmotility disorder. It occurs when the nerves responsible for properly moving the esophagus muscles and relaxation of the LES become damaged. People with achalasia have trouble swallowing solid and liquid foods and frequently throw up undigested food or saliva. Because of this, they are at risk of aspiration while lying down. Chest pain, heartburn, trouble belching, frequent hiccupping, and weight loss may also occur. It is usually diagnosed with manometry.

Achalasia treatments include using a balloon to expand the LES (pneumatic balloon dilatation), surgery to loosen the LES muscle (surgical myotomy), or botulinum toxin (Botox) injections to relax the muscle.

KEY POINTS TO REMEMBER

1. SLE can cause esophageal dysmotility, in which the esophagus muscles do not move food or liquid normally through the esophagus.

2. Esophageal dysmotility can cause difficulty swallowing, heartburn, and chest pain. If severe, it can cause stomach contents to go into the lungs when lying down.

3. Esophageal dysmotility is diagnosed by an upper GI study, esophagram, barium swallow, or esophageal manometry. EGD excludes other problems.

4. Esophageal dysmotility can be treated with medicines that decrease stomach acidity or drugs that affect the esophagus muscles. However, the most essential part of the treatment is to do everything in table 15.2.

Stomach

SLE rarely affects the stomach. Stomach (gastric) ulcers and stomach inflammation (gastritis) are common in SLE. However, they are often due to medications, *H. pylori* infection, or other factors (chapter 28).

Gastroparesis is a condition in which the stomach does not empty its contents normally. *Gastro-* refers to the stomach, and *-paresis* to paralysis. Diabetes is the most common cause of gastroparesis. However, SLE can also cause it.

Gastroparesis causes nausea, vomiting, abdominal pain, bloating, and feeling full too quickly (called early satiety). Potential causes include SLE affecting the nerves that help the stomach work properly (autonomic dysfunction, chapter 13) or causing the muscles in the stomach's lining not to work correctly due to inflammation or damage. Gastroparesis tends to occur in those who have had severe SLE, and in those who have had SLE a long time. Therefore, permanent damage (rather than inflammation) is usually the cause, and immunosuppressants do not help most patients.

Its treatment is similar to that of diabetic gastroparesis. Medications that can help the stomach muscles work better include metoclopramide, domperidone, erythromycin,

Table 15.2 Improving Esophageal Dysmotility and GERD

- Eat smaller, more frequent meals.
- Take small bites of food and small sips of liquids at a time.
- Eat food slowly. Put the fork down after each bite. Pick it back up after completely swallowing.
- Use xylitol lozenges or gum before eating (increases saliva flow).
- Avoid substances that relax the LES (such as caffeine, tobacco, chocolate, peppermint, high-fat food, and alcohol): they worsen GERD.
- Avoid highly acidic foods like soda, citrus juices, tomatoes, and wine.
- If possible, stop drugs that worsen GERD (table 28.1).
- Avoid tight clothing and belts (they increase pressure on the stomach).
- Maintain normal weight (abdominal fat puts pressure on the stomach).
- Do not lie down for at least two to three hours after eating or drinking.
- Avoid exercise and bending at the waist for one to two hours after eating.
- Maintain good posture. Sit and stand upright.
- Elevate the head of the bed on six- to eight-inch blocks or furniture risers.

azithromycin, and cisapride. Anti-nausea drugs are sometimes necessary. Severe cases may require inserting a tube into the stomach to allow gas and stomach contents to empty and inserting a feeding tube into the small intestine.

Intestines

Inflammation of the intestines can be due to different problems in SLE. These include mesenteric vasculitis, inflammatory bowel disease (IBD), and blood vessel inflammation (vasculitis) in the intestinal walls.

In lupus enteritis (*enter-* from the Greek for "intestine," and *-itis* for inflammation), SLE causes inflammation of the walls of the intestines. It occurs in around 5% of SLE patients. It is most common in anti-SSA positive patients who have low C3 or C4 complements (chapter 4). Lupus enteritis can affect either the small intestine or the large intestine. All patients tend to have abdominal pain, and most have nausea, vomiting, and diarrhea. The inflammation can involve the veins, arteries, or muscles of the walls of the intestines.

Those with large intestine enteritis can have intestinal pseudo-obstruction (*pseudo-* means "false"). Intestinal obstruction is a condition in which there is an anatomical blockage (caused by cancer or scar tissue, for example). However, in lupus-related enteritis, there is no true anatomical obstruction (hence a pseudo-obstruction). Instead, the inflamed intestinal wall muscles cannot move digested food through the intestines.

Abdominal CT usually shows intestinal wall swelling in lupus enteritis. Some patients have extra fluid around the abdominal organs (called ascites). The doctor will usually drain the liquid and send it to the lab for analysis to ensure it is not due to something unrelated to lupus, such as infection or cancer. Lupus enteritis tends to return if treated only with steroids, so other immunosuppressants are usually needed to prevent flares during steroid tapering.

Inflammatory bowel disease (IBD) includes two conditions: Crohn's disease and ulcerative colitis. IBD can cause many symptoms, including abdominal pain, anemia from blood loss, bloating, and diarrhea. These conditions are diagnosed by colonoscopy, in which a flexible camera is inserted through the anus so that the doctor can look for inflammation inside the intestines. Small biopsies are done to send to the lab for analysis.

A 2016 Israeli study showed that SLE patients were twice as likely to have IBD as the general public. SLE can also cause intestinal wall inflammation (enteritis and intestinal vasculitis) and can look similar to IBD. The distinction is important because they are caused by different genes, and there are also treatment differences. Biopsies are usually needed to tell which it is.

Another autoimmune disease called celiac disease (also called nontropical sprue and gluten-sensitive enteropathy) can affect the small intestine. Someone with celiac disease develops difficulty absorbing gluten-containing foods (especially common in wheat products). This can cause a wide variety of problems, including diarrhea, stomach upset, weight loss, anemia, and iron and vitamin deficiencies. A 2006 study found that 2.4% of celiac disease patients also had SLE. This is a much higher percentage than that of SLE in the general population.

The diagnosis of celiac disease (CD) begins with blood tests for autoantibodies, primarily anti-tissue-transglutaminase-IgA (chapter 4). Anti-gliadin antibody is unhelpful in diagnosing celiac disease in non-lupus patients but not in SLE patients.

A small bowel biopsy obtained during an EGD (see the esophagus section) is the most accurate test. However, sometimes the biopsy results in SLE patients can look like CD yet be due to something else—in other words, the biopsy is a false positive. Conditions

---

LUPUS IN FOCUS

Not all wheat and gluten sensitivities are due to celiac disease

Celiac disease (CD) is an autoimmune disease with positive blood antibodies and an abnormal small intestine biopsy.

Wheat allergy (WA) is an allergic reaction (not autoimmune) to wheat that can cause a rash and tingling sensations beginning minutes to hours after eating. It is diagnosed by blood and skin allergy tests.

Nonceliac gluten sensitivity (NGS) causes bloating, "brain fog," and other intestinal symptoms beginning hours to days after ingestion (delayed symptoms compared to wheat allergy). The diagnosis is made when CD and WA have been excluded. NGS is not thought to be an autoimmune reaction to gluten (therefore, "nonceliac"), but rather to a sugar byproduct of gluten or another substance found in gluten-containing products.

CD and NGS are treated with a gluten-free diet (such as avoiding wheat, barley, and yeast), while a WA is treated by avoiding only wheat products.

LUPUS IN FOCUS

Gluten-free diets have not been shown to decrease lupus flares

One of the most common internet myths is that eating a gluten-free diet decreases inflammation and flares in lupus patients. Gluten-free diets have been shown to reduce inflammation only in celiac disease (CD). Avoiding wheat decreases allergic reactions in those with wheat allergies (WA). Many people just feel better while eating a gluten-free diet. This may be due to other reasons, such as eating less carbohydrates that can cause stomach upset. However, no medical studies link gluten with lupus flares. Nonetheless, if you feel better eating a gluten-free diet, it is OK to do so if you have SLE.

that can cause a false positive small bowel biopsy in SLE include autoimmune enteropathy and combined variable immunodeficiency (chapter 22). A gastroenterologist with a special interest in CD should evaluate SLE patients to ensure a correct diagnosis. They should discuss the biopsy results with the pathologist and get specialized help from a gastrointestinal pathologist.

Drugs commonly used to treat lupus can also mimic CD with similar biopsy results. These include non-steroidal anti-inflammatory drugs (NSAIDs), mycophenolate mofetil, azathioprine, and rituximab. A trial period of not taking these may be needed (if possible) to see if the symptoms resolve.

Celiac disease is treated by avoiding gluten-containing foods.

Protein-losing enteropathy (PLE) is a rare SLE complication in which the intestines cannot absorb proteins well. Protein (especially albumin) is vital for healthy nutrition and for keeping fluids inside blood vessels. Low blood albumin levels from PLE cause fluid leakage from blood vessels into the soft tissues, creating swollen feet, ankles, and legs. The medical term for this swelling is "edema." Edema worsens while the person walks, sits, and stands (due to gravity pulling fluid down) and improves after the patient lies down. About 50% of people will also have severe diarrhea. Other causes of a low albumin level and edema must be excluded. These more common causes include medications, circulation problems, obesity, and disorders of the heart, liver, and kidneys.

Protein-losing enteropathy is diagnosed with a particular test called the alpha-1 antitrypsin fecal clearance test. Alpha-1 antitrypsin is a large protein that is increased in the stool in PLE. The person collects all their stool over 24 hours and gives a blood sample. Then the lab calculates the alpha-1 antitrypsin clearance. An extremely elevated level is consistent with PLE. It is treated with immunosuppressants.

KEY POINTS TO REMEMBER

1. SLE does not generally involve the stomach by direct inflammation.

2. Celiac disease (CD) is an autoimmune disorder related to gluten sensitivity (found especially in wheat).

3. CD causes the body not to absorb nutrients properly, causing diarrhea, stomach upset, and anemia.

4. CD may be suspected in anti-tissue-transglutaminase-IgA-positive individuals but is best diagnosed during EGD with a duodenal mucosa biopsy.

5. Anti-gliadin is not useful in SLE for diagnosing CD.

6. CD is treated by avoiding gluten.

Peritoneum

The abdominal contents are surrounded by a lubricated sac called the peritoneum (figure 15.1), just as the heart is covered by the pericardium, and the lungs are surrounded by the pleura. These lubricating sacs are called serosae (the plural of serosa). Serosal inflammation is an SLE classification criterion (chapter 1).

SLE patient autopsies show that 70% had inflammation of the peritoneum (peritonitis) at some time. However, doctors do not identify it very often due to its nonspecific symptoms. Peritonitis typically causes abdominal discomfort and sometimes can cause increased fluid in the abdomen (called ascites). Doctors treat it with immunosuppressants.

Ascites occurs in about 10% of SLE patients. In addition to lupus peritonitis, ascites can be caused by lupus nephritis (kidney inflammation), liver disease, enteritis, mesenteric vasculitis, and protein-losing enteropathy. Non-lupus causes include infections, heart failure, and cancer. Doctors need to consider all these possibilities in SLE patients.

KEY POINTS TO REMEMBER

1. The serosa surrounding the abdominal contents is called the peritoneum. It can become inflamed from SLE (peritonitis).

2. 70% of SLE patients have had peritonitis per autopsy studies. Doctors usually miss it because it causes nonspecific symptoms.

3. Peritonitis should be considered in any SLE patient with abdominal pain. It is treated with immunosuppressants.

Intestinal Blood Vessels

Vasculitis occurs when there is inflammation of blood vessels (chapter 11). It causes narrowing of the blood vessels, which decreases blood flow. The organs that depend on those blood vessels for nourishment and oxygen undergo damage, pain, loss of function, and even death when vasculitis creates decreased blood flow. The mesenteric arteries (*mes-* means "middle"; *-enteric* means "related to intestines") supply blood to the stomach and intestines. One of the most dangerous complications of SLE occurs when these develop vasculitis (mesenteric vasculitis), resulting in abdominal pain, fever, vomiting, bloody diarrhea, and even perforation (a hole) in the organ walls. It usually occurs in people who have severe SLE and other organs affected at the same time (for example, arthritis, pleurisy, or lupus nephritis). Fortunately, it is rare, affecting 1% to 2% of SLE patients.

An arteriogram can diagnose mesenteric vasculitis. Dye is injected into the arteries, and x-rays are taken to view the arteries. Vasculitis appears as abnormal dilations (bulging areas) and constrictions (narrowing). Magnetic resonance angiography (MRA) is now used more often. MRA looks at the arteries using an MRI machine and no radiation.

Surgery is required to remove any dead bowel from mesenteric vasculitis. Immunosuppressants are also necessary. Cyclophosphamide and rituximab (Rituxan) have had the best results in studies. Up to 50% of patients die unless treated quickly. Fortunately, early diagnosis and treatments are improving.

Some mesenteric artery blockages are due to blood clots from antiphospholipid antibodies (chapters 4 and 9). These can also cause severe intestinal problems and even death to part of the bowel. These people are treated with blood thinners, such as heparin and warfarin (Coumadin).

KEY POINTS TO REMEMBER

1. Mesenteric vasculitis occurs when the blood vessels that supply blood to the stomach and intestines become inflamed from SLE.

2. Mesenteric vasculitis causes abdominal pain, vomiting, diarrhea, and bloody feces.

3. Mesenteric vasculitis is diagnosed with an arteriogram x-ray or MRA.

4. Mesenteric vasculitis is treated with immunosuppressants, such as steroids, rituximab, and cyclophosphamide. Surgery can remove dead bowel tissue.

5. Mesenteric vasculitis has a high death rate, but this is improving with earlier diagnosis and treatment.

Liver

The liver is in the upper right side of the abdomen, underneath the rib cage. It performs many jobs, including producing energy for the body, essential proteins, hormones, and bile (which helps with digestion). It is also crucial for removing toxic products from the bloodstream.

The liver can be affected by lupus in many ways. The most common is an enlarged liver, called hepatomegaly (*hepato-* means "liver," and *-megaly* means "enlargement"), found in about 25% of SLE patients. Hepatomegaly can often be felt on physical exam or seen on imaging studies (such as ultrasound, CT, or MRI). Fortunately, hepatomegaly is rarely significant. Patients with hepatomegaly often also have an enlarged spleen (splenomegaly, chapter 9). In this case, the combination is called hepatosplenomegaly, often abbreviated HSM in doctors' notes.

Liver blood test abnormalities are quite common in SLE. The liver blood tests (also called liver enzymes, liver function tests, or LFTs) include AST, ALT, alkaline phosphatase, and bilirubin (see chapter 4 for details). LFTs are checked regularly in SLE patients to ensure nothing is wrong with their liver, either from SLE itself or from drug side effects. The most common reasons for elevated liver enzymes are drugs (especially non-steroidal anti-inflammatory drugs, or NSAIDs), alcohol, and fatty liver. Fatty liver occurs most commonly in SLE patients who are obese, on steroids, or have diabetes.

There are other potential causes of elevated LFTs that need to be excluded. "Hepatitis" means liver inflammation (*hepato-* means "liver," and *-itis* means "inflammation"). Hepatitis can be due to drugs, viral hepatitis B and C, alcohol, obesity, diabetes, or even genetic disorders. When someone has unexplained elevated LFTs, the doctor will often stop any drug that could irritate the liver to see if the levels return to normal. Other tests, such as imaging studies (such as ultrasound or CT scan) and blood tests for viral hepatitis B and C, may also be performed.

Muscle inflammation can also cause elevated LFTs because muscle cells also contain AST and ALT. Therefore, muscle enzymes, such as creatine phosphokinase (CPK, chapter 4), are usually measured to exclude muscle problems.

If the doctor excludes the above possibilities, one potential cause is lupus hepatitis, due to SLE affecting the liver. A liver biopsy can diagnose lupus hepatitis. This is done by numbing the skin and tissues overlying the liver and then inserting a thin biopsy needle to remove a small sample of liver tissue. It is then examined under a microscope. When liver biopsies are done on people with SLE, lupus hepatitis is the second most seen abnormality (fatty liver being the most common).

Lupus hepatitis occurs in 5% to 10% of SLE patients. It may be more common in children than adults. The inflammation is commonly mild, causing no significant problems other than the elevated LFTs. LFTs tend to increase from lupus hepatitis when SLE is more active in other body parts and decrease when SLE is better controlled. Lupus hepatitis responds well to immunosuppressants and hydroxychloroquine.

On rare occasions there can be enough inflammation in lupus hepatitis to cause significant problems. These include hepatomegaly (enlarged liver), upper right abdominal discomfort, ascites (excessive fluid in the abdomen), jaundice (yellowish discoloration of the eyes and skin due to excessive bilirubin in the blood), and cirrhosis. Cirrhosis, in which irreversible scarring and damage occur, is the most severe consequence of hepatitis. If cirrhosis becomes severe, the liver stops working, putting the person at risk for death, and organ transplantation may be needed. One of the potential consequences of cirrhosis is portal hypertension (explained below).

Note that autoimmune hepatitis (AIH), a separate autoimmune disease that attacks the liver, can occur in some SLE patients. A liver biopsy can help figure out if someone has lupus hepatitis or AIH. AIH patients are also often positive for autoantibodies such as anti-smooth muscle or liver/kidney microsomal-1 antibodies (chapter 4). While lupus hepatitis rarely causes cirrhosis, AIH often does and needs aggressive immunosuppressant treatment to prevent cirrhosis. If someone with SLE has AIH, it is called an overlap syndrome (chapter 2)

Hepatic vasculitis occurs when the arteries that supply blood to the liver are inflamed, causing abdominal pain and elevated LFTs. It is rare and is treated with immunosuppressants.

Antiphospholipid antibody syndrome (APS, chapter 9) can cause blood clots in the liver. The most common APS complication is Budd-Chiari syndrome in which the large veins that drain the liver become obstructed by blood clots. Blood backs up into the

Other autoimmune liver diseases

Autoimmune hepatitis (AIH) and primary biliary cholangitis (PBC), mentioned in chapter 2, are organ-specific autoimmune diseases distinct from lupus, although they do occur more commonly in SLE patients than in the general population. AIH occurs twice as often in SLE patients than PBC. In SLE patients with elevated liver enzymes, 5% to 10% have AIH. PBC occurs more frequently in people who have Sjögren's. AIH is also called lupoid hepatitis, but it is not caused by lupus. See the main text regarding *lupus* hepatitis, which is not the same as *lupoid* hepatitis (or AIH).

liver, which enlarges (hepatomegaly). The pressure in the blood vessels of the liver increases (called portal hypertension), and the liver can stop functioning normally.

With portal hypertension, the increased pressure in the blood vessels can cause higher blood pressure in nearby blood vessels. If this occurs in the blood vessels of the lower esophagus, portal hypertension can cause swollen veins inside the esophagus, called esophageal varices. Esophageal varices are fragile and can potentially bleed, creating a dangerous situation requiring urgent medical help. People with esophageal varices are usually monitored closely by EGD. If the varices are large and at risk of bleeding, the doctor can treat them in various ways to decrease this risk.

APS can cause other liver problems, such as clogging of smaller liver blood vessels that are not visible on imaging studies. If a large liver artery is affected, part of the liver can die. This is called liver infarction. APS involving the liver is treated with blood thinners (chapter 9).

Another potential cause of portal hypertension in SLE, other than cirrhosis and Budd-Chiari syndrome, is noncirrhotic portal hypertension, also called nodular regenerative hyperplasia (NRH). In non-lupus patients, cirrhosis is the most common cause of portal hypertension. However, in NRH, liver biopsies do not show cirrhosis; hence "noncirrhotic." Instead, the biopsies often show microscopic collections of cells (nodules) packed together (nodular), squeezing the surrounding liver cells (therefore, "nodular regenerative hyperplasia"). Liver MRI or CT can sometimes help diagnose NRH. It can improve with immunosuppressants and hydroxychloroquine.

KEY POINTS TO REMEMBER

1. Hepatitis refers to any inflammation of the liver.

2. Lupus hepatitis (liver inflammation due to lupus) occurs in 5% to 10% of SLE patients. It is essential to exclude other causes of hepatitis, such as drugs, hepatitis B or C infection, alcohol, fatty liver, and other autoimmune liver diseases.

3. Hepatitis is suggested by elevated liver function tests (LFTs, especially AST and ALT).

4. Muscle inflammation can also cause elevated LFTs.

5. Usually, drugs that can irritate the liver (such as NSAIDs and methotrexate) are stopped first. Additional blood studies, liver ultrasound, CT scan, and sometimes even a liver biopsy may be needed to determine the cause of hepatitis.

6. Lupus hepatitis is usually mild and rarely progresses to cirrhosis. Autoimmune hepatitis (AIH) is different from lupus hepatitis. AIH frequently causes cirrhosis.

7. Vasculitis of the liver's blood vessels is extremely rare, but it is dangerous when it occurs.

8. Antiphospholipid antibody syndrome may cause liver blood clots, requiring blood thinners.

Gallbladder

Gallbladder involvement by SLE is extremely rare. It is estimated that less than 1 out of 1,000 SLE patients develop gallbladder inflammation. The gallbladder is attached to the liver and is a sack that stores bile, a substance that is produced by the liver and is important for digesting food. After eating a meal (especially a fatty meal), the gallbladder squeezes bile into the intestines to aid digestion.

Gallbladder inflammation is called cholecystitis. *Cholecyst-* comes from the Greek for "gallbladder," and *-itis* means "inflammation." Most cases of cholecystitis are due to gallbladder stones. "Acalculous cholecystitis" (*a-* from the Greek for "without" and *-calculous* for "stone") refers to inflammation of the gallbladder by any disease not associated with gallbladder stones. Since it usually happens quickly, it is often called acute acalculous cholecystitis (AAC). Common causes include infections, cancer, and hardening of the arteries. SLE is a rare cause of AAC.

Patients with lupus-AAC are usually quite sick with active SLE in other organs and have lab abnormalities such as low C3 or C4 complements and high anti-dsDNA. Most (but not all) patients have active lupus nephritis (kidney inflammation) during the episode. They usually have belly pain, fever, and elevated LFTs. Around half of the patients with lupus-ACC will have increased pain when breathing in while the doctor pushes under the right ribcage (Murphy's sign).

AAC is diagnosed using either an ultrasound or a CT scan. The doctor also needs to exclude infection. The cause of lupus-AAC is vasculitis (blood vessel inflammation) in the gallbladder wall. Therefore, it is usually treated with immunosuppressants. Fewer than 10% of lupus-ACC patients die. However, around 30% of ACC patients die when it is due to non-lupus problems, such as infection.

Pancreas

The pancreas is an organ that lies in the upper abdomen just in front of the spine. The pancreas is vital for producing hormones (such as insulin, which lowers blood glucose, or sugar, levels) and secreting them into the blood. The pancreas also makes important food digestion enzymes. It secretes these substances directly into the

LUPUS IN FOCUS

Amylase and lipase elevations

Mild amylase elevations occur in 30% to 45% of SLE patients who do not have pancreatitis. In pancreatitis, the amylase and lipase are usually at least three times higher than the upper limits of normal. I have cared for one SLE patient incorrectly labeled as having "pancreatitis" based upon mild elevations of amylase and lipase. She had abdominal pain due to medication but not pancreatitis.

small intestine. Pancreas inflammation is called pancreatitis and occurs in up to 4% of SLE patients, more commonly in children. SLE patients who are at increased risk of developing pancreatitis include those with high triglyceride levels (a type of fat measured on cholesterol blood tests, chapter 21), pleurisy (chapter 10), psychosis (chapter 13), and Sjögren's disease (chapter 14), and those who are positive for SSA (Ro) antibodies.

Pancreatitis symptoms include nausea, vomiting, and abdominal pain in the upper mid-abdomen, which often radiates (spreads) to the back. Blood tests show elevated amylase and lipase levels (enzymes produced by the pancreas). Pancreatitis typically causes amylase and lipase levels to be over three times higher than the upper limits of normal. Cases of subclinical pancreatitis, in which SLE patients have remarkably elevated amylase and lipase levels yet not have any pancreatitis symptoms, are rare. "Subclinical" is a medical term meaning that a condition is occurring, but it is not causing any actual symptoms.

Although SLE can cause pancreatitis, there are other potential causes. These include gallbladder stones, alcohol, trauma, high triglyceride levels, high calcium levels, and genetic disorders. SLE drugs such as azathioprine, steroids, diuretics, and NSAIDs can also cause pancreatitis. Therefore, pancreatitis in someone with lupus and taking steroids or azathioprine presents difficult treatment decisions for doctors.

Treatment often requires hospitalization. The person is not allowed to eat or drink anything to enable the pancreas to rest. Intravenous (IV) fluids are given. A tube is sometimes inserted through the nose down into the stomach so that stomach contents can continuously be suctioned out, allowing the pancreas to rest.

Lupus pancreatitis is usually due to vasculitis (blood vessel inflammation) of the pancreas blood vessels. Therefore, immunosuppressants are generally needed once other causes have been excluded. Plasmapheresis (plasma exchange) and IVIG have been used for severe cases. If a patient has antiphospholipid antibodies, blood clots in the pancreas could be the cause, and blood thinners may be needed.

Pancreatitis is a potentially severe problem with an elevated risk of dying. Severe pancreatitis occurs more often in children with SLE than in adults. While 60% of lupus pancreatitis patients died in the past, better treatments have decreased this to around 16% (range of 3% to 20%, depending on the study).

1. Pancreatitis is rare in SLE.

2. Pancreatitis causes nausea, vomiting, or abdominal pain, often radiating to the back.

3. Pancreatitis requires hospitalization, IV fluids, not eating or drinking, and draining the stomach with a nasogastric tube to rest the pancreas.

4. Some SLE drugs (especially azathioprine and steroids) can cause pancreatitis and may need to be stopped.

5. Common causes of pancreatitis are alcohol and gallbladder stones.

6. SLE pancreatitis is treated with immunosuppressants; blood thinners may be needed if antiphospholipid antibodies are present.

7. SLE pancreatitis can have a high mortality rate, especially in children.

8. Mildly elevated amylase and lipase levels are common in SLE and usually do not indicate a significant pancreas problem.

Nausea, Vomiting, Abdominal Pain, and Diarrhea

Nausea and vomiting (N/V) in SLE patients are most commonly due to medications. They typically begin soon after starting the medication, making it easy to identify. In this case, the medication should be stopped, or the dosage decreased. But N/V can sometimes occur after someone has been on a medication for a while. In that case, several medicines may need to be stopped, then reintroduced one at a time to figure out which one is causing the problem.

N/V occurs in around 8% of SLE patients during lupus flares. It could be related to inflammation around the abdominal organs (peritonitis), inflammation of any GI tract organs, or even vasculitis (blood vessel inflammation). When due to SLE, it usually resolves after immunosuppressant treatment.

N/V can also be due to other problems such as stomach ulcers, gastritis, and duodenitis (chapter 28).

Around 10% of SLE patients will have abdominal pain during SLE flares due to lupus-induced peritonitis, pancreatitis, cholecystitis, or enteritis. These conditions respond to immunosuppressants. Still, figuring out the cause of abdominal pain can be quite complicated, requiring many tests and the involvement of other specialists, such as gastroenterologists.

Diarrhea is most commonly due to medications (and addressed similarly as above) or infection. Difficulty absorbing nutrients from food (malabsorption) can also cause diarrhea (as in celiac disease). Protein-losing enteropathy is a rare lupus problem and is discussed above.

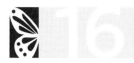

Eyes

Jonathan Solomon, MD, *Contributing Editor*

Most SLE patients develop a close relationship with their eye doctors (ophthalmologists and optometrists). This is usually because the eyes need to be monitored and examined regularly while taking hydroxychloroquine (Plaquenil). In addition, up to half of SLE patients may develop dry eyes from Sjögren's disease and other causes requiring the assistance of an eye doctor.

The most common problems involving the eyes in SLE patients are related to dysfunctional tear syndrome (dry eyes) and Sjögren's disease (see chapter 14). Sjögren's can cause dry eyes, lacrimal (tear) gland swelling, keratoconjunctivitis sicca (inflammation of the cornea and conjunctiva of the eye from dryness), and blepharitis (swelling or inflammation of the eyelids). Other eye parts can also be involved (figure 16.1). We have organized this chapter by the parts of the eye, starting at the front and moving back. Discussions of glaucoma, cataracts, and eye surgery conclude the chapter.

Eyelids

The eyelids are folds of skin above and below the eye. Their primary purpose is to protect the eye. While the outer part of the eyelids is covered with very thin skin, the underparts have a moist surface called the conjunctiva, similar to the wet surfaces inside the mouth, nose, and vagina.

Periorbital is the area around the eyes, including the eyelids. Periorbital edema is a condition in which the skin around the eyes, including the eyelids, swells and becomes puffy. This occurs in around 5% of SLE patients. One potential cause of periorbital edema is angioedema. Angioedema can occur due to SLE, genetic disorders, or allergic reactions (see chapter 8). Another potential cause is nephrotic syndrome (chapter 12).

The outer surface of the eyelids is skin. Cutaneous lupus, especially discoid lupus erythematosus (DLE), can affect the eyelids. DLE of the eyelid (also called periorbital DLE) occurs in 6% of SLE patients. If it occurs by itself, with no other DLE lesions, it can be hard to diagnose. The typical appearance of scaly redness of the eyelid is similar to that of other problems, such as blepharitis (below), psoriasis, and eczema. Incorrect treatment due to an initial misdiagnosis can result in permanent eyelid damage. For

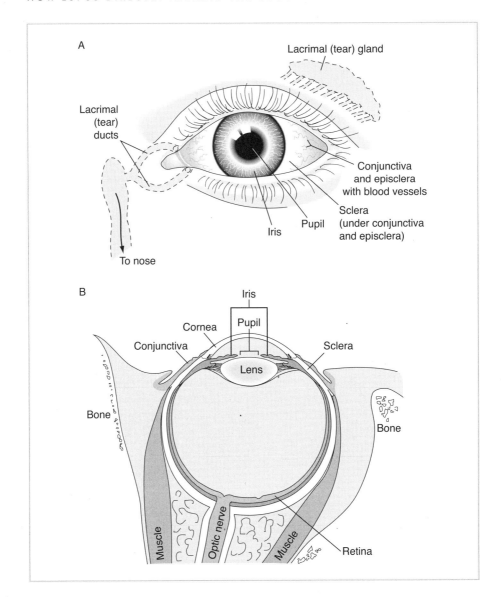

Figure 16.1 The eye

example, if periorbital DLE is not treated properly, it can leave permanent pigment changes that can cause cosmetic concerns.

A much more common eyelid problem in SLE is blepharitis (*blephar-* from the Greek for "eyelid, and *-itis* for "inflammation of"). Blepharitis causes tenderness, redness, and swelling of the eyelid, as well as blurry vision, the sensation of having a foreign body sensation, and itchiness. In SLE patients, it is most commonly due to dry eye from Sjögren's overlap (chapter 14).

Lacrimal Gland (Tear Gland)

The lacrimal tear gland is in the upper, outer part of the eyeball, closest to the ear. If you look in a mirror, pull up on the upper outer eyelid, and shine a bright light (use your smartphone flashlight), you can see it. It is a whitish, yellow area sitting behind the pink, moist skin next to the upper outer eyeball. SLE patients with Sjogren's can develop inflammation lacrimal gland inflammation. This can lead to swelling of the gland and decreased production of tears and dry eyes. See chapter 14 for treatment.

Cornea

The cornea is the clear covering at the front of your eye. It allows light to enter the eye so that you can see. The most common problem of the cornea in SLE patients is dry eye, usually due to Sjögren's. Another term for dry eye, which you may see in your eye doctor's notes, is "keratoconjunctivitis sicca" (KCS, chapter 14). Other potential causes of dry eyes include medications (such as blood pressure medication, anti-depressants, and over-the-counter allergy medications), smoking, and improper eyelid closure. If not treated appropriately (table 14.3), KCS can lead to inflammation and damage to the clear part of the eye, causing vision problems.

SLE also increases the risk of developing a rare condition called keratoconus (*kerato-* from the Greek for "cornea," and *-conus* for "cone-shaped"). It occurs in around one of every 1,500 people. Keratoconus is a problem where the cornea is weakened, causing the front of the eye to bulge forward in a cone shape, which in turn causes problems with vision. Management can include special contact lenses, UV-light therapy, and even corneal transplantation.

Sclera

The sclera is the white outer part of your eye. It surrounds and connects to the cornea and is quite thick. It is responsible for keeping the round shape of the ball of your eye. This is similar to how the hard rubber of a basketball keeps the ball round.

Scleritis is inflammation of the sclera and is rare in SLE, occurring in only 1% of patients. Scleritis causes the white of the eye to become red and painful. The pain can be deep and severe, "like a toothache," according to some. It is usually treated with anti-inflammatory drugs, such as nonsteroidal anti-inflammatory drugs (for example,

---

LUPUS IN FOCUS

Intolerance or sensitivity to light: photophobia

The term for when the eyes are sensitive to light is "photophobia." If you develop photophobia, it is essential to see your eye doctor right away. The leading causes of severe photophobia in SLE patients are migraine headaches, Sjögren's dry eyes, and uveitis.

indomethacin, chapter 36), steroid eye drops, and immunosuppressants (table 22.1). Episodes of severe scleritis can sometimes leave a permanent area of bluish discoloration to the sclera.

Episcleritis is inflammation of the thin layer of tissue covering the sclera. It occurs in up to a quarter of adult SLE patients but is rare in SLE children. Like scleritis, episcleritis causes the sclera to become red, with swollen-appearing blood vessels visible. It can also cause a "gritty" sensation and watering of the eyes with tenderness to the touch. Episcleritis is a mild problem and usually resolves on its own. However, like scleritis, episcleritis can signify that lupus is more active systemically and may require treatment changes.

The Iris and Uvea

The iris is the portion of our eye that has color. It is what makes someone blue-eyed or brown-eyed. Its purpose is to adjust the amount of light that enters the back of the eye by changing the size of the pupil (the central, circular dark opening) and helps you focus. The iris squeezes the pupil smaller (constricts) when you look at something close up or in bright light. It relaxes to allow the pupil to get larger (dilate) when looking at things close up or in darkness. Anything that affects the iris and prevents it from controlling the size of the pupil will cause difficulty with focusing and blurred vision.

Inflammation of the iris is called iritis. The iris is part of a section of the eye called the uvea. Sometimes doctors use the term "anterior uveitis," which is the same thing as iritis. It is called anterior because inflammation of the uvea can also occur in the back (posterior) part of the eye. If inflammation occurs in the back part of the uvea, it is called posterior uveitis, which is different from iritis.

Iritis causes eye discomfort and blurred vision, especially with light exposure, which causes the iris muscles to constrict and squeeze the pupil. This causes pain in the inflamed iris (similar to the way that an inflamed joint, arthritis, causes pain when it is moved). Often there is redness of the eye where the sclera meets the cornea. It is essential to treat iritis quickly. Over time, uncontrolled inflammation can cause scar tissue to develop, leading to permanent vision problems. Doctors usually treat iritis with steroid eye drops and drops that dilate the pupils. This helps calm down the inflammation and minimize the scar tissue. Steroid drops have little to no side effects in areas of the body away from the eye. However, they can cause side effects such as elevated pressures in the eye (called ocular hypertension and, in severe cases, glaucoma) or clouding of the lens (called cataracts). As with scleritis, your rheumatologist must know if you have developed iritis. Your lupus treatment plan may need to be changed.

All types of uveitis are rare in SLE. Posterior uveitis from SLE is less common than anterior uveitis (iritis). To diagnose posterior uveitis, the eye doctor must look inside the eye. There is even a rarer form of uveitis called "intermediate uveitis." It involves the uvea located between the anterior and posterior portions. Both posterior and intermediate uveitis cause blurred vision, sometimes "floaters," and less frequently red-eye or eye pain. They are treated similarly to anterior uveitis. Sometimes, injections of steroids inside the eye are required.

Retina

The retina is located in the back of the eye. Light contacts the retina and forms an image. This is what makes us able to visualize what we see. After dry eye, which is the most common eye problem in SLE, lupus retinopathy (damage to the retina) is second. It occurs in 10% of SLE patients, especially those in whom SLE is severe.

In retinopathy, the doctor may see something called cotton-wool spots or small areas of bleeding (retinal hemorrhages) in the back of the eye on the retina. SLE patients with lupus retinopathy are at increased risk of central nervous system lupus (chapter 13).

Lupus retinopathy can occur from SLE inflammation or from decreased blood flow. Knowing the cause of the retinopathy is important as it dictates the best treatment. For example, immunosuppressants would be needed for inflammation (such as vasculitis, see below) or blood thinners for decreased blood flow related to antiphospholipid (aPL) antibodies.

Retinopathy can be severe if there is active blood vessel inflammation (retinal vasculitis), and people with lupus retinal vasculitis tend to have severe SLE. Treatment for retinal vasculitis includes immunosuppressants, plasmapheresis, or plasma exchange (chapter 38). Unfortunately, people with retinal vasculitis are usually left with some permanent vision loss from permanent retina damage. Even so, if identified and treated early, restoration of near-normal vision is possible.

Lupus retinopathy (retinal damage) due to retinal blood vessel abnormalities is called a "retinal vasculopathy." Up to 77% of patients with retinal vasculopathy are positive for aPL antibodies, which can cause blood clots in the vessels and decreased blood flow. Retinal vasculopathy from aPL antibody blood clots requires blood thinners such as heparin and warfarin (Coumadin).

Retinal artery occlusion (RAO) occurs when one of the larger arteries of the retina is completely blocked. The retinal arteries are the blood vessels that supply essential nutrition and oxygen to the retina. RAO usually causes the loss of vision in one eye. If a smaller blood vessel is blocked, the vision loss may be partial. The retina is an extension of the central nervous system. So, when RAO occurs and a part of the retina dies (retinal infarction), it is considered a type of stroke (chapter 13 and 21).

There are many potential causes of RAO in SLE, and treatment is directed toward the cause. For example, immunosuppressants are used for active SLE inflammation, blood thinners are used for aPL antibodies, and measures are taken to minimize hardening of the arteries (chapter 21) if due to peripheral vascular disease.

LUPUS IN FOCUS

Cotton-wool spots

In some SLE patients, spots on the retina look like little specks of cotton. The retina in the back of the eye is made up of several layers, one of which contains tiny nerves. If a small blood vessel that feeds these nerves becomes damaged from lupus (vasculopathy), blood flow stops, and a small nerve fiber layer area dies. This dead area appears as the "cotton-wool."

RAO can also occur from small pieces of blood clots that may have traveled to the artery from a different part of the body (called an embolus, chapter 9). An embolus can come from one of the large arteries in the head and neck (carotid arteries) or from the heart. The doctors will examine the carotid arteries and heart, usually with a machine that uses sound waves (ultrasound machine or echocardiogram, chapter 11) to see if they are the source of an embolus. If so, treatment is directed at minimizing future emboli (plural of embolus) from occurring. This may involve surgery on the carotid artery or the use of blood thinners.

The retinal veins drain blood away from the retina. When a vein becomes blocked, it is called a retinal vein occlusion (RVO). Usually, patients with RVO have blurred vision. However, a few fortunate patients may not have any vision problems.

RVO is less likely to be related to active lupus inflammation and is more often due to peripheral vascular disease (chapter 21). It is treated by controlling blood pressure, sugar (glucose) levels, cholesterol, and weight while also not smoking, eating a healthy diet, and regularly exercising. Blood thinners may be needed if aPL antibodies are present. Some cases of RVO can be treated with various types of eye injections and laser treatments. These are beyond the scope of this book.

Unfortunately, blood thinners and lifestyle changes do not reverse the damage that has already occurred from RAO or RVO. However, these measures can help slow down and prevent additional areas from developing RAO and RVO.

If lupus retinopathy affects the central retina, the macula, then it is known as a maculopathy. Lupus maculopathies are much more likely to cause problems with vision, but they are rare. Diabetes and age-related macular degeneration are much more likely causes of maculopathy and retinopathy in SLE patients than lupus itself.

Hydroxychloroquine (HCQ, Plaquenil) can also cause a maculopathy (a type of retinopathy). However, if you get the proper screening tests each year (chapter 30), you can pretty much guarantee that you will not develop vision problems from HCQ. It is usually safe for people with lupus retinopathy, diabetic retinopathy, or age-related macular degeneration to take HCQ, but they must get the proper eye tests done every year.

LUPUS IN FOCUS

"Doctor, I stopped my Plaquenil. It was making my vision blurry."

Although hydroxychloroquine (HCQ, Plaquenil) can potentially cause retinopathy (chapter 30), it is uncommon and takes years to occur. As long as you faithfully get the annual eye tests recommended in chapter 30, your eye doctor would notice something before you would. Blurred vision and other eye symptoms are much more commonly due to other problems such as dry eyes, cataracts, or prescription glasses changes. Steroids are much more likely to cause eye side effects than HCQ. If you develop eye problems, the proper response is NOT to stop HCQ. Instead, call and see your eye doctor immediately and remind them to send your rheumatologist a note about your problem.

Choroid

The choroid is a layer of blood vessels and connective tissues (supporting tissue, like collagen) behind the retina. As a result, it is hard to see without special diagnostic devices. The choroid is vital in supplying oxygen and nutrients to the outer layer of the retina.

In lupus choroidopathy, SLE causes inflammation of the choroid and damage to the choroid blood vessels. It is very rare, with fewer than 50 cases described in the medical literature. It causes blurred vision and usually occurs in patients with severe active SLE. It is treated with immunosuppressants. Some patients regain their vision, while others are left with some blurred vision.

Most patients with lupus choroidopathy also have high blood pressure, which makes it worse. But since high blood pressure can cause choroidopathy, it is not always possible to distinguish between choroidopathy from SLE and choroidopathy due to high blood pressure. High blood pressure must be controlled adequately with blood pressure medications (chapter 21).

Optic Nerve

The optic nerve is located in the back of the eye. It is responsible for transmitting information from the light contacting the retina to the brain to be interpreted into visual pictures. Optic nerve inflammation (optic neuritis or optic neuropathy) occurs in 1% of SLE patients. It is a form of central nervous system lupus (chapter 13) and causes blurred vision or even blindness. It is sometimes seen in a multiple-sclerosis-like involvement from SLE or as a part of neuromyelitis optica spectrum disorders (chapter 13). Optic neuropathy can be due to direct inflammation of the nerve, inflammation of the covering around the nerve, or vasculitis (inflammation of the blood vessels). Immunosuppressants are useful for treatment. There have also been cases reported of aPL antibodies causing blood clots in the blood vessels that feed the optic nerve. In these cases, lifelong blood thinners such as warfarin (Coumadin) need to be used. Approximately 50% of people with SLE optic neuropathy fully recover their eyesight. Unfortunately, the other half has some permanent vision loss.

The optic nerve can also be involved by benign intracranial hypertension (pseudotumor cerebri, see chapter 13). Methotrexate is a drug commonly used to treat lupus. It can cause optic neuropathy, but only rarely, and the condition usually goes away when the medication is stopped. Patients who take daily folic acid or weekly folinic acid (leucovorin, chapter 32) are unlikely to get this complication.

Ocular Muscles (Eye Muscles)

There are six muscles around and behind the eye that enable you to look up, down, left, and right. Anything that interferes with how these muscles work can cause vision problems, such as double vision, or diplopia (*diplo-* from the Greek for "double" and *-opia* meaning "sight").

A 1995 study done in a hospital in Los Angeles, California, found eye muscle problems in 30% of SLE patients sick enough to be admitted. Half of them were due to stroke. Out of 33 patients, 2 had eye muscle inflammation (ocular myositis). Some other nerve problem causes included meningitis, Guillain-Barré syndrome, sixth cranial nerve palsy, and intracranial hypertension (chapter 13). Some others had electrolyte abnormalities (problems with sodium and water balance), low oxygen levels, and even hysteria—reminders that non-lupus causes always need to be considered. The muscles that move the eye can also be affected if the arteries that supply them are inflamed (orbital vasculitis, discussed below). Immunosuppressants are needed if SLE inflammation is the cause.

Internuclear ophthalmoplegia (INO) is a condition in which the lower part of the brain (brain stem), which is responsible for controlling eye muscle movement, is affected. A 1998 Spanish study found INO in 1.5% of their SLE patients. INO causes double vision when looking to the right or left, affecting the eye that moves to the mid-line (toward the nose). For example, if someone whose right eye is affected by INO is asked to look to the left, the left eye would move easily, while the right eye would lag and have difficulty moving toward the nose, resulting in double vision. All their patients had just one eye affected, and 75% of the patients' INO was due to active SLE inflammation. All but one fully recovered with immunosuppressant therapies. One patient had permanent double vision due to a stroke.

A droopy upper eyelid is called ptosis. It is usually due to problems with the muscles that open the eyelids. This can be caused by myasthenia gravis or third cranial nerve palsy from lupus (see chapter 13). Horner's syndrome is a rare cause of ptosis in SLE patients (one Japanese case). We will not discuss it.

Ocular Orbit

The orbit is the space around and behind the eyeball. It includes the bony walls of the skull and surrounds the eye. It is filled with the eye muscles, nerves, blood vessels, fat, and connective tissues (such as collagen). Lupus inflammation in the orbit can affect any or all of these structures. If it primarily affects the muscles, it is called ocular myositis or orbital myositis. If it mainly affects the blood vessels, it is orbital vasculitis. When it involves the fat, it is called orbital panniculitis. It is not uncommon to have inflam-

---

LUPUS IN FOCUS

Another cause of a bulging eye (proptosis) in lupus patients

SLE patients are at increased risk of having Graves' disease (chapter 17), an autoimmune thyroid disease that can cause proptosis by causing a build-up of fat inside the ocular orbit. The condition is called thyroid eye disease (TED) or Graves' ophthalmopathy. It is diagnosed by checking thyroid function tests, such as TSH, and stimulating TSH receptor antibodies (chapters 4 and 17). Sometimes, taking too much thyroid hormone (like Synthroid) can mimic proptosis. Too much thyroid hormone can cause the eyelids to be raised too high (lid lag) and the person to have an intense stare. In this case, the TSH level will be low, and CT or MRI of the involved orbits will not demonstrate TED. It is reversible by lowering the dose of Synthroid. TED can be permanent in 40% of patients after treatment of their Graves'.

mation occurring in more than one part of the orbit, in which case, it can go by several different terms, including "orbital inflammation," "orbital pseudotumor," and "orbital inflammatory syndrome." These problems typically respond to immunosuppressants.

These are rare complications of SLE. They can cause blurred vision, eye pain, or a bulging eye. A bulging eye, called proptosis, is caused by swelling of the structures inside the orbit. When the swelling goes down after successful treatment, the bulging decreases. In orbital panniculitis, the inflamed fat can lead to the loss of fatty tissues surrounding the eye, causing the eyeball to sink back into the eye socket. This condition is called enophthalmos and unfortunately is permanent when it occurs.

Glaucoma

Glaucoma is an eye disease that causes damage to the optic nerve (which connects the eye to the brain). It is often due to high pressure within the eye. There are two main types of glaucoma: angle-closure glaucoma and open-angle glaucoma. In simple terms, while angle-closure glaucoma causes problems quickly, open-angle glaucoma usually doesn't cause any problems for many years. When you hear someone in the United States say that they have glaucoma, it is likely to be open-angle glaucoma. SLE does not cause open-angle glaucoma.

Acute angle-closure glaucoma can cause red eyes (pink eye), decreased vision, headaches, nausea and vomiting, severe eye pain, and the appearance of a halo around lights. Acute angle-closure glaucoma due to SLE is extremely rare. Only four cases have been reported, and these were associated with either central nervous system vasculitis (chapter 13) or choroiditis. It is treated with immunosuppressants. Thalidomide (chapter 35) and surgery have been used as well.

Steroids are the most common cause of glaucoma in SLE patients. Those at increased risk for steroid-induced glaucoma include the very young (under 10 years old), the elderly, people of African ancestry, and diabetics. People with high myopia (severe nearsightedness) are also at increased risk for this complication. People with high myopia can see things very close to them much more easily than farther away.

Glaucoma-suspect patients are at particularly high risk for glaucoma when taking steroids. Of these 30% will develop elevated pressure in the eyes, usually within four weeks of oral steroid treatment.

While steroid eye drops, steroid creams applied to the eyelids, and steroid injections in the eyes have the highest chances of causing or worsening glaucoma, oral steroids and systemic steroids are less likely to do so. People susceptible to developing steroid-induced glaucoma tend to develop it within the first few weeks of steroid use.

A daily dose of prednisone less than 10 mg usually doesn't cause glaucoma, even after a year of treatment. However, 75% of people who take more than 15 mg daily develop elevated pressure after one year.

Most people with steroid-induced glaucoma do not notice any problems at first. Most of the time, it is diagnosed by the eye doctor during a routine eye examination. The treatment of choice is to stop or lower the steroid dose. If the steroid is stopped, the pressure inside the eye can return to normal within a few weeks. Persistently elevated pressure is possible, though. If it is not caught and treated appropriately, it can lead to irreversible optic nerve damage and vision loss.

Pink eye

To many nonmedical people, "pink eye" is a highly infectious type of eye infection. However, there are many other possible causes for "pink eye," such as dry eye, scleritis, episcleritis, uveitis, iritis, and glaucoma. Each of these has a different treatment. If an infectious cause is treated with steroid drops, the infection can worsen. If an inflammatory cause (such as uveitis) is treated with antibiotics instead of steroids, eye damage and blindness may occur. If you develop eye redness, call and see your eye doctor immediately to get a correct diagnosis and treatment.

Cataracts

The lens of your eye lies just behind the pupil and iris. It looks like and functions like a tiny lens of a magnifying glass. It is a clear, dense, oval-shaped structure that focuses the incoming light on the retina and allows you to see near images more clearly.

If the lens becomes cloudy, causing less light to enter the eye, it is called a cataract. Although lupus inflammation does not cause cataracts, they occur much more often in lupus patients than in the general population because of steroids, such as prednisone. They are more likely to occur in patients who take larger doses and for more extended periods, but even tiny amounts over the years can cause cataracts. Lupus patients who smoke, have had lots of sun exposure, do not eat well, don't exercise much, are overweight, and have diabetes get cataracts more easily. While steroid-induced glaucoma can resolve after stopping the steroid, cataracts are permanent. People with cataracts will often note difficulty reading small print. They also have trouble driving at night and reading road signs, as well as being bothered by glare from oncoming headlights.

When vision interferes with the safety and activities of daily living, cataract surgery is the treatment of choice.

Eye Surgery

Vision correction procedures such as **photorefractive keratectomy (PRK)**, **small incision lenticule extraction (SMILE)**, **refractive lens exchange (RLE)**, and **laser-assisted in-situ keratomileuses (LASIK)** surgery have become popular methods to improve eyesight. They reduce the need to wear glasses or contact lenses. In 2002, the American Academy of Ophthalmology and the FDA listed autoimmune diseases such as SLE as a relative contraindication for getting LASIK. In other words, some people with these disorders may not do well with LASIK surgery. More recently, experienced surgeons have shown that patients whose SLE is under reasonable control with medications can safely undergo laser vision correction.

An important contraindication is if someone has severe dry eyes. However, if dry eye is mild, laser vision correction procedures may be performed safely. Your eye doctor

Usually continue your lupus drugs before and after eye surgery

Usually, rheumatologists recommend that patients stop immunosuppressants (except for prednisone) before surgery. An exception is eye surgeries, during which they should be continued. A potential complication after eye surgery is eye inflammation; these drugs decrease this complication.

should perform multiple tests to assess your relative risk before attempting surgery. You must understand that you may be at higher risk for complications from LASIK when you have SLE, especially if you have dry eyes.

KEY POINTS TO REMEMBER

1. By far, the most common problem in the eyes due to SLE is dry eyes from Sjögren's (chapter 14).

2. Iritis (rare in SLE), also called anterior uveitis, can cause blurred vision, red eyes, and difficulty tolerating light. Steroid eye drops treat iritis.

3. Episcleritis is common in SLE. Scleritis is uncommon. These problems cause red eyes and eye discomfort. Doctors treat scleritis with steroid eye drops and immunosuppressants.

4. Lupus retinopathy is an abnormality in which SLE affects the retina in the back of the eye. It can be caused by active inflammation (vasculitis) and treated with immunosuppressants. It can also be caused by blood clots (due to aPL antibodies) and treated with blood thinners.

5. Optic neuritis is a type of CNS lupus (chapter 13) that causes blurred vision and even blindness. It is treated with immunosuppressants.

6. People with SLE can get laser vision correction procedures (LASIK, PRK, SMILE, RLE) if they do not have severe dry eyes.

The Endocrine Gland System

Caitlin O. Cruz, MD, FACP, *Contributing Editor*

The exocrine system (*exo-* means "outside") consists of glands that secrete fluids outside of the body (including sweat and tears) and can be affected by Sjögren's disease (chapter 14). The endocrine (*endo-* means "within") glands secrete hormones inside the body. Hormones are chemical messages that endocrine glands produce. They are meant to travel through the body to other body parts, giving them instructions for what to do. For example, when it gets dark outside, the pineal gland (an endocrine gland in the brain) secretes the hormone melatonin that goes to other parts of the brain, causing sleepiness. Many organs (skin, kidneys, intestines, liver, pancreas, heart, and more) function as endocrine glands and secrete hormones. While lupus can affect these organs and cause problems with hormone production, the endocrine gland affected most by SLE is the thyroid. This chapter focuses on thyroid involvement by SLE.

The thyroid gland (figure 17.1) is a soft gland underneath the Adam's apple (which is most prominent in men) in front of the windpipe cartilage (or trachea). The thyroid secretes thyroid hormones, which help regulate body metabolism (how our bodies use calories or energy). The thyroid also secretes a hormone called calcitonin, which is important for how our bodies use calcium. It is not affected by lupus, so we will discuss only thyroid hormone production in this chapter.

Some SLE patients can develop auto-antibodies that are directed at the thyroid gland and affect thyroid hormone levels. The thyroid can become either overactive in hyperthyroidism (*hyper-* means "over") or underactive in hypothyroidism (*hypo-* means "under").

Depending on the study, between 13% and 50% of SLE patients also have an autoimmune thyroid disease (AITD). In 2018, 10 large studies looked at over 10,000 SLE patients. They showed that they were six times more likely to have subclinical hypothyroidism (defined below) and three times more likely to have hyperthyroidism than the general population. Due to the high risk of AITD in lupus patients, rheumatologists check thyroid function tests.

Dr. Cruz contributed to this article in her personal capacity. The views expressed are her own and do not necessarily represent the views of the Naval Medical Center Portsmouth, the Uniformed Services University, or the United States government.

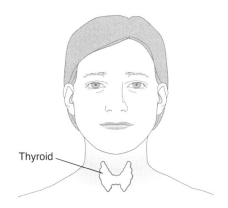

Figure 17.1 Location of the thyroid gland in the neck, below the Adam's apple area

---

LUPUS IN FOCUS

Triggers for developing Hashimoto's

Some of the genes that cause lupus can also cause Hashimoto's. It is common for both to occur in the same family. Microchimerism (chapter 3) could also be a trigger. Microchimerism has been seen in some Hashimoto's patients in whom cells of a fetus (baby) from an earlier pregnancy are found in the thyroid gland.

Hashimoto's Thyroiditis

Hypothyroidism occurs in up to 15% of people who have SLE. It is usually caused by Hashimoto's thyroiditis (also called chronic autoimmune lymphocytic thyroiditis), named after Hakaru Hashimoto, the Japanese doctor who first described it. Antibodies to thyroglobulin and thyroid peroxidase (chapter 4) can cause this type of AITD. When inflammation (thyroiditis) begins in Hashimoto's, most people do not even notice. However, the gland can sometimes enlarge (called a goiter). The patient may notice a small area of soft tissue swelling below the Adam's apple. If the swelling occurs quickly—which is rare—the thyroid becomes tender and painful. If the pain is severe, the thyroid may have to be surgically removed (called a thyroidectomy). During this early phase of active inflammation, 5% to 10% of people with Hashimoto's develop hyperthyroidism where the thyroid secretes too much thyroid hormone and have some of the symptoms described below under Graves' disease.

As the inflammation of Hashimoto's persists, thyroid tissue and cells are destroyed, and the gland shrinks. The gland makes fewer thyroid hormones, causing hypothyroidism. The hypothyroidism of Hashimoto's thyroiditis is diagnosed by finding an elevated TSH level in the blood (chapter 4). Most rheumatologists test for TSH regularly since hypothyroidism is such a common problem, so it is usually identified and treated before problems start.

Initially, most people with Hashimoto's have such mild hypothyroidism that treatment is unnecessary. This is called subclinical hypothyroidism. In this condition the

TSH level is elevated, but the T4 hormone (specifically free T4 level) is normal. In most labs, the normal upper level of TSH is around 4.5 to 5.0 mU/L (milliunits per liter). Experts generally agree that everyone with subclinical hypothyroidism and a TSH of 10 mU/L or higher should be on a thyroid hormonal supplement. Some would argue that people over 65 with subclinical hypothyroidism and a TSH less than 7 mU/L should not be treated. Older people have an increased risk of side effects from thyroid supplements (brittle bones and heart problems). In addition, it is thought that slightly elevated TSH levels can be considered normal in older individuals.

Some experts recommend that people younger than 65 who have subclinical hypothyroidism take a thyroid supplement if their TSH is 7 mU/L or higher, even if they feel fine. However, not everyone agrees with this approach and would treat with a supplement only if hypothyroid symptoms occur.

As more thyroid tissue is lost over time, the TSH level gradually rises, and the thyroid gland cannot produce enough thyroid hormone (T3 and T4). When the free T4 level becomes lower than normal, the condition is called overt hypothyroidism. Hypothyroid symptoms include hair loss, cold and clammy skin, fatigue, mental sluggishness, weight gain (even though the appetite is less than normal), weakness, and feeling cold while others feel warm. These symptoms usually go away with thyroid hormonal treatment. Treatment is generally needed for the rest of the person's life.

Hypothyroidism can cause severe brain and nerve problems if not found and treated early. Fortunately, this is rare in SLE patients who are followed regularly by a rheumatologist.

A small number of people with Hashimoto's who are treated quickly still do not get entirely better on thyroid supplementation. These patients tend to have very high thyroid peroxidase antibody (anti-TPO) levels and continue to have profound fatigue and a poor quality of life. Some thyroid experts believe that they feel bad because of the effects of anti-TPO on other body organs. In other words, autoimmune disease is causing problems with other organs outside of the thyroid gland. In 2019, a team of thyroid experts in Norway performed a study that showed that total thyroidectomies (surgical removal of the thyroid gland) performed on this group of patients caused a dramatic drop in their anti-TPO. They felt better and had more energy and a better quality of life. Since thyroidectomy can have significant complications (such as permanent vocal cord paralysis), this approach is controversial.

LUPUS IN FOCUS

The risk for hypothyroidism with Hashimoto's thyroiditis

Hashimoto's thyroiditis patients with subclinical hypothyroidism have a 5% chance each year of getting worse and needing thyroid supplements. For example, two years after diagnosis, around 10% of patients will need supplements; most will eventually require lifelong thyroid supplements. However, Hashimoto's hypothyroidism in small children and women who develop it after childbirth occasionally reverts to normal. These individuals can stop their treatment but still require regular thyroid function testing.

Graves' Disease

Another autoimmune thyroid disease that can occur with SLE, but not as often, is Graves' disease, a disorder first described by Dr. Robert Graves, an Irish surgeon. It is associated with thyrotropin (or TSH) receptor antibodies. Graves' disease usually causes an enlarged thyroid gland (goiter) and hyperthyroidism. The symptoms of hyperthyroidism include anxiety, increased frequency of bowel movements, shortness of breath, weight loss while eating more, heart palpitations, heat intolerance, warm skin with increased sweating, and muscle weakness. Medications such as methimazole or propylthiouracil can calm down the increased thyroid activity. Some people with Graves' disease are treated with nuclear iodine-131 to keep it from being overactive. After treatment, the thyroid gland stops working, and patients must take a lifelong thyroid supplement. Others may require surgical removal (thyroidectomy).

Thyroid Function Tests in Sick Lupus Patients

It is essential to be careful about how thyroid function tests (TFTs) are interpreted in SLE patients who are ill. Steroids, such as prednisone, can cause the TSH to be lower than usual. Although a low TSH usually indicates an overactive thyroid (hyperthyroidism), this is not always the case if someone is on prednisone, especially someone taking 20 mg or more daily.

Patients with high lupus disease activity can often have low TSH levels along with low T3 and T4 thyroid hormone levels. At one time doctors thought that this high disease activity would cause the thyroid function to be abnormal and that it would improve when the patient got better. We now believe that systemic inflammation from severe lupus can cause the brain to make less TSH. In lupus, the lower TSH levels cause the thyroid gland to produce less T3 and T4 than they normally would. This may be a way for the body to protect itself during periods of severe stress and illness. Finding low TSH, T3, and T4 levels in someone with active lupus is probably not helpful in making a diagnosis. It is best to wait until they are doing better (and are not on very high doses of steroids).

KEY POINTS TO REMEMBER

1. Endocrine glands secrete hormones directly into the body, as opposed to exocrine glands (chapter 14), which secrete substances outside the body.

2. Many organs (such as the skin, liver, pancreas, and kidneys) also function as endocrine glands.

3. Lupus-induced inflammation of these organs can disrupt their release of important thyroid hormones.

4. Approximately one-fourth of everyone with SLE will develop autoimmune thyroid disease.

5. Hashimoto's thyroiditis is common and is diagnosed by finding positive anti-thyroglobulin or anti-thyroid peroxidase antibodies.

6. Many people with Hashimoto's thyroiditis have to take lifelong thyroid supplements due to permanent hypothyroidism.

7. Another autoimmune thyroid problem is Grave's disease, which causes an enlarged thyroid gland, hyperthyroidism, and goiter.

8. Graves' disease is treated with either medication to calm down the thyroid gland or with nuclear iodine-131 treatments (which destroy the thyroid gland). Sometimes, the thyroid gland is removed surgically.

9. People with Graves' disease usually need to take a thyroid supplement for the rest of their lives after iodine-131 treatment or after surgical removal of the thyroid gland.

10. Thyroid function tests must be interpreted with caution in sick lupus patients and those who take steroids. A low TSH level may not be important.

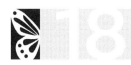

The Reproductive System and Pregnancy

Julie Nusbaum, MD, *Contributing Editor*

SLE does not typically cause significant inflammation or damage to reproductive organs, such as the uterus (womb), ovaries, or testicles (testes). It can, however, potentially cause problems with the breasts, endometriosis, fertility (men and women), menstruation, menopause, and pregnancy. Issues can also arise after giving birth. Women can even pass antibodies into their babies, causing a condition called neonatal lupus. These problems will be discussed in this chapter.

Chapter 41 is devoted to measures that women with SLE can take to deal with pregnancy problems and prepare for a successful pregnancy. All women who plan on becoming pregnant should read this chapter and chapter 41 to prepare for pregnancy to the best of their abilities.

Lupus Breast Involvement (Lupus Mastitis)

SLE inflammation of the breast (lupus mastitis) is rare, with fewer than 30 reported cases (including four in men). It can occur in patients with SLE or with only discoid lupus (cutaneous lupus). It is usually noted as one or several lumps under the skin of the breast, which are frequently tender. The overlying skin can be healthy or affected, as in lupus profundus (see chapter 8). Lupus mastitis also commonly causes tiny calcium deposits. Since breast lumps and small calcium deposits can occur in both lupus mastitis and breast cancer, a mammogram (an x-ray used to look for breast cancer) is not sufficient to identify the problem. A biopsy of the affected area is needed. Lupus mastitis usually shows fat inflammation (lupus panniculitis) or blood vessel inflammation (vasculitis). Other conditions, such as diabetes and lymphoma, can mimic lupus mastitis.

The best treatment is unknown, but it can probably be treated similarly to lupus profundus (chapter 8).

Endometriosis and Lupus

The uterus, also known as the womb, is the female organ that carries a fertilized egg from fertilization to birth. The inner uterine lining thickens and becomes enriched with blood approximately once a month in anticipation of a fertilized egg. When this does not

Successful lupus pregnancies are increasing

A 2019 United States study evaluated close to 100,000 SLE pregnancies between 1998 and 2015. Between 2013 and 2015, there were almost half as many fetal deaths as in 1998 to 2000, and maternal deaths markedly decreased also. Today, 80% to 90% of pregnant SLE women will have a successful live birth.

happen, menstruation (menses or period), in which the uterine lining is shed, occurs. If this inner uterine tissue begins to grow abnormally outside of the uterus, the condition is known as endometriosis. The most common problems experienced by women with endometriosis are abdominal pain, pelvic pain, and heavy menstrual cycles.

The exact cause of endometriosis is not entirely understood. However, immune system abnormalities and genetics seem to play a role. Several studies have suggested that women with endometriosis may be at increased risk of developing autoimmune disorders, such as lupus. Women with endometriosis are positive for antinuclear antibodies (the blood screening test for SLE) more often than women without endometriosis. Two large studies in 2016 evaluated over 130,000 women, including close to 3,000 SLE patients. One of these studies showed that endometriosis patients were 40% more likely to develop SLE. The other study showed a two-fold increased risk of SLE developing in women with endometriosis compared to the general population.

Menstrual Cycles, Fertility, and Menopause in SLE

Irregular menstrual cycles can also occur in SLE, especially when lupus is more active. In women with SLE the timing and duration of menstrual cycles, as well as the amount of blood flow, can vary. A 2019 study showed that SLE patients were almost twice as likely to have heavy menstrual cycles (menorrhagia) than other women. The reason is unknown, but it may be related to the stress the body goes through during lupus flares. When SLE is less active, menstrual cycles tend to be more regular.

When lupus is highly active, it may be difficult to become pregnant. However, overall fertility in women with well-controlled lupus is similar to the general population.

Women with decreased kidney function from lupus nephritis (kidney inflammation) can have difficulties becoming pregnant. Fertility can improve after kidney transplantation in patients with complete kidney failure (end-stage renal disease).

Another problem in women with SLE that can make it more challenging to have children is waiting until an older age for pregnancy. Women who develop SLE in their early twenties may delay pregnancy, or their doctor may advise them to wait until their lupus is under better control. The ability to become pregnant decreases with age.

Cyclophosphamide, a strong immunosuppressant for severe SLE, can cause infertility. The ovaries are the reproductive organs in women that produce eggs, and cyclophosphamide can decrease or halt egg production. It can also cause ovary tissue destruction. Older cyclophosphamide dosing regimens (high monthly doses for 7 months

NSAIDs and fertility

Nonsteroidal anti-inflammatory drugs (NSAIDs), such as ibuprofen (Motrin) and naproxen (Naprosyn), are often used for joint pains, headaches, and fevers. NSAIDs may possibly cause temporary, mild infertility. If you have trouble getting pregnant, try not taking any NSAIDs while trying to get pregnant.

followed by doses every 3 months) often resulted in infertility, especially in women over 30. However, newer cyclophosphamide dosing (EuroLupus regimen, chapter 12) uses much lower doses and does not interfere with fertility. When total cyclophosphamide doses are kept to less than 7000 mg, the chances for infertility are low. The EuroLupus regimen uses a total of 3000 mg.

The medicine leuprolide (Lupron) helps prevent female infertility when given 10 to 14 days before high-dose cyclophosphamide. Menstrual cycles will temporarily cease after leuprolide is started, and the ovaries temporarily stop making eggs. Resting eggs are less likely to be damaged by cyclophosphamide. Leuprolide is most likely not needed for the EuroLupus dosing.

The best method to preserve female fertility with cyclophosphamide is to "freeze" eggs or embryos (fertilized eggs), a process called ovarian cryopreservation. This process involves stimulating the release of an egg from the ovary. This can take a few weeks to complete. Since cyclophosphamide is usually given for very severe SLE, it is rarely practical to delay cyclophosphamide treatment to freeze eggs. Still, patients should be aware of this option. See chapter 41 for more on ovarian cryopreservation.

One rare cause of infertility in SLE women is a genetic condition called trisomy X (or triple X), in which women have an extra X chromosome. Most women have two X sex chromosomes (XX), and most men have an X and a Y (XY). Women with trisomy X have a higher risk of SLE since some of the genes associated with lupus are on the X chromosome (chapter 3). While 1 out of 1,000 women in the general population has trisomy X, 1 out of every 400 SLE women has it. Some trisomy X women are infertile because the ovaries can stop working at a young age.

Menopause is when estrogen levels decrease, menstrual cycles cease, and the ability to bear children stops. Women treated with high doses of cyclophosphamide or those with kidney failure are at increased risk of early-onset menopause. This can be another reason for reduced fertility.

Other immunosuppressants (table 22.1) do not appear to cause infertility.

Men and Fertility

SLE can affect the testicles (the male reproductive organs). Men with SLE tend to have smaller testes, increased sperm DNA damage, decreased ejaculate volume, and poor sperm quality. This does not mean they are infertile. Antiphospholipid syndrome is a very rare cause of infertility in men with SLE (APS, chapter 9).

A 2019 study showed that almost half of male SLE patients had sexual problems, including erectile dysfunction (ED). ED refers to difficulty achieving a sufficient erection for sexual intercourse. This may be due to accelerated atherosclerosis (hardening of the arteries, chapter 21), which can occur at a younger age in SLE. Atherosclerosis can reduce blood flow through the arteries of the penis. Treatment is aimed at preventing arteriosclerosis from getting worse. Medications such as Viagra and Cialis can help. Sexual problems from depression and other psychological stressors are also commonly experienced by SLE patients.

Erections depend on the parasympathetic nervous system (discussed in chapter 13). ED can occur if these nerves are damaged from lupus (dysautonomia, chapter 13). If you get dizzy when you stand or have other symptoms suggestive of dysautonomia, ask your doctor to have you evaluated. Drugs such as blood pressure medications and antidepressants are other common causes of ED, and your doctor may be able to adjust them.

Cyclophosphamide therapy can damage the cells in the testicles responsible for making sperm and cause infertility. After puberty, it can take as little as 100 mg/kg of cyclophosphamide to cause sperm production problems. Total doses over time of 6 grams or higher can cause permanent loss of sperm production (permanent infertility). This was a potential problem with the older high doses. However, the newer low-dose EuroLupus regimen uses a total of only 3000 mg. For a 190 pound (86 kg) man, this amounts to 35mg/kg of cyclophosphamide, well below the 100 mg/kg threshold, and it dramatically reduces infertility risks.

Just as women can freeze eggs, men can freeze their sperm (sperm cryopreservation). Since cyclophosphamide is typically started urgently for severe SLE, there is rarely time to plan for sperm cryopreservation, and many insurance companies do not cover the costs.

Men treated with cyclophosphamide should wait three months before trying to have a baby with their partner. Those who take thalidomide should wait one month. Men can safely take methotrexate while trying to have a baby, though the official package insert states otherwise. Newer studies show that pregnancy and fetus problems do not occur from men taking methotrexate.

Recommendations for women are more complicated and are discussed later in this chapter and in chapter 41.

LUPUS IN FOCUS

Klinefelter syndrome as a cause of male SLE infertility

Men with Klinefelter syndrome are at much higher risk for developing SLE (chapter 3). Over 90% of men with Klinefelter syndrome are infertile. Since up to 75% of Klinefelter syndrome men do not know they have it, infertile SLE men should be assessed for Klinefelter syndrome as a possible reason. Reproductive techniques can help them have children.

1. Irregular menses can occur when SLE is more active.

2. It can be more difficult for women with SLE with kidney disease or those having a flare to become pregnant. Other than that, most SLE women have normal fertility rates compared to other women their age.

3. High-dose cyclophosphamide can cause male and female infertility. However, the low-dose EuroLupus regimen does not.

Lupus Flares and Pregnancy

Lupus can become more active during pregnancy, probably due to hormonal changes. This increases the risk of pregnancy complications such as kidney problems, seizures, high blood pressure, or miscarriage.

Many body changes occur during pregnancy, some of which can mimic lupus flares. It is crucial for both the doctor and patient to keep this in mind so that steroids are not inappropriately used. Up to 75% of pregnant women develop chloasma (called the mask of pregnancy), which causes pigment changes on the cheeks in the same regions as the lupus butterfly rash, although chloasma is usually darker colored. Other changes mimicking lupus include red-colored palms (palmar erythema), facial flushing, hair loss, sore gums (pregnancy gingivitis), joint pains, fluid build-up in the knees, fluid retention, fatigue, shortness of breath, anemia, mildly low platelet counts, mildly elevated urine protein (less than 300 mg per day, chapter 4), and a high ESR (chapter 4).

Around one out of five pregnant SLE women will have a mild to moderate lupus flare, while severe flares occur in only about 6% of pregnancies. Certain factors may predict who is at increased risk for severe flares (table 18.1). Lupus nephritis (kidney inflammation) onset during pregnancy is one of the biggest concerns. This tends to occur more often in patients with a history of nephritis or patients with a low C4 level.

Women with severe, active SLE have higher chances of pregnancy complications. Women can significantly reduce this risk by having lupus well controlled for at least six months before pregnancy.

Women with the following problems should not become pregnant until these symptoms are resolved or improved and after consultation with their doctor:

LUPUS IN FOCUS

Pregnancy complications before SLE onset

Chapter 2 describes a preclinical stage of SLE, when the immune system is overactive before the affected person feels anything wrong. Women in this preclinical stage are two to three times more likely to have pregnancy complications (such as preeclampsia and slowed fetal growth).

- active lupus nephritis (kidney inflammation)

- severe chronic kidney disease (serum creatinine greater than 2.8 mg/dL)

- myocarditis (heart inflammation)

- congestive heart failure

- severe interstitial lung disease (with a forced vital capacity of less than 1 liter on pulmonary function tests)

- significant pulmonary hypertension (systolic pulmonary artery pressure greater than 50 mm Hg).

- have had severe preeclampsia or HELLP syndrome previously (discussed below)

Someone with active, severe lupus nephritis while pregnant has a 50% chance of losing her baby and a 75% chance of preterm birth. There are multiple ways that lupus affects the kidneys (chapter 12). Patients with proliferative lupus nephritis (Classes III and IV) are at the highest risk for pregnancy complications, while those with mesangial (Class II) and membranous (Class V) lupus nephritis can do as well during pregnancy as SLE patients without nephritis, as long as other active lupus problems are not present.

Although it is rare to die during pregnancy, the chances are particularly increased in lupus nephritis patients.

Sometimes a kidney biopsy is needed during pregnancy. In the couse of 11 years at Johns Hopkins Hospital, Baltimore, Maryland, 11 pregnant SLE patients had a kidney biopsy. All the biopsies were successful with no complications. This shows that kidney biopsies can be safely done. In addition, most biopsy results affected these women's treatment in meaningful ways.

Mildly active SLE does not affect pregnancy as much as severely active SLE. For example, mild lupus problems such as mouth sores, mild arthritis, or rash probably do not affect pregnancy much. However, severe arthritis, low platelet counts, and severe cutaneous (skin) lupus can. Active lupus must be treated during pregnancy, with the aim of low disease activity or remission, to improve the chances for a successful outcome.

Women with an increased risk of lupus flares during pregnancy (table 18.1) should regularly see their rheumatologist during pregnancy (such as monthly). All SLE pregnancies are considered high-risk, and patients should consider seeing a high-risk obstetrician.

Factors that can cause pregnancy complications like preeclampsia, eclampsia, premature birth, intrauterine growth restriction, and miscarriage are listed in table 18.2. Some of these, like not stopping hydroxychloroquine, are preventable.

Table 18.1 Factors That Can Increase Lupus Flares during Pregnancy

- Active lupus during the 6 months before pregnancy
- Severe disease in the past (especially lupus nephritis)
- If it is the first pregnancy
- High anti-ds DNA levels
- Low complement (C3 and C4) levels
- Younger age

Table 18.2 Factors That Increase SLE Pregnancy Complications

- SLE not being in reasonable control for 6 months before conception
- First pregnancy
- Active lupus during pregnancy
- Having a history of lupus nephritis, myocarditis, CNS lupus, or pulmonary hypertension
- Having protein in the urine, low C3, low C4, high EC4d, low vitamin D, or low platelets
- C3 or C4 not increasing during pregnancy (they normally should increase)
- Having positive anti-ds DNA, anti-thyroid peroxidase (TPO) antibodies, anti-SSA, or anti-SSB
- Older maternal age
- Being overweight (BMI > 25 kg/m²)
- High cholesterol, high blood pressure, or needing a blood pressure drug during pregnancy (even if the drug normalizes the blood pressure readings)
- Positive aPL antibodies (anticardiolipin antibodies, lupus anticoagulant, beta-2 glycoprotein I antibodies, or antiphosphatidylserine antibodies); lupus anticoagulant causes the highest risk
- Being African American or Hispanic
- Stopping hydroxychloroquine

Preeclampsia is a condition in which high blood pressure and protein in the urine occur. When seizures (epilepsy) also occur the condition is called eclampsia. Preeclampsia and eclampsia increase the risk of fetal developmental delays, miscarriage, and fetal death. These are treated with blood pressure medicines, magnesium infusions, and delivering the baby as soon as possible. Delivery of the baby is the only cure.

Since preeclampsia causes increased protein in the urine (proteinuria), it can look similar to lupus nephritis. But while nephritis is treated with immunosuppressants, preeclampsia is treated with blood pressure drugs and by delivering the baby.

Clues for preeclampsia include blood uric acid levels higher than 5.5 mg/dL, normal anti-dsDNA, and normal or elevated C3 and C4 complement levels. Lupus nephritis usually has low C3 or C4 levels, and the anti-dsDNA level may be elevated. The urine sample may also show the presence of red blood cells and cellular casts (chapter 4), which do not occur in preeclampsia. Preeclampsia usually does not happen before 20 weeks of pregnancy, while lupus nephritis can flare at any time. A 24-hour urine calcium measurement of less than 195 mg/dL is also most suggestive of preeclampsia.

Another problem in SLE pregnancy is HELLP syndrome. HELLP stands for hemolysis, elevated liver enzymes, and low platelets. "Hemolysis" refers to anemia (decreased red blood cells, RBCs) due to RBC destruction. It can be challenging to differentiate HELLP from a lupus flare because both conditions may cause hemolytic anemia, elevated liver enzymes (ALT and AST, chapter 4), and low platelets. Figuring out the difference is crucial because treatment for a lupus flare would be immunosuppressants, while the treatment of HELLP is to deliver the baby as soon as possible.

A condition called intrahepatic cholestasis of pregnancy can mimic HELLP. It causes elevated liver enzymes, high bilirubin levels, and itching. It is treated with medicines that decrease blood bilirubin levels.

If lupus is under excellent control for six months before a women becomes pregnant, the likelihood of a successful pregnancy is near normal. But if lupus is active within three months of getting pregnant, the woman is four times more likely to lose the baby. Therefore, it is crucial to use reliable birth control methods (chapter 41) until a woman has planned the pregnancy with her doctor's advice.

Important steps may need to be taken before becoming pregnant. Some medications used for lupus, for example, are not safe in pregnancy and will need to be changed.

A critical step in decreasing the risk for lupus flares during pregnancy is to take hydroxychloroquine (HCQ, Plaquenil) throughout pregnancy. Stopping it increases the chances of lupus flares, miscarriages, and losing the baby.

Taking hydroxychloroquine decreases the risk of preeclampsia by as much as 90%. A 2019 French study evaluated 84 pregnant SLE patients. Most of them took HCQ and low-dose aspirin during pregnancy, and 94% of them had successful pregnancies.

Low doses of aspirin (such as 81 mg daily) during pregnancy reduces the risk for preeclampsia, low birth weight, and preterm birth. One study suggested that 150 mg of aspirin a day may be superior to 81mg in preventing preeclampsia, and so some doctors recommend this higher dose.

SLE sometimes improves during pregnancy. This may be because the fetus and placenta produce steroids, such as cortisone and progesterone. These can enter the mother's bloodstream during the second and third trimesters, decreasing lupus disease activity.

While many medications should not be taken during pregnancy, other drugs are safe. For this reason, it is vital to inform the rheumatologist immediately when becoming pregnant or planning to become pregnant. A woman's obstetrician should not stop any lupus medications without consulting the rheumatologist. Hydroxychloroquine (Plaquenil), chloroquine, steroids (such as prednisone), azathioprine (Imuran), tacrolimus, colchicine, TNF blockers (such as certolizumab, Cimzia), and cyclosporine can be taken during pregnancy. Some experts consider Benlysta safe for pregnancy.

High dose steroids increase the risk for high blood pressure, diabetes, preeclampsia, premature birth, and a pregnancy complication called premature rupture of the membranes. If lupus is under reasonable control, steroids should be tapered to the lowest possible dose under the direction of the rheumatologist. Steroids should be tapered gradually and not stopped abruptly to avoid adrenal insufficiency (chapter 26) and lupus flares.

Methotrexate, leflunomide (Arava), thalidomide, and mycophenolate (CellCept and Myfortic) should not be taken during pregnancy. They can potentially cause miscarriage or birth defects. Some experts consider leflunomide safe during pregnancy.

Cyclophosphamide is usually not used during pregnancy because it can cause birth defects, especially in the first trimester. It may, however, be needed for severe SLE problems. There are cases of women using cyclophosphamide during the second and third trimesters with no issues. Most organs in the fetus have already developed by the third trimester. When cyclophosphamide has to be used, SLE is usually life-threatening, and the chances of having a good outcome from the pregnancy (having a healthy baby) are much lower.

COX-2 inhibitors and pregnancy

NSAIDs that inhibit an enzyme called cyclo-oxygenase-2 (meloxicam and cele-coxib) have not been studied well in pregnancy. It is probably best to avoid them.

Non-steroidal anti-inflammatory drugs (NSAIDs), such as naproxen and ibuprofen, are usually safe during the first two trimesters (chapter 36). NSAIDs are often used to treat fever, joint pains, and headaches.

In rare cases, NSAIDs may cause problems with the amount of amniotic fluid in the womb (oligohydramnios). This can result in fetal kidney problems.

A condition called patent ductus arteriosus, which reduces oxygen in the baby's blood, can occur if NSAIDs are taken after the 20th week. NSAIDs should thus be stopped before then if they are not absolutely needed. If they are required, then the lowest possible doses should be used.

There have been conflicting studies regarding NSAIDs and miscarriages. The largest study (65,457 pregnancies) showed no increase in miscarriages from NSAIDs during pregnancy. Other studies that suggest possible increased risks have been criticized for not being well done.

NSAIDs may make it more difficult for a fertilized egg and embryo to adhere to the inside of the womb, thereby reducing successful fertilization. It may make sense to avoid NSAIDs when trying to become pregnant, especially for women who have had difficulty getting pregnant.

KEY POINTS TO REMEMBER

1. Most lupus flares during pregnancy are mild. Only 6% of women have a severe flare.

2. SLE flares increase pregnancy complications such as preeclampsia, eclampsia, and miscarriages.

3. See tables 18.1 and 18.2 for factors that increase SLE pregnancy complications.

4. All women with any of these risk factors should consider seeing their rheumatologist monthly during pregnancy, and all pregnant SLE patients should consider seeing a high-risk obstetrician.

5. Hydroxychloroquine (Plaquenil) and low-dose aspirin reduce SLE complications and increase the chances of healthy births.

6. Hydroxychloroquine, steroids, tacrolimus, cyclosporine, and azathioprine (Imuran) can be taken during pregnancy. Benlysta may also be safe to take.

7. Methotrexate, leflunomide (Arava), thalidomide, and mycophenolate (CellCept and Myfortic) should not be taken during pregnancy. Cyclophosphamide can be considered for severe SLE during the third trimester.

8. NSAIDs (other than celecoxib and meloxicam) can generally be taken up to the 20th week.

9. The best way to increase the likelihood of a safe, successful pregnancy is to have lupus well controlled for six months before becoming pregnant and then during pregnancy.

10. Read chapter 41 thoroughly to best prepare for a successful pregnancy.

Ethnicity and Pregnancy Outcomes

A recurrent theme in SLE is that ethnicity and socioeconomic factors play a role in lupus severity (chapter 19). Socioeconomic factors refer to a person's situation in terms of income, social class, and educational level, among others. It should be no surprise that ethnicity and socioeconomic factors play significant roles in SLE pregnancies. A large study called the **PR**edictors of Pregnancy Outcome: Bio**M**arkers **i**n Antiphospholipid Antibody **S**yndrome and **S**ystemic Lupus **E**rythematosus" (PROMISSE) , which evaluated pregnancy outcomes in around 400 SLE patients, showed that non-Hispanic, white women with SLE, with no risk factors for poor pregnancy outcomes (table 18.2), had successful pregnancies 92% of the time. Only 4% of their pregnancies resulted in the death of their fetus or baby. This is similar to the general population.

However, women with African ancestry had poor fetal outcomes 27% of the time, and those with Hispanic heritage 21%. The outcomes were even worse in women of African and Hispanic origin who required blood pressure medication and were positive for lupus anticoagulant or had active lupus during pregnancy. Overall, women with African heritage were two to three times more likely to have pregnancy complications than non-Hispanic white women. Hispanic women also had increased difficulties, but not as much as those with African ancestry.

Not graduating high school and having a family income in the bottom 50% of the population were associated with poor pregnancy outcomes, even while receiving monthly expert care from rheumatologists and high-risk obstetricians. How much of this is due to genetics versus health care disparities (chapter 19) is unknown. Still, the question itself points out that we need to be especially diligent in recognizing racial/ethnic, medical, psychological, and socioeconomic factors that may decrease a woman's

---

LUPUS IN FOCUS

Hashimoto's thyroiditis and pregnancy

Hashimoto's thyroiditis commonly occurs in SLE, and most patients have positive anti-thyroid peroxidase (TPO) antibodies. TPO antibodies increase the risk of preterm delivery. If Hashimoto's causes overt hypothyroidism (high TSH and low free T4; chapter 17), taking a thyroid supplement reduces pregnancy complications. However, those with subclinical hypothyroidism do not benefit from thyroid medication. See chapter 17 about subclinical hypothyroidism.

chances of a healthy pregnancy. Read and practice everything in chapter 41 to ensure you have the best opportunities for a successful pregnancy.

Antiphospholipid Antibody Syndrome and Pregnancy

Antiphospholipid (aPL) antibodies (such as anticardiolipin auto-antibody, lupus anticoagulant, and beta-2 glycoprotein I) can potentially cause miscarriages, eclampsia, preeclampsia, HELLP syndrome, and other pregnancy complications (chapter 9). The large PROMISSE study mentioned above showed that lupus anticoagulant (LAC) was a more significant predictor of pregnancy complications than the other aPL antibodies. APL antibodies increase pregnancy complications 12-fold in those with African ancestry, 10-fold in Hispanic women, and 3-fold in non-Hispanic white women.

These antibodies can cause blood clots in the placenta (the organ connecting the fetus's umbilical cord to the mother's blood supply). The blood clots interrupt blood flow between the mother and fetus, potentially causing death and miscarriage of the fetus.

Most experts recommend that women with aPL antibodies take a small dose of aspirin (such as 81–162 mg a day) during pregnancy. This can thin the blood and possibly prevent these problems.

Miscarriages before the 10th week of pregnancy (early miscarriages) are common. Up to 30% of pregnancies in healthy women result in early miscarriage. These are usually due to genetic abnormalities in the embryo (the term for an unborn baby before the 11th week of pregnancy). Because early miscarriages are common, aPL antibodies are generally not considered responsible for one or two early miscarriages. But if a woman with aPL antibodies has three or more early miscarriages (and there were no embryo genetic abnormalities), she may be diagnosed with antiphospholipid antibody syndrome (APS). Women are also diagnosed with APS if the fetus dies for unknown reasons (such as no genetic abnormalities) after 10 weeks or if severe eclampsia, preeclampsia, or placenta problems occur before 34 weeks.

Stronger blood thinners should be used in women with pregnancy problems due to APS. Standard therapy is heparin and low-dose aspirin. Keeping the blood thin with these medicines increases the chances of a healthy pregnancy and birth. If a woman takes warfarin (Coumadin) for APS before pregnancy, the medication is changed to heparin during pregnancy because warfarin can cause fetal abnormalities. It is also essential to continue hydroxychloroquine (Plaquenil) to prevent blood clots and increase the likelihood of live birth rates.

Using this approach (heparin and/or aspirin), a large 2018 study of 264 women showed that 85% of the women with APS had a successful pregnancy. Although minor bleeding problems occurred in 45% of the pregnancies, only 3% had any major bleeding. These happened soon after delivery.

Unfortunately, even using the standard therapy of heparin plus aspirin during pregnancy, some women with APS will still have unsuccessful pregnancies. Women who are triple positive for aPL antibodies, meaning they have lupus anticoagulant, cardiolipin antibody, and beta-2 glycoprotein antibody, are especially at high risk. Women with APS and more than four pregnancy losses are also at high risk of not responding well to treatment. We do not know the best way to treat these high-risk women. Some experts recommend trying (in addition to heparin, aspirin, and hydroxychloroquine) IVIG (chapter 35), low dose steroids, or a statin (such as pravastatin or fluvastatin). However, in 2020, the 16th International Congress on Antiphospholipid Antibodies Task Force recommended caution in their use due to the weakness of the research behind them.

Around 44% of women with lupus anticoagulant (LAC) and SLE will have pregnancy complications like preeclampsia, miscarriages, and stillbirths. LAC appears to involve placenta inflammation and damage at three to four months into pregnancy. An immune system molecule called tumor necrosis factor-alpha (TNF-α) also participates in this damage. Theoretically, blocking the effects of TNF with drugs called TNF-inhibitors (TNFi's) may decrease this damage.

Certolizumab (Cimzia, chapter 33) is a TNF-inhibitor FDA-approved for rheumatoid arthritis, an autoimmune disease related to SLE. It does not cross into the baby's bloodstream before the third trimester. Doctors hoped that giving certolizumab to women with SLE and LAC would be safe and help increase live births. This resulted in the **Improve Pregnancy in APS with Certolizumab Therapy (IMPACT)** research study, in which LAC-positive women with SLE and a previous pregnancy complication were given certolizumab starting in the ninth week, followed by 400 mg two weeks later, then again two weeks later. Then it was given every four weeks after that with the last dose given on the 28th week.

In November 2020, preliminary results showed that only 13% of the patients who received certolizumab developed a complication (much lower than the usual 44%). After this study is completed, we will see if certolizumab could help our patients.

KEY POINTS TO REMEMBER

1. If a woman is positive for aPL antibodies and has had any of the following, she may have APS: a blood clot, three or more miscarriages before the tenth week, a stillbirth after ten weeks (in the absence of genetic abnormalities of the embryo or fetus); or severe preeclampsia, eclampsia, or placenta problems before week 34.

2. Women whose APS causes pregnancy problems are more likely to have a successful pregnancy if they take hydroxychloroquine, heparin, and low-dose aspirin.

3. Pregnant women who have aPL antibodies but do not have APS may decrease their chances of miscarriage by taking daily low-dose aspirin and hydroxychloroquine.

Neonatal Lupus

Heart Problems

When a woman is positive for anti-SSA (also called anti-Ro), these antibodies can go through the placenta and enter the fetus. If these antibodies contact the heart, skin, liver, or other organs, they may cause inflammation. The result is neonatal lupus. Suppose they create inflammation in the heart's electrical system. A type of neonatal lupus called fetal heart block or congenital heart block (CHB) can occur. Fortunately, only 2% of pregnancies in anti-SSA-positive women result in CHB. In women who have already had a baby with CHB, this risk jumps to 18%.

LUPUS IN FOCUS

High anti-SSA levels may be more likely to cause neonatal lupus than lower levels

Very high levels of anti-SSA may be more likely to cause neonatal lupus (heart, skin, and other organs) than mildly elevated levels. Currently (2023), the Surveillance and Treatment tO Prevent fetal atrioventricular Block Likely to Occur Quickly (STOP BLOQ) study is evaluating the risk of mild elevations versus high levels of anti-SSA. Anti-SSA positive women can sign up at stopbloq.org.

LUPUS IN FOCUS

Hydroxychloroquine helps prevent neonatal lupus

Hydroxychloroquine reduces neonatal lupus (congenital heart block and cutaneous neonatal lupus) by 50% to 86% (depending on the study). It also markedly decreases congenital heart block deaths.

While anti-SSA is the most common reason for neonatal lupus, it rarely occurs in anti-RNP-positive women.

SSA antibodies can also cause other heart problems, though not as often. If they cause heart muscle inflammation, it is called myocarditis. If this inflammation results in severe heart muscle scarring, it is called endocardial fibroelastosis. Babies with endocardial fibroelastosis usually require a heart transplant.

CHB must be diagnosed quickly. All women with anti-SSA antibodies should consider having fetal heart monitoring starting around the sixteenth week of pregnancy (detailed in chapter 41). This can be set up by a high-risk obstetrician.

Three forms of CHB range from first-degree to third-degree, With third-degree being the most severe.

The best management of first-degree heart block is not known. Some experts recommend steroids, while others recommend close monitoring and treating only if it worsens.

If second-degree CHB is detected, steroids such as dexamethasone or betamethasone (typically 4 mg daily) may be given to the mother to try to prevent worsening. Dexamethasone and betamethasone are used instead of prednisone because they pass through the placenta and into the fetus. The steroids are typically continued through the 26th week. Even with steroid treatment, many babies will still progress to third-degree CHB.

IVIG (chapter 35) is also sometimes used for second-degree CHB.

Third-degree heart block does not respond to steroids. One out of five fetuses with third-degree CHB will die in the womb or within one year after birth, and 70% will require a pacemaker immediately after birth.

Children born with CHB are at high risk for permanent heart muscle damage (cardiomyopathy), heart failure, and strokes as they get older. Follow-up with a cardiologist throughout life is important.

After delivery, all babies born to women with SSA antibodies should have an electrocardiogram (ECG, chapter 11). A pediatric cardiologist should see any baby with heart problems after birth. If myocarditis (heart muscle inflammation) or pericarditis (fluid or inflammation around the heart) occurs, steroids may help.

KEY POINTS TO REMEMBER

1. Neonatal lupus develops in 2% of anti-SSA-positive women.

2. One form of neonatal lupus is congenital heart block, which can be potentially treated if caught early.

3. Women positive for anti-SSA should consider weekly fetal heart monitoring from the sixteenth to the twenty-eighth week (some experts recommend the eighteenth to the twenty-sixth week). Later the frequency can be decreased to every other week.

4. If second-degree heart block is detected in the fetus, steroids or IVIG may help.

5. If a woman has a baby with neonatal lupus CHB, there is an 18% chance of it recurring in later pregnancies.

6. Hydroxychloroquine can reduce the risk of CHB recurrence by more than 50%.

Neonatal Lupus of the Skin and Other Organs

The other common form of neonatal lupus is cutaneous neonatal lupus (cNL), which causes a rash after birth. This happens due to the reaction of SSA antibodies with the baby's skin. The rash is rarely evident at delivery. It requires exposure to ultraviolet (UV) light for the rash to develop, as is the case in UV light–induced cutaneous lupus (chapters 3 and 8). This may occur soon after birth or weeks to months later (the average is six weeks). The babies of mothers taking HCQ tend to develop cNL approximately two months later than babies whose mothers did not take HCQ.

The rash of cNL is similar to subacute cutaneous lupus (chapter 8) in appearance and skin biopsy. However, biopsies are rarely needed. It causes circular-shaped red areas, especially on the face (particularly around the eyes) and scalp. The most important part of treatment is sunscreen and avoiding UV light, especially the sun.

While SSA antibodies disappear from the baby's system within six to eight months. 10% of babies are still anti-SSA positive at nine months. The cNL disappears within eight to nine months in most babies. Up to one-third of cNL babies will have permanently dilated blood vessels under the skin (telangiectasias), dark or light pigment changes, or skin thinning. This can become a cosmetic and self-esteem issue.

Women with a cNL baby have a 50% chance of having a baby with neonatal lupus in a subsequent pregnancy. CHB occurs in 18% of pregnancies, while 30% have a recurrence of cNL. Therefore, the mother with a cNL baby needs to take extra precautions during later pregnancies. These include getting the proper fetal heart monitoring starting at 16 weeks, having an ECG performed on the baby after delivery, and protecting the baby from UV light. Taking hydroxychloroquine during pregnancy reduces the risk of recurrence.

Table 18.3 Additional Neonatal Lupus Problems

- Decreased red blood cells, platelets, or white blood cells
- Mildly elevated liver enzymes (AST, ALT) in 15%–50% of cases: usually resolve by 6–8 months
- Enlarged liver, liver inflammation (hepatitis), jaundice; occur in 9% of neonatal lupus babies
- Hydrocephalus (swollen brain), macrocephaly (large brain): occur in 20% of neonatal lupus babies
- Brain MRI abnormalities are common but rarely problematic

LUPUS IN FOCUS

Increased autoimmune disease in neonatal lupus children

In one study, 6 out of 49 children with neonatal lupus (NL) developed an autoimmune disease, compared to none of their 45 siblings. These diseases included type I diabetes, juvenile idiopathic arthritis, psoriasis, nephrotic syndrome (a kidney disease), and Hashimoto's thyroiditis. A larger 2019 Swedish study monitored 119 children with neonatal congenital heart block (CHB). They developed autoimmune disease more than five times more often than normal.

Neonatal lupus is not limited to the heart and skin. There are some less common complications (table 18.3). Most of these are mild and tend to resolve without any long-lasting effects (especially those that involve the blood and liver).

If neurologic issues occur, most are mild and resolve. However, some can persist, causing disability problems.

There may be an increased risk of learning disabilities and attention deficit disorder in children with neonatal lupus. However, this association is not certain.

KEY POINTS TO REMEMBER

1. Taking hydroxychloroquine during pregnancy decreases the risk of neonatal lupus by half.

2. Cutaneous neonatal lupus (cNL) causes a red rash, particularly on the face and scalp. It is more noticeable after ultraviolet (UV) light exposure.

3. Sunscreen should be applied to babies with cNL, and they should be kept out of UV light.

4. The disappearance of SSA antibodies in the sixth to eighth month usually results in cNL going away.

5. Neonatal lupus can cause hepatitis or low blood cell counts. These also resolve by the eighth month. Neurologic involvement is usually mild and resolves but occasionally persists.

6. If a mother of a cNL child becomes pregnant again, she has around an 18% chance of having a baby with fetal heart block and a 30% chance of having a baby with cNL.

Problems after Pregnancy

Lupus Flares

The fetus's part of the placenta produces steroids (such as cortisol and progesterone) that enter the mother's body and can decrease lupus activity during pregnancy. After delivery, when this source of steroids abruptly stops, lupus flares can develop close to 30% of the time. Most are mild to moderate, and the mild flares rarely require treatment. Only 2% of women will have a severe flare after delivery.

Women not taking HCQ have an increased chance of flaring 3 to 12 months after giving birth.

KEY POINTS TO REMEMBER

1. Up to 30% of women with SLE may flare during the first few weeks after giving birth. These flares are rarely severe.

2. Hydroxychloroquine helps prevent lupus flares after pregnancy.

Blood Clots from Antiphospholipid Antibodies

Women who are positive for aPL antibodies are at increased risk for blood clots after pregnancy. After delivery, many mothers spend so much time caring for the baby that

LUPUS IN FOCUS

Autism and learning disabilities in children of SLE patients

Several studies suggest that children born to mothers with SLE who are positive for antiphospholipid antibodies (especially lupus anticoagulant) have higher rates of learning disabilities, delayed speech, attention deficit hyperactivity disorders (ADHD), and autism.

Children born to mothers with SSA antibodies may be at increased risk for ADHD.

It would be a good idea for women with SLE who are aPL or SSA antibody positive to pay especially close attention to their children's development. Have a low threshold for formal evaluation if you suspect any developmental delays.

their level of physical activity decreases. This is a prime setup for blood clots. The blood clots of primary concern are deep venous thromboses (DVT), which are blood clots that form in the legs' veins. The other problem is pulmonary emboli (PE, chapter 9), which are blood clots that initially form in other body parts (such as the legs) and travel to the lungs. A PE is potentially deadly.

The American College of Rheumatology guidelines for reproductive health management recommends that all women with APS (including those who have never had a blood clot) continue blood thinners (such as heparin or warfarin) 6 to 12 weeks after delivery.

After delivery, some doctors treat women who have aPL antibodies and are at lower risk for DVT and PE with low-dose aspirin plus intermittent pneumatic compression. This involves a device with air-filled bags covering the legs like long boots. These bags go through regular cycles of filling up with air and squeezing the legs, followed by periods of relaxation. This helps keep the blood traveling through the veins, decreasing the risk for blood clots.

KEY POINTS TO REMEMBER

1. Women with APS may be at increased risk of developing blood clots (DVT or PE) in the weeks following delivery.

2. Continuing heparin or warfarin should be considered during this time (approximately the first six weeks after delivery). However, not all doctors agree.

3. Low-dose aspirin (such as 81 mg daily) plus intermittent pneumatic compression is an alternative for lower-risk patients.

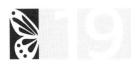

Prognosis, Special Populations, and Health Care Disparities

Titilola Falasinnu, PhD, and Julia F. Simard, ScD, *Contributing Editors*

Most lupus patients today live long average lifespans, thanks to better therapies. My clinic now has many SLE patients in their 70s, 80s, and 90s. This was unheard of a couple of decades ago. I'll never forget the "Thank You" card I received from one of my patients in 2020. She is one of my many patients who religiously follow my "Lupus Secrets" (chapter 44). Part of her note said, "Dr. Thomas . . . none of my family ever lived past 60 years old [many family members had died of severe SLE]. . . . With your help, I plan on living as long of a healthy life with my lupus as possible." What makes this card even more noteworthy is that she was 73 years old when she wrote this!

Even so, there are certainly people with severe disease who die much too young. There will also always be those with mild illness who unexpectedly develop severe complications.

"Prognosis" is the medical term describing how a disorder affects a person and whether it may shorten their lifespan. SLE patients should learn as much as possible about lupus, its potential complications, and what they can do to avoid bad outcomes. While SLE can seem overwhelming, people who arm themselves with knowledge are empowered with a degree of control over a disease that sometimes seems uncontrollable.

Lupus is seldomly the sole cause of death in SLE patients. Infections, blood clots, strokes, and heart attacks are more common causes (chapters 21 and 22). People with SLE should learn how to prevent these complications if possible and how to manage them if they occur. This way, they can go a long way toward taking control of their lives.

Other factors are also associated with doing poorly from SLE. These include whether you take your medicines, age, income, sex, health insurance, and even where you live (table 19.1). This chapter discusses these in detail.

Prognosis

"Prognosis" comes from the Greek word for "to know beforehand," or "foresee." Almost everyone diagnosed with an illness wants to know what is in store for them in the future (their prognosis). How will it affect my life? How long will I live? Since SLE affects every person differently and can affect any body part, determining an individual's prognosis can be difficult. However, there are some general predictors, and much of this chapter is devoted to these.

Table 19.1 Factors Associated with Worse SLE Problems

Factors often under your control

- Not taking drugs as prescribed
- Unhealthy habits (such as smoking, eating poorly, not exercising, being overweight)
- Not getting care by a lupus expert or at a teaching center
- Seeing a rheumatologist who is difficult to communicate with

Factors not under your control

- Non-Caucasian race
- Hispanic ethnicity
- Genetics
- Male sex
- Childhood-onset SLE
- Older people get more severe organ damage due to aging
- Poor insurance coverage
- Geography (areas lacking rheumatologists and low-income regions)

Note: This table does not include lupus lab tests or specific organ system problems.

There are many aspects to the prognosis of SLE. Chapters 5 to 18 discuss how lupus affects the body and what can happen with and without proper treatment. However, other factors not directly due to lupus's inflammation, also affect prognosis (chapters 21 to 28).

Death (mortality) is one part of prognosis. Will SLE cause someone to die earlier than expected? This chapter covers life expectancy in SLE patients. When SLE patients know which problems can potentially kill them, they can learn how to reduce their risks.

Unfortunately, some people are afraid of taking medicines because of potential side effects. Of the patients I have seen die from SLE, most either refused to take their lupus drugs or did not have adequate insurance. The people who refused to take their medicines often wanted to take herbal supplements, or "natural" remedies. They were also usually afraid of potential drug side effects. If people understand what SLE does if it is not treated appropriately, they can be more motivated to trust their doctors and accept the recommended therapies. Ensure honest conversations with your doctor on herbal supplements, diet, and lupus medications. Read chapter 39 about complementary medicine.

To realize how important it is to treat SLE, it helps to understand what happened to people before treatments were available. Before modern medicine, people with SLE did poorly. How long SLE patients lived can be divided into several periods.

The first period would be before the availability of any treatments, including antibiotics. In 1935, Dr. P. Klemperer (creator of the term "connective tissue disease") said that none of his SLE patients lived past four and a half years after diagnosis. Some doctors reported average life expectancies as low as four to seven months after diagnosis. Around half of the SLE patients died of severe infections during.

LUPUS IN FOCUS

SLE, immunosuppressant drugs, and infections

Before antibiotics, steroids, and other lupus drugs were available, up to 60% of SLE patients had an infection at the time of death. This is important to recognize. Some people with SLE do not take their lupus drugs because they are afraid they will cause infections. But infections are also caused by the abnormal lupus immune system. This emphasizes the importance of controlling lupus inflammation using medications, preventing infections, and treating any infection as soon as possible.

SLE patients lived longer after antibiotics became available in the mid- to late 1930s. During this time, but before steroids and antimalarials, around 50% of patients survived two years after diagnosis. Approximately 20% made it to five years. These statistics illustrate the importance of preventing infections in the first place (chapter 22).

Another reason for such high death rates (besides the lack of treatments) is the difficulty in diagnosing SLE. The first blood test to help diagnose lupus (the LE cell, chapter 2) was not available until 1948. Before that, many people with SLE, probably the majority, were not diagnosed until after they died, and an autopsy was performed.

The importance of diagnosing SLE earlier is a repetitive theme that continued over time. Each newly discovered lab test (such as ANA and most recently CB-CAPS, chapter 4) and each newly developed set of classification criteria (such as the 1982 and 1997 ACR criteria) were followed by earlier diagnoses, earlier treatment, and longer survival.

The first useful lupus drugs were antimalarials (initially quinacrine, then chloroquine) and steroids in the 1950s. After steroids and antimalarial drugs became available, at least 50% of SLE patients lived five years or longer.

In the 1950s to 1960s, lupus nephritis was responsible for 70% of deaths in SLE. In the early 1960s, fluid pills (diuretics) and dialysis machines became available for kidney disease. Survival increased to more than 90% at two years. Cyclophosphamide became available in the 1980s to treat lupus nephritis (kidney inflammation) and other severe SLE problems. After that, death from nephritis dropped considerably.

In the new millennium, research studies continued to show improving life expectancies. In 2010, SLE patients' average life expectancy in Spain was 61 years old, compared to 42 years in 1981. A 2019 Canadian study showed that in the 1970s, SLE patients had a death rate 13 times higher than the general population. In 2013 it dropped down to two times higher. Recent studies show that 93%–98% of SLE patients (depending on the population studied) are still alive ten years after diagnosis.

As previously mentioned, another reason for longer lifespans is doctors' ability to diagnose lupus earlier during milder periods of disease activity. For example, mildly low blood counts can be found during routine checkups, and workups can show SLE as the cause even while the person feels perfectly normal. Treatment at this early, mild stage of the disease can keep them from feeling poorly and prevent progression to severe forms of SLE and permanent organ damage.

Unfortunately, 2%–8% of SLE patients still die within 10 years of diagnosis. Most of these deaths are due to lupus (most commonly lupus nephritis), cardiovascular disease (heart attacks, strokes, and blood clots), infections, and cancer.

SLE patients who learn how to prevent and reduce risk from these conditions can significantly improve their survival chances. The rest of this chapter and later chapters go into more detail about these issues.

The Four Most Common Causes of Death in SLE Patients

Systemic Lupus

Better therapies have resulted in much longer lives for SLE patients. If someone with SLE dies from lupus itself, lupus nephritis (and its complications) is the most common cause. Neuropsychiatric lupus (chapter 13) is the second most common cause of SLE disease-related deaths. However, lupus affecting the heart, lungs, or severely low blood counts can also result in death. Most commonly, it is a combination of factors.

Early research suggests during the first five years after diagnosis with lupus, death tended to occur mostly from infections or lupus itself. After that, death was more often due to cardiovascular disease or infection. Although death from lupus itself can occur at any time, the treatment of lupus has improved significantly, reducing this possibility. SLE patients should stay vigilant in managing their disease and regularly see their doctor throughout their lives.

Cardiovascular Disease

"Cardiovascular" refers to the heart and blood vessels. When doctors talk about cardiovascular disease (CVD), they generally refer to heart attacks, strokes, and blood clots. CVD and infections are the two most common causes of death after the first five years of having SLE.

While CVD is the most common cause of death in people without lupus, people with SLE are three times more likely to die from CVD and at younger ages. SLE patients should work with their primary care providers to reduce their CVD risk factors and lower their risk of premature death (chapter 21).

Infections

The immune system of SLE patients has more difficulty fighting infections. In the 1930s and 1940s, before either antibiotics or steroids became available, up to 60% of people with SLE had a severe infection when they died. Today, SLE patients are five times more likely to die of infection than people without SLE.

Another reason for these increased infections is that patients with moderate to severe SLE may need medications that suppress the immune system (immunosuppressants, table 22.1). The immune system is vital for fighting infections. Most infections are preventable and treatable. These measures include getting all recommended vaccines (especially COVID-19, flu, and pneumonia shots), practicing proper hygiene and social distancing, and seeing a physician at once at the first signs of any infection. Read chapter 22 for more details.

LUPUS IN FOCUS

Fewer SLE patients are hospitalized or die in the hospital than in the past

I remember how incredibly busy I was in the early 1990s caring for SLE patients in the hospital during my rheumatology training. We seemed to always have several patients with SLE in the hospital simultaneously. Often, there would be one or two who were very sick in the intensive care unit. Over the years, we gradually saw fewer hospitalized patients. Around 2010, my rheumatology group (and the large group in the county next to ours) stopped going to hospitals. Instead, patients were sent to one of the nearby large medical center hospitals if needed.

A 2017 study from the University of California confirmed our experience. It showed that while 40% of their hospitalized rheumatology patients had SLE in 2005, this figure had dropped to 31% by 2013 (a 25% decrease over eight years). While 4% of those patients died in 2005, none died in 2013. This is a sign that SLE treatments are improving.

Cancer

SLE patients have an increased chance of getting certain cancers and dying from them than people without SLE. Possible reasons include increased risk for human papillomavirus–induced cancers, smoking, and some lupus medications. The inability of the lupus immune system to adequately rid the body of cancer cells may also play a role. These topics are discussed in chapter 23. Proper screenings for cancer and maintaining good lifestyle habits can help reduce their risk.

KEY POINTS TO REMEMBER

1. The overwhelming majority of SLE patients survive 10 years or longer after diagnosis.

2. The improved life expectancy (compared to earlier in the 20th century) is largely due to diagnosing SLE at earlier (milder) stages, improved lupus treatments, antibiotics, infection preventive measures (vaccines), and better management of high blood pressure, diabetes, and high cholesterol.

3. The most common causes of death in SLE are lupus disease activity, cardiovascular disease (such as blood clots, heart attacks, and strokes), infections, and cancer.

4. Adhering to SLE therapy (taking medications, seeing doctors as directed, and getting recommended medical tests) lowers the chances of premature death.

5. SLE patients should be careful about preventing and treating infections and heart attacks. They should keep up with their cancer screenings.

6. Read "The Lupus Secrets Checklist" (chapter 44), for a simplified list of things to do to live longer and better with your lupus.

Different SLE Issues in Different Groups of People

Some people with SLE have issues (table 19.2) that increase their risk of doing poorly. A person's age, sex, race, ethnicity, and socioeconomic status can significantly influence how SLE affects them. So will health care access, which, unfortunately, is not equal worldwide or within a single community. Such health care disparities influence how someone with SLE will do. There are other factors, such as age and gender, that are also influential and not under you control. But there are also some that you can partly or fully control, such as taking your medications as prescribed.

Table 19.2 SLE Differences in Particular Groups of People

Race/Ethnicity/Geographical area	
African ancestry	• Lupus occurs 2 to 3 times more often than in Caucasians
	• Remission achieved less often, and more slowly
	• Worse outcomes related to low income and poor health care
	• Increased racism and childhood stress contribute to worse SLE
	• SLE problems that occur more often than in Caucasians include nephritis, discoid lupus, low platelet counts, neuropsychiatric lupus, serositis, more severe disease, pregnancy complications, lower remission rates, and higher death rates
	• More anti-RNP and anti-Smith antibodies
	• Nephritis is more severe and doesn't do as well compared to Caucasians
	• Mycophenolate works better than cyclophosphamide for nephritis
	• Usually require the higher doses of mycophenolate (starting dose of 3 grams total per day)
	• Increased uncontrolled high blood pressure that increases death rates
	• Medicaid patients have higher death rates than Asians and Hispanics on Medicaid
	• Family members are more likely to develop SLE than those of Caucasian families
Afro-Caribbean ancestry	• See above under "African Ancestry"
	• Possibly the highest rates of lupus nephritis = 78% of SLE Afro-Caribbeans
	• Afro-Caribbean SLE women have high death rates (80% alive after 5 years)

(continued)

Asian ancestry	• Develop SLE at younger ages
	• Higher rates of SLE than Caucasians
	• More nephritis than Caucasians (as high as 69% in Chinese)
	• Arthritis, antiphospholipid syndrome, and neuropsychiatric SLE may be more common
	• SLE children with nephritis tend to respond to treatment similar to whites
	• Have more side effects on mycophenolate. Lower starting doses recommended (such as 1.5 grams daily)
	• Medicaid Asians have lower death rates than Caucasians, people of African ancestry, and Native Americans
	• Need 3 eye tests yearly on hydroxychloroquine instead of 2 as in other patients: VF 24-2 or 30-2 plus an SD-OCT plus a VF 10-2
European ancestry	• SLE occurs less often than in other races
	• Nephritis is less frequent (in 10%–38% of SLE Caucasians)
	• Respond better to azathioprine for nephritis than Blacks
	• Lower death rates
Hispanic ethnicity	• Higher rates of SLE, lupus nephritis, more severe disease, and higher death rates than Caucasians
	• Worse outcomes related to low income and poor health care
	• Nephritis is more severe and does not do as well compared to Caucasians
	• May have less neuropsychiatric lupus
	• Pregnancy complications are higher than in Caucasians
	• Mycophenolate works better than cyclophosphamide for nephritis
Indigenous Peoples	• Native Americans and Alaskans have higher rates of SLE than Black, Asian, and White Americans
	• Worse disease and higher death rates than Caucasians
	• Native American family members are more likely to develop SLE than white and Black SLE patients and have an earlier age of onset compared to Blacks, whites, and Hispanics
Mestizos (Latin American mixed race)	• Earlier age of onset than Latin American Europeans
	• More likely to have myositis (muscle inflammation), autoimmune hemolytic anemia, nephritis (lupus inflammation), severe disease, anti-RNP, anti-Smith, and anti-Ro antibodies

Table 19.2 *(continued)*

Pacific Islanders	• Have higher rates of SLE, lupus nephritis, severe disease, and death rates than Caucasians
	• May have higher rates of the antiphospholipid syndrome
Puerto Ricans	• Less lupus nephritis (25%)
Saudi Arabians	• More nephritis (63% of SLE Saudis)
Gender	
Men	• Much less likely to have SLE than women
	• Average age of onset is mid-40s and older (but occurs at all ages)
	• SLE occurs more often in men with Klinefelter's syndrome (chapter 3)
	• Have more lupus nephritis, discoid lupus, fevers, weight loss, serositis, low blood counts, blood clots, heart attacks, vasculitis, neurological problems, more severe disease, and higher death rates than women
Women	• Much more likely to develop SLE than men
	• Most likely to develop SLE between puberty and menopause
	• Less severe disease and lower death rates than men
	• More likely to develop Raynaud's phenomenon, sun sensitivity, mouth ulcers, and nose ulcers than men
Age	
Less than 1	• SLE is very rare
	• The highest death rates, close to 50%
1 to 18	• After puberty, much more likely in girls than in boys
	• More severe SLE than adults (80% have major organ involvement, especially nephritis and neuropsychiatric) and higher death rates
Onset after 50 (late-onset)	• More Sjögren's, pleurisy, arthritis, and higher death rates than younger adults
	• Less cutaneous lupus, fevers, lymphadenopathy, low blood cell counts, Raynaud's, nephritis, and neuropsychiatric lupus than younger adults
	• Less severe disease: 20% having major organ involvement
	• More permanent organ damage from aging organs
	• Increased uncontrolled high blood pressure that increases death

Note: The higher and lower statements in this chart are in comparison to the average SLE patient, unless stated otherwise.

Issues Fully or Partly under Your Control

Adherence to Treatment

"Adherence" describes how well patients stick to the management recommended by their health care providers. Some health care providers use the word "compliance," but "adherence" is the preferred term. The importance of adherence and recommendations on how to improve adherence are discussed in detail in chapter 29.

Lifestyle Choices

Smoking and obesity increase the risk of SLE inflammation, more permanent organ damage, and earlier death from lupus (chapters 3 and 5). Obese SLE patients are at a higher risk of lupus nephritis than are those of healthy body weight. Although stopping smoking and losing weight is difficult, reversing these two significant problems can make a considerable impact.

Eating a healthy diet is essential. Evidence is building that a diet rich in omega-3 fatty acids (fatty fish, flaxseed, chia seed, and walnuts, chapter 38) can decrease inflammation. In contrast, Western diets rich in omega-6 fatty acids and saturated fats (red meats, butter, premade foods) increase inflammation. Researchers think that the high-sugar, high-fat Western diet may cause unhealthy changes to our DNA (epigenetics, chapter 3). These DNA changes can persist, at least for a while, even after changing the diet. A 2019 US research study of 456 SLE patients showed that those who ate higher amounts of omega-3 fatty acids than omega-6 fatty acids tended to have less active lupus. They also had less depression and insomnia (chapter 27), fewer symptoms of fibromyalgia, and a better quality of life.

Type of Medical Care

SLE is one of the most complex diseases to understand and care for. Proper care of an SLE patient involves listening to and examining the patient, ordering and evaluating many tests regularly, and prescribing drugs that require a high level of knowledge and experience to use correctly. But proper care does not end there. The doctor should regularly ask whether the patient is avoiding ultraviolet light, make sure vaccines are up to date, and monitor issues that can cause heart attacks and strokes. While most rheumatologists are trained to care for lupus patients, some specialize in the disease. Your rheumatologist may invite doctors from other medical specialties to help manage your lupus. These other specialties include, for example, hematology, pulmonary, nephrology, and neurology, which deal with blood cells, lungs, kidneys, or the brain, respectively.

Researchers from Rush University came up with 20 quality measures of good lupus doctors (table 19.3). I added some important items to this list as well. They showed that academic lupus clinics scored higher on those 20 measures than general rheumatology clinics. These measures include sunscreen recommendations, vaccinations, heart attack prevention strategies, antiphospholipid antibody testing, bone density x-rays in high-risk patients, and using medications to lower steroid doses. This does not mean that all SLE patients should go to academic centers. There are rheumatologists in the community who specialize in lupus and supply outstanding care equal to or better than some academic centers. Checking this list of quality measures is one way you can eval-

Table 19.3 Excellent SLE Care Quality Measures

- Conduct ANA, CBC, sCr, eGFR, and UA labs at diagnosis.
- Conduct anti-ds DNA, C3, C4, and antiphospholipid antibodies labs within 6 months of diagnosis.
- Recommend sunscreen use daily.
- Prescribe pneumococcal pneumonia vaccines and yearly influenza (flu) vaccines.
- Conduct bone density x-ray if patient is on steroids longer than 3 months (7.5 mg or higher of prednisone daily).
- Recommend calcium and vitamin D treatment if on steroids longer than 3 months (7.5 mg or higher of prednisone daily).
- Discuss risk and benefits of any new medicine.
- Conduct baseline tests for new drugs.
- Monitor drugs for possible side effects (such as CBC and LFTs regularly).
- Prescribe osteoporosis medicine if patient is on 10 mg daily of prednisone or more for 3 months or longer.
- Look for SLE complications every 3 mo (UPCR, eGFR, CBC, LFTs, C3, C4, anti-dsDNA).
- For Class III or IV lupus nephritis, treat with steroids and immunosuppressants within 1 month of diagnosis.
- Prescribe BP treatment in lupus nephritis patients if BP is higher than 130/80 on two occasions.
- Prescribe ACEi or ARB medication if increased urine protein.
- Assess risk of heart attacks and strokes, and counsel about preventative measures (like diet, not smoking, exercise, and maintaining a healthy weight, BP, cholesterol, and sugar levels).
- Test for anti-SSA, anti-SSB, and antiphospholipid antibodies at pregnancy.
- Treat antiphospholipid syndrome during pregnancy if present.
- Counsel patient about birth control and pregnancy issues.
- Prescribe an antimalarial medication for all SLE patients.*
- Ensure all patients on chloroquine or hydroxychloroquine get the correct eye tests yearly. Some patients can wait 5 years before yearly eye exams.*
- Treat vitamin D deficiency.*
- Adjust treatment regularly, aiming for remission or low disease activity, and off steroids or on prednisone doses less than 6 mg daily.*
- Ensure cancer screenings are up to date.*
- Offer human papillomavirus vaccine (such as Gardasil) to high-risk patients.*
- Offer shingles vaccine (Zostavax and Shingrix) to high-risk patients.*
- Offer COVID-19 vaccines to all patients.*

Source: Adapted from S. Arora et al., "Does Systemic Lupus Erythematosus Care Provided in a Lupus Clinic Result in Higher Quality of Care Than That Provided in a General Rheumatology Clinic?" *Arthritis Care Res.* 70:1771 (December 2018).

Notes: * = additional recommendations. ACEi = angiotensin converting enzyme inhibitor, ANA = antinuclear antibody, ARB = angiotensin receptor blocker, BP = blood pressure, CBC = complete blood count, eGFR = estimated glomerular filtration rate, LFTs = liver function tests, LN = lupus nephritis, mo = months, sCr = serum creatinine, UA = urinalysis, UPCR = urine protein to creatinine ratio, vit = vitamin.

uate your lupus care. If you have any questions about that care, the list can be a good way to introduce the issue for discussion with your doctor.

Patient-doctor communication is critical. It is important to see someone you trust and with whom you communicate well. A 2017 California study showed that patients with poorly rated communications with their physicians were more likely to have ongoing organ damage than those who had good communications. This does not necessarily mean that these physicians were not good doctors. People are naturally less likely to understand and follow health care instructions if they do not have a good relationship and communicate well with their health care provider. This study showed that it is essential to see a rheumatologist with whom you can communicate well.

Issues Not Under Your Control

Race and Ethnicity

There is still a lot to learn about why some people get SLE more often and severely than others. We know that SLE is partly genetic, but environment also plays a role. Some races and ethnic groups stand out in terms of the frequency of developing SLE and its severity. For example, SLE occurs more commonly in people of Asian, Native American, Alaska Native, Hispanic, and African ancestry than in whites. In the United States, it occurs approximately three times more often in people of African descent and Native Americans than in whites.

Age at onset appears to vary between patients of different races and ethnic groups. Asians and Native Americans tend to develop SLE at a younger age than whites, Hispanics, and Black people.

SLE complications and manifestations may vary by race and ethnicity, too. Black people with SLE also tend to have more discoid lupus, low platelet counts, anti-Smith and anti-RNP antibodies, neuropsychiatric lupus, and serositis (such as pleurisy) than white patients. Hispanic patients may have lower rates of neuropsychiatric lupus (chapter 13), and Asian and Pacific Islander patients may have higher rates of antiphospholipid syndrome (chapter 9).

The severity of SLE and how often it goes into remission and low disease activity also vary. Black people, Hispanics, Pacific Islanders, and indigenous peoples (such as Native Americans and Alaskans) tend to have more severe SLE disease problems than whites. A study of Latin American Mestizo (European and indigenous mixed ethnicity) SLE patients showed they were more likely to have myositis (muscle inflammation), autoimmune hemolytic anemia, nephritis (lupus inflammation), and more apt to be positive for anti-RNP, anti-Smith, and anti-Ro antibodies than most SLE patients.

One study evaluated SLE in different ethnic populations (primarily Hispanic, African American, and white). Called the LUMINA study, it included SLE patients mainly from Alabama, Texas, and Puerto Rico. Among the findings was that lupus nephritis was more common in non–Puerto Rican Hispanic and Black patients (up to 60%) than in white and Puerto Rican patients (25%). Non–Puerto Rican Hispanics and Black patients also had higher death rates. The LUMINA study also found that low income and inadequate health insurance may play a bigger role in having more severe SLE than ethnicity. Similar findings appeared from an extensive Canadian ethnicity study.

At the Johns Hopkins Lupus Center, white patients were more likely to achieve low disease activity than Black patients, in whom it took longer to go into low disease activity, especially if they had lupus nephritis or low C3 or C4 complement levels (chapter 4). SLE patients who take longer to go into remission (or low disease activity) are more likely to develop permanent organ damage.

Worldwide, there is a lot of variability in the occurrence of lupus nephritis (LN), one of the most important SLE complications. While only 15% to 38% of white SLE patients (depending on the population or region studied) develop LN, it occurs much more often in other racial and ethnic groups (as high as 78% in Afro-Caribbeans). It should be noted that people of Hispanic and African origins have higher rates of kidney disease in the general population than those of other races and ethnicities.

Disparities have also been noted in the severity of LN and response to treatment. For example, patients of African and Hispanic backgrounds tend to have more severe Class IV LN (diffuse proliferative LN, chapter 12) than whites. A study of lupus patients sponsored by the US Centers for Disease Control (CDC) showed that young Black SLE women were up to seven times more likely to go into kidney failure and require dialysis than white women. These differences are likely influenced by genetics and social factors, including problems related to health care access.

Despite significant advances in survival, death rates are still much higher in Black patients than whites, especially in the first few years after diagnosis. Fortunately, the chances of dying from kidney failure in Black SLE patients dropped by 40% from 1999 to 2014, and in Hispanics it dropped almost 50%.

Stress contributes to lupus and lupus flares and affects some groups more than others. A 2016 study showed that a patient's experiencing childhood trauma was associated with worse active lupus than patients without childhood trauma. Those with childhood traumas had more depression and a lower ability to function physically. Black and Hispanic SLE patients were more likely to have experienced childhood trauma than white patients.

A CDC-sponsored Georgia study found that 80% of Black women with SLE experienced racism and that these patients had worse lupus disease activity and more permanent organ damage than those who had not. Vicarious racism, which is hearing about racism toward one's own race or seeing it (such as on the news), also causes stress and anxiety and has been associated with higher lupus disease activity.

LUPUS IN FOCUS

SLE is the sixth most common reason for hospital readmissions

Needing to be readmitted to the hospital within 30 days after discharge is one measurement for treatment success. A 2014 study showed that SLE was the sixth leading cause for the need for readmission within 30 days of discharge. Only sickle cell anemia, gangrene, hepatitis, white blood cell disorders, and kidney failure did worse. One out of every six SLE patients needed readmission within 30 days. SLE groups most likely to be readmitted were younger patients (one out of every four 20-year-olds), African American and Hispanic patients, and Medicare and Medicaid patients.

A 2016 Harvard University study evaluating over 40,000 SLE Medicaid patients showed that the Native American patients had the highest risk of dying within a given time period, followed by Black and then white patients. Native Americans had a 40% higher death rate than whites. This dismal result for Native Americans is similar to findings for indigenous patients in other locations such as Canada, South America, and Australia, where they had more severe lupus and higher death rates than non-indigenous citizens.

A 2018 Vanderbilt University study showed that African American SLE patients were two to four times more likely to have heart attacks, strokes, high blood pressure, and infections than white SLE patients. This reinforces the importance of vigilant prevention measures for these complications. These include controlling high blood pressure, not smoking, good nutrition and exercise, getting vaccines, and having good hygiene to prevent infections.

Studies comparing the medicines azathioprine (AZA, Imuran) and mycophenolate mofetil (MMF, CellCept) suggest that different ethnicities respond to them differently. People of African and Hispanic ancestry with lupus nephritis do better with MMF than AZA. People of African heritage also tend to require higher MMF doses than whites. The effects on the immune system differ between the races when similar amounts are used. Why some medications would work better in some ethnicities is not entirely understood. Hopefully, it will become clearer in the future, so doctors can use genetic testing to inform medical treatments (called "precision medicine") when possible.

Asians develop higher MMF drug levels than whites when given similar doses and get more side effects at full doses, so Asian patients may need lower doses. Although many do well with the standard 2–3 grams daily of MMF, they should initially consider lower doses, such as 1.5 grams daily (in divided doses).

Another ethnic difference occurs in Asians on hydroxychloroquine (Plaquenil) and chloroquine. Although rare, damage to the back of the eye (the macula area of the retina) can occur with long-term use of hydroxychloroquine (the condition is called antimalarial retinopathy or antimalarial maculopathy). Regular screening tests can find the problem early. Everyone needs two tests yearly—preferably a visual field (VF) 10-2 and an SD-OCT (chapter 30).

The VF 10-2 test looks for damage in the macula center, which is usually damaged earliest and most severely by antimalarial retinopathy. However, in about half of Asians with antimalarial retinopathy, the condition affects the outer retina instead of the central portion. This is missed by a VF 10-2 test but is picked up by either a VF 24-2 or a VF 30-2. Therefore, Asians need three eye tests yearly—an SD-OCT, a VF 10-2, and either a VF 24-2 or 30-2.

Cultural beliefs also affect how SLE patients do. For example, some ethnic groups may place a higher trust in home remedies or non-Western medicine practices. They may be less likely to take their prescribed drugs.

Sex and Gender

Although most SLE patients are female, about 10% are male. Sex hormones and lupus-associated genes on the X-chromosome help explain this difference. Men with Klinefelter's syndrome (with the sex genes XXY) are 14 times more likely to develop lupus than men with the usual XY sex genes (chapter 3).

Great news: SLE hospital deaths are decreasing

Although patients with SLE have high readmission rates, an analysis of close to 2 million SLE patient admissions showed that SLE hospital deaths fell by 30% between 1996 and 2008. From 2008 to 2016, they were similar to the levels of people who do not have lupus.

Unfortunately, Asian/Pacific Islander SLE patients had a 79% higher hospital death rate than white patients, implying significant health care disparities. Although Black and Hispanic SLE patients also had higher rates than whites, they were not nearly as high as Asian/Pacific Islanders. Black Americans only had a 0.03% higher death rate than whites in this database. We hope this is a positive trend for Black Americans, but we are deeply concerned about why the rate was high in Asian/Pacific Islanders.

While women commonly develop SLE during the childbearing years, men are usually diagnosed with SLE during middle age and older. Both men and women can also develop it in childhood and adolescence.

Men appear to have more lupus nephritis (kidney inflammation), discoid lupus, fevers, weight loss, serositis (such as pleurisy), low blood counts, blood clots, heart attacks, vasculitis (blood vessel inflammation), and seizures than women. Women are more likely to have Raynaud's phenomenon, arthritis, sun sensitivity, mouth ulcers, and nose ulcers compared to men. Most studies show that men with SLE tend to have more severe disease and more permanent organ damage and are more likely to die prematurely.

Black men tend to be more likely to have a sudden onset of severe SLE than most SLE patients. It is not unusual for a very healthy Black male to become sick with rapid major organ damage and end up in the intensive care unit. On the other end of the spectrum, white women are more likely to gradually add lupus problems over time. Of course, there are always exceptions.

Age at Onset

SLE in children (chapter 20) tends to be more severe than in adults. At the other end of the spectrum are people who develop SLE after menopause (or generally after age 50). This is called late-onset lupus and occurs in about 10% to 15% of SLE patients.

SLE onset in females and males varies by age. Many more women than men develop SLE during childbearing years (between puberty and 50 years old). This probably has a lot to do with the high levels of female hormones (such as estrogen) in women of this age. A greater percentage of people with childhood-onset and late-onset lupus are male, compared to those who develop it during childbearing years. Approximately 25% of pre-puberty SLE patients are men while only 9% of those developing SLE between puberty and 50-years old are men.

People with late-onset SLE tend to have milder disease and less frequent flares than those who develop SLE at younger ages. However, lung involvement may be more common than in younger patients. Of late-onset SLE patients, 20% have major organ involvement

LUPUS IN FOCUS

SLE is one of the leading causes of death in young women

In 2018, an evaluation of US death certificates showed that after excluding accidents and suicides, SLE was the seventh top cause of death in women aged 15 to 24. It is eleventh for ages 25 to 44. In Black and Hispanic women, SLE is the fifth top cause of death in the 15–24 age group and sixth in the 25–34 age group.

(compared to 50% of women with SLE onset in childbearing years and 80% of children with SLE).

We do not know if menopause causes SLE to become less severe. Women who develop SLE before menopause tend to have milder SLE after going through menopause. But note that this may not be a consequence of menopause. A large 2006 Canadian study showed that lupus disease activity generally improves over time without any direct effects of menopause. One problem with such research studies is that women with the most severe SLE may die younger than women with milder lupus. Since those with less disease are more likely to make it to menopause, it could appear as if SLE becomes less serious as women age.

While SLE is milder in late-onset SLE patients, the toll on older individuals is relatively high. The aging organs are more susceptible to damage from lupus inflammation, and severe, uncontrolled high blood pressure is more common. The latter is a significant source of permanent damage to aging organs like the kidneys and brain.

Socioeconomic Status and Insurance Coverage
Socioeconomic status is complex. It includes housing, education, employment, income, and more. Numerous studies have suggested that lower socioeconomic status, often represented by low income, plays a significant role in disease activity and mortality. Lower incomes tend to correlate with fewer insurance options, less disposable income (for medications and medical tests), and more difficulty with transportation, among many other things. It is not surprising that this would translate into more severe SLE and a higher chance of dying. A 2020 study of close to 2 million hospitalized SLE patients showed that those without insurance had a 36% higher chance of dying than those with private insurance or Medicare. A 2017 study showed a lower chance of permanent SLE organ damage in patients who could exit from poverty into a higher income bracket.

Although socioeconomic factors are not necessarily permanent, they can be difficult to change. Someone in a low socioeconomic position who develops severe SLE may find themselves in a vicious cycle of poverty and poor health care. When a person is very sick, it becomes difficult, if not impossible, to work or study, and this may have nothing to do with their motivation. It is harder for SLE patients with low incomes to get well. Certainly, the US health care system needs improvement to provide all Americans with good health care.

Income also interferes with health care when it comes to access to technology. As we wrote this chapter in 2022, the world was in the middle of the COVID-19 pandemic. Many doctor visits were through telehealth, while most of society practiced social distancing

LUPUS IN FOCUS

Survival of younger SLE patients compared to older

A 2014 Boston, Massachusetts, study showed that the 10-year survival rate in SLE patients diagnosed at less than 50 years of age was an impressive 98%, while those diagnosed after age 50 years was 90%.

and stayed home. Telehealth encounters use webcams and videos that require personal computers, electronic tablets, and smartphones. Unfortunately, not everyone has access to these devices, reducing the chances for telehealth visits in lower income groups.

Problems with health technology can develop for reasons other than access. For example, digital health wearable devices enable people to track data such as activity level, quality and quantity of sleep, and heart rate. Their usage may be influenced by more than just availability or cost. A 2018 study found that Black and Hispanic participants whose income was twice as high as that of a lower-income group used the devices around 50% more often when they were provided at no cost. This suggests that other factors, not just being able to afford the device, are at play.

Geographic Location

A 2001 study showed that different US regions had higher SLE mortality rates than others. The highest death rate was in the Southwest (especially Southern California through southeastern New Mexico). Louisiana, Arkansas, and Alabama also had higher death rates. The lowest SLE death rates were clustered around the Northeast (particularly New Hampshire and Vermont). Washington, Minnesota, Illinois, and Ohio had relatively low death rates.

A 2018 research study that evaluated the causes of deaths of all US citizens from 1968 through 2013 showed that death related to SLE was higher in the South and West and lowest in the Northeast (similar to the above study). In the South, non-Hispanic whites, in particular, had higher death rates. In contrast, Hispanic and Black SLE patients had higher death rates in the West.

These geographic differences may also be related to differences in factors, such as ultraviolet B (UVB) light exposure, poverty rates and demographics, and regional differences in care. Several studies have found geographic differences in the quality of SLE health care and prescription drug practices. Also, the Northeast and Mid-Atlantic have the highest concentration of rheumatologists. In contrast, the Southwest and the Western Mountain region have the lowest.

Note that it is difficult to reach any firm conclusions on why these geographical differences occur. They are included here out of interest.

Differences in SLE also seem to occur in urban and rural areas, with several studies showing higher rates of SLE in urban areas. Patients living in a metropolitan area in Greece were diagnosed with SLE at younger ages, and they had higher rates of malar (butterfly) rash, sun sensitivity, mouth sores, and arthritis than patients from rural areas.

Multiple studies worldwide have shown high disease activity and flares after periods of high pollution, including in Brazil, the United States, and China. Studies from Canada and Taiwan even showed higher numbers of newly diagnosed patients during periods of high pollution periods than periods of low pollution. A Chinese study found that people living at elevations above 6,600 feet (2,000 meters) developed SLE earlier on average and with worse organ involvement (brain, kidneys, and low blood counts) than those living at lower elevations. Differences in environmental factors may play a role and call for more studies in examining geography, UV exposure, altitude, pollution, and more.

The country you live in and its health care system's ability to care for complex SLE patients make a big difference in survival. The 10-year survival rate of people with SLE is 97% in high-income countries (such as the United States). However, it is only 79% in middle and low-income countries (such as South Africa and Ghana). This is an example of health care disparities on a global level.

Some countries lack a health care structure that is adequate for the needs of their citizens. In 2018, there was only 1 rheumatologist in sub-Saharan Africa per 820,000 inhabitants. That same year, Ghana had only 2 rheumatologists in the entire country of 31 million people. This is overwhelmingly inadequate compared to the United States, where, in 2019, there was 1 rheumatologist per 66,000 people.

Another issue is that diagnostic tests are expensive, adding another barrier to proper diagnosis and treatment. Doctors who supply invaluable services (such as pathologists trained to evaluate kidney biopsies) are few and far between. The situation in poor countries is dire for SLE patients.

KEY POINTS TO REMEMBER

1. Older people may have a lower risk for severe major organ involvement from SLE, whether they developed lupus at an older age or younger age, but their aging organs tend to develop a more significant amount of permanent damage.

2. Men with SLE have more severe disease and higher death rates than women.

3. African American, Hispanic, Asian, and indigenous patients have more severe diseases than their white counterparts. Part of this is related to genetics, poverty, and inadequate health insurance.

4. Hispanic and Black patients may respond better to mycophenolate than cyclophosphamide for lupus nephritis.

5. Patients of African ancestry often require higher doses of mycophenolate than whites. Asian patients may need lower doses due to a higher risk of side effects.

6. Asian patients need three different hydroxychloroquine (and chloroquine) eye screening tests yearly (VF 10-2, SD-OCT, plus a VF 24-2 or VF 30-2) instead of two tests as in other races.

7. Patients can improve their health and outcomes by adhering to treatment recommendations, eating healthy, exercising regularly, not smoking, maintaining a normal body weight, and learning and abiding by "The Lupus Secrets" (chapter 44).

8. Health care disparities exist worldwide and need to be addressed to improve care for all SLE patients.

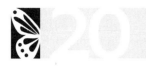

Lupus in Children and Adolescents

Matthew A. Sherman, MD, and Sangeeta Sule, MD, PhD, *Contributing Editors*

With proper care, most children and adolescents with SLE now have an excellent prognosis. This is the view of lupus experts today, and it's essential to bear in mind if any child or adolescent for whom you care is diagnosed with this disease. Most people react to such a diagnosis by searching for "lupus" on the internet, but that can bring up a lot of scary stuff, and figuring out what information is trustworthy, correct, and current can be a challenge. In addition, childhood lupus has unique features, which may not even turn up in that search. This chapter covers these unique features in young children and adolescents, up to age 18. Our goal is to describe the essential characteristics of childhood lupus, supply guidance, and discuss the management of this lifelong condition.

This chapter is written for the guardians of children with SLE as well as for the patients themselves who are old enough to understand. Portions of it are occasionally directed toward one or the other group.

A note about language: we use "child," "children," and "childhood" broadly to refer to young children and adolescents. Where there are differences, we refer to the specific age group. Systemic lupus erythematosus (SLE) in children is known as juvenile or pediatric SLE (pSLE). The terms "lupus," "SLE," and "pSLE" will be used throughout this chapter. "SLE" can be used to refer to systemic lupus in both children and adults, while "pSLE" is used only with children less than 18. "Lupus" itself includes all types of lupus, such as SLE, cutaneous lupus (chapter 8), drug-induced lupus (chapter 1), and neonatal lupus (chapter 18).

One out of five SLE patients develop it before they are 18 years old. In most cases, children develop SLE after 10 years old, particularly during adolescence. It is very unusual for children younger than 5 to develop SLE.

It is still not entirely clear what causes SLE. As with other autoimmune diseases, it is due to a complex mix of factors (chapter 3). Genetics likely play a significant role, and children with SLE are more likely to have genes that may cause SLE. This is called having a high genetic burden. Those with a high genetic burden tend to develop SLE at a younger age and have more severe disease. At this time, rheumatologists are unable to test for these high-risk genes.

Like adults, some children are more likely to develop SLE if they have African American, Asian, Hispanic, or indigenous (such as Native American or Alaskan) ancestry.

SLE is more common in females than males, although the extent of this difference changes with age. Before puberty, 25% of pSLE patients are boys. After puberty, this

LUPUS IN FOCUS

What is proper care for those with pSLE?

The optimistic statement at the beginning of this chapter about the excellent prognosis in children with SLE hinges on the words "with proper care." What that means and what family members should do are as follows:

- Follow up routinely with a pediatric rheumatologist (if possible)
- Obtain recommended labs and other evaluations
- Adhere to all medications
- Practice non-medication therapies, such as wearing sunscreen, eating healthy, and exercising
- Get all recommended vaccinations
- Learn and doing everything in "The Lupus Secrets" (chapter 44)

LUPUS IN FOCUS

Seeing a pediatric rheumatologist

Most pediatric rheumatologists are located near large cities, often in large pediatric medical centers, some of which are academic, or teaching hospitals. If you live in an area without a pediatric rheumatologist, you may have to rely on your local pediatrician, hopefully with the help of a nearby adult rheumatologist. However, it is ideal if you can travel to see a pediatric rheumatologist.

The 2019–2020 COVID-19 pandemic made telehealth using secure video encounters commonplace. We hope that this continues after the pandemic. If so, then a remote pediatric rheumatologist using telemedicine may become an essential member of your child's health care team.

decreases to around 10%. The most likely reason is that during childbearing years women are more likely to develop SLE due to the effects of female hormones (such as estrogen) on the immune system.

Diagnosing Pediatric SLE

SLE is diagnosed similarly in children and adults using several different sets of criteria, which were designed mainly for research purposes (chapter 1). Most patients satisfy at least one of these sets of criteria. But since they were devised primarily for SLE adults, they may not account for some differences in children.

A 2017 United Kingdom study showed that the 2012 SLICC criteria identify children with SLE better and sooner than the ACR 1997 criteria. A later US study showed that the EULAR/ACR 2019 criteria also identified pSLE patients better than the ACR criteria. All these sets of criteria are described in detail in chapter 1.

Child-onset SLE can be a challenging diagnosis because lupus can affect many different body parts. Vague lupus problems such as fever, fatigue, enlarged lymph nodes, mouth sores, joint pain, and low blood counts are common early on in pSLE. These features may resemble other childhood illnesses, including infections (especially viruses) and cancer. All possibilities must be considered before diagnosing pSLE.

It is also not unusual for children to have only one or two symptoms—such as joint pains or low platelet counts—for months or years before other problems, such as a malar rash, develop. Further, the way that SLE presents in adolescents is more likely to resemble the way it does in adults, while in younger children it can appear differently. Although diagnosing pSLE is daunting, after a prolonged period of wondering what is going on, it can be, in a way, a source of relief to finally have the correct diagnosis.

Specific Features of pSLE

Although most of the issues discussed in chapters 6 through 18 also pertain to pSLE, there are important differences.

In general, children have more severe SLE with disease activity in more body parts causing more damage than in adults. Children are also more likely to be hospitalized for SLE. Vague symptoms such as fever, fatigue, enlarged lymph nodes, and involvement of the kidneys, brain, and blood cells are more common in children. Many of the long-term problems from pSLE result from lupus activity in the kidneys and brain, often present within the first year following the diagnosis. Adults are more likely to have lupus problems such as pleurisy, dry mouth and dry eyes, and Raynaud's phenomenon.

Some of the specific features of pSLE are outlined below. Unless otherwise noted, "more" or "less" indicate comparisons between pSLE patients and adult SLE patients. Further information about each condition can be found in the chapter noted in the heading.

Autoantibodies (Chapter 4)

Almost all pSLE patients have a positive antinuclear antibody (ANA) blood test result. Anti-dsDNA, anti-histone, and anti-ribosomal-P antibodies are more often positive in pSLE compared to adult-onset SLE.

Anti-dsDNA also tends to be higher in adolescents than in younger children. The significance of this is that anti-dsDNA positivity and how high it is often mirrors disease severity. Overall pSLE patients have more severe disease than adult-onset SLE patients.

Anti-Ro/SSA is seen in up to 50% of pSLE patients and anti-La/SSB in around 20%. Anti-SSA and anti-SSB-positive adult SLE patients have a higher risk for dry mouth and eyes from Sjögren's disease (chapter 14). Although we do not often see dryness in anti-SSA—and anti-SSB–positive children, a study from Cincinnati Children's Hospital in Ohio showed that 35% of pSLE patients had salivary gland ultrasound findings, which is similar to what we see in adult Sjögren's patients; 82% of these abnormal salivary gland patients were anti-SSA positive. This is interesting because Sjögren's disease is underdiagnosed in pSLE. Children usually do not have dry eyes or dry mouth and tend to present with salivary gland inflammation, instead. If your child is anti-SSA positive, ask your doctor to examine the salivary glands (especially the parotid glands) for swelling and inflammation by physical exam and ultrasonography. If abnormal, read chapter 14. Special focus should be on performing daily healthy oral health habits (flossing, using prescription high fluoride toothpaste, and so on; table 14.5) to reduce the risk of premature cavities and tooth loss.

Musculoskeletal Conditions (Chapter 7)

Joint pain, arthritis, and tendon inflammation are common in children. Up to 80% of those with pSLE may develop arthritis, which is often present at diagnosis or develops within the first year. Fortunately, this form of arthritis does not typically cause joint damage. Whereas adults with lupus arthritis may have prominent joint pain, some children with lupus arthritis do not. Therefore, it is important to look for hints of arthritis, such as trouble walking, avoidance of a favorite activity, or difficulty getting around in the morning. Even if it isn't apparent, a pediatric rheumatologist can find joint swelling on physical exam.

Cutaneous Lupus (Chapter 8)

The malar, or "butterfly," rash may be seen in over half of children with SLE. Discoid lupus, a type of rash that often scars, is relatively rare in children. When it occurs, it can do so by itself without the involvement of other body areas. Because sun exposure can cause a rash and lupus flares, it is critical for children to cover up and wear sunscreen on exposed areas.

Mouth sores are more common in children. These typically form on the roof of the mouth and are usually painless. For that reason, they are often first noticed by a medical provider. Alopecia (hair loss) also happens often in pSLE.

Blood and Lymph System Issues (Chapter 9)

Most pSLE patients have blood cell count problems at some point. Leukopenia (low white blood cells) is common, and the lymphocytes (a type of white blood cell) are most often affected. Anemia (decreased red blood cells) is particularly common. The breakdown of red blood cells by autoantibodies is called autoimmune hemolytic anemia (AIHA) and occurs more often in pSLE. Anemia may also happen due to long-term inflammation or from iron deficiency. These are treated differently than AIHA (chapter 9). Thrombocytopenia (low platelet counts) is also more common in children.

Fewer than half of children produce antiphospholipid (aPL) antibodies (chapters 4 and 9). Although aPL antibodies increase the risk for blood clots (called antiphospholipid syndrome, or APS), APS is not very common in pSLE.

Macrophage activation syndrome (MAS) (chapter 9), a severe lupus problem, occurs in less than 10% of pSLE. It occurs much more commonly in children than in adults. MAS is due to a hyperactive immune system leading to low blood counts and inflammation in multiple organs, especially the liver, spleen, and lymph nodes. Fever is one of the most common symptoms. Ferritin, a protein involved in iron metabolism, is characteristically quite elevated. Although it may develop at any point, MAS is more likely to be present at pSLE diagnosis. MAS requires prompt treatment with immunosuppressants (table 22.1).

Lung (Chapter 10) and Heart (Chapter 11) Issues

Lung and heart involvement are more common in SLE adults than in pSLE. Adolescents are more likely to have these problems than younger children. Overall, up to 30% of pSLE patients develop inflammation of the lining of the lungs (pleuritis) and/or the heart (pericarditis). Other lung and heart problems occur much less often.

Although abnormal PFTs (pulmonary function tests, chapter 10) are often asymptomatic, up to 70% of those with pSLE may have abnormal PFTs. Sometimes a CT scan is necessary to determine whether there is lung inflammation (called interstitial lung disease).

Children with SLE have an increased risk of lung infections such as pneumonia and the flu. Getting vaccinations is essential.

Lupus Nephritis (Chapter 12)

Lupus nephritis is significantly more common in children. It is often present at the initial SLE diagnosis or within the following year. The most severe form is proliferative (also known as Class III and Class IV) lupus nephritis. Over half of children with pSLE will develop this type of nephritis (much more common than in adults), and around 10%–20% of children may develop kidney failure within 10 years of diagnosis. The risk is highest for Class IV and for those of African American, Asian, and Hispanic ethnicities. Younger children tend to be less likely to develop kidney involvement than adolescents. It is important to recognize that children with lupus nephritis are at higher risk for long-term complications. This includes early-onset strokes, heart attacks (chapter 21), and infections (chapter 22). They may also need higher doses of steroids for long periods, which increases the risk of osteoporosis (chapter 24), avascular necrosis (chapter 25), and adrenal insufficiency (chapter 26).

Neuropsychiatric Lupus (Chapter 13)

Neuropsychiatric SLE (NPSLE) occurs more often in pSLE. For those children with NPSLE, the majority will do so within the first year or two of pSLE diagnosis. As in adults, NPSLE may present without other signs of lupus activity. It is an important diagnosis to make promptly because it is one of the most severe problems of SLE and is associated with an overall worse prognosis. As in adults, the evaluation includes checking the blood and spinal fluid, taking images of the brain, and an assessment by a mental health provider, such as a psychiatrist. Fortunately, most children respond well to treatment, which typically includes high doses of steroids (chapter 31) and cyclophosphamide (chapter 32).

Chapter 13 describes the NPSLE categories involving the central nervous system (CNS, the brain and spinal cord) and the peripheral nervous system (PNS, nerves elsewhere). In children, the CNS is more often affected than the PNS. Common presentations include memory problems, headaches, altered mood, and seizures. Memory problems (cognitive dysfunction) may be subtle and hard to identify. It may present as trouble with schoolwork, concentration, or memory. Other factors, such as steroids or depression, may also contribute.

Psychosis occurs in over 10% of pSLE patients. This typically causes hallucinations (seeing or hearing things that are not there). Many children with hallucinations do not let others know about them. It is critical for those with pSLE to understand that these are never normal and share them with family members, guardians, and health care providers if they experience them.

Gastrointestinal Issues (GI, Chapter 15)

Autoimmune hepatitis (liver inflammation) occurs more commonly in pSLE and can precede the diagnosis of lupus. Abdominal pain occurs in approximately 20% of children. A few of the lupus-related causes are peritonitis (inflammation of the lining around the abdominal contents), ascites (excess fluid in the abdomen), and pancreatitis (pancreas inflammation). Drugs, especially steroids and non-steroidal anti-inflammatory drugs (NSAIDs), are one of the most common causes of GI issues in pSLE.

KEY POINTS TO REMEMBER

1. Children with SLE tend to have more severe major organ involvement than adults, especially the kidneys and brain.

2. Younger children with lupus arthritis may not complain of pain. Take note if your child avoids playing or has difficulty getting around in the morning.

Treating Childhood Lupus

Just about every medical student hears the adage "Children are not little adults." Although there are many similarities between children and adults, there are important differences in anatomy, physiology (how the body works), lab results, medication doses, and coping with illness. Moreover, family members or guardians are much more intimately involved because children are too young to participate fully in their care.

Many of the principles of treating adults with SLE apply to children. The treatment goal is remission; if that is not possible, the aim is to lower lupus activity and prevent disease progression. Most pSLE patients need antimalarial drugs (chapter 30) plus immunosuppressants (table 22.1) at first to induce remission. This is called induction therapy. It is then followed by more prolonged immunosuppression to maintain remis-

LUPUS IN FOCUS

The first drug approved to treat pSLE

A significant advancement for pSLE occurred in 2019 when the Food and Drug Administration (FDA) approved intravenous (IV) belimumab (Benlysta) for pSLE patients aged five years and older. This study, called PLUTO (Pediatric LUpus Trial Of belimumab), found that pSLE patients who received belimumab in addition to standard therapy, such as hydroxychloroquine and methotrexate, did better compared to those taking placebo plus standard treatment. They also tolerated it well. In 2022, it was approved for pediatric lupus nephritis.

sion, called maintenance therapy. Treatment is continued for years until the lupus activity is considered quiet enough to begin to slowly taper the immunosuppressants. Even then, certain medicines such as hydroxychloroquine (an antimalarial drug, chapter 30) are continued to prevent the return of lupus activity. Virtually every pSLE patient should be treated with an antimalarial because of their protective effects against lupus flares, blood clots, and even early heart disease.

Refer to chapters 29 through 39 to learn more about different SLE treatments. An excellent way to start would be to read chapter 29 (general treatment), chapter 30 (antimalarials), and chapter 38 (nonmedical treatments) and then to look up your current medications in the index and read about them too.

Medications are generally chosen based on lupus severity and which body parts are involved. Most pSLE patients have major organ involvement, such as lupus nephritis or neuropsychiatric lupus, which require immunosuppressants. Almost every pSLE patient will need steroids at some point (chapter 31). Children in whom pSLE occurs before puberty are more likely to require higher doses. Although steroids are highly effective, they have many undesirable side effects.

While these side effects are similar to those in adults, there are some differences. Due to requiring steroids longer and at higher doses, children have higher risks of developing such conditions as cataracts (chapter 16), diabetes, avascular necrosis, and osteoporosis with broken bones. The latter two are discussed later in this chapter.

Unique to children, steroids adversely affect growth. Specifically, steroids interfere with bone growth plates, the part of bones that make children grow. Children may wind up shorter than expected by an inch or more, depending in part on the dose and duration of steroids. Poorly treated pSLE can also cause shorter adult height.

Although certain immunosuppressants, such as cyclophosphamide (chapters 18 and 32), may have negative effects on fertility and pregnancy, both females and males exposed to cyclophosphamide earlier in life, especially before puberty, are less likely to have their fertility affected. Methods exist to preserve fertility, such as using hormones or egg preservation for females and sperm preservation for males.

It is crucial for sexually active adolescents with pSLE to practice safe sex. They need to understand the impact of medications they may be taking on pregnancy and a developing baby. Some, such as methotrexate, mycophenolate, and thalidomide, may cause devastating effects or stillbirth. Others, such as ibuprofen and other NSAIDS are safe during only part of pregnancy. Note, though, that not all forms of birth control are safe for females with lupus. Be sure to figure out a safe and proper birth control method with your medical providers. Chapter 41 covers these topics in detail.

The most common reason those with pSLE do poorly is poor adherence to their medications. This is especially true during adolescence when children become more independent and even rebellious. Medicines may taste bad. It can be hard to remember and even annoying to take them. They may have unwanted side effects, and children often must take them without having any say in the matter.

Although pSLE patients will have to deal with lupus their entire lives, they should not feel held captive by it. The best way for those with pSLE to try to stay in control is to take their medications regularly—and this is particularly true even when they are feeling well. Many SLE drugs do not start working at once; they take time to build up in the body before taking full effect. Frequently, SLE patients stop taking their medicine once they feel well because they don't think that they need them, even though it is the medications that keep them feeling well. If they are stopped, lupus flares can develop and require even more steroids, with their undesirable side effects.

Fostering a greater sense of independence at a young age may also help adherence. Although children with SLE have little say in doctor visits, medications, or blood work, there are ways to include them in decisions about their treatments. For example, ask them what type of sunscreen, pill organizer, or medication reminder they would like to use.

Sometimes in addition to immunosuppressants, other medications are needed to address complications from lupus or side effects of medications. These may include antihypertensives for high blood pressure, statins for high cholesterol, blood thinners to prevent blood clots and strokes, and calcium and vitamin D for bone health. Lupus can also be better controlled by wearing sunscreen, eating well, exercising regularly, getting enough sleep, and managing stress. And remember, in addition to your rheumatologist, other providers, such as physical and occupational therapists, social workers, and mental health specialists can help. It takes a team to treat lupus, and you are the quarterback. Always let your providers know how they can help you stay healthy.

It is important to mention clinical trials. Adult SLE treatments are guided by research studies in which patients are given different treatments to determine if they are safe and effective. The randomized controlled trial is regarded as the best kind of study. In this type of research, patients are randomly divided into groups in which one is given the treatment and the other is given a placebo (fake medicine). These patients do not know which group they're in. Very few studies like this exist for pSLE because lupus is relatively rare in children. Family members also may be reluctant to enroll their child in research because they think their child may get a placebo rather than the actual treatment or because they think their child may have to remain in the clinical trial no matter what. That is not the case. A patient may withdraw from taking part in a study for various reasons, such as if their disease worsens or they experience side effects. Although there are some pediatric studies, most pSLE treatments are based on adult studies or on the expert opinion of pediatric rheumatologists.

The Childhood Arthritis and Rheumatology Research Alliance (CARRA) puts together consensus treatment plans (CTPs) that provide different ways of treating certain diseases that have not otherwise been investigated with a randomized controlled trial. This way, all patients receive treatment rather than a placebo, and the different treatment options can be compared. For now, there is a lupus CTP for proliferative lupus nephritis.

It is crucial to enroll children with SLE in clinical research studies or CTPs to find the best possible treatments. Consider asking your pediatric rheumatologist if there are any studies available.

KEY POINTS TO REMEMBER

1. SLE is a lifelong disease requiring lifelong treatment.

2. Antimalarial drugs, such as hydroxychloroquine, should be taken by all pSLE patients throughout their lives, if possible.

3. It is essential to take lupus medications regularly to get lupus under control and prevent flares. Steroids are often needed to control SLE if other medicines are not routinely taken. Steroids have many unwanted side effects.

4. Immunosuppressants are usually necessary to control lupus and avoid steroids.

5. Treating lupus also includes wearing sunscreen daily, eating a healthy diet, exercising regularly, and getting enough sleep (chapters 38 and 45).

Complications and Prognosis

Managing lupus is often a balancing act between addressing the inflammation and limiting treatment side effects. Children with SLE can experience many of the same complications as adults, but significant differences exist. Children with more active disease are more likely to suffer more organ damage and have a higher risk of death than adults. Children generally develop more damage over time as well. Certain lupus problems, such as nephritis and neuropsychiatric involvement, as well as exposure to certain medications, such as prednisone and cyclophosphamide, are associated with more damage in pSLE. This is not to suggest that prednisone or cyclophosphamide is harmful in and of itself, but that children requiring treatment with them generally have more severe lupus.

In contrast, antimalarial drugs such as hydroxychloroquine are protective against lupus damage. This is why it is so important to take this drug regularly if prescribed. Table 20.1 lists factors that increase permanent organ damage in pSLE.

The SLICC/ACR Damage Index (SDI) is a research tool that measures SLE organ damage. Though helpful, it does not account for pediatric-specific problems, such as impaired growth and delayed puberty. Children with SLE, especially females, may be shorter than their peers. Puberty is often delayed. Females have their first period around one year later than expected, and periods may occur irregularly, if at all, depending on how active their lupus is. For these and other reasons, the Pediatric Rheumatology International Trials Organization (PRINTO) came up with the Pediatric-SLE Damage Index (Ped-SDI) as a more comprehensive method of measuring pSLE organ damage.

Thanks to earlier diagnoses and improved treatments, children with SLE are doing better than ever. Nowadays, the risk of death within the first 10 years after diagnosis is

Table 20.1 Factors That Increase Organ Damage in Pediatric SLE

- Delay in diagnosis
- African American or Hispanic ethnicity
- Lupus nephritis Classes III and IV (chapter 12)
- Neuropsychiatric lupus (chapter 13)
- High-dose steroids
- Recurrent lupus flares
- Not taking hydroxychloroquine and other medications regularly

much lower (less than 5%) than in the past. Earlier in the disease course, infection and severe lupus activity are the most common causes of death, while end-stage kidney disease (the need for dialysis or kidney transplant) and cardiovascular disease pose a greater risk later on. In addition, demographic factors such as non-white ethnicity (predominantly African and Hispanic) and lower socioeconomic status tend to be associated with worse outcomes. This remains a highly active area of study. While part of the difference in outcomes may be due to health care disparities, genetic factors likely also play a role (chapter 19).

Chapters 21 through 28 review some of the more common complications that may occur in SLE. They may happen to children, so it is important to read any relevant chapters in full. Some of the distinctions in children are discussed below.

Cardiovascular Disease (Chapter 21)

One of the most concerning long-term complications of SLE is cardiovascular disease. This includes heart attacks, strokes, blood clots, and hardening of the arteries (atherosclerosis). These conditions typically occur in older adults. However, those with SLE, including children, are at high risk of these occurring at a younger age. This is partly due to inflammation and using steroids. Hypertension is common in lupus nephritis, and blood pressure medicine is usually needed. Medications called statins are also sometimes used to treat elevated cholesterol. The risk for cardiovascular disease continues into adulthood. One study found that pSLE patients who went on to suffer strokes and heart attacks had them at the average ages of 20 and 39, respectively.

Infections (Chapter 22)

Infections are not uncommon in SLE and should be considered whenever a patient presents with what looks like a lupus flare. Moreover, infection is the leading cause of death for children with SLE. The reason is twofold: patients with lupus have an abnormal immune system and immunosuppressants suppress the immune system. The only way to lessen lupus inflammation is to calm down the overactive immune system.

Antimalarials such as hydroxychloroquine reduce infection risks—this is yet another reason that almost every pSLE patient should take antimalarial medication.

Vaccinations are one of the most effective ways to prevent serious infections. Children with SLE should receive all routine vaccines.

Avoiding most live vaccines while on immunosuppression is important because those with a weakened immune system could get infected. Live vaccines include measles, mumps, and rubella (MMR), varicella (chickenpox), herpes zoster (shingles), oral polio, rotavirus, and yellow fever. Of these, MMR and varicella are routine childhood vaccines. They should be administered, if possible, four weeks before starting immunosuppression.

Every year, it is also beneficial to get the influenza vaccine (flu shot). While the intranasal version is a live vaccine, the intramuscular version injected in the arm or thigh is a killed vaccine and is safe.

It is also recommended that children be vaccinated against pneumococcus. This bacterium can cause potentially severe infections such as pneumonia, bacteremia (infection in the bloodstream), and meningitis (infection around the brain and spinal cord).

You should discuss vaccines with your doctor. See chapter 22 for in-depth information.

Cancer (Chapter 23)

It is important for pSLE patients to get the human papillomavirus (HPV) vaccine. HPV is a sexually transmitted disease. Due to alterations in how the immune system works, those with SLE are at higher risk for this infection. What's more, those with SLE are more likely to develop HPV-related cancers, such as in the cervix, genital areas, mouth, anus, and throat. The HPV vaccine offers protection against the forms of this virus that most commonly cause cancer and is recommended for females and males starting at nine years old to protect them later in life. This type of cancer is in large part preventable by getting the vaccine. Ask your doctor for this vaccine.

Osteoporosis (Chapter 24)

Decreased bone density (weak or brittle bones) is common in SLE. Osteopenia and its more severe form, osteoporosis, occur in around 20–40% of pSLE patients. Children with SLE before puberty are more likely to have decreased bone density. Between 5 and 10% of children with SLE may suffer a fracture from weak bones. The bones become strongest during adolescence, and it is key to improve bone health during this time to reduce the risk of fractures later in life. As in adults, the back bones (vertebrae) that protect the spine are the most common fracture type in children.

The most common method to measure bone density is the DEXA scan (chapter 24). Bone density is reported as a Z-score, which compares the patient's bone density to the average bone density of someone the same age, height, and sex. The lower the Z-score (the more negative), the higher the risk for fractures. A Z-score between –1 to –2 suggests that a child is at risk for low bone density, and a Z-score less than –2 is consistent with low bone density. A child with a Z-score less than -2 plus certain types of fractures meets a diagnosis of osteoporosis.

Specific factors have been found that place pSLE patients at higher risk for poor bone health. Vitamin D is essential for healthy bones, and those with SLE generally have lower vitamin D levels than their peers. Those who have had SLE longer, have needed steroids for a longer time and/or at higher doses, have lupus nephritis, and are less physically active are more likely to develop weaker bones.

Calcium and vitamin D are essential parts of the diet for strong bones. Certain foods, such as dairy, are rich in calcium and vitamin D (chapter 24). The recommended

---

LUPUS IN FOCUS

The importance of healthy bones in children

One out of every two adults older than 50 is at high risk for broken bones from osteoporosis. Children and young adults who build up the most bone density before 20 years old are at a lower risk for broken bones from osteoporosis when they are older. Therefore, all children should follow the recommendations in this section regarding diet and exercise to build strong bones.

daily amounts of calcium and vitamin D vary by age, and sometimes supplements are necessary. Improving the vitamin D level may also help the immune system (chapter 38). Although many experts, including the American Academy of Pediatrics, recommend regular sun exposure to increase vitamin D production, those with SLE should not follow this recommendation, since all sources of ultraviolet light, especially the sun, may cause lupus flares. Exercise is another way to keep bones healthy. Specifically, weight-bearing activities, such as running, rather than lower impact exercise, such as swimming or bicycling, strengthen the bones. One study showed that jumping, hopping, or skipping for 10 minutes only 3 days a week improved bone density. Sometimes, medications called bisphosphonates are needed (chapter 24).

Avascular Necrosis of Bones (Chapter 25)

Avascular necrosis (AVN) is one of the most dreaded complications of steroids. AVN occurs when part of a bone dies due to poor blood supply. It may cause pain, joint damage, and difficulty walking. Although the bone may recover if detected early, AVN sometimes causes significant damage if it goes undiagnosed by a certain stage. In some instances, joint replacement surgery is needed. Around 5%–10% of children with SLE may have AVN, and for some reason, it is more common in those with SLE than in others who take steroids for other diseases. AVN is more frequent in adolescents, those with more severe illness, and those on more prolonged use and higher doses of steroids. The hips and knees are most often involved.

KEY POINTS TO REMEMBER

1. Heart attacks and strokes occur much earlier in adults who have had pSLE.

2. Infection is the most common cause of death in pSLE. Make sure to get all proper vaccines.

3. Strongly consider getting an HPV vaccine to prevent cancer types that occur more commonly in SLE.

4. Keep bones healthy by eating foods rich in calcium and vitamin D and doing weight-bearing activities. Sometimes calcium and vitamin D supplements may be needed.

Coping with a Lifelong Illness

Like having any chronic illness, having lupus is difficult and demanding, and it affects multiple aspects of life. Children with SLE often have decreased quality of life. Growing up is already hard enough; it is even more challenging with pSLE. It is no wonder that 30–50% of those with pSLE have depression or anxiety. Over 10% may consider suicide. Children with SLE who are depressed are also more likely to have worse medication adherence, miss more days of school and appointments, and suffer from worse pain and disability.

Recognizing depression early and seeking professional help is essential. Familiarize yourself with the symptoms of depression (chapter 13). Possible warning signs in

pSLE affects the ability to work as an adult

Childhood SLE is often severe, leading to problems in adulthood. A 2021 Netherlands study looked at adults who had SLE for an average of 20 years and developed it as children. Although their education levels were similar to the general Dutch population, around half stated that SLE affected their education. Half ended up changing their plans for what type of work they wanted to do. Around half were disabled. Of those who finished their education, only 44% had a paid job, and of those who did work, approximately 60% worked only part-time.

This illustrates a great unmet need to better support people with pSLE in achieving their educational and employment goals. Proactively guiding teenagers and young adults with pSLE toward vocations they can do and enjoy is important.

children include withdrawing from friends and family, anger, sleep and appetite changes, fatigue, difficulty concentrating, and trouble keeping up with school or household chores. Take the self-home test for depression (chapter 13) and let your doctor know if you score high. Let your parent, guardian, or doctor know as soon as possible if you have thoughts of suicide. If you don't feel comfortable doing that, call the Suicide and Crisis Lifeline at 988. If you live outside of the United States, check if your country has a similar service.

Teasing and bullying from other children are possible. This is often related to drug side effects, such as weight gain and acne from steroids. The book *Easing the Teasing* by Judy S. Freedman (Contemporary Books, 2002) is a great resource with tools that may help deal with teasing.

SLE presents many challenges to success at school. Over one-third of pSLE patients find that it has affected their school experience. At the same time, though, even though they are more likely to miss school days, in general, children with chronic illnesses do not seem to do more poorly than their peers. There are several keys to getting the most out of school.

First, depending if you are comfortable doing so, consider sharing with others (friends, teachers, nurses, principals, guidance counselors, or social workers) that you have SLE. Many people may not have heard of lupus, and you can be the one to teach them about it and how it affects you. It is prudent to supply a letter to your teacher, guidance counselor, and nurse that explains what lupus is and how it may affect your education. It may also be helpful to schedule a meeting with these individuals to discuss any specific concerns.

Legally protected accommodations are available for children with difficulties or learning impairments that may interfere with school. These government protections include the 504 plan (table 20.2) and the Individuals with Disabilities Education Act (IDEA). If you think that your child may qualify, even if only during lupus flares, it is essential to reach out to your health care team and school about obtaining one of these plans.

Table 20.2 School Accommodations: 504 Plans and the Individuals with Disabilities Education Act

- Make up missed work and tests without penalty
- Extra time for assignments and tests; modified writing assignments
- Preferential seating
- Visual, verbal, and technology helps
- Modification of textbooks and other materials (such as audio-visual)
- Permission to leave the class to go to the bathroom
- Have extra time to get to the next class
- Schedule less demanding activities in the mornings (if arthritis is a problem)
- Modified physical education
- No forced outdoor recess (sun protection)
- Extra breaks and rest periods during the day
- Leave class when needed to see the school nurse
- Regular access to the school counselor
- Behavior management support and access to a social worker.
- Occupational therapy, physical therapy, or speech therapy
- Have ultraviolet filters or screens on lights (or switch them to LED bulbs)
- Have hand sanitizer to use regularly to prevent infections
- Use of an elevator
- Transportation to and from school

Source: Partially adapted from the Lupus Foundation of America, lupus.org/resources/assistance-at-school-for-children-with-lupus

It is also likely that at some point, you may not feel well from lupus while at school. For this reason, **it is important to meet with the school nurse to put together an individualized health care plan (IHP) and an emergency care plan (ECP).** The IHP covers what may be necessary for your child's health care, including medications, during school. The ECP explains what to do when your child experiences a specific problem related to lupus and whom to call.

Children may react to and cope with SLE differently depending on their age and level of development. Older children and adolescents may better process and express their feelings. Younger children may benefit from techniques such as pretend play. Be sure to use language proper for their level. Consider obtaining children's books about lupus to enhance their understanding. Consider using the techniques in table 20.3 to prepare a young child for their first appointment.

Talking to others with pSLE also helps with coping. While most children won't know someone else with SLE, many others are out there, just a click away among internet support groups. For example, the Lupus Foundation of America has online groups under

Table 20.3 Preparing Your Child for Doctor Visits

Before the doctor visit

- Discuss upcoming visit in a positive way with non-frightening language.
- Reassure them they did not do anything wrong; it is not their fault they have lupus.
- Explain to them that the doctor will check them over and help them feel better.
- Consider talking about blood draws, shots, or intravenous drugs. Add that although they may be uncomfortable, they are needed to help them feel better.
- Ask your child if they have any questions for the doctor, write them down, and encourage them to ask those questions at the visit.

Role play with your child

- Look at the eyes, ears, and mouth using the light from a smartphone.
- If your child has a doctor's or nurse's kit, use the stethoscope to listen to the heart and lungs.
- With your child lying down, gently press on their abdomen with your hand.
- Practice the exam: Have them lift their arms above their heads, shake them around. Push on their wrists and fingers. Do the same with their legs, ankles, and toes.
- Encourage your child to examine their stuffed animal, doll, or other toy.

a system called LupusConnect. There are specific groups for teenagers, young adults, parents of children with lupus, and neonatal lupus parents.

For many, it is vital to include a mental health provider, such as a psychologist or, in some cases, a social worker, as part of the health care team. While arming yourself with knowledge about lupus is essential, it cannot be overstated just how important it is to develop healthy coping skills and a reliable support network. Also, you can consider the resources at www.lupusencyclopedia.com/patient-resources. Resources specifically for children and families are toward the bottom of the website page.

A note to the parents and guardians: You and your family are indispensable participants in your child's journey. Everyone, in some way, will have to adapt to this diagnosis. It may be stressful for you, any other children, other caretakers, and for other relatives. Be proactive about taking care of yourself. Your child with lupus will do better when you address your own wellness. Also, figure out ways that the entire family can contribute to helping your child with lupus. And don't forget to ask for help if you need it. Having a child with a chronic illness is difficult, and others in your community and health care team are there to help.

KEY POINTS TO REMEMBER

1. Due to the burden of pSLE, decreased quality of life and depression are common. Children with depression often do worse over time than their peers.

2. Learn the signs of depression and speak openly about them with your family.

3. Children with SLE often have trouble with school. Meet with their teachers, principal, guidance counselor to ensure they receive any accommodations available through the Individuals with Disabilities Education Act or a 504 plan. Don't forget to include your rheumatologist in this process.

4. Coping strategies differ by age and development. Speak to your child with lupus in language they understand. Consider children's books about lupus and internet support groups. Engage a mental health provider early if there are any concerns.

5. Parents and guardians: taking care of a child with a chronic illness may be very stressful. Be sure to ask for help and make time for yourself and others in your family.

Transitioning to an Adult Rheumatologist

Adolescents mature into young adults between 17 and 21 years. This is also the time when they commonly leave their pediatric rheumatologist and begin seeing a rheumatologist who cares for adults (though some pediatric rheumatologists continue to see their patients until they finish college). Transferring care from a pediatric to an adult rheumatologist is called transitioning, which is an ongoing process, often started years earlier when the patient begins to do many of the tasks previously taken care of by their parents or guardians. Adolescents and young adults with SLE need to transition successfully. Many pSLE patients have worse lupus activity and are more likely to be hospitalized during the transition. This is especially true just after switching to an adult rheumatologist.

Every young adult may handle this transition differently. While some adapt to it with ease, for others, it may be difficult. Transitions are more effective if the last visit with a pediatric provider is soon followed by a visit with an adult provider. A study showed that 25% of pSLE patients did not see an adult provider within one year of the last visit with their pediatric rheumatologist. Patients who do not see an adult provider within this time frame are less likely to seek medical attention and are less likely to take their medications. Even after setting up care, about 10%–50% of patients do not make it to a second visit with their new rheumatologist. Some pediatric lupus centers have specialized transition clinics where pediatric rheumatologists and adult rheumatologists work together, often with specially trained nurses and social workers, to facilitate a smoother transition.

This is also a period when anxiety or depression may worsen, making the transition process even harder. Other challenges include limited access to local rheumatologists. There are disparities in health care (chapter 19) for minorities and those of lower socioeconomic status who already suffer from SLE in higher numbers. High unemployment rates in young adults with SLE and an associated absence or loss of health care access result in inadequate medical care. Lower levels of maturity due to chronic and sometimes disabling illness and the rebelliousness and vulnerability of adolescence also interfere with the transition process.

The first step for a smooth transition is to talk to your pediatric rheumatologist about transitioning care to an adult rheumatologist—the earlier, the better. This will allow more time to plan, develop skills, and find an adult provider. Even though most patients will not transition until they are around 18, some pediatric rheumatologists will bring up transitioning when they are as young as 12. This is the age that children are turning into adolescents and becoming more responsible. Therefore, it is proper for them to begin helping with some of their medical care tasks. Some rheumatology practices have adolescent clinics that have certain expectations of their patients. They encourage their patients to practice more self-management responsibilities.

Many transition readiness assessments are available. They take the form of questionnaires that families and providers fill out to determine how ready they are to be self-sufficient. It is best to fill one out early on as a baseline and then every so often to find areas that may need more work before transition. Two options include the quizzes at www.gottransition.org and the "Transition Readiness Assessment Questionnaire" at https://www.rheumatology.org/Portals/0/Files/Transition-Readiness-Assessment -Questionnaire.pdf.

It is essential to plan ahead. Make a timeline with your family and pediatric rheumatologist that includes a specific date at least one year in advance of when you plan to transfer to an adult provider. This should allow enough time to find an adult rheumatologist nearby, develop self-management skills, obtain alternative health care, and hopefully get lupus activity under best control. There are times when transferring to an adult rheumatologist may not be ideal, such as during a lupus flare, an episode of depression, a period of financial or social insecurity, or before obtaining health insurance. Choose a moment when things are most stable. Table 20.4 below lists other recommendations to help ensure a successful transition.

Parents and guardians should keep a folder with relevant medical records, including medical notes, labs, imaging, and biopsy results. The new adult rheumatologist will appreciate having these documents to review and keep for reference. It is beneficial to encourage your child to become an active participant in their health care. Allow them to take part in decision-making, call in drug refills, and keep track of and schedule appointments. These are invaluable skills that your child will one day need when they see a rheumatologist by themselves. During their final year with the pediatric rheumatologist, help build independence by offering them to be with the doctor by themselves on occasion or at least for part of the visit.

Your child is considered an adult when they turn 18. You should discuss how much they would like for you to be involved in their health care at that point. You will need to sign a form from the doctor allowing you to take part.

As the patient enters young adulthood, it's up to them to take medications regularly and see their rheumatologist. Get the most out of your doctor visits (table 20.5). Keep in mind that you are in control of your lupus in many ways and that you have a team of people who care about you and are eager to help.

Table 20.4 Transitioning to an Adult Rheumatologist: Success Tips

- Ask your pediatric rheumatologist to recommend an adult rheumatologist nearby.

- Find an adult primary care provider (internal medicine or family practice): see them at least yearly.

- Make sure that your insurance is active.

- If you have Medicaid, be aware that benefits often end at 19 years old.

- If going to college, check if health insurance is available through the school.

- If you are starting a job, check if health insurance is provided.

- Check The Affordable Care Act (https://www.healthcare.gov/).

- If you are not sure about health care options, ask if your clinic has a social worker who may be able to help.

- Plan ahead.

    Request a copy of your medical records from each doctor visit.

    Keep an up-to-date list of your drugs and any allergies on your phone.

    Take your medicine regularly and request refills before you run out.

    If you are unsure why you are taking certain drugs, ask your rheumatologist.

    Let your rheumatologist know if you are having trouble taking drugs or having side effects. There is always something they can do to help.

    Arrive at least 30 minutes before appointments. If you are late, even a few minutes, the adult rheumatologist may not have time to see you and may require rescheduling.

    Adult rheumatology visits are often 15 minutes (compared to 30 minutes with pediatrics).

    If unable to make an appointment, call the office at least 24 hours in advance.

    Bring a list of questions, your most recent medical records, list of medications and allergies, and something to take notes with.

- Review chapter 43 for tips for getting the most out of your visit.

- It is understandable if you feel apprehensive about this transition. Don't be afraid to ask for help. Some offices have additional helpful resources (for example, social workers).

- Learn about your lupus and review chapter 44, "The Lupus Secrets," to do everything you can to help.

LUPUS IN FOCUS

Keeping copies of medical records is essential

As a rheumatologist who cares for adults, I (Donald Thomas, MD) cannot overemphasize the importance of keeping copies of all your child's medical records. When I get a new patient with pediatric-onset lupus, they arrive with no records most of the time. It is often impossible to get copies of the biopsies, labs, imaging studies, and doctors' notes, especially if their diagnosis occurred 10 to 20 years ago. These patients can be challenging to treat as I have to guess what happened.

Ensure that your child has the best future possible by collecting all records from the initial diagnosis. If your child has had lupus for some time and you have not collected records, it is not too late. You may have to pay for copies if they are extensive (it can take up a lot of staff time), but it is well worth it for your child's future.

Table 20.5 Getting the Most from Doctor Visits

Stay organized and prepared

- Find out from staff beforehand what office times are least busy.
- Wear clothing that are easy to remove for a physical exam (chapter 43).
- Arrive at least 15 minutes early.
- Be courteous to all staff (chapter 43).
- Bring a current referral if required by your insurance (usually with HMOs).
- Find out from the staff beforehand what office times are least busy.
- Take all personal medical records kept at home (like doctor notes, labs, biopsies, test results, x-rays, and so on).
- Take an up-to-date list of medicines (table 29.6, or all pill bottles) and drug intolerances to all doctor visits to make sure their list is correct.
- Write down your primary concerns and a few questions. Do not make the questions long.
- Hand the list to your doctor as soon as they enter the room (chapter 43).
- Answer all questions honestly.
- Take notes about your doctor's recommendations during the visit.
- Ask the doctor to legibly write down their instructions for you.
- Always say "I don't understand" if your doctor says something that doesn't make sense.
- Verbally ask all specialists to send copies of notes and test results to your rheumatologist and primary care provider.
- Discuss staff and billing issues with the office manager, not the doctor (chapter 43).
- If a patient portal is available, enroll in it to obtain online access to your health information and easily contact your provider.

Prepare answers to the "2-minute check-in" before your visit

- How has the past week been?
- How active is your lupus right now?
- What major areas is your lupus affecting your life?.
- What is the most important thing you want from the visit?

Source for the 2-minute check-in: Kathleen Kenney-Riley, "Adolescents with Lupus: Discordance & Relationships Between Functional Status and Quality of Life," American College of Rheumatology Annual Conference, November 2020.

1. Transition from a pediatric to an adult rheumatologist should be planned years in advance.

2. Transition readiness questionnaires can help keep track of areas that need more practice.

3. As they mature, adolescents should become more active and independent in their medical care.

4. Before transitioning, it is important to figure out what health insurance options may be available.

5. Transitioning is a team process involving the patient, family members, doctors, and others, such as social workers.

Neonatal Lupus

Neonatal lupus (NL) is discussed primarily in chapters 18, and 41. NL is not the same as pSLE. While pSLE is a life-long disease, NL generally is not. Most NL manifestations, such as rashes, low blood cell counts, and liver inflammation, resolve within the first year. One critical exception is when the heart is involved. Unfortunately, some infants may develop permanent damage to the electrical system that causes the heart to beat, resulting in congenital heart blockage and requiring a pacemaker. These children will need to see a pediatric cardiologist regularly.

PART III

Other Complications of Lupus and Their Treatments

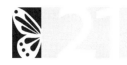

Heart Attacks, Strokes, and Blood Clots

Mariana J. Kaplan, MD, *Contributing Editor*

I ask that all my lupus patients have a primary care doctor and see them regularly. This is as important as seeing a rheumatologist regularly, even if someone is young and feels perfectly fine. Why?

- After the first few years of SLE diagnosis, cardiovascular (CV) problems (heart attacks, strokes, and blood clots) are a top cause of death in developed countries.

- These problems occur at a younger age in SLE patients than they do with their peers. Throughout this chapter, comparisons of problems occurring more or less often refer to people of the same age and sex in the general population (unless noted otherwise).

- Primary care doctors and cardiologists (heart doctors) help prevent these problems by treating the CV risk factors of high blood pressure, high cholesterol, diabetes, obesity, lack of exercise, poor diet, and smoking.

If you are serious about living a long, normal life with your SLE, you should make it a priority to prevent these complications.

· · · ·

Cardiovascular (CV) events include problems with the heart and blood vessels. *Cardio*- refers to the heart, and "-vascular" refers to the body's blood vessels. CV events are a top cause of death in SLE patients in the United States. More than one out of every three people with SLE die from a CV event.

Chapter 11 discussed how SLE could attack the heart and blood vessels, causing inflammation and damage. This chapter focuses on how people with lupus develop heart and blood vessel problems for other reasons as well. These CV problems occur in people who do not have lupus as well, and they are the most common causes of death in the United States. But they occur at a much younger age in SLE patients.

This is an excellent point to define some medical terms associated with hardening of the arteries. Doctors describe hardening of the arteries using both "arteriosclerosis" and "atherosclerosis." *Arterio*- refers to the blood vessels called arteries, and *-sclerosis* means

Dr. Kaplan contributed to this article in her personal capacity. The views expressed are her own and do not necessarily represent the views of the National Institutes of Health or the United States government.

LUPUS IN FOCUS

Major adverse cardiovascular events (MACE)

"MACE" stands for "major adverse cardiovascular events" and is becoming widely used in research. While we stick with "CV events" in this book, it's worth knowing what this new medical term means.

"scarring" or "hardening of"—therefore, "arteriosclerosis" is literally "hardening of the arteries." The Greek word *athero-* means "paste." Atherosclerosis refers to the buildup of a paste-like substance called plaque within the hardening blood vessels. As plaque builds up (figure 21.1), it decreases blood flow. Organs with clogged arteries get less blood flow. This lack of blood results in inadequate amounts of nutrition and oxygen. If a blood vessel that feeds the heart muscle gets completely blocked, the person can have a heart attack. If a blood vessel that feeds the brain gets blocked, it is called a stroke or cerebrovascular accident, or, sometimes, a "heart attack of the brain" (see chapter 13).

Arteriosclerosis in the heart muscle arteries (coronary arteries) is known as coronary artery disease (CAD). Cerebrovascular disease is when it occurs in the brain's blood vessels (chapter 13). And peripheral vascular disease is when it occurs in arteries in other organs. Two major areas of PVD are in the legs and in the neck.

SLE patients who develop arteriosclerosis (or atherosclerosis) develop CV disease, cerebrovascular disease, and peripheral vascular disease at a younger age (or "faster") than others. This has been termed "accelerated arteriosclerosis" and "accelerated atherosclerosis." Some of the causes of arteriosclerosis are similar in lupus patients and in the general population. These include high blood pressure, diabetes, obesity, high cholesterol, and smoking cigarettes. In addition, however, direct inflammation from lupus plays an important role. This chapter discusses types of CV events and their causes and gives recommendations to decrease CV events.

Types of CV Events

Coronary Artery Disease (Angina and Heart Attacks)

Coronary artery disease (CAD) occurs when the insides of the heart's arteries narrow due to plaque, causing less blood flow. When the heart muscle works harder (such as during exercise, walking, or stress), it requires more oxygen and nutrition and thus more blood flow. In CAD the heart muscle cannot get enough oxygen.

This can cause a type of chest pain called angina. Angina is often felt under the breastbone as a pressure-like discomfort. Sometimes it will travel (or radiate) to the arm (usually the left), neck, or jaw. It gradually resolves once the person rests or takes angina medications (such as nitroglycerin). Other symptoms (besides chest pain) include nausea, shortness of breath, jaw pain, and arm pain without chest pain.

If a coronary artery is completely blocked, part of the heart muscle loses blood supply and thus oxygen and nutrients. That section of heart muscle begins to die, causing symptoms similar to angina, but they are usually more intense and prolonged. Heart muscle

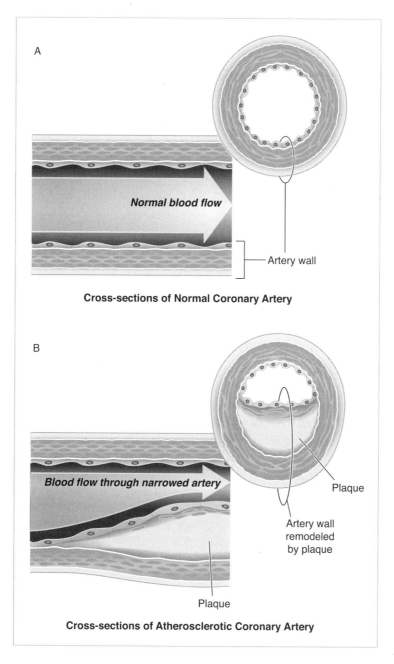

A

Normal blood flow

Artery wall

Cross-sections of Normal Coronary Artery

B

Blood flow through narrowed artery

Plaque

Artery wall
remodeled
by plaque

Plaque

Cross-sections of Atherosclerotic Coronary Artery

Figure 21.1 Normal artery (A) and artery with plaque (B) due to atherosclerosis

death due to blood flow loss is called a myocardial infarction (or heart attack). "Myocardial" refers to the muscle (*myo-*) of the heart (*-cardio*), and "infarction" is the medical term describing the death of tissue due to the lack of oxygen because of a blocked artery.

SLE patients develop CAD, have heart attacks, and die from heart attacks younger than people without SLE (table 21.1). Patients who have had lupus nephritis (kidney inflammation) are especially at high risk for CV events. Ethnicity also plays a role, with Black people having the highest rates of heart attacks.

Table 21.1 Cardiovascular (CV) Issues in SLE: By the Numbers

Treatment-resistant high blood pressure
- 2 times more likely in SLE patients

CV events in general
- 2–4 times more likely in SLE; CV events can occur 2 years before SLE diagnosis
- 6 times more likely in Black SLE patients than in whites
- 18 times more likely during first 10 years after an SLE diagnosis in Black patients than in whites
- average age of first CV event in SLE patients: 48

Hardening of the arteries and dying from it
- 30% more likely in patients with cutaneous lupus than in the general population

Coronary artery disease (CAD, blocked arteries of the heart) and heart attacks
- occur in 1 out of 3 SLE patients by 45 years old
- CAD occurs 20 years earlier in SLE
- 10 times more likely in SLE: nonfatal heart attacks
- 17 times more likely in SLE: CAD deaths
- 50 times more likely in female 35–44 year-old SLE patients: heart attacks

Carotid atherosclerosis
- occurs in 33% of SLE patients over 5 years compared to 4% in non-SLE people
- 200% more likely in lupus nephritis

Congestive heart failure (CHF)
- 4 times more likely in SLE

Strokes
- 8 times more likely in SLE

Blood clots
- 3–4 times more likely in SLE

Aortic aneurysms (chapter 9)
- 6 times more likely in SLE

Note: All comparisons in this chart are to the general population.

CAD can be diagnosed using various tests. These include ECG (electrocardiogram, also called an EKG), a stress test (where an ECG is checked while a person exercises), and an echocardiogram (see chapter 11). It is essential that a person experiencing unexplained chest pain go to an emergency room (ER) at once for evaluation. Blood tests can show if there is an increase in certain enzymes (troponins) due to heart muscle damage, and if the person is evaluated quickly enough, doctors can use medications that open clogged arteries and prevent permanent heart damage. It can be a fatal mistake to experience chest pain and then wait to see if it goes away instead of immediately going to the hospital.

Heart Rhythm Problems (Arrhythmias)

The heart has a network of nerves called the cardiac conduction system. Each heartbeat and squeezing of the heart muscle relies on electrical impulses traveling along this nervous system. There are four heart chambers containing blood surrounded by heart muscle: two atria and two ventricles. The cardiac conduction system makes sure that the two atria squeeze blood simultaneously, followed by the two ventricles. It also ensures that the heart does this effectively (which we measure as the heart rate or how many times the heart beats in a minute).

Proper regulation of this sequence of the atria and the ventricles squeezing (or constricting) ensures that the right amount of blood enters the lungs, absorbing oxygen, then goes into the aorta and then throughout the body.

If the heart's electrical activity becomes abnormal, the heart can beat too quickly or too slowly. The order in which the atria and the ventricles beat in relationship to each

---

LUPUS IN FOCUS

Prolonged QT intervals

Different sections of each heartbeat on an ECG are labeled with a letter (P through T). One section is the QT (or QTc) interval. This is the length between the Q and the T of each heartbeat. A longer QT section is called a prolonged QT interval. This increases the risk of arrhythmias. As many as 15% of SLE patients have a prolonged QT interval, which is often due to an earlier episode of heart muscle inflammation (myocarditis) due to SLE or decreased blood flow from coronary artery disease.

The public became more aware of the term "prolonged QT interval" during the COVID-19 pandemic. Hydroxychloroquine (HCQ, Plaquenil) was studied as a possible treatment for COVID. Some patients who took it developed prolonged QT intervals and arrhythmias. However, these patients were treated with higher doses of HCQ (600 mg to 1,200 mg daily) than we use in lupus. Significantly long QT intervals from HCQ on standard doses are unusual. When it does occur, it is usually reversible by stopping the medication. Anti-SSA (Ro) antibodies may increase the risk of a prolonged QT interval. SLE patients should have their ECG checked. If a prolonged QT interval develops, consultation between a cardiologist and a rheumatologist is a good idea.

other can also be affected. If any of these abnormalities occur, blood flow through the lungs and body decreases. The condition in which the heart's electrical conduction system works incorrectly is called an arrhythmia (*a*- means "absence of"). Therefore, an arrhythmia is the absence of a normal beating rhythm of the heart muscle. Some common types of arrhythmias include atrial fibrillation, atrial flutter, supraventricular tachycardia, sick sinus syndrome, bradycardia (slow heartbeat), and tachycardia (fast heartbeat). The nonmedical term for arrhythmia is "irregular heartbeat."

People with SLE have an increased risk of having arrhythmias. Although lupus inflammation damage (chapter 11) or autonomic nerve involvement (chapter 13) can cause them, they usually develop from coronary artery disease causing reduced oxygen and nutrient supply to the electrical conduction system. Arrhythmias can also occur when the heart muscle becomes thicker or larger than normal due to coronary artery disease, high blood pressure, or valvular heart disease (chapter 11).

Arrhythmia can produce palpitations, where the person notices the heart beating prominently or quickly in the chest. Other symptoms are related to not enough oxygen flowing from the lungs and to the rest of the body. These include chest pain, lightheadedness, dizziness, and shortness of breath. Severe arrhythmia can cause someone to pass out or even die.

An ECG is usually required for diagnosis. An ECG device called a Holter monitor can be worn for twenty-four hours or longer to pick up arrhythmias. Benign (minor) arrhythmias are common and need no treatment. Medication may be needed to treat more significant arrhythmias. In severe cases, the person may need a pacemaker or defibrillator implanted under the skin of the chest. These small devices have wires that go to or near the heart. If they detect a bad arrhythmia, they can send electrical signals to the heart, creating a normal heart rhythm.

Electrical cardioversion can help treat arrhythmias. In this procedure electricity-generating paddles, placed on the chest, send an electric shock to the heart, causing it to beat properly. Some people can have a surgical procedure called ablation, where part of the electrical network is blocked (ablated) to prevent excessive, unwanted electrical impulses.

Congestive Heart Failure

Congestive heart failure (CHF) occurs when the heart muscle cannot pump blood adequately ("failure") to the body. As a result, blood backs up into the lungs or into the veins, causing fluid to leak. If it leaks into the lungs, it causes shortness of breath. This shortness of breath tends to worsen with exertion, which brings on fatigue. When the person lies down, more fluid collects in the lungs, causing worse shortness of breath. A person with CHF will often learn to sleep in a reclining chair to breathe more easily. If the leakage occurs in the soft tissues of the legs, the result is a type of swelling called edema. Gravity pulls this fluid down to the ground, and the edema increases the longer someone is standing and sitting. Edema is typically worse toward the end of the day than when a person first gets out of bed.

CHF is a severe problem and is one of the most common causes of death in older people, although it can occur in anyone (even babies) with a severe condition that prevents the heart from working correctly. Potential causes include high blood pressure (HBP, also called hypertension), coronary artery disease, myocarditis (chapter 11), arrhythmias, and valvular heart disease (chapter 11). Doctors treat CHF by identifying the heart condition and then treating it, by, for example, controlling HBP or using diuretics (water pills) to remove excess fluid from the body. Some drugs for CHF help the heart muscle squeeze harder. A person with severe CHF may require oxygen. Although CHF can result in death, it can also be managed well for many years if mild.

People with SLE are more likely to develop CHF than the general population. Lupus nephritis and being male increase this risk.

Sudden Cardiac Death

If the heart stops working abruptly, this is called sudden cardiac death. This is most commonly due to a massive heart attack (from coronary artery disease) or a severe arrhythmia. Sudden cardiac death occurs more commonly in SLE patients than the general population and at younger ages. Follow the recommendations under the Preventing CV Disease section below to reduce your chances of this happening.

Peripheral Vascular Disease

When arteriosclerosis (atherosclerosis) occurs in blood vessels outside of the heart (coronary artery disease) or brain (cerebrovascular disease), it is called peripheral vascular disease (PVD) or peripheral artery disease (PAD). Both mean the same thing. Blockage of peripheral arteries can cause problems with the organs that the blocked arteries supply. Arteriosclerosis in the legs can cause muscle cramping or leg muscle pain with walking (claudication). It can cause the feet to be cooler than usual. The feet and toes may have a bluish discoloration due to less oxygen. Leg PVD is treated by treating the causes of arteriosclerosis (discussed later in this chapter). Surgery and medicines can help open up the arteries.

If PVD occurs in the kidney, there can be decreased kidney function. A low eGFR on blood tests (chapter 4) signifies reduced kidney function. The blood pressure can become elevated due to this reduced blood supply. PVD can also develop in the intestines and cause damage there (called bowel ischemia), leading to abdominal pain and bleeding from the rectum.

Another type of PVD is carotid artery disease. The carotid arteries are the large neck arteries that supply blood to the brain. If plaque from atherosclerosis clogs these arteries, it is called carotid artery stenosis, where "stenosis" means "narrowing of." This can potentially cause less brain blood flow. Mild involvement usually does not cause any symptoms. However, mild carotid artery disease can worsen over time. So, even mild involvement needs to be taken seriously and managed to prevent its worsening (see the section on Preventing CV Disease below).

If the arteries are moderate to severely blocked, the brain may not get enough oxygen and nutrients, leading to confusion, memory problems, or decreased vision. Most worrisome, carotid artery stenosis can also cause cerebrovascular accidents (CVA, strokes) or transient ischemic attacks (TIA; see chapter 13 to learn more about strokes).

Sometimes, a piece of plaque can become loose (called an embolus) and travel to the brain, causing a TIA or CVA. This can even occur with very mild carotid artery disease. If an embolus travels to the arteries of the eyes, it can cause temporary loss of sight (amaurosis fugax), which is a type of ministroke or TIA. *Amaurosis* comes from

Know your numbers!

Many SLE patients do not have their CV risk factors (such as high blood pressure and cholesterol) treated adequately. Many non-rheumatologists do not realize that lupus dramatically increases the risk of CV events, especially in women younger than 60.

One of the best habits you can get into is to know your numbers. Regularly ask your doctors to measure your blood glucose, HbA1C, and lipid profile. Try to fast (no food, just water and medicines) at least eight hours before labs so that your results are dependable. Keep a diary of your numbers (blood pressure, blood glucose, HbA1C, total cholesterol, LDL cholesterol, and HDL cholesterol). Then ask your doctor (usually your primary care doctor or cardiologist) what your goal is for each one. If your number is not at goal, ask, "What can we do to get this to goal?"

Include diet, exercise, and weight management in your treatment. But if those are insufficient, be open to taking medications, even if that means taking four different blood pressure medicines daily. It is well worth it to take a bunch of pills if doing so keeps you from becoming bedridden from a stroke. We know patients in this situation who wish they had been obsessive about normalizing their numbers.

Not all doctors specialize in managing these problems. If you feel you are not getting adequate help, tactfully ask your doctor, "Since I have lupus, I know that I am at high risk for heart attacks and strokes. Who is a good doctor, such as a cardiologist, in our area who specializes in preventing these?"

the Greek word for "darkening of" and *fugax* means "fleeting." In other words, there is a fleeting (temporary) dimming of vision in one eye. This can be a vital clue to carotid artery disease. A carotid artery ultrasound can find the plaque buildup to diagnose carotid artery disease. This is important because the person with amaurosis fugax is at high risk of a CVA if the condition is left untreated. In addition to treating the causes of arteriosclerosis (discussed below), surgery to open the artery can also be performed.

PVD can also result from the walls of the arteries becoming dilated and thin. This is known as an aneurysm (chapter 11). Aneurysms usually occur in the body's largest artery (the aorta) and in the brain's blood vessels. The danger of aneurysms is that they can potentially burst, which can be deadly. Surgery and medication may be needed to decrease the chances of it rupturing.

Cerebrovascular Disease

Chapter 13 discusses cerebrovascular disease in detail. While cerebrovascular disease can be due to the direct influence of lupus inflammation, it can also be due to other causes, including arteriosclerosis. Doctors call arteriosclerosis of the brain cerebrovascular disease—*cerebro-* refers to the brain.

Blood Clots (Thrombi and Emboli)

Chapter 9 discusses the problem of blood clots from antiphospholipid syndrome. Blood clots are also more common in people who have diabetes or HBP, as well as those who are obese, take steroids or smoke. SLE patients with these problems have a higher risk of blood clots.

Causes of Accelerated Arteriosclerosis in SLE

Diabetes

Diabetes mellitus is a disease in which glucose (a type of sugar) is elevated. We will call it diabetes for short throughout this book. Diabetes damages blood vessels, causing arteriosclerotic plaque. People with SLE are at increased risk of developing diabetes and insulin resistance (a cause of diabetes, discussed below) due to their increased risk of obesity and taking steroids. There are several ways to diagnose diabetes (table 21.2).

We can identify people at risk of diabetes so they can take steps to prevent it. Those at increased risk include people who are non-white (especially those with African, Asian, and Hispanic ancestries) or obese; those who are prediabetic, have had gestational diabetes (diabetes during pregnancy), or have a family history of diabetes (especially diabetes type 2); and those who have polycystic ovarian syndrome or metabolic syndrome (discussed below). Lifestyle changes by at-risk individuals, such as weight loss, incorporating a diabetic diet, exercising regularly, and not smoking, can reduce this risk.

Prediabetes is a condition in which the body cannot handle glucose (sugar) properly and develops insulin resistance. Insulin is a hormone produced by the pancreas (an abdominal organ), which causes the body's cells to absorb blood glucose for energy. When these cells stop responding appropriately to insulin (insulin resistance), they use up less glucose, resulting in higher blood glucose levels.

Prediabetes is diagnosed by having (on two different occasions) a HbA1C of 5.7% to 6.4% or a fasting glucose level of 100 to 125. In addition, prediabetes can cause problems similar to those caused by diabetes, such as nerve damage (peripheral neuropathy) and CV disease. Prediabetics who are less than 60 years old, have a BMI of 35 kg/m or higher, or have had gestational diabetes should consider taking a drug called metformin (a diabetes drug), which may have anti-inflammatory benefits in lupus (chapter 37).

Obesity

Overweight people are at increased risk of arteriosclerosis, diabetes, HBP, and high cholesterol. SLE patients are at increased risk of obesity from steroids and decreased calorie

Table 21.2 How Diabetes Is Diagnosed

Hemoglobin A1C	≥6.5%
Fasting glucose	≥126 mg/dL
Blood glucose (either non-fasting or fasting)	≥200 mg/dL
Two-hour plasma glucose	≥200 mg/dL

417

use (from doing less activity). Fatigue and pain can result in less movement, resistance to exercise, and subsequent weight gain.

Around one-third to one-half of people with SLE are obese. Obesity is a medical condition of excessive body fat to the point where it has adverse health effects. The usual criterion for obesity (emedicine.medscape.com/article/123702-overview) is having more than 33% body fat in women and more than 25% in men.

Various measurements (table 21.3) can diagnose obesity—most commonly, the body mass index (BMI), the waist circumference (WC) measurement, and the weight:hip ratio (WHR).

Online calculators or doctor's office charts can figure out your BMI. BMI is measured by the formula (weight in pounds $\times$ 703) $\div$ (height in inches $\times$ height in inches). Suppose someone is 4 feet 8 inches (or 56 inches) and weighs 150 pounds. This person can calculate their BMI: $(150 \times 703) \div (56 \times 56) = (105,450) \div (3,136) = 33.6$. In general, a person with a BMI of 25 or higher is considered overweight. A BMI of 30 or higher is obesity. A BMI of 40 or higher is extreme obesity (or morbidly obese). A BMI of 50 or higher is super morbid obesity.

Most people who are 10% to 20% heavier than their ideal body weight are considered overweight if that extra weight is not from muscle (as in athletes). Overweight people are at greater risk of CV disease than those with a healthy weight. People with morbid obesity and super morbid obesity are at the highest risk for CV disease, diabetes, high blood pressure, degenerative arthritis, nerve damage (peripheral neuropathy), and early death.

BMI has limitations as a diagnostic tool. For example, athletic people can have a high BMI due to increased muscle. Using BMI alone could incorrectly classify them as obese or overweight, even though they are healthy and have low body fat.

Table 21.3 Obesity Definitions

SLE women who have been on steroids or do not exercise regularly	
BMI	$\geq$26.8 kg/m^2
WC	>33.4 inches
WHR	>0.80
SLE women who have not been on steroids and do exercise regularly	
BMI	$\geq$30.0 kg/m^2
WC	>35 inches
WHR	$\geq$0.85
SLE men	
BMI	$\geq$30.0 kg/m^2
WC	>40 inches
WHR	$\geq$1.0

Note: BMI = body mass index; WC = waist circumference; WHR = waist to hip ratio

On the opposite end of the spectrum are people with reduced muscle mass. This includes the elderly, ill people, people who have been on steroids, SLE patients, and non-exercisers. They can have a normal BMI (18.5 to 24.9), yet be overweight or obese. They have too much fat compared to muscle. Reduced body muscle is called sarcopenia (*sarco-* from the Greek word for "flesh" and *-penia* meaning "lack of").

Sarcopenia is common in SLE. SLE patients with sarcopenia can appear to be normal in weight (even skinny) and yet be medically obese. Sarcopenia occurs in most people treated with steroids, such as prednisone, which causes muscle breakdown and increased fat. They may have a normal BMI but may be obese or overweight. SLE patients who do not move around or exercise due to pain and fatigue can have reduced muscle mass and increased fat. A 2011 study suggested that a BMI of 26.8 or higher more accurately predicts obesity in women with SLE than a BMI of 30.

Another way to diagnose obesity is by waist circumference (WC). To calculate your WC, stand up relaxed without wearing a top. With your fingers, find the soft part above your hipbones. Exhale slightly and then wrap a tape measure around this area at approximately the level of or just above the belly button. Make sure it is snug but not compressing the skin. Place one finger on the tape at the point where the zero end of the tape hits your waist measurement and read the measurement. Repeat two more times. Use an average of the two numbers that are closest to each other. A WC of greater than 35 inches in women and 40 inches in men increases the risk of CV disease. In women with SLE a WC more than 33.4 inches (instead of 35 inches) more accurately diagnoses obesity. This is especially true if you have been on steroids or do not exercise regularly.

Measuring the waist-to-hip ratio (WHR) can also diagnose obesity. To calculate WHR, measure your waist circumference in inches and your hip circumference at the widest part of your buttocks. Then divide the number for your waist size by the hip size. Normal WHR in women is 0.8 or less, and in men is 0.95 or less. Women are considered obese if the WHR is 0.85 or higher; for men, the figure is 1.0 or higher. However, women with SLE and a WHR greater than 0.8 are more likely obese, especially those who have been on steroids or those who do not exercise.

Like women with SLE, men with SLE who have been on steroids or do not exercise regularly should probably use lower numbers. There has not been a study in men with lupus, to our knowledge, to answer this question.

A more accurate measure of body fat is dual-emission x-ray absorptiometry (DXA, pronounced "DECKS-uh"). DXA is commonly used to diagnose osteoporosis by measuring bone density (chapter 24), but it is also helpful for measuring body fat. Many rheumatologists, endocrinologists, and radiology offices have DXA machines. A 2012 study showed that while 26% of a large group of people were obese according to their using BMI, 64% of them were obese using the more accurate DXA scan. Note, though, that most insurance companies do not cover the use of DXA scans to diagnose obesity.

Hypertension (High Blood Pressure)

High blood pressure (HBP, also called hypertension) causes repetitive damage to the body's arteries, increasing the risk of arteriosclerosis. It is also one of the leading causes of strokes, heart attacks, blood clots, and kidney disease. SLE patients are at higher risk of HBP from steroids, obesity, and lupus nephritis (chapter 12).

Blood pressure (BP) is measured by your doctor using an inflatable cuff filled with air (called a sphygmomanometer) placed on your upper arm. When it compresses the blood in the arm's arteries, a stethoscope is used to listen to the blood flowing in the arteries below the cuff. When the cuff is slowly deflated, the first audible sound when blood flows back through the arteries is the systolic BP, which is the top number of your BP reading. The point at which the blood flow stops making noise is the diastolic BP, the bottom number. You have HBP if your systolic BP is ≥ 130 mm Hg (abbreviation for millimeters of mercury) or a diastolic BP ≥ 80 mm Hg.

Home BP readings are thought to be more accurate for BP assessments than those in doctors' offices, which are often higher due to the increased stress of the visit. A high-quality BP machine for home use can be purchased in most drugstores. Everyone with SLE should have one. To ensure it is a good machine, take it to your doctor's office visit and compare what you get on your machine with what your doctor gets when using a sphygmomanometer and stethoscope. Then, keep a log of BP readings at home and take it to each doctor's visit.

There are cases in which your BP is always normal at home (and you are not on BP medicine), but high at the doctor's office. This is called white coat HBP. It occurs because of the stress of going to the doctor's office. Chapter 39 describes the fight-or-flight response to stress, and this is a classic example. While this stress response usually should not cause HBP, it probably occurs in people who have CV abnormalities that predispose them to HBP (such as stiffer artery walls). You can think of it as a mild form of HBP that occurs only during stress. People with white coat HBP are twice as likely to die from CV disease than the general population.

We do not treat white coat HBP with medications, but with diet, exercise, and weight loss and by avoiding substances that increase BP (such as cigarettes). Practicing daily mindfulness, including when you are at the doctor's office, may also help (chapter 39).

HBP patients who are on BP treatment cannot have white coat HBP. They can, however, have a white coat effect. Unlike white coat HBP, which increases the risk for CV death, having a white coat effect does not. Make sure to always bring a log of your home

LUPUS IN FOCUS

A blood pressure of 120/80 is not normal!

In 2017, the American College of Cardiology (in conjunction with the American Heart Association) changed the definitions of normal BP and high BP. Large studies showed that middle-aged individuals had a higher risk for CV events starting at a BP of 120/80 and higher. Someone with a BP of 130/80 or higher was 50% more likely to have a CV event (139/89 doubled the risk). Therefore, 130/80 and higher became the definition of hypertension.

These new definitions were then applied to 1,532 Canadian SLE patients. Over an average of 11 years, those with a BP of 130–139/80–89 mmHg were 2.5 times more likely to have a CV event. The ideal BP for most people is 119/79 and lower.

BP readings to your doctor visits. This reduces the risk of unnecessary BP drug increases if you have the white coat effect.

The opposite of white coat HBP occurs when BP readings are high at home yet normal at the doctor's office. In someone not diagnosed with HBP, this is called masked HBP. In someone already treated for HBP, it is called masked uncontrolled HBP. The American College of Cardiology recommends treating both with BP drugs if lifestyle changes do not normalize the home BP readings.

HBP that is hard to control is known as treatment-resistant HBP (TRH). We say that someone has TRH if they need four or more drugs to control their HBP or have HBP while taking three. SLE patients are more likely to have TRH, which triples the risk for death. It occurs most commonly in Black SLE patients with low kidney function, high cholesterol, and active systemic inflammation. This chapter's recommendations on preventing CV events (below) can also help prevent TRH.

Another BP problem is BP variability (BPV), in which the BP varies significantly at each doctor's office visit. Studies in non-lupus patients show that BPV increases CV events and deaths. In 2019, a study at Vanderbilt University, in Nashville, Tennessee, showed that SLE patients had BPV more often than found in the general population. It occurred more often in patients with more inflammation. Hydroxychloroquine (Plaquenil) decreased BPV. In 2020, Johns Hopkins Lupus Clinic, in Baltimore, Maryland, showed that if the diastolic BP (bottom number) varied by 9 mmHg or more at different visits, that patient had a higher chance of a CV event. Again, hydroxychloroquine decreased variability.

Abnormal Cholesterol

Our bodies need cholesterol. Millions of individual cells make up the body, and a thin cellular membrane surrounds each one, keeping it intact. Cholesterol is an essential part of cellular membranes, helping protect the inner portions of cells from the outside world. Cholesterol is also needed for sex hormones, such as estrogen and testosterone. In addition, some types of cholesterol protect us by absorbing excess fat from the body and bloodstream.

However, too much cholesterol can accumulate if you eat too many saturated fats or if your body produces too much (usually a genetic condition). Excess cholesterol can cause blood vessel problems. Cholesterol is a primary plaque component that clogs up arteries in atherosclerosis. SLE patients can develop high cholesterol from steroids or from obesity. Your doctor may label this problem "dyslipidemia" or "hyperlipidemia" in your medical records. *Dys-* means abnormal, *hyper-* means elevated, and *-lipidemia* refers to fats and cholesterol in the blood.

There are many different types of cholesterol your doctor can measure. Low-density lipoprotein (LDL) cholesterol is a "bad" cholesterol that helps form plaque. High-density lipoprotein (HDL) cholesterol is "good" cholesterol (most of the time). HDL removes excess cholesterol that produces plaque and takes that cholesterol to the liver, where it can be disposed of. You want low levels of LDL and high levels of (HDL), (except as noted below, in proinflammatory HDL).

A complete cholesterol test (also called a lipid panel, lipid profile, or cholesterol panel) is a blood test that measures the cholesterol and triglycerides (a type of fat) in

When is HDL, or "good" cholesterol, not so good?

Around 45% of SLE patients have an abnormal type of HDL called proinflammatory HDL, in which lupus inflammation converts good cholesterol HDL to abnormal proinflammatory HDL. Instead of decreasing atherosclerotic plaque and inflammation the way that normal HDL does, proinflammatory HDL increases plaque and inflammation.

Lupus inflammation also changes other cholesterols into bad forms through a process called oxygenation, in which extra oxygen atoms are added to substances in the body. Material that undergoes oxygenation is oxidized, and SLE inflammation causes both HDL and LDL to be oxidized. Just as SLE produces antibodies that attack different body parts, it does so with cholesterol. Around one out of every three SLE patients has antibodies directed at cholesterol. These antibodies increase oxidized LDL levels. Oxidized LDL and oxidized HDL increase hardening of the arteries, heart attacks, strokes, and blood clots.

Doctors usually cannot distinguish between good HDL, proinflammatory HDL, and oxidized HDL. These distinctions are not made in ordinary lab results and do not appear on lab slips. They are measured only in research studies (2023). Thus harmful HDLs can be included along with the good HDL in the total HDL reading. SLE patients can be told their cholesterol is fantastic because the HDL is high, while they may actually have a high amount of proinflammatory HDL or oxidized HDL, increasing the risk of heart attacks and strokes (rather than lowering it). Since this information is primarily in the lupus research literature, most doctors are unaware of this fact.

These bad HDL variants do not always cause high HDL results. SLE patients with low or normal HDL levels can also have proinflammatory or oxidized HDL present. This primarily occurs in those who have low good HDL levels.

A 2010 study showed that SLE patients who exercised regularly had significantly lower amounts of proinflammatory HDL and less atherosclerosis. SLE patients should exercise regularly to help prevent this cause of death.

your blood. It is best to fast for eight hours for an accurate reading. The normal values for the different cholesterol tests vary by age, gender, and race.

Cholesterol is one type of body fat; Triglycerides are another. When doctors measure cholesterol, the test results usually also give a triglyceride level. High triglycerides (hypertriglyceridemia) are not as strongly associated with CV disease as high cholesterol. However, as discussed below, having hypertriglyceridemia increases the chances for metabolic syndrome.

Metabolic Syndrome

Suppose someone has three or more of these problems: prediabetes, HBP, abdominal obesity, high triglycerides, and low HDL cholesterol. That person is said to have metabolic syndrome. This person is particularly at increased risk of diabetes and CV disease. They are also at increased risk for fatty liver disease, cirrhosis, liver cancer, kidney disease, polycystic ovarian syndrome (a sex hormone disorder in women), sleep apnea (chapter 6), and gout (arthritis due to uric acid). To lower these risks, people with metabolic syndrome should work hard at lifestyle changes such as weight loss, eating well, and exercise. It is possible to reverse some of these with aggressive lifestyle changes, reducing CV disease and diabetes risk.

Smoking Cigarettes

Smoking cigarettes is a major contributor to atherosclerosis. Smoking causes plaque buildup in arteries, increasing blood clots, heart attacks, and strokes. These can occur even without other risk factors such as high cholesterol and high BP. Cigarettes have dangerous chemicals that have profound adverse effects. Smoking also directly damages blood vessels and increases abnormal cholesterol levels, making it easier for plaque to form. The chemical nicotine in cigarettes causes the body's blood vessels to constrict, decreasing blood supply to organs such as the brain, heart, and kidneys. Nicotine also increases heart rate. The muscle cells of the faster-beating heart require more oxygen and nutrients than blocked arteries may be able to provide. This can lead to angina or a heart attack.

Second-hand smoke refers to exposure to harmful chemicals from cigarette and cigar smoking by someone near you. You can breathe in enough of these chemicals for them to harm you. Second-hand smoke increases the risk of heart attacks, strokes, and deaths by 30%. People with SLE should not allow anyone to smoke around them.

Immune-Related Effects of SLE

SLE and other diseases that cause systemic inflammation (such as rheumatoid arthritis, Sjögren's, psoriatic arthritis, and gout) cause arteriosclerosis more often and at a younger age than usual.

Blood vessel inflammation increases atherosclerosis. Lupus inflammation can promote early-onset heart disease. For example, abnormal neutrophils (a type of white blood cell, chapter 3) and interferons (a type of cytokine, chapter 3) involved with lupus inflammation and disease activity promote atherosclerosis.

SLE patients with less disease activity have a lower chance of developing coronary artery disease than those with high disease activity. A 2010 study showed that people with SLE with active disease developed coronary artery disease four times more often than those in remission. Therefore, we know that in addition to controlling BP, cholesterol levels, weight, diabetes, and cigarette smoking, it is essential to control lupus inflammation.

People with lupus nephritis have an exceptionally high risk of accelerated arteriosclerosis. This may be due to the increased amounts of lupus-related inflammation, the HBP that occurs with lupus nephritis, and the use of high-dose steroids. Kidney disease also raises homocysteine levels, which may increase atherosclerosis (discussed below).

Another lupus complication associated with arteriosclerosis is vasculitis. This is not surprising because vasculitis is due to lupus directly attacking and causing inflammation and damage to blood vessels.

People with CLE (such as discoid lupus) without the systemic form are also more likely to have CV disease and die than the general population. Although we can see just a small area of inflammation affecting the skin in these individuals, there may also be enough systemic inflammation to harden the arteries.

Antiphospholipid (aPL) antibodies also increase the risk of heart attacks and strokes. This is probably related to the tendency for these antibodies to cause blood clots in arteries. One type of aPL (beta-2 glycoprotein I antibody, chapter 4) can bind to oxidized LDL. These combination particles can transform white blood cells into foam cells, which contribute to plaque buildup inside arteries with atherosclerosis.

APL antibodies may play an important role, even in people who do not have SLE. A 2018 Swedish study looking at non-SLE people who had a first heart attack showed that 1 out of 10 was positive for aPL antibodies (specifically anticardiolipin and beta-2 glycoprotein I antibodies). Yet, these antibodies occurred in only 1 out of 100 people who had never had a heart attack.

Doctors prescribe blood thinners such as warfarin (Coumadin) to treat heart attacks or strokes due to antiphospholipid antibody syndrome (see chapters 9, 11, and 13).

Vitamin D Deficiency

Vitamin D deficiency is more common in SLE patients and in those with more severe and active disease. SLE patients with low vitamin D are more likely to develop arteriosclerosis and have CV events than SLE patients with normal levels. One small study suggested that SLE patients may end up with less arteriosclerosis by taking vitamin D.

Steroids

SLE patients who have received high dose steroids or taken steroids for a long time have a higher chance of CV events. It is not clear whether the steroids cause the blocked arteries or whether the use of steroids simply reflects the higher severity of lupus inflammation (patients with more severe disease are more likely to take steroids).

Steroids are a double-edged sword. Using low-dose steroids for a short time can decrease disease activity and thus blood vessel inflammation. But when high-dose steroids are used for longer periods, they increase weight gain, diabetes, high BP, and elevated cholesterol, all of which increase arteriosclerosis.

Hyperhomocysteinemia

Homocysteine is a protein, specifically an amino acid. High levels are called hyperhomocysteinemia and are associated with atherosclerosis and HBP. Potential causes of hyperhomocysteinemia in SLE include vitamin deficiencies (specifically folic acid, vitamin B-12, or vitamin B-6), cigarette smoking, and kidney disease. Homocysteine damages blood vessels when present in high amounts, increasing the risk of arteriosclerosis. Adding folic acid, vitamin B-12, and vitamin B-6 supplements can reduce homocysteine. However, some studies show that these supplements do not reduce heart attacks and strokes. Therefore, some experts do not recommend these vitamin supplements for hyperhomocysteinemia.

A 2017 medical literature review concluded that daily folic acid supplementation can lower the risk of CV events and lower BP in people with HBP or hyperhomocysteinemia. This effect was seen mainly in people who do not have a history of CV disease. Some doctors, therefore, treat patients having HBP or hyperhomocysteinemia with daily folic acid.

Genetics

People with family members with heart attacks and strokes at younger ages (men younger than 50 and women younger than 60) are at increased risk of arteriosclerosis due to their genes. The genetics of arteriosclerosis is complex and extends beyond just elevated cholesterol levels, HBP, and diabetes. The bottom line is that if you have family members with arteriosclerosis, elevated cholesterol levels, HBP, or diabetes, then you are at increased risk of arteriosclerosis as well. Unfortunately, you have no control over this risk factor.

Preventing CV Disease

While treating strokes and heart attacks is beyond the scope of this book, we will discuss measures you can take to decrease the risk of their occurrence. Early prevention is essential. While you cannot do anything about your genetics, you can control other risks.

We recommend that SLE patients regularly see a primary care provider (family practice or internal medicine) or a heart specialist (cardiologist). Primary care doctors are specially trained to assess and manage CV disease risk factors. Your doctor should check you regularly for high cholesterol, high BP, and diabetes. If any of these occur, you should get treatment.

Doctors should treat SLE patients more aggressively for these problems than people without SLE. For example, the proper treatment of a 30-year-old female with elevated cholesterol and who is overweight but has no other risk factors for CV disease may be diet, exercise, weight loss, and no medications. However, a 30-year-old obese female SLE patient with high cholesterol should probably take cholesterol-lowering drugs in addition to practicing healthy lifestyle habits.

A group of cholesterol-lowering drugs called statins also has anti-inflammatory properties. While it has not been proven that statins reduce lupus inflammation, research shows that statins can reduce heart attacks and strokes in lupus patients with high cholesterol.

SLE patients should take the following measures to help prevent accelerated arteriosclerosis.

Adhere to Your SLE Treatment

The number one cause of not having lupus under control is not adhering to a prescribed treatment regimen. A high percentage of SLE patients do not take their medications or use sunscreen regularly. Poor adherence increases lupus flares, hospitalizations, heart attacks, and strokes.

Hydroxychloroquine (HCQ, Plaquenil) is the most important lupus medicine. HCQ decreases lupus severity, increases lifespan, and contributes significantly to successful lupus pregnancies. Multiple studies have shown that HCQ decreases total cholesterol and LDL ("bad") cholesterol. It also decreases the risk of diabetes and improves sugar (glucose) levels. HCQ can also lower antiphospholipid antibody levels, reducing blood clot risks.

Since HCQ lowers cholesterol, helps with diabetes, and reduces blood clots, it may also help prevent other CV events, as shown by a 2017 Italian study of 189 SLE patients. When taken with low-dose aspirin, CV events and death rates fell even further.

Mycophenolate mofetil (MMF, CellCept), another lupus drug, may also provide CV protection. A 2019 study showed that MMF improved CV event prediction labs, such as proinflammatory HDL levels, after three months of use. MMF reduces high BP in lupus mice. Research also shows reduced atherosclerosis in both lupus mice and human organ transplant recipients on MMF. Kidney transplant patients had an impressive 20% reduction in CV deaths while taking MMF. However, extensive studies on MMF and CV events have not been done in SLE humans.

Many of the biologics used to treat other systemic autoimmune diseases also help SLE (chapter 33). However, some biologics (TNF inhibitors) can increase total cholesterol and LDL levels. Tocilizumab (chapter 32) does the same. How this affects the risk for CV problems is not completely understood.

When TNF inhibitors and abatacept (Orencia, also a biologic) were studied in rheumatic diseases other than SLE, there were fewer CV events, CV disease occurrence, and less artery plaque formation. When methotrexate is used in combination with biologics, there also seems to be a reduction in CV events. One Spanish study using rituximab (Rituxan) in SLE showed that it may reduce triglyceride and LDL cholesterol. However, rituximab's effects on CV events are unknown.

Low-Dose Aspirin

Platelets are blood cell fragments that help blood clot. They play an essential role in forming blood clots that cause strokes and heart attacks. Aspirin interferes with platelet clumping and therefore decreases plaque production and blood clots. Aspirin may also help reduce inflammation involved in arteriosclerotic plaque. Thus, taking aspirin in small doses, such as 81 mg a day, can help prevent CV events, such as heart attacks, blood clots, and strokes.

Two 2017 Italian studies looked at SLE patients who used hydroxychloroquine (HCQ, Plaquenil) and low-dose aspirin (81 mg daily). While those patients taking either HCQ or aspirin had fewer CV events and deaths, those who took both HCQ and low-dose aspirin had the least. More extensive studies are needed. In the meantime, we recommend that our SLE patients take HCQ and low-dose aspirin if there are no reasons not to.

A few SLE patients may not respond well to aspirin (called aspirin resistance). In other words, it may not effectively thin out the blood. Patients with aspirin resistance are at higher risk of CV events. Potential causes of aspirin resistance include obesity, metabolic syndrome, genetics, taking enteric-coated aspirin (the pill coating helps them dissolve slower), and taking proton pump inhibitors (PPIs, chapter 28). We currently do not have a way to figure out aspirin sensitivity, and it deserves more study. In the meantime, to reduce this possibility, take immediate-release aspirin (especially chewable forms) rather than enteric-coated, avoid PPIs, maintain normal body weight, and practice lifestyle habits that prevent metabolic syndrome.

Since aspirin thins out the blood, it can increase bleeding. These include bleeding from a stomach ulcer or bleeding in the brain if you have head trauma (such as falling and hitting your head). Bleeding from aspirin can occur for a variety of reasons (table 21.4). Although many people with SLE should take aspirin to decrease the like-

LUPUS IN FOCUS

Naproxen, the NSAID drug of choice in SLE

Nonsteroidal anti-inflammatory drugs (NSAIDs, chapter 36) are commonly used for pain and mild lupus inflammation, especially arthritis and serositis. NSAIDs can increase blood pressure, cause decreased kidney function, increase fluid retention, and damage the insides of blood vessels. All of these can lead to heart attacks and strokes.

Naproxen is different and does not appear to increase these risks. Therefore, naproxen (Naprosyn) is our NSAID of choice.

Another choice is celecoxib (Celebrex) when dosed at 200 mg a day or less. While some studies suggest it may increase CV events, one large study showed that it did not.

For mild pain not caused by inflammation, acetaminophen (Tylenol), which is not an NSAID, can be used—it does not increase CV events.

NSAIDs can counteract the protective effects of low-dose aspirin. If someone takes both aspirin (for heart attack and stroke prevention) and an NSAID, the NSAID should be taken at least two hours after the aspirin.

Table 21.4 Factors That Increase Bleeding Risks from Aspirin

A previous bleeding episode

Older age

Chronic liver disease

Pancreatitis

Alcoholism

Cigarette smoking

Diabetes

Cancer

Stomach ulcers

Steroids (such as prednisone)

Selective serotonin uptake inhibitors (chapter 27)

NSAIDs (chapter 36)

Blood pressure–lowering drugs

lihood of CV events, your doctor should help you figure out if the potential benefits outweigh the potential risks.

Diet

A healthy diet can reduce CV risks (chapter 38). Eat a diet low in fat and cholesterol while high in omega-3 fatty acids, fiber, whole grains, fruits, and vegetables. The most often recommended diets for the prevention of CV disease are the Mediterranean diet, the DASH diet (**d**ietary **a**pproaches to **s**top **h**ypertension), and vegetarian diets.

Best dietary practices depend upon whether someone has problems such as obesity, diabetes, HBP, high cholesterol, or kidney disease. Consider asking your doctor to refer you to a dietician to teach you how to eat correctly based on your situation.

Some supplements may help prevent CV disease. As discussed earlier, folic acid may be helpful in people with hyperhomocysteinemia or HBP.

Fish oil (omega-3 fatty acids) supplements may help lower cholesterol (especially triglycerides) and may help reduce HBP and CV disease. The Food and Drug Administration has gone as far as to say that there is credible evidence for these supplements to make this qualified health claim.

Alcohol

Studies show that alcohol has potential health benefits when used in moderation. Alcohol can increase good HDL cholesterol and decrease CV problems such as strokes and heart attacks. A 2018 study of close to 600,000 alcohol drinkers (averaged 6 servings weekly) showed a lower risk of heart attack deaths. Chapter 38 discusses healthy alcohol habits and the dangers of too much alcohol.

Exercise

Lack of exercise is another risk factor for atherosclerosis and CV events. Regular exercise has many health benefits beyond preventing CV disease (chapter 7). Everyone should exercise regularly to improve their overall health and increase their chances of living a long life.

Aerobic exercise helps decrease weight and BP, control glucose, and elevate HDL. Strengthening exercises are also important. The added muscle mass helps the body use more calories and thus support a healthy weight. As noted above, having too little muscle (sarcopenia) and too much fat are significant problems.

Read chapter 7 for exercise recommendations.

Not Smoking

Fortunately, this is one of the risk factors that people can eliminate. The Centers for Disease Control reports that 15 years after quitting cigarettes, that person has the same risk for heart disease as if they had never smoked. Therefore, quitting smoking can make a big difference. Chapter 38 discusses smoking cessation.

Diabetes

The actual treatment of diabetes is complex, involving diet, exercise, and medications. Diabetic SLE patients should work closely with their primary care doctor or with a diabetic specialist (endocrinologist).

Obesity

Losing excessive weight can be very challenging. Successful long-term weight loss generally comes from adopting healthy lifestyle habits of proper diet and exercise. Working with your primary care provider to design a suitable weight loss program can help. Legitimate programs such as Weight Watchers and Noom also give excellent guidance. For those who cannot lose weight on their own and have medical problems related to obesity, weight loss surgery (such as gastric bypass and sleeve gastrectomy) is an option. People with BMIs of 35 and above have a much higher long-term success rate of losing weight through weight loss surgery than people who exercise and diet alone. See chapter 38 for more advice.

High Blood Pressure (HBP)

Regular exercise combined with a proper diet can help lower BP in HBP patients. One helpful diet is the DASH diet. You can easily find it on the internet or ask your doctor. SLE patients with HBP should take BP-lowering medicines if diet and exercise are insufficient. BP goals vary depending on age and the likelihood of developing heart attacks or strokes. Many experts recommend that the BP be kept around 120–125 mm Hg (millimeters of mercury) for the top number (systolic) and less than 80 mm Hg for the bottom number (diastolic) on blood pressures measured at home. For BPs taken in the doctor's office, an acceptable top number is up to 130 mm Hg with a bottom number less than 80 mmHg. Slightly higher numbers may be acceptable in people 65 years old and older. You should work closely with your primary care provider or cardiologist.

High Cholesterol

A diet low in fat and cholesterol helps decrease total cholesterol and LDL (bad cholesterol). Regular aerobic exercise increases HDL (good cholesterol) and most likely decreases dangerous proinflammatory HDL. In addition, low amounts of alcohol help increase HDL, while hydroxychloroquine decreases both total cholesterol and LDL. Many people with SLE should consider taking medications, especially statins (table 21.5). Some lupus experts recommend that everyone with SLE take a statin. A small 2018 Polish study showed that taking a statin (simvastatin) lowered antiphospholipid antibodies (specifically IgG cardiolipin and IgG beta-2 glycoprotein I antibodies) in SLE. Antiphospholipid antibodies (chapter 9) play a role in blood clots and other CV events; lower levels have been linked to lower blood clot risks.

Statins are generally safe. Headaches and upset stomach are the most common side effects. These are usually mild and resolve when people stop the medicine. Your doctor will want to regularly check liver blood tests to ensure you do not develop liver irritation from the statin. A few people get muscle pain or weakness from statins. If so, they should see their doctor right away to find out if it is due to the statin or another reason. People with severe liver disease and pregnant women should not take statins.

Table 21.5 Statins That Improve Cholesterol

atorvastatin (Lipitor)

fluvastatin (Lescol)

lovastatin (Mevacor)

pitavastatin (Livalo)

pravastatin (Pravachol)

rosuvastatin (Crestor)

simvastatin (Zocor)

Statins and SLE

Studies suggest that statins may decrease cardiovascular disease and deaths in SLE patients with high cholesterol. One study even showed that atorvastatin reduced the hardening of the arteries. A large 2019 study looked at the records of over 61 million Americans and found over 37,000 lupus patients. Those lupus patients who took a statin had fewer heart attacks.

Everyone with abnormal cholesterol should eat a cholesterol-healthy diet. Diets including soy, fiber, nuts, vegetables, legumes, whole grains, fruits, fatty fish, soybean oil, canola oil, chia seed, flaxseed, coffee, cocoa, red wine, and tea are beneficial. Examples of good diets include the Mediterranean diet and the DASH diet, as well as vegetarian, low-carbohydrate, and low trans-fatty acid diets. Over-the-counter supplements that can help include omega-3 fatty acids (fish oil), green tea extracts, berberine, and red yeast rice supplements. Be careful with red yeast rice because it can cause side effects and interact adversely with some drugs. Talk to your doctor before taking it.

KEY POINTS TO REMEMBER

1. CV events such as heart attacks, strokes, and blood clots are among the most common causes of death in SLE.

2. Accelerated arteriosclerosis (also atherosclerosis) occurs in SLE, meaning it occurs faster and at earlier ages.

3. The reasons that people with SLE develop accelerated arteriosclerosis include diabetes, obesity, HBP, abnormal cholesterol levels, lupus inflammation of blood vessels, lupus nephritis, antiphospholipid antibodies, high homocysteine levels, lack of exercise, a family history of CV disease, steroids, and smoking.

4. SLE patients should follow up regularly with a primary care provider (internal medicine or family practice doctor) or cardiologist to check and treat CV risk factors such as diabetes, high cholesterol, obesity, and HBP.

5. A high HDL, or good cholesterol, reading in SLE is not necessarily good. Lupus inflammation can create proinflammatory and oxidized HDL that can cause heart attacks and strokes. This is especially a concern in those who do not exercise regularly.

6. Eating correctly, exercising regularly, not smoking cigarettes, and maintaining a healthy weight can decrease CV events.

7. Take 81 mg of aspirin a day, if approved by your doctor, to reduce CV events.

8. Taking hydroxychloroquine (Plaquenil) decreases blood clots, heart attacks, strokes, and death from CV events (especially if taken with low-dose aspirin).

9. Keep your BP below 120/80. Check your BPs regularly at home, keep a log, and take them to all doctor visits.

Infections

George C. Tsokos, MD, *Contributing Editor*

Infections are among the top three causes of death in SLE patients, and most are preventable. Vaccines, antibiotics, and doing everything you can to control lupus through measures that do not require immune system suppression can significantly reduce infection deaths.

Infections occur when disease-causing organisms, or germs, get into the body, use the body for nourishment, reproduce, and cause damage. The immune system should detect these invaders and attack them to protect us. This battle between the germs and the immune system can cause pain, heat, redness, and swelling (signs of inflammation). For example, strep throat, an infection from streptococcus bacteria, can cause pus and redness in the throat and fever.

While infections are often mild and readily treatable, some can spread throughout the entire body or severely injure a major organ (such as the lungs from pneumonia) and can lead to death.

Why People with SLE Get Infections

Infections are among the top causes of death in 20% to 50% of all SLE patients. SLE patients are more prone to infections than people without SLE for several reasons. One is the nature of the condition itself. The lupus immune system may not be able to fight off infections normally. Before lupus drugs and antibiotics were available, most SLE patients died from infectious complications.

The second has to do with immunosuppressant drugs (immunosuppressants for short, table 22.1). While these can work miracles in controlling lupus, they can also lower the immune system's ability to fight off infection. People taking these drugs need to be vigilant with preventing infections.

Note that the antimalarial drugs hydroxychloroquine (Plaquenil) and chloroquine are not immunosuppressants. They are some of the safest and most essential lupus drugs. Antimalarials lower the risk of infections—as much as 60% lower than people who do not take an antimalarial. Part of this decrease in infections is due to their reducing lupus disease activity.

The final reason for increased infections is that lupus can damage body parts that protect us. For example, the skin and lungs play vital roles in keeping invading organisms

LUPUS IN FOCUS

Lupus can cause false-positive infection results

Lupus can cause incorrect infection test results. The lupus immune system can produce abnormal antibodies against many different things. Many of the tests for infections require the detection of antibodies against that particular germ. Lupus can sometimes produce antibodies detected by these tests even though the person was never infected. When a medical test suggests something is going on, but the test result is inaccurate, it is called a false positive.

A typical example is the false-positive syphilis test, which is one of the SLE classification criteria (chapter 1). A false-positive syphilis test means that while the positive results of RPR or VDRL (chapter 4) tests suggest a syphilis infection, in fact the more accurate FTA-ABS syphilis test show that there is no such infection. Lupus can do this with other infections, including cytomegalovirus, rubella, toxoplasmosis, Lyme disease, HIV, and COVID-19.

Table 22.1 Immunosuppressants

steroids (such as prednisone and methylprednisolone)

> weak immunosuppression: prednisone less than 20 mg a day

> strong immunosuppression: prednisone 20 mg a day or more

methotrexate

> weak immunosuppression: less than 0.4 mg/kg/week (dose used in most patients)

> strong immunosuppression: 0.4 mg/kg/week or more

leflunomide (Arava)

> weak immunosuppression (per the American College of Rheumatology)

azathioprine (Imuran)

> weak immunosuppression: less than 3.0 mg/kg/day (dose used in most patients)

> strong immunosuppression: 3.0 mg/kg/day or more

mycophenolate mofetil and mycophenolic acid (CellCept and Myfortic)

cyclophosphamide

calcineurin inhibitors (cyclosporine, tacrolimus, and voclosporin)

biologics (such as belimumab, anifrolumab, rituximab, abatacept, tocilizumab, and certolizumab)

Janus kinase inhibitors (JAKi) such as tofacitinib (Xeljanz), baricitinib (Olumiant), and upadacitinib (Rinvoq)

Note: Antimalarials (hydroxychloroquine, Plaquenil, chloroquine, quinacrine) do not suppress the immune system. Patients on weak immunosuppression may be able to get the measles, mumps, and rubella (MMR) vaccine and Zostavax if needed.

out of the body. If a person has an open sore from cutaneous lupus or pneumonitis affecting the lungs (chapters 8, 10), that person has lost part of this protection. The person with decreased saliva from Sjögren's overlap (chapter 14) has also lost an essential protective element. Saliva is crucial for maintaining healthy bacteria in the mouth. When there is less saliva, harmful organisms (such as the fungus *Candida albicans*) increase, causing infections such as thrush and periodontitis.

Besides the lupus immune system not working properly, two other conditions can occur where the immune system does not perform well against infections. The first is if the spleen does not work properly, and the second is when there is an immunodeficiency disorder. These will be discussed next.

The spleen is an essential part of the immune system that lupus can destroy in a process called autosplenectomy (chapter 9). In addition, surgical removal, or splenectomy, may be needed to treat severe thrombocytopenia (low platelets) from SLE. Either way, the lack of a functioning spleen is called asplenia (absence of a spleen) or hyposplenism (an underactive spleen, chapter 9). People with asplenia are at increased risk for severe infections from pneumococcus, *Hemophilus influenzae*, and meningococcus bacteria. Infection can be quick in onset, severe, and potentially deadly. People with lupus with functional asplenia should get vaccinated against pneumococcus (discussed below), H. influenzae, and meningococcus (table 22.2).

Some asplenic patients should take daily antibiotics. They should also keep an emergency supply of antibiotics at home, work, and school. These antibiotics can be taken immediately for any infection symptoms (table 22.3).

Asplenic patients should take great care in preventing tick bites and seek immediate medical attention if infection symptoms occur. Animal bites, especially dog bites, can cause infection with a deadly bacterium called *Capnocytophaga canimorsus*. Any animal bite should be cared for by a medical professional immediately.

LUPUS IN FOCUS

Opportunistic infections

SLE patients can get opportunistic infections. These are infections that healthy people rarely get and usually occur in people with bad immune systems. For example, people with acquired immunodeficiency syndrome (AIDS) caused by the human immunodeficiency virus (HIV) have lower levels of a type of white blood cell called a CD4+ T-cell. These lower levels can also develop in some SLE patients with antibodies against CD4+ T-cells. As a result, their risk of getting similar opportunistic infections as AIDS patients increases. Examples include tuberculosis, *Pneumocystis jirovecii*, toxoplasmosis, *Candida*, Streptococcus pneumoniae, herpes zoster, and human papillomavirus. Strong immunosuppressants (especially mycophenolate, cyclophosphamide, and steroids) further increase the risk for opportunistic infections.

Table 22.2 Preventing Infections in Asplenia (Lupus Autosplenectomy, or Surgical Removal)

Vaccines needed:

Pneumococcal vaccines

H. influenzae type b vaccine (Hib)

Meningococcal vaccines (MenACWY, MenB-4C or MenBFhbp)

Take daily prophylactic antibiotics if:
- you are under 16 years old or over 50
- you have had severe infection after a previous vaccine for that bacteria
- you have another immunocompromising condition:
  - immunodeficiency disorder
  - take immunosuppressants (table 22.1)

Keep an emergency supply of antibiotics at home, work, school, and while traveling.

Seek medical attention immediately for infection symptoms, tick bite illness (possible babesiosis), and after animal bites (especially dogs).

Table 22.3 Infection Symptoms

Infection Type	Possible Symptoms
Systemic	Fever, chills, sweats, fatigue, muscle and joint pains, headaches, swollen glands in multiple areas (lymphadenopathy)
Skin (such as cellulitis)	Red, hot skin (especially if it spreads out), wound pus or foul smell
Sinuses (sinusitis)	Sinus or nasal congestion, runny nose, facial pain, headache
Lungs and upper airways (such as pneumonia and bronchitis)	Cough, sputum, chest pain, shortness of breath
Brain (such as meningitis and encephalitis)	Headache, stiff neck, difficulty thinking, seizures, vomiting, confusion
Bladder and kidneys (cystitis and pyelonephritis)	Urination pain, frequent or urgent urination, lower abdominal pain, flank pain
Throat and mouth infection (such as pharyngitis and thrush)	Swollen neck glands, sore throat, trouble swallowing, painful swallowing, white patches in the mouth, red and sore tongue
Gastrointestinal tract (such as from food poisoning or parasite infection)	Nausea, vomiting, stomach pain, diarrhea, bloating

Primary Immunodeficiency Disorders

Immunodeficiency disorders increase infection risk. Primary immunodeficiency disorders are genetic. They can be inherited from parents or caused by genetic mutations. People with lupus are at higher risk of primary immunodeficiency than the general population.

Secondary immunodeficiency disorders are the most common cause of increased infections in SLE patients. This is partly due to the disease itself since the abnormal lupus immune system increases infection risks. Another type of secondary immunodeficiency is due to immunosuppressants. This section discusses some of the primary immunodeficiency disorders.

Very rare lupus-associated immunodeficiencies (T-B-NK+ SCID, Wiskott-Aldrich syndrome, autoimmune polyendocrinopathy candidiasis, ectodermal dystrophy, autoimmune lymphoproliferative syndrome, and idiopathic CD4(+) lymphocytopenia) are not covered.

Hypogammaglobulinemia

Gamma globulins are also called immunoglobulins or antibodies. They are produced by white blood cells called B-cells (or B-lymphocytes). Hypogammaglobulinemia occurs when B-cells produce fewer gamma globulins (*hypo-* is from the Greek for "lack of," and *-emia* is from the word for "blood"). It is diagnosed by a blood test called the serum protein electrophoresis (SPEP). While immunosuppressants are the most common cause of hypogammaglobulinemia in SLE, it can also occur due to primary immunodeficiencies. There are several different classes of gamma globulins (or immunoglobulins), each of which is designated by a letter (A, E, G, or M). The most common types of deficiency are IgA deficiency, IgG subclass deficiencies, and common variable immunodeficiency, which are discussed below.

Selective IgA Deficiency

IgA refers to "immunoglobulin A." Selective IgA deficiency (sIgAD) is one of the most common immunodeficiencies: it occurs in 1 out of every 500 people. There is a much higher risk of having it if another family member does. Selective IgAD is diagnosed by finding normal IgM and IgG levels but low IgA levels on a quantitative immunoglobulins lab test. The doctor must also exclude other causes of low IgA (such as immunosuppressants).

Most non-lupus patients with sIgAD have no problems from it, although some will have allergies or autoimmune disorders, including lupus-like symptoms.

Only a minority of people with sIgAD have increased infections. These include infections of the ears (otitis media), sinuses (sinusitis), airway passages (bronchitis), lungs (pneumonia), and intestinal infection due to a parasite called *Giardia lamblia* (giardiasis, which occurs from infected water). If infections recur, they are usually treated by antibiotics, although IVIG (intravenous immunoglobulin, chapter 35) treatments are sometimes needed.

Patients with severely low IgA levels can have severe reactions to blood product transfusions and IVIG preparations containing IgA. Measuring and finding positive IgA antibodies can help identify at-risk patients. Special precautions are needed before giving these treatments to IgA-antibody-positive patients.

Selective IgG Subclass Deficiencies

Immunoglobulin class G (IgG for short) is further divided into subclasses (1 through 4). If the total IgG level is normal, but one of the subclasses is low, this is called a selective IgG subclass deficiency.

Selective IgG2 subclass deficiency is more common in SLE than in the general population. This deficiency can increase the risk for infections of the ears (otitis media), sinuses (sinusitis), airway passages (bronchitis), lungs (pneumonia), and meninges (meningitis, infection around the brain).

Selective subclass deficiencies of IgG1, IgG3, and IgG4 are unusual in SLE and do not occur more commonly than in the general population. Around 80% of selective IgG1 deficiency patients have recurrent sinus, upper airway, or lung infections. Most patients with IgG3 or IgG4 deficiencies do not have increased infections and are not considered to have an immunodeficiency disorder. In other words, most of these patients' immune systems are not negatively affected by lower-than-normal immunoglobulin levels. However, some IgG3 and IgG4 deficient patients do get recurrent sinus, upper airway, or lung infections and are considered to have an immunodeficiency disorder.

If infections are infrequent in patients with a selective IgG subclass deficiency, they can be treated with antibiotics as needed. Some of our patients frequently get the same types of infections, so we give them a supply of antibiotics to keep on hand. Taking an antibiotic daily for prevention or IVIG treatments may be needed in those with more frequent infections.

Common Variable Immunodeficiency

Common variable immunodeficiency (CVID) refers to a group of genetic immunodeficiency problems that cause low IgG, IgM, IgA, and sometimes IgE levels. It is significantly more common in people from a British Isles heritage than in the general population. Like the previously discussed hypogammaglobulinemias, CVID cannot be diagnosed in someone already taking a medicine that can cause low gamma globulin levels. The low levels can be due to the drug and not due to CVID.

In addition to finding low immunoglobulin blood levels, it is also essential to demonstrate that the person does not respond to vaccinations. A normal immune system produces enough gammaglobulins (or antibodies) to have an excellent response to a vaccine, such as the flu shot. To test whether someone does not respond to vaccines due to CVID, the doctor usually gives either a pneumonia, tetanus, or diphtheria vaccine and then measures blood levels of IgG antibodies to the vaccine several weeks later. If the immunization IgG levels are very low (usually less than 200 mg/dL), this is additional evidence for CVID.

Having CVID increases the risk of many different infection types. It is usually treated with IVIG (intravenous immunoglobulin, chapter 35) via an infusion into a vein. However, IVIG can also be injected under the skin (subcutaneous), making these treatments more convenient. Other than infections, other problems in people with CVID include lung diseases, intestinal problems, asthma, increased allergies, large lymph nodes, enlarged spleen, liver disease, stomach cancer, and non-Hodgkin lymphoma.

Approximately 25% of people with CVID also develop an autoimmune disease such as lupus. People with both SLE and CVID may have a smaller risk of developing lupus nephritis (kidney inflammation) than other SLE patients. IVIG therapy for CVID can help reduce lupus disease activity in some patients.

Selective IgE Deficiency

IgE is essential in fighting viruses and parasites and for allergic responses. During allergy season many people have high IgE levels from pollen allergies. IgE also helps identify cancer cells and get rid of them.

While about 3% of the total population has selective IgE deficiency (sIgED, where IgE is low while IgA, IgM, and IgG are normal), it occurs in about 10% of patients with rheumatologic autoimmune diseases such as lupus.

People with sIgED may get more infections of the upper respiratory tract (sinusitis, colds), the breathing tubes (bronchitis), and from *H. pylori* infection of the stomach (chapter 28). Infections are treated when they occur with standard antibiotics.

There is some controversy as to whether sIgED is a primary immunodeficiency or not. We include it here since it does seem to be associated with increased risks for the infections listed above.

Complement Deficiencies

Complement deficiency is a rare primary immunodeficiency in SLE. Complement comprises 30 or so proteins that act together to destroy invading organisms (germs, bacteria, and others). Complement, along with white blood cells, are the first responders in fighting infections. Complement proteins are essential immune system components.

People without certain complement proteins, particularly those responsible for the direct destruction of germs, have an increased risk for infections such as *Streptococcus*

LUPUS IN FOCUS

Which SLE patients are at the highest risk for infections from immunodeficiency?

Some specialists teach the "rule of 500s." Patients with an absolute neutrophil count less than 500/microL, an absolute lymphocyte count less than 500/microL, or a total IgG serum level less than 500 mg/dL are at increased risk for infections. Offending medicines should be stopped or lowered in dose.

pneumoniae, Hemophilus influenzae, and meningococcus and should be vaccinated against these.

People who lack some complement proteins (specifically C1q, C1r, C1s, C2, C3, and C4) can develop lupus. More than 75% of people who completely lack C1q, C2, or C4 develop lupus. These people are usually young.

Effects of Infections

Infection symptoms depend upon the body area infected (table 22.3). Some symptoms (such as fever and fatigue) are common with most infections. Some symptoms commonly seen in infections also occur in other disorders. For example, allergies can cause cold-like sneezing, cough, and runny nose. Blood clots in the lungs can cause pneumonia-like cough, chest pain, and shortness of breath. The treatments for these differ drastically from infection treatments. Therefore, it is essential to see a physician for evaluation.

Severe infections can damage major organs (such as the lungs or the brain), involve multiple organs, or spread through the bloodstream. Bacteremia (*-emia* refers to blood) occurs when bacteria are in the blood. In SLE patients, it usually occurs in those with severe active disease and who are on steroids. These situations are potentially deadly.

If an infection is powerful enough to cause a body-wide reaction, threatening organ function, we call it sepsis. Signs of sepsis include an increased respiratory rate, increased heart rate, decreased blood pressure, low platelet count, difficulty thinking, abnormal liver blood tests, and reduced kidney function. Septic shock occurs if the blood pressure drops enough so that medicines are required to keep the blood pressure up (vasopressors). Septic shock has a high death rate. Sepsis is becoming one of the most common causes of infection-related admissions to the hospital for SLE patients.

Severe infections also increase the risk for lupus flares. It is important to monitor SLE closely during and after severe infection and treat it promptly if a lupus flare occurs.

Infections and Treatments

Fevers and chills in someone with lupus could signal an infection. Although fever can happen due to lupus itself, this should not be assumed. Treating infection is vastly different from treating lupus fever.

In addition to fever and chills, other symptoms of an infection depend on the area in which it occurs (table 22.3). Infections should be assessed and treated promptly by

LUPUS IN FOCUS

Steroids can decrease fever from infections

Severe infections cause fever in most people. However, steroids, such as prednisone, can reduce temperature response to infections. If you have other symptoms suggesting infection (table 22.3) but you do not have a fever, do not dismiss infection as a possible cause. Make sure to see your doctor.

your primary care provider and, if not available (after hours), by emergency room (ER) or urgent care center doctors. Your primary care provider may also ask you to see your rheumatologist if there is a possibility that your lupus may be causing your symptoms. Sometimes, it can be challenging to determine if symptoms are due to lupus or infection, and you may be treated for both.

Certain people are at higher risk of getting infections than others. They include people with lung disease (such as chronic obstructive lung disease, emphysema, and interstitial lung disease), congestive heart failure, chronic kidney disease, lupus nephritis, or diabetes, as well as those who are over 65 years old, and anyone who has been previously hospitalized for a severe infection. Although all immunosuppressants increase infection risks, steroids (such as prednisone) are the biggest problem, especially at doses above 7.5 mg a day. The higher the dose (especially above 15 mg a day), the higher the risk. Doses less than 5 mg a day can be problematic as well. This is why doctors should use other drugs (including other immunosuppressants) to get patients off steroids.

Even so, if a patient with an infection is on steroids, the steroids should not be stopped. This is especially true for someone who has been on steroids for a significant amount of time and who develops adrenal insufficiency (chapter 26). In this case, it would be dangerous to stop the steroid. There are times when the steroid dose should be increased to replicate what the body normally does during infection (produce more steroids for the stressful event). But if a steroid had only recently been added to a patient's regimen, a doctor may decide to discontinue its use during the infection.

The chances for infection are greater when lupus is active. Simply having active lupus inflammation means that the immune cannot fight off infections as well. If that person is also on steroids, they are at greater risk. For example, someone who has active lupus arthritis, fatigue, and mouth sores and is taking prednisone 5 mg a day has a much higher chance of getting an infection than someone in remission. This is why it is important to do everything possible to get lupus under control (table 22.4).

Some infections that are common among lupus patients deserve special mention. One is thrush, which is a yeast infection from *Candida albicans*. It is described in chapter 14. Several other infections are described below.

COVID-19

In March 2020, a pandemic was declared involving a novel coronavirus labeled **coronavirus disease 2019** (COVID-19 for short) due to **severe acute respiratory syndrome coronavirus 2** (SARS-CoV-2). The virus is spread primarily by aerosolized water droplets (from people talking, breathing, sneezing, and coughing). It causes numerous potential symptoms, most of which are similar to the common cold and flu, along with some unusual symptoms, such as the loss of taste and smell. Since the pandemic began, over 1,125,365 Americans have died from COVID-19, and around 80% have been infected at least once (as of April 2023).

SLE patients have been disproportionately affected. They are more likely to get infected, and once infected, they have worse outcomes, such as hospitalization and death. They are less likely to have a good response to the COVID-19 vaccines and the vaccines tend to wear off faster. Patients on immunosuppressants (especially rituximab) have done worse with all these measures.

Table 22.4 Preventing Infections

Vaccinations to get:

- Influenza ("flu") shot every September/October.
- Pneumococcal vaccines for all SLE patients.
- Shingrix (shingles vaccine): FDA-approved for all immunosuppressed adults and anyone over 50.
- Gardasil HPV vaccine (if 9 to 45 years old).
- Hepatitis B vaccines if you are 19 to 59 years old. If 60 or older, get them if you have risk factors (such as diabetes or fatty liver).
- Meningococcal vaccine if you have asplenia, complement deficiency, or live in a college dorm or military barracks.
- Tetanus-diphtheria every 10 years.
- Receive vaccines before starting immunosuppressants, if possible

Other precautions:

- Take hydroxychloroquine or chloroquine regularly.
- Take vitamin D if your level is low.
- Get 8 hours of sleep nightly, practice UV protection, learn to control stress, eat an anti-inflammatory diet, exercise regularly, do not smoke (chapter 38).
- Maintain physical (social) distancing for COVID-19 and other respiratory infections.
- Wear a mask in public during COVID-19 and flu season.
- Wash hands frequently during flu and cold season.
- Wear gloves.
- Cover your cough or sneeze.
- Avoid contact with sick people.
- Urinate right after sexual intercourse if female (reduces urinary tract infections, UTI).
- Wipe front to back after bowel movements if female (reduces UTIs).

LUPUS IN FOCUS

Stopping immunosuppressants during infections

No professional medical groups have published guidelines on stopping immunosuppressants during infections. Most immunosuppressants (other than steroids) do not substantially increase infection rates. No studies prove that stopping immunosuppressants during infections makes a difference.

Some specialists stop immunosuppressants in patients if they require hospitalization, have a fever greater than 102°F, or are highly immunosuppressed (on chemotherapy, had a kidney transplant, or have an immunodeficiency disorder) and have a fever greater than 101°F. Others will stop immunosuppressants during any type of infection. No approach is proven to be best.

Our knowledge about COVID-19, the emergence of new strains, how to prevent infection, and how to treat it is constantly changing. But in general, the most important thing people can do is to prevent infection in the first place. This is done through social distancing, hand washing, avoiding crowded places, wearing masks, getting vaccines, and using other preventative treatments (see Preventing Infections section below).

Because CDC recommendations for vaccines change as new variants of the virus emerge, we recommend that you talk to your doctors, especially your rheumatologist. Many of the drugs used to treat lupus (especially rituximab, mycophenolate, steroids, and methotrexate) decrease vaccine responses, so it is important to stop some of these after vaccines (if not at high risk for flaring, table 22.6).

For the latest research and updates on COVID-19, including vaccine schedules, and what drugs should be stopped for vaccines, visit lupusencyclopedia.com/4th-covid -vaccines and rheumatology.org/covid-19-guidance.

Shingles (Herpes Zoster)

If you develop a band of burning, painful red rash on one side of the body, often accompanied by small blisters, you could have shingles. Shingles (also called herpes zoster) is due to the virus that causes chickenpox (called varicella zoster virus) and that continues to live in the nerves next to the spinal cord after someone is infected with the chickenpox virus (usually as a child). When the immune system becomes less effective at keeping the virus under control, it can multiply and attack one of these nerves, causing pain and rash in the skin area to which the nerve gives sensation.

Shingles occurs much more commonly in SLE patients than in the general population. Even young SLE patients are up to 3 times more likely to get shingles than a healthy 75-year-old. Shingles should be treated as soon as possible with antiviral drugs that target the herpes virus. These include acyclovir (Zovirax), famciclovir (Famvir), and

---

LUPUS IN FOCUS

JAK inhibitors and anifrolumab (Saphnelo) significantly increase the risk of shingles

Janus kinase inhibitors (JAKi, chapter 32) are a group of drugs that may help some SLE patients. These drugs, which include tofacitinib (Xeljanz), baricitinib (Olumiant), and upadacitinib (Rinvoq), are FDA-approved to treat other rheumatic diseases, such as rheumatoid arthritis and psoriatic arthritis. JAKi increase the risk of developing shingles two to six times more than normal. Anifrolumab (Saphnelo, chapter 34), which is a biologic, was FDA-approved to treat SLE in August 2021. It increases the risk of developing shingles approximately three times more than normal. Fortunately, these outbreaks tend to be mild and usually respond well to antiviral drugs.

Patients should be vaccinated for shingles, preferably with Shingrix, before they begin a JAKi or anifrolumab if this is possible.

valacyclovir (Valtrex). They can help prevent permanent damage to the nerve, which can cause long-lasting, severe pain in some people.

Shingles usually affects just one side of the body in a band of skin going from the back (near the spine) to the front of the body, or down one arm, or down one leg. However, in people on immunosuppressants, shingles can sometimes occur in numerous nerves simultaneously and appear in multiple body areas. This is called disseminated zoster and may need intravenous (IV) antiviral medications.

Postherpetic neuralgia is a condition in which pain persists after the shingles rash heals. There may also be numbness, increased sensitivity, and itching. This painful complication is more common in older people. Drugs that decrease nerve pain may be needed.

The complications of shingles vary depending on the nerves involved. Some severe problems include blindness, stroke, paralysis, and even death. Shingles also increases the chances of having a heart attack. I have had an immunosuppressed patient become paralyzed from shingles and another die from shingles (it attacked her brain); both were unvaccinated. Getting Shingrix is the best prevention.

Herpes simplex

Another type of herpes virus infection is *Herpes simplex* virus (HSV). This virus is spread by direct contact with an infected person and lives inside your body your entire life. It causes painful open sores, most commonly on the lips (called herpes labialis; *labia-* from the Latin word for "lips") or on the genitals (genital herpes). When it occurs on the lips, it often begins as a burning sensation followed by itchy bumps that become open, painful sores. In addition to being painful, the sores can be cosmetically embarrassing. Nonmedical people often call them "cold sores" or "fever blisters." Stress, illness, and dry, chapped lips can cause them to occur. Genital herpes can be sexually transmitted and shows these symptoms on the genitals. People with SLE are more likely to have HSV than the general population.

Patients on immunosuppressants can develop more frequent and severe episodes if infected with *Herpes simplex*. It is essential to get treatment right away if you have an attack while on an immunosuppressant. The quicker an anti-herpes drug is used, the easier it is to treat. If the outbreaks occur more often, you may want to take a shingles antiviral drug daily to prevent the attacks. Anti-herpes drugs include acyclovir (Zovirax), famciclovir (Famvir), and valacyclovir (Valtrex).

Human Immunodeficiency Virus (HIV)

Human immunodeficiency virus (HIV) is transmitted by sexual contact or through blood contact (such as sharing needles). HIV primarily attacks white blood cells, especially a type of T cell called CD4+ T, which leads to severe immunosuppression and risk for deadly infections in most people if not treated. Human immunodeficiency virus infection causes acquired immunodeficiency syndrome (AIDS); together, they are called HIV/AIDS.

Distinguishing between SLE and AIDS/HIV can occasionally be challenging. Both can cause positive ANA, antiphospholipid antibodies, sun sensitivity, arthritis, rashes, swollen glands (lymphadenopathy), major organ involvement (heart, lungs, kidneys, brain), and low blood counts. SLE can even cause a false positive HIV blood test result.

SLE patients may be less likely to get HIV/AIDS, and HIV-infected individuals are less likely to develop SLE. The antibodies formed by SLE patients (notably anti-RNP) may help protect the person from HIV infection. SLE patients can still be infected with HIV, but possibly at lower rates.

Since HIV/AIDS results in fewer T-cells, white blood cells that play a major role in SLE, SLE often becomes inactive after HIV infection.

As with all infections, immunosuppressants for SLE can potentially lead to worse outcomes in HIV-infected patients, making them even more vulnerable to infections.

On the other hand, the drugs used to treat HIV/AIDS can increase the number of T cells, causing the immune system to become more active and with it SLE. SLE can even appear for the first time due to this increased T cell activity in someone treated with anti-HIV drugs. Well-coordinated care between a rheumatologist and an infectious disease expert is needed in SLE patients infected with HIV.

Other Viral Infections

Not all infections are treatable. For example, most virus infections, such as sinus infections, bronchitis, and colds, do not respond to antibiotics. Your doctor may not recommend any treatment except over-the-counter drugs to help you feel better. Unnecessary overuse of antibiotics leads to organisms becoming resistant to them, making infections more difficult to treat over time. Taking vitamin C and Echinacea (an herb from the purple coneflower) have not been shown to be effective against the common cold. People with SLE should not take Echinacea because it can worsen lupus.

One possible treatment for the common cold is to use over-the-counter zinc acetate lozenges (such as Cold-EEZE); they may decrease symptom duration. Zinc lozenges work best if used immediately at the beginning of cold symptoms and then used regularly (such as every few hours). Note that supplements containing zinc gluconate and zinc sulfate do not appear to be effective.

Preventing Infections

If you have lupus, it is important to prevent infections in the first place (table 22.4). Preventative medicine is always better than waiting until bad things happen and then treating them after the fact.

One of the most important ways to prevent infections is to take care of your lupus, using all the therapies available to keep it under control without suppressing the immune system. All SLE patients should be taking hydroxychloroquine (Plaquenil) or chloroquine daily if not intolerant. These are the safest drugs for SLE. They do not suppress the immune system and can help decrease the need for stronger medications, especially steroids. Patients with mild SLE taking hydroxychloroquine regularly are less likely to evolve into a more severe form of SLE.

Not smoking is also important. Cigarettes contain chemical substances that increase immune system activity, increasing lupus flares. One such chemical is hydrazine, which can actually cause a lupus-like autoimmune reaction. Other cigarette substances (carbon monoxide, cyanide, and hydroquinone) can cause cell damage, DNA abnormalities, and increased immune system activity. Another way that smoking may increase lupus disease activity is by preventing hydroxychloroquine from working correctly.

Smoking also damages the lungs and the passageways leading to them, increasing the chance of infections such as bronchitis and pneumonia. Smokers are more likely to get more severe infections that last longer, and they are more likely to die.

Avoiding ultraviolet (UV) light exposure and taking vitamin D regularly are also important for a healthy immune system (chapters 35 and 38).

Staying up to date on vaccines is crucial. In the United States you can help prevent over sixteen infections with vaccines.

Unfortunately, many people do not get vaccinated. The Centers for Disease Control (CDC) estimates that more than 45,000 adult Americans die every year from vaccine-preventable infections. Most of these deaths are from influenza, COVID-19, and pneumonia.

There are two general types of vaccines. One is comprised of live, attenuated vaccines, meaning that the germs in the vaccine are live but in a significantly weakened state (table 22.5). People who take immunosuppressants should not receive these vaccines that contain live organisms since they can have strong, long-lasting effects. The other type does not have live organisms. It includes vaccines such as "inactivated" vaccines, which are made of killed germs and mRNA (messenger RNA) vaccines (such as many of the vaccines for COVID). We will not go into deep details on these, but do note that inactivated and mRNA vaccines are safe for patients on immunosuppressants.

Specific vaccinations are discussed below.

Inactive Vaccines

COVID-19 Vaccines. COVID-19 vaccines have greatly reduced hospitalizations, intensive care unit admissions, and deaths. All lupus patients should keep up to date with their vaccines.

Because vaccine recommendations keep changing as new strains develop and research progresses, you should ask your doctor for the latest recommendations. If you take an immunosuppressant, you can refer to lupusencyclopedia.com/4th-covid-vaccines and cdc.gov/coronavirus/2019-ncov/vaccines/recommendations/immuno.html.

Also ask your doctor if you are considered immunocompromised. Note that SLE patients can have other immunocompromising conditions (such as asplenia and hypogammaglobulinemia) in addition to taking immunosuppressants. Those who are not immunocompromised should follow recommendations for the general public.

Pneumonia Vaccines. Everyone with SLE should be vaccinated against *Streptococcus pneumoniae* (pneumococcus for short). Pneumococcus is the most common bacteria causing pneumonia in the United States. However, with effective vaccines, it has become less common.

A 2014 Dutch study showed that SLE patients were 13 times more likely to develop serious pneumococcal infections than the general public. Even SLE patients who were not taking immunosuppressants had higher rates of pneumococcal infection. Therefore, lupus experts recommend that all SLE patients get pneumococcal vaccines.

As of 2022, the pneumococcal vaccine PCV13 (Prevnar 13) is no longer recommended, and the regimen was simplified. Instead, SLE patients of all ages should get a PCV15 (Vaxneuvance) followed one year later by a PCV23 (Pneumovax) or get a PCV20

Do vaccines cause lupus flares?

In our opinion, yes, but only rarely. We have seen only a few cases of convincing vaccine-induced flares in SLE patients during our careers (a total of over 60 years).

We can look at more solid evidence. Some Chinese epidemiologists reviewed 18 excellent studies regarding vaccines and SLE in 2016. Only 32 out of 1,966 (1.6%) SLE patients had a flare after the flu shot, and all flares were mild. These studies included patients with low to moderate disease activity. You may be quick to think, "That means close to 2% of SLE patients will flare after a flu shot." However, this is incorrect. Think about it: If you monitor 1,966 SLE patients who are not in a vaccine study, how many do you think will flare? That is the nature of SLE—it causes flares. To determine if there is a relationship between flares and vaccines, you would have to do a study comparing two SLE groups; half would get a vaccine, while the other half would get a placebo. That way, you could see whether the vaccine group gets more flares.

(Prevnar 20). If someone gets a Prevnar 20, they do not need a follow-up Pneumovax. If someone receives Pneumovax initially, this should be followed up one year later with either a Prevnar 20 or a Vaxneuvance.

Unfortunately, some people with SLE do not respond well to pneumococcal vaccines. This is especially the case for those with very low lymphocyte counts (chapter 9), hypo-gammaglobulinemia (discussed above), and those on immunosuppressants.

Influenza (flu) Vaccines. Influenza is a viral infection that can attack many different organs, but especially the lungs. It is a major source of illness and death. In non-tropical countries, flu season most commonly occurs during winter months. This generally means October to March in the Northern Hemisphere (in countries such as the United States) and April to September in the Southern Hemisphere (Australia, for example). Tropical countries can have active influenza all year.

Every fall before the flu season occurs, everyone should get the flu vaccine (flu shot). Patients with rheumatic diseases such as SLE are twice as likely to be hospitalized and die from the flu than the general population. Yet, less than 30% of SLE patients get their flu shot.

The CDC recommends getting the flu shot in September or October (before the end of October). They do not recommend getting it in July or August (primarily in older people) because it may start to wear off before the flu season ends. But if you forget your flu shot in September or October, you should get it as soon as possible up through the end of the flu season (as late as January through March) to have at least some protection.

There are several types of flu vaccines. FluMist (live-attenuated influenza vaccine) is a nasal spray, but since it contains live virus (discussed below), it should be avoided in patients on immunosuppressants (table 22.1). Inactivated flu vaccines, or flu shots, are not live vaccines. They come in a trivalent form, which protects again three different strains of flu (*tri-* means three) and a quadrivalent form, which provides immunity against four (*quadri-* means four). If the quadrivalent is not available in your area, it is recommended to get the trivalent form.

There is also a high-dose flu shot, which contains four times more flu proteins (also called antigens) than the regular flu shot. It provides a more robust immune response (and protection) in patients 65 and older. It has not been studied extensively in younger immunosuppressed patients. However, some experts recommend the high-dose flu shot for their immunocompromised patients.

The flu shot never causes the flu, though some people mistakenly think it does. One reason for this misperception is that flu shots are given during the time of year when respiratory conditions (allergies, colds, the flu, bronchitis, and sinusitis) typically occur, so if someone develops one of these problems soon after the flu shot, it is easy to blame the shot, even though in reality, this is simply a coincidence. Another reason is that some people get a flu-like syndrome as a side effect of the shot. This is not actually the flu—it can be a side effect of any vaccine—but it can feel like the flu. Symptoms can include muscle and joint achiness and a low-grade fever that can last for a few days. Doctors consider this a mild reaction. Taking acetaminophen (Tylenol) can help alleviate these symptoms.

The Advisory Committee on Immunization Practices recommends that people who have experienced hives (an allergic itchy rash) from eggs should receive flu shots. People with more significant allergic reactions should also receive a flu shot. However, they should be observed for 30 minutes afterward in a facility able to treat severe allergic reactions (just in case). The amount of egg protein in today's vaccines is miniscule.

The main reason to not get a flu shot is if you had an actual severe allergic reaction to a flu shot in the past.

HPV Vaccine. Human papillomavirus (HPV) infection occurs through sexual contact and can cause cancer. These HPV-associated cancers are more common in SLE. See chapter 23 for more about preventing HPV-related cancers and catching them in the early stages while they are still potentially curable.

LUPUS IN FOCUS

What to do if you get a severe complication from a vaccine

The chances of a severe reaction to vaccines are very low. Because vaccines prevent the spread of infectious diseases, the US government requires people to get vaccinations under certain circumstances (such as children attending public schools and military personnel).

While the benefits of vaccinations outweigh the risks, the government recognizes that severe reactions can occur, and so it established the National Vaccine Injury Compensation Program. Reactions such as shoulder injuries, passing out, severe allergic reactions, and nerve and muscle damage (Guillain-Barre syndrome) are listed in the program's "Vaccine Injury Table." Anyone with a reaction listed in this table can receive compensation. If you believe you suffered a severe vaccine complication, go to www.hrsa.gov/vaccine-compensation/index .html, call 1-800-338-2382, or email vaccinecompensation@hrsa.gov.

Tetanus and Diphtheria Vaccine. People should also get a tetanus-diphtheria toxoid vaccine (Td vaccine) every ten years. Diphtheria infection can cause pneumonia, nerve problems, heart damage, and death.

Tetanus is a bacterial infection that attacks the nervous and muscle systems of the body, causing paralysis and a high death rate. Tetanus is rare in the US due to vaccines. Tetanus toxin shots are also used for "dirty" puncture and trauma wounds to prevent infection.

Hepatitis A and B Vaccines: Hepatitis A and hepatitis B are viral infections. As their names suggest, their primary target is the liver. Although mild infections can occur, they can also be severe. In the worst cases, liver failure and death can occur. Hepatitis B can even cause permanent liver damage (cirrhosis) and liver cancer.

SLE patients with autoimmune hepatitis, fatty liver disease, or whose ALT or AST levels (chapter 4) are more than double the upper limits of normal should receive hepatitis A and hepatitis B vaccines.

As of 2022, it is recommended that everyone aged 18 to 59 get the hepatitis B series vaccines. If you are pregnant, it is recommended that you wait until after pregnancy. Those aged 60 and older who have risk factors (ask your doctor) should also get it. Children aged 2 to 18 years old should get the hepatitis A vaccine series. If 19 or older, it is recommend for those with additional risk factors (ask your doctor).

Meningococcal Vaccine. Neisseria meningitidis is a bacterium that particularly likes to infect the meninges (lining of the brain). It can be prevented with a meningococcal vaccine. SLE patients who should receive the meningococcal vaccine include those with hyposplenism (surgical or functional), those with a complement protein deficiency, and those who live in a college dorm or military barracks.

. . . .

It is safe to get any number of vaccines mentioned above on the same day. Live vaccines (table 22.5), however, need to be given at least 28 days apart, one at a time. You can get one live vaccine (such as for yellow fever) and multiple inactivated vaccines on the same day.

Live Vaccines

As mentioned above, patients on immunosuppressants generally should not receive most live vaccines (table 22.5). However, it is fine to get the Zostavax vaccine if you are on certain lupus drugs, such as methotrexate and azathioprine. If a live vaccine is recommended, and you are on an immunosuppressant, read the section below about that vaccine first to ensure it is safe for you. Also, always double check with the doctor who treats your lupus.

If a live vaccine is recommended and you are planning to start an immunosuppressant for which the vaccine is contraindicated, it is recommended that you start the drug at least a month after the vaccine. For example, suppose you need to get the yellow fever vaccine, your only drug is hydroxychloroquine, and you are about to start on mycophenolate mofetil (MMF). In this case, if you can wait an entire month before starting the MMF, it is preferable to get the vaccine right away. If your disease activity

Table 22.5 Vaccines with Live, Attenuated Organisms

Adenovirus type 4, 7 (oral)

BCG (Bacille Calmette-Guérin, tuberculosis)

Dengue tetravalent live vaccine

FluMist (nasal flu vaccine)

MMR (measles, mumps, rubella)

OPV (oral polio)

RV (rotavirus)

Typhoid (oral form)

Vaccinia (smallpox)

VZV (varicella-zoster virus, varicella, chicken pox)

Yellow fever

Zostavax (varicella zoster virus, herpes zoster, shingles)

Note: These vaccines should be avoided by people taking most immunosuppressant medications.

LUPUS IN FOCUS

Can live vaccines be safe with immunosuppressants?

The recommendation to not give live, attenuated vaccines (such as Zostavax) to people receiving immunosuppressants is based primarily on the theory that live germs, though weakened, could potentially cause infection in the vaccinated person. However, studies have shown that the MMR vaccine can be given safely to children on methotrexate or biologics. Other studies show that patients on some biologics (specifically TNF inhibitors) can receive Zostavax safely. Zostavax can be given with weak immunosuppressants (see the Zostavax section).

In general, the CDC recommends not giving live vaccines to immunosuppressed patients, even though there is no evidence that they are harmful. The CDC's stance is to be as risk-averse and safe as possible. More studies are being done on this topic.

---

is severe and you cannot wait a month for MMF, then it is recommended to not get the vaccine.

Once you are on an immunosuppressant, it is possible to get a live vaccine, but only if the drug is stopped. We usually consider this only for patients in remission and at low risk of flaring. In this situation, the doctor would usually stop the immunosuppressant, then give the vaccine once the drug is out of the patient's system and when their suppressed immune system is most likely working better (this time varies by drug). Then the drug can be restarted a month after the vaccine.

Shingles vaccine. There are two shingles vaccines: the recombinant zoster vaccine (called Shingrix) and Zostavax (a live vaccine). Shingrix is most effective and the preferred vaccine. It is FDA-approved for people 50 years and older and for immunosuppressed patients 18 and older.

Shingrix is given in a two-part series, two to six months apart. If it is later than six months after the first shot, the second should still be given at the first opportunity. However, its effectiveness at that scheduling is unknown. If the second shot is given accidentally within a month of the first, it is recommended to get a third shot two to six months later.

If you get shingles, it is important to get your Shingrix after the attack is over. The best timing is not known. Since a shingles attack boosts the immune system's response to the shingles virus, many experts recommend that people with normal immune systems wait a year before getting the vaccine. There is no consensus regarding immunosuppressed patients.

Shingrix is such a potent vaccine that it is not surprising that pain, swelling, and redness occur at the injection site in 8 of 10 people. In 1 out of 10, this reaction is severe enough to temporarily cause difficulty using the arm. Many people get headaches, body pains, fever, chills, stomach upset, and malaise. These are generally mild and subside in one to three days after the injection.

Zostavax is also FDA-approved for people 50 years old and older. Although it is a live vaccine, the Centers for Disease Control states that it is safe for those on weaker immunosuppressants (table 22.1). The American College of Rheumatology has added leflunomide (Arava) to this list. The European League Against Rheumatism and a Canadian "Executive Summary" group have stated Zostavax is safe for patients receiving immunosuppressants, including biologics.

If you have had the Zostavax, you should still get the Shingrix because Shingrix is more effective, and Zostavax wears off after five to seven years.

People born in 1980 and later most likely received the varicella-zoster virus (VZV) vaccine to prevent chickenpox when they were children. Because the vast majority of people born before 1980 have been infected with chickenpox, the CDC does not recommend VZV blood testing in this age group. They should get a shingles vaccine without testing. They should be tested and vaccinated against VZV if negative. VZV vaccine is also a live vaccine.

Measles, Mumps, Rubella Vaccine. Although the measles, mumps, and rubella (MMR) vaccine is a live-attenuated vaccine, a Dutch study showed no significant complications in immunosuppressed children receiving MMR while on immunosuppressants, such as methotrexate and TNF inhibitors (Humira and Remicade). The European League Against Rheumatism has therefore stated that MMR can be given to patients on weak immunosuppressants (table 22.1) if they are at increased risk of getting measles (such as when traveling).

Yellow Fever Vaccine. People who travel to some areas of South America and Africa need to be vaccinated against yellow fever (a tropical infection with a high death rate). The yellow fever vaccine (a live vaccine) can cause live virus to circulate in the body, leading to infection in immunosuppressed people. Since no adequate studies assessing this potential risk exist, the European League Against Rheumatism recommends against yellow fever vaccines for immunosuppressant patients.

Other Vaccine Issues

After a live vaccine, someone could theoretically infect someone else with the virus. The risk for immunosuppressed people who are in contact with the vaccinated individual is minimal, but it is possible.

All close contacts of immunosuppressed SLE patients should receive all recommended vaccines. We call this "cocooning" or the cocoon strategy. If the immunosuppressed person's loved ones all vaccinate themselves, they surround that person with extra protection, like the cocoon around a developing butterfly.

But there are special precautions with live vaccines. For example, it is recommended that close contacts not get the oral polio vaccine (OPV), Zostavax, or FluMist. Each of these has safer non-live vaccine alternatives. These include Shingrix for shingles, enhanced-potency inactivated polio vaccine (eIPV) for polio, and multiple influenza vaccines.

Some live vaccines are safe for close contacts because they are not transmitted. These include the oral typhoid vaccine, yellow fever, measles, mumps, and rubella. Mumps and rubella vaccines can be spread through breast milk, but this is rare.

If a close contact receives the oral polio vaccine (OPV), the immunosuppressed person should avoid contact for four weeks. With the vaccinia vaccine, contact should be avoided for two weeks. If someone develops a rash after the varicella (chickenpox) or Zostavax (herpes zoster) vaccine, contact should be avoided until the rash has resolved. Infants getting the rotavirus vaccine can excrete rotavirus in their feces for several weeks, so immunosuppressed patients need to avoid fecal-soiled items for four weeks. Everyone else should practice strict handwashing with soap and water after possible fecal exposure.

If a woman receives a biologic (chapter 33) during the last four and a half months of pregnancy, the medication can enter the baby's circulation and persist for the first six months after birth. The European League Against Rheumatism recommends that babies not be given a live-attenuated vaccine during their first six months if the mother was treated with a biologic during the third trimester.

No vaccine is 100% effective. In other words, you can still be infected after a vaccine. If infection occurs, it is usually less severe than it would have been without the vaccine.

LUPUS IN FOCUS

Do you refuse vaccines?

Many people, unfortunately, refuse vaccines. There are many myths about vaccines, such as their causing autism. They do not. Nor do you get the flu from flu shots—another myth. The internet is full of misinformation. The Centers for Disease Control and Prevention has some excellent and medically accurate information at www.cdc.gov/vaccinesafety/concerns/index.html.

One important reason for vaccines is to protect the ones you love. (See "cocooning" above.) This is why flu and COVID-19 vaccines are a requirement of employment at many health care facilities: so that we protect our patients.

Do not get vaccines while lupus is severely active or if you are on 20 mg a day or more of prednisone (or 16 mg methylprednisolone). You are less likely to respond to vaccines if you are on high-dose steroids. If you are, wait until you are on lower doses. Ask your rheumatologist if it is safe before getting any vaccinations.

Some immunosuppressants may prevent the immune system from responding adequately to a vaccine. For a vaccine to work, the immune system needs to recognize the vaccine's components. Then the immune system's B-cells (a type of white blood cell) respond by making antibodies directed toward the organism for which the vaccine is intended. For example, after a person gets the Pneumovax vaccine, the B-cells make antibodies directed toward the pneumococcal bacteria. If a person vaccinated with Pneumovax becomes infected with the pneumococcal bacteria, these B-cells recognize the bacteria because of the vaccine and produce a lot of that antibody to fight against the infection. However, some immunosuppressants can prevent these important reactions.

The medication rituximab (RTX, Rituxan) reduces B-cells and thus vaccine responses. We are seeing this especially with COVID-19 vaccines in RTX-treated patients. Many have little to no antibody response after the vaccines.

It is best to get vaccines at least four weeks before starting RTX. Once someone is on RTX, live vaccines should be avoided. Inactivated vaccines should be given two to five weeks before the person's next RTX dose to work best. This causes the most difficulties for patients receiving RTX in late summer or early fall, just before flu shot season. If the next RTX treatment is in February, the optimal time for the flu shot is January, when the flu season is already in full force. If you are scheduled for RTX in summer or early fall, discuss options with your doctor. If you are at low risk for lupus flares, delaying RTX treatment so that a flu shot can be given at a time it could work better could be a good idea.

If possible, all vaccines should be given before starting immunosuppressants. However if an immunosuppressant is needed for SLE, it is often not realistic to wait two to four weeks before starting immunosuppression.

If you are interested in learning in-depth about any vaccine, look into the Immunization Action Coalition at www.immunize.org/askexperts. They answer many interesting and not-so-common vaccine questions.

LUPUS IN FOCUS

Timing immunosuppressants for COVID-19 and other vaccines

A 2017 study showed that when rheumatoid arthritis (RA) patients whose disease was under excellent control skipped methotrexate (MTX) for two weeks after their flu shots, the vaccine worked better and without significant RA flares. It did not matter when the last MTX dose was given before the shot. For example, getting the flu shot two days after the previous MTX dose, then skipping two weeks' of MTX worked as well as when the last dose was a week before the shot. Based on this study, I recommend that SLE patients on MTX and in remission skip their next one to two weeks of MTX after all vaccines.

Table 22.6 provides information about timing drugs for COVID-19 vaccines. Some rheumatologists also adopt these recommendations for other vaccines.

Table 22.6 Timing Drugs for COVID-19 Vaccines

Stop for 1–2 weeks after vaccination, if not at risk of lupus flares:

    abatacept SQ (Orencia SQ)

    azathioprine (Imuran)

    belimumab (Benlysta)

    cyclophosphamide pills

    cyclosporine

    JAK inhibitors (Xeljanz, Olumiant, Rinvoq)

    leflunomide (Arava)

    methotrexate (Otrexup, Rasuvo)

    mycophenolate (CellCept, Myfortic)

    tacrolimus

    voclosporin (Lupkynis)

Ask your doctor about:

    anakinra (Kineret)

    sulfasalazine

    TNF inhibitors (adalimumab, etanercept, infliximab, golimumab, certolizumab)

    tocilizumab (Actemra)

Do not stop:

    chloroquine

    hydroxychloroquine (Plaquenil)

    IVIG

Follow special instructions for

    Abatacept IV (Orencia)

        Give vaccine 4 weeks after Orencia IV (i.e., the entire dosing interval), and postpone subsequent IV Orencia by 1 week (i.e., a 5-week gap in total)

    Acetaminophen, paracetamol (Tylenol)

        Don't take 24 hours before; OK to take afterward.

    Cyclophosphamide (CYC) IV

        Time CYC approximately 1 week after vaccine dose, when feasible.

    Nonsteroidal anti-inflammatory drugs (NSAIDs)

        Don't take 24 hours before; OK to take afterward.

    Prednisone

        Do not stop. Work with your doctor to be on the lowest dose possible.

    Belimumab, IV

        No formal recommendation (as of April 2023); previously recommended to be given midway between infusions.

    Rituximab (RTX, Rituxan)

        Schedule vaccine approximately 4 weeks before the next RTX. If in low disease activity or remission, try to delay RTX as long as possible (for example, if you get it every 4 months, try to wait 5–6 months).

Source: Modified from the American College of Rheumatology "COVID-19 Vaccine Clinical Guidance Summary for Patients with Rheumatic and Musculoskeletal Diseases," rheumatology .org/Portals/0/Files/COVID-19-Vaccine-Clinical-Guidance-Rheumatic-Diseases-Summary.pdf (August 2022 revision).

Additional Prevention Strategies

Physical (social) distancing is the practice of staying far enough away from others to decrease contact with infected respiratory droplets. The greater the distance, the lower the chances of spreading infections such as COVID-19, colds, and influenza. The Centers for Disease Control recommends at least six feet of separation.

You should wash your hands frequently (for at least 20 seconds) after touching public surfaces where infected persons may have been. Use a sanitizer with at least 60% alcohol. Soap and water are also effective. Wear gloves in public areas or where there may be infected surfaces. When removing gloves, don't touch their outer surfaces. Having short, clean fingernails and avoiding artificial nails also help.

If you cough or sneeze, cover your mouth or nose. Because viruses such as COVID-19, influenza (the flu), and the common cold enter the body through the moist skin (mucosa) of the eyes, nose, and mouth, it is essential not to touch these areas. The American Academy of Ophthalmology even advised against contact lenses during COVID-19 to decrease how often people touch their eyes. It is also important to regularly disinfect and clean surfaces that infected people may touch.

Many experts recommended universal mask-wearing in public during the COVID-19 pandemic. This helps protect the mask wearer as well as those around them. People can potentially infect others even if they feel well (asymptomatic infection) and do not know they are infected. Since so many SLE patients are immunosuppressed, they are at increased risk of infection and severe complications and so masks are strongly recommended.

Preventing Specific Infections

Prevention of a few possible infections deserve special mention. This includes endocarditis (heart valve infection), prosthetic joint infections (after total joint replacements), and urinary tract infections.

Preventing Heart Valve Infections

Subacute bacterial endocarditis (SBE) is an infection of the heart valves. It can cause severe heart valve damage, leading to congestive heart failure and death. High-risk patients should receive antibiotics during dental procedures, such as teeth cleaning, when bacteria can enter the blood and infect particular kinds of heart valves. Rheumatologists used to recommend that most SLE patients take antibiotics during dental procedures to prevent SBE. However, the American Heart Association has relaxed these recommendations because most patients are at low risk for SBE but at high risk of antibiotic side effects. They now recommend antibiotics only for people who have had congenital heart surgery, SBE, a heart valve replacement, or for those with the most severe heart valve damage.

Preventing Joint Replacement Infections

Some SLE patients end up with joint replacement surgery due to SLE complications. For example, avascular necrosis (chapter 25) and osteoporotic fractures (chapter 24) can sometimes require joint replacement. As lupus care improves and most of our patients live to be over 60 years old, many patients will get joint replacement surgery for osteoarthritis, also called degenerative joint disease (due to the aging process).

The joint replacement hardware is always at increased risk of infection. Infected joint replacement hardware is complicated to treat, often requiring removal and more surgeries. It is essential to take measures to prevent this from happening. Any manipulation of the gums can cause bacteria to enter the bloodstream and potentially go to a joint replacement and infect it. This is primarily a concern in people with poor oral hygiene, where bacteria are more abundant in the gums and tissues surrounding the teeth. It is recommended to be diligent about good dental hygiene and ensure that mouth infections are treated immediately. The American Academy of Orthopedic Surgeons no longer recommends antibiotics during dental procedures in joint replacement patients.

Preventing Urinary Tract Infections (UTIs)

Urinary tract infections (UTIs) are common in women. Their urethra (the tube through which urine passes to exit the body) is much shorter than in men, allowing easier access for bacteria to enter the urinary bladder from the vaginal area. Having bacteria in their urine (called bacteriuria) is common for women. Most of the time, this is not an infection, especially if there are no symptoms, such as pain on urination, frequent or urgent urination, lower abdominal pain, flank pain, or fever. This is called asymptomatic bacteriuria.

Since we obtain a urine sample at almost every lupus clinic visit, and since bacteriuria is so common, we follow up with phone calls asking patients if they have UTI symptoms. If not, we ask them to drink plenty of fluids, consider drinking sugar-free cranberry juice, take a cranberry supplement, or take a D-mannose supplement (used for UTI prevention) to decrease the risk of the asymptomatic bacteriuria turning into a UTI. Studies suggest that cranberry and D-mannose may help prevent bacteria from adhering to the bladder and urethra walls.

It is essential that asymptomatic bacteriuria not be treated with antibiotics. Antibiotic overuse increases the problem of antibiotic-resistant bacteria. In addition, women with asymptomatic bacteriuria are more likely to get antibiotic side effects than to reap any potential benefits.

Contamination with bacteria from the rectal area and infection related to sexual intercourse are two of the most common ways women develop UTIs. Methods to prevent

LUPUS IN FOCUS

Bacteriuria, lupus inflammation, and lupus flares

A 2020 research study suggests that bacteriuria may worsen SLE. One-third of the SLE women in the study had bacteriuria, as well as more lupus inflammation, more flares, and higher anti-dsDNA antibodies and lower C3 and C4 complement levels (disease activity measures) than the SLE women without bacteriuria. They also had elevated antibodies against a bacterial protein (amyloid Curli) bound to a type of bacterial DNA (bacterial extracellular DNA). The researchers proposed that this bacteria DNA could mimic human DNA, triggering the lupus immune system to be active.

Women with SLE should take steps to prevent bacteriuria, such as taking cranberry and D-mannose supplements, urinating immediately after intercourse, and wiping front to back after a bowel movement. Could these measures reduce lupus disease activity? We do not know for sure; additional research is needed.

these include wiping from front to back after bowel movements and urinating right after sexual intercourse to flush out bacteria. Spermicidal gels and intrauterine devices (chapter 41) may increase the risk of UTIs.

Specific Infections and Immunosuppressants

Some infections can be particularly severe in someone on immunosuppressants. This section covers some of the most important ones.

Tuberculosis (TB)

Tuberculosis (TB) is a potentially deadly bacteria that tends to attack the lungs. Like CO-VID-19, it is most commonly spread by respiratory droplets from the infected person.

Although some people infected with TB do not get very sick, the TB bacteria can live in their bodies for the rest of their lives. If they start taking immunosuppressants (especially TNF inhibitors, high-dose steroids, or leflunomide), the TB bacteria can reproduce, causing a severe and sometimes deadly infection. Therefore, those treated with these medicines should get a TB test before starting the medication. As of 2020, it has been recommended that anyone who starts a biologic (except for anifrolumab, belimumab, rituximab, and anakinra) or leflunomide should have a TB test before beginning the drug.

Both skin tests and blood tests can diagnose TB infections. The skin test is performed by injecting a small amount of PPD (purified protein derivative), a liquid that contains inactive components of TB, underneath the skin of the forearm. Then two to five days later, the amount of swelling under the skin (called induration) is measured by a medical professional. If this measurement is 5 mm or more in immunosuppressed patients, it is considered positive, meaning that they were probably exposed to TB in the past.

Blood tests for TB are known as interferon-gamma release assays. One is called the QuantiFERON-TB Gold In-Tube (QFT-G); the other is the T-SPOT.TB.

Some countries give BCG vaccines (Bacille Calmette-Guérin) to lower TB risk. Because BCG can cause a positive skin TB test (PPD) result, the blood tests (T-SPOT.TB or QFT-G) should be done in BCG-vaccinated patients.

If any of the skin or blood tests is positive, the next step is to ensure no active TB infection by taking a chest x-ray (CXR). If the CXR does not show active TB, the person is considered to have latent TB, meaning that that they have probably been exposed to TB in the past and could have TB still living in their bodies. Recommended treatment is a TB antibiotic, such as isoniazid, rifapentine, or rifampin, for three to nine months (depending upon the chosen antibiotic). During this period, they can receive the immunosuppressant as well. Some experts recommend waiting to start the immunosuppressant one to two weeks after the antibiotic.

Once on the immunosuppressant, most people who initially tested negative for TB do not need to be tested again. However, people at increased risk of infection should be tested regularly. People in this category include those who live in or visit areas with high TB rates, such as India, Cambodia, Indonesia, Nigeria, Sub-Saharan Africa, the Philippines, Pakistan, Bangladesh, South Africa, Vietnam, China, Haiti, the Dominican Republic, and Mexico.

If someone needs active TB treatment, then biologics (especially TNF inhibitors) should be avoided until the infection is treated and resolved. Steroid treatment increases the risk of doing poorly from TB. It should be avoided or used in the lowest doses possible. Antimalarial medications are safe. The safety of other immunosuppressants is not well known.

Hepatitis B

Hepatitis B can live silently in someone's body for years, then become active when they take certain immunosuppressants. Hepatitis B can cause jaundice (yellow eyes and skin), cirrhosis (liver scarring and liver failure), and liver cancer. If not treated, it is a potentially deadly infection in immunosuppressed patients.

Hepatitis B blood testing (with blood tests HBsAg, anti-HBc, and HBsAb) should be done in all patients before starting TNF inhibitors, rituximab, and abatacept. As of 2023, belimumab (Benlysta), tocilizumab (Actemra), and anifrolumab (Saphnelo) did not have this recommendation. Some people are at higher risk for hepatitis B; they include men who have sex with men, IV drug users, and health care workers exposed to blood products and needle sticks. They should also be tested before starting methotrexate, leflunomide (Arava), and high-dose steroids.

HBsAg-positive people should receive anti-hepatitis B medication before starting immunosuppressants. Anti-hepatitis B antiviral therapies are usually very effective at keeping the virus under control. However, they do not completely eliminate hepatitis B virus from most patients (in stark contrast to hepatitis C treatments, mentioned below, which cure almost all patients). Therefore, antiviral therapy is needed throughout immunosuppressant therapy.

Hepatitis C

Hepatitis C is a virus that primarily infects liver cells. The hepatitis C virus is usually transmitted through exposure to infected blood, IV drug use, blood transfusions, and needle sticks. However, sexual contact, mother to fetus transmission, tattooing, and body piercing can also result in infections. The CDC recommends that all adults be tested for hepatitis C. Regular testing should be done in those with increased risk for infection (such as IV drug users).

Hepatitis C infection can cause the immune system to become overactive. Just like an HIV infection, it can look exactly like SLE and can produce many of the same antibodies seen in SLE and in problems such as arthritis and other organ involvement. This is why rheumatologists usually test everyone with possible SLE for hepatitis C. Treating and curing hepatitis C results in the lupus-like disease disappearing.

SLE patients have a higher chance of being infected with hepatitis C than the general population. This is probably due to their immune system not protecting them properly. Since hepatitis C causes the immune system to become more active, SLE may worsen if infected.

Hepatitis C infection does not appear to worsen on immunosuppressants. Like hepatitis B, untreated hepatitis C infection can cause jaundice, cirrhosis, and liver cancer. However, the antiviral drugs cure over 95% of hepatitis C patients.

Progressive Multifocal Leukoencephalopathy (PML)

Although PML is a very rare infection complication, we discuss it since it is specifically mentioned as a potential side effect for some lupus drugs. These include rituximab and belimumab (Benlysta). PML is due to the JC virus (named after John Cunningham, the first person in whom the virus was isolated). JC is a common infection, which occurs in 85% of all adults. In people with abnormal immune systems, this virus can attack the brain and is potentially deadly.

Brain infection from JC virus is exceedingly rare in people with normal immune systems. PML can occur in SLE patients who do not take immunosuppressants as well as in those who do, but that is very rare in SLE. One large study found PML in 1 SLE patient out of every 20,000 per year.

Testing for JC virus in patients is not recommended since most adults are positive for JC virus, but it is exceedingly rare to get PML from it. Common symptoms of PML include difficulty thinking, paralysis, difficulty walking, and double vision. However, many other problems can also occur. Although it can cause similar issues as in CNS lupus (chapter 13), brain MRI and a spinal tap (chapter 13) can tell the difference. There are no known, effective treatments. It is essential to stop, or at least lower, any immunosuppressant amounts, especially steroids.

Pneumocystis Pneumonia (PCP)

PCP is a potentially deadly pneumonia due to *Pneumocystis jirovecii* (formerly *P. carinii*) bacteria. It occurs primarily in severely immunosuppressed people. Prophylactic antibiotics (antibiotics that help prevent infection) should be taken to prevent PCP under certain circumstances. The most common is when high-dose steroids (20 mg a day of prednisone or higher) are used with another immunosuppressants (especially cyclophosphamide or mycophenolate) for more than a month. Another reason for prophylactic antibiotics is if there is severe lymphocytopenia (low lymphocyte count), especially if the lymphocyte count is less than 200–350 cells/microL.

One of the most commonly used drugs for PCP prophylaxis is trimethoprim-sulfamethoxazole (TMP-SMX, Bactrim). However, this can cause a high risk of dangerous side effects and lupus flares in SLE patients. Therefore, we do not recommend it (see end of this chapter). Instead, we recommend dapsone or atovaquone. Dapsone may be a good choice for patients with significant cutaneous lupus (especially bullous-forms, chapter 8). If someone is intolerant of dapsone and atovaquone, TMP-SMX could be used as long as the patient makes sure to contact their doctor immediately if any lupus flare symptoms or side effects occur.

Measles

Measles deserves special attention since the number of infections in the United States has increased since 2008. There was an especially severe outbreak in 2019. A decrease in vaccination rates is to be blamed. There were few infections during 2020 and 2021 due to physical isolation during the COVID-19 pandemic.

To put into perspective how bad measles is, before vaccines (1963), measles killed over 2 million people worldwide. Most were small children. It is so infectious that if someone with measles is in a room and leaves, the virus can remain in the air for two hours. If 100 unvaccinated people entered the room, 90 would get infected.

Measles infected almost everyone before measles vaccines (MMR) were available. People born before 1957 are considered to have natural immunity. Everyone should have two MMR vaccines in their lifetime. If someone cannot locate a vaccine record, they have two options. The first is to get a blood test for measles. If the IgG result is low, they should get vaccinated. The second is to go ahead and get the vaccine without checking labs. People at highest risk for infection (health care workers, college students, and foreign travelers) should especially consider vaccination as adults.

Postexposure Prophylaxis

Postexposure prophylaxis (infection prevention) refers to treating someone at high risk for a bad outcome after infection exposure. We will list some important ones by infection type.

Influenza Exposure

SLE patients at high risk for flu complications include those who take immunosuppressants, those 65 years old and older, those with a body mass index (BMI) of 40 and greater, pregnant women up to two weeks after delivery, Native Indians, Alaska Natives, and those with chronic lung, heart, kidney, or liver disease. If someone in one of these categories is exposed to influenza and has not been vaccinated, an antiviral medication (such as oseltamivir and zanamivir) can be helpful if taken within 48 hours of contact. Contact your doctor immediately if this situation applies to you. Also, if you are in one of these categories, and if an unvaccinated close contact is exposed to someone infected with influenza, they should be treated within 48 hours to lower the chances of infecting you. Even taking one of these antiviral medications before known exposure (such as during a community influenza outbreak or in a long-term care facility with an outbreak) can help.

An alternative, which is especially good for people allergic to flu vaccines, is to immediately take an antiviral medication during any episode of fever or respiratory symptoms during flu season.

Chickenpox and Shingles Exposure

Varicella is the virus that causes chickenpox and shingles. People who have not had chickenpox or have not been vaccinated are at high risk of infection if exposed to chickenpox or shingles. Someone with shingles in multiple skin areas (disseminated zoster) or with chickenpox can infect others through respiratory droplets (similar to colds, the flu, and COVID-19). Face-to-face contact increases infection risk.

Typical shingles, which affects just one skin area (called a dermatome), does not spread through respiratory droplets. The affected area must be touched to spread infection (such as through hugging). Infection risk occurs up to two days before shingles are visible on the skin and continues until all open sores have crusted over. If an exposed person has not had chickenpox, shingles, or one of the shingles or varicella vaccines, they should contact a health care provider for postexposure prophylaxis. This treatment is complicated, depending upon immunosuppression, pregnancy status, and time since exposure. Vaccines, antiviral medications, or intravenous immunoglobulin (IVIG) can be used. The specifics are beyond the scope of this book.

Measles Exposure

People born after 1956 who do not have a history of measles infection or vaccination should immediately contact their physician for treatment if exposed to measles, especially if they are on an immunosuppressant or are pregnant. A measles vaccine within 72 hours of exposure or intravenous immunoglobulin (IVIG) within 6 days is usually given.

Consider daily yogurt during and after antibiotics

Antibiotics kill invading organisms but kill good bacteria as well. This could negatively impact our microbiome (chapter 3). The microbiome is composed of the organisms that naturally live in (and on) us. They interact with the immune system and may be instrumental in it working correctly. Some experts recommend eating yogurt with "active and live cultures" daily while on antibiotics (and continuing afterward). This may help replenish healthy bacteria in the gut microbiome. Probiotics (products containing healthy bacteria) may decrease diarrhea from antibiotics, and yogurt is a natural probiotic source. We do not recommend taking probiotic supplements (such as in capsules) because some could potentially worsen lupus disease activity. However, probiotic-rich foods such as yogurt do not cause lupus flares.

Other Infection Exposures

Other infection exposures that may need postexposure prophylaxis include exposures to blood (such as needle sticks from another person), hepatitis B, HIV, meningococcus (meningitis), animal and human bites, deer tick bites (Lyme), and puncture wounds (tetanus prevention). Management of these infection exposures in SLE patients is similar to that of the general public and is beyond the scope of this book. A prompt physician assessment is recommended for these situations.

Sulfa (Sulfonamide) Intolerance

On a final note, it is important to mention antibiotics that SLE patients should avoid—namely, sulfonamide ("sulfa") antibiotics. They should be included as a drug intolerance on an allergy list that they always carry with them (along with an up-to-date medication list, chapters 5 and 44), even if they have never taken them before. Sulfonamide antibiotics—such as Septra, Bactrim, trimethoprim-sulfamethoxazole, Gantrisin, and sulfadiazine—can cause lupus to flare, and people with lupus have a high chance of being allergic to them as well.

KEY POINTS TO REMEMBER

1. Infections are among the top three causes of death in SLE.

2. SLE patients are prone to infections due to their altered immune systems and immunosuppressants.

3. You can improve your chances of not needing stronger immunosuppressants by taking hydroxychloroquine, not smoking, taking vitamin D (if deficient), and avoiding UV light (table 22.4).

4. Everyone should get a flu shot every fall.

5. All SLE patients should get pneumococcal pneumonia vaccines.

6. If someone accidentally receives Pneumovax first, it should be followed by either Prevnar 20 or Vaxneuvance one year later.

7. Taking an antimalarial (Plaquenil or chloroquine) lowers infections; taking steroids increases infections.

8. Always list sulfa antibiotics (such as Bactrim and Septra) as a drug intolerance; they can cause lupus flares.

9. Shingrix is 95% effective against shingles and is FDA-approved for people 50 years old and older as well as immunosuppressed patients 18 and older.

10. Get the tetanus-diphtheria vaccine every 10 years.

11. Avoid live vaccines (table 22.5) if taking immunosuppressants, although it is OK to get the Zostavax and MMR if on a weak immunosuppressant (table 22.1).

12. Do not get vaccinated if your SLE is very active or on 20 mg or more of prednisone a day.

13. Get all vaccines at least four weeks before starting immunosuppressants, if possible.

14. If you develop a fever or any symptoms of an infection, call your primary care physician or go to an emergency room or urgent care center for assessment and treatment as soon as possible.

Cancer

Sasha Bernatsky, MD, PhD, *Contributing Editor*

Cancer is the fourth most common cause of death (after lupus, cardiovascular events, and infections) in SLE according to many studies from developed countries, including the United States. Many cancers are potentially preventable, and many can be detected at early, curable stages.

SLE patients tend to get diagnosed with cancer at a younger age than their peers. This may be because they see doctors and get blood and urine tests frequently.

They have a higher risk of some cancers than others, partly due to their abnormal immune system. A healthy immune system protects the body not only from infections but also from potentially cancerous cells that our bodies regularly produce. A normal immune system recognizes and removes these abnormal cells. In SLE, however, the immune system is not as effective at policing the body and removing cancerous or precancerous cells. This results in increased cancer risk.

A weak immune system is also less effective at fighting against some cancer-causing viruses. For example, human papillomavirus (HPV) causes several types of cancer, and these occur more often in SLE.

This chapter discusses the links between cancer, lupus, the drugs used to treat lupus, and how cancer treatments may affect lupus.

Specific Cancers and SLE

Lymphoma

Lymphoma is a group of cancers affecting lymphocytes (a type of white blood cell, chapter 9). Even though rare, people with systemic autoimmune diseases have an increased chance of developing lymphoma, especially non-Hodgkin's lymphoma (NHL). The risk for NHL is highest for Sjögren's disease (chapter 14). Overall, around 5% of Sjögren's patients have lymphoma, but the percentage increases over time. After 20 years of illness, close to 20% of Sjögren's patients develop lymphoma.

The risk is much less in SLE than in Sjögren's. However, SLE patients are still five times more likely to get lymphoma than the general population. This increased risk is probably due to B-cells (also called B-lymphocytes) being overactive in SLE. Consequently, they not only produce lupus autoantibodies, such as antinuclear antibodies, but can also become cancerous. In combination with an abnormal immune system that is less efficient at removing them, there is a higher risk of some evolving into lymphoma.

SLE patients with Sjögren's overlap are at particularly higher risk of lymphoma. One study suggested that SLE patients with low blood counts or lupus lung disease may be at increased risk as well.

Lymphoma may cause lymph gland enlargement. Typically, a person with lymphoma has swelling in areas with many lymph nodes. These include the armpits, anywhere in the neck, just above the elbow (epitrochlear lymph nodes), and the groin. Other lymphoma symptoms include weight loss, fever, and night sweats.

However, the most common cause of swollen lymph nodes in people with SLE is lupus inflammation (lymphangitis), not lymphoma. Infection is also a common cause of lymph node swelling.

A biopsy may be needed to discriminate between lupus, lymphoma, or something else. A surgeon uses local anesthesia to numb the area around a lymph node and removes it for examination under a microscope. Most biopsy results show benign (noncancerous) lupus lymphangitis. Hydroxychloroquine and immunosuppressants (table 22.1) can help lupus lymphangitis.

Lymphoma is considered a type of blood cancer. Other blood cell cancers include leukemia (white blood cell cancer) and multiple myeloma (see chapter 9). Although both occur more often in SLE, they are rare. Blood cancers (lymphoma, leukemia, or multiple myeloma) tend to be less severe (overall) in SLE patients than most cancer patients, and they have a higher chance of going into remission. Frequent blood work and physical exams on SLE patients may identify blood cancers at earlier stages than usual.

Cyclophosphamide, used to treat severe SLE, increases the risk for lymphoma and other blood cell cancers.

Lung Cancer

Lung cancer is the number one cause of cancer deaths in the United States. Lung cancer occurs around 1.4 times more often in SLE patients than in the general population. Between 70% and 85% of these lung cancers develop in smokers. SLE patients who smoke are six times more likely to get lung cancer than nonsmokers. This is another crucial reason why people with lupus should not smoke. Some rare lung cancers occur more commonly among people with lupus for unknown reasons.

If you have a 20-pack-year history of smoking or more—meaning that you smoked a pack a day for 20 years or 2 packs a day for 10 years—consider a yearly low-dose chest CT scan starting at age 50. This can help catch early, curable stages of cancer.

Cervical, Vaginal, and Vulvar Cancer

Human papillomavirus (HPV) is transmitted sexually and can live inside us our entire lives. Over time, HPV virus can turn infected cells into cancer, such as cervical cancer, anal cancer, throat cancer, and some skin cancers.

SLE women have higher rates of HPV infections. For example, a 2007 United Kingdom study showed that SLE women were five times more likely to be infected with the cancer-causing strain called HPV-16 than the general population.

A Danish study that followed 576 SLE patients over 38 years found that they were 27 times more likely than non-SLE patients to develop HPV-associated cancer of the anus, 9 times more likely to develop vulvovaginal cancer, and twice as likely to develop mouth cancer and non-melanoma skin cancers (squamous cell and basal cell).

There are several reasons why SLE patients get HPV-associated cancer more often. Higher rates of HPV infection play a crucial role. The abnormal lupus immune system may not be very good at fighting HPV, and it may have a more challenging time getting rid of cancerous cells as they form.

Some vaccines reduce HPV infections. The HPV quadrivalent (*quadri-* means four) vaccine (called Gardasil) protects against four strains (types) of HPV—strains 16 and 18, which cause 70% of cervical cancers, 90% of anal cancers, and a high number of vaginal, vulvar, and throat cancers; and strains 6 and 11, which cause 90% of genital warts. Gardasil reduces genital warts and cervical, anal, vulvar, and vaginal cancers, which occur more often in SLE.

It is most useful to get Gardasil before sexual activity. In women who have never been infected by HPV, Gardasil lowers the chances of cervical cancer by close to 100%. In a large population with many HPV-infected individuals, it reduced the risk by around half.

The American Cancer Society recommends Gardasil at 9 years of age or soon after that up to age 26. The Centers for Disease Control (CDC) recommends Gardasil for people aged 27 to 45 if they are at risk of infection. An example would be a 40-year-old who divorces after being married for many years and then starts dating and having sexual relations again. Some even recommend it for high-risk patients older than 45.

The cervix is in the back of the vagina at the uterus (or womb) entrance. It is through the cervix that sperm travels to fertilize an egg. Cancer of the cervix is almost always due to HPV. The Pap smear (short for Papanicolaou, the last name of the doctor who developed it) and testing for HPV can find early cervical cancer. Pap smear and HPV testing are performed during a pelvic exam by taking a specimen of cells and fluid from the cervix for evaluation in the laboratory. Since the Pap smear was introduced in 1941, deaths from cervical cancer have decreased a lot because cervical cancer is curable at early stages.

In the United States, it is common for women to begin having Pap smears and HPV tests 3 years after starting sexual activity or at 21, whichever comes first. Most women should have these tests every 3 years until they are 30, then every 2 years. However, women at increased risk (such as those on immunosuppressants and those infected with HPV) should be screened yearly.

While cyclophosphamide (CYC) increases the risk of cervical cancer, hydroxychloroquine (HCQ, Plaquenil) lowers the risk by about half. SLE patients taking HCQ also tend to have less severe forms of cervical cancer when it does occur.

Cancers of the vagina and vulva (the skin flaps surrounding the vagina) appear to occur more frequently in SLE, but they are rare. Regular visits to your gynecologist and an annual pelvic exam will help catch these at an early stage.

LUPUS IN FOCUS

Alcohol and breast cancer

Drinking as little as three servings of alcohol a week increases the risk for breast cancer, especially in those with a sister who had breast cancer and those who carry the breast gene called BRCA2. Taking folic acid daily may lower this risk.

Breast, Ovarian, and Uterine Cancer

Cancers sensitive to estrogen (a female hormone), including breast, uterine (endometrial), and ovarian cancers, may occur less often in SLE than in the general population for several reasons. They may take estrogen hormones (which increase the risk) less often due to doctors not prescribing estrogen as often for birth control and menopausal symptoms (such as hot flashes), fearing they may increase lupus activity. Estrogen decreases on its own when some SLE women stop producing eggs (stop ovulating) prematurely (chapter 18). Also, taking NSAIDs (such as ibuprofen and naproxen) for lupus-associated pains and hydroxychloroquine may reduce breast cancer risk.

Nonetheless, breast, ovarian, and uterine cancers occur in SLE women. They should undergo mammograms and pelvic exams regularly. When caught early, they are potentially curable.

Other Cancers

Liver cancer occurs more commonly in SLE than in the general population. It can cause pain in the right upper area of the abdomen just under the ribs, as well as jaundice (where the eyes and skin turn yellow). Usually, it is discovered by the doctor finding an elevation in liver function blood tests. This is usually followed by imaging studies such as an ultrasound or CT scan.

We do not know if lupus patients develop colon cancer more or less often than others.

A Californian study showed increased lymphoma and more kidney, thyroid, lung, and liver cancers in SLE patients. Kidney cancer can cause pain on the side of the lower chest, lower back, or upper abdominal area, as well as blood in the urine (hematuria, chapter 4). Thyroid cancer is usually discovered when the doctor feels a swollen area in the thyroid during examination. Someone may notice some difficulty swallowing or hoarseness from pushing on the esophagus (tube leading to the stomach) or the trachea (windpipe).

The Californian study also found fewer cases of prostate cancer, a male sex hormone–driven cancer, in SLE men. Men with SLE may have an imbalance of estrogen and testosterone (a male hormone). In addition, taking NSAIDs (chapter 7) for SLE pains may reduce prostate cancers.

There are several skin cancer types, and malignant melanoma is the most dangerous. It is unusual in SLE, although the drug abatacept (Orencia) may slightly increase the risk.

An Iceland study showed an increased occurrence of squamous cell carcinoma (a type of skin cancer) in SLE. The other two types of skin cancer (squamous cell carcinoma and basal cell carcinoma) are often lumped together as non-melanoma skin cancers.

Non-melanoma skin cancers may occur in people who take tumor necrosis factor inhibitors (TNFi, chapter 33). TNFi include drugs such as certolizumab (Cimzia), adalimumab (Humira), etanercept (Enbrel), and infliximab (Remicade). They are most often used for rheumatoid arthritis overlap with lupus (called rhupus). Other immunosuppressants that may increase the risk for these cancers include azathioprine, methotrexate, mycophenolate, cyclosporin, and tacrolimus. These risks are highest with ultraviolet light exposure. Hopefully, lupus patients lower their risk through diligent UV protection.

Discoid lupus erythematosus (DLE) patients have a small chance of their DLE turning into squamous cell carcinoma (3%). Avoiding ultraviolet light (chapter 38) and not smoking lowers this risk.

Lupus Drugs and Cancer

Cyclophosphamide (CYC) is the only immunosuppressant used in SLE that has significant evidence for increased cancer risks. CYC has been linked to lymphoma, blood cancers, some skin cancers, and cervical cancer. Doctors avoid CYC unless there are no other options—it can be life-saving for severe SLE.

On the other hand, some drugs used for lupus may lower some cancer risks. Hydroxychloroquine may lower the risk for cervical and breast cancer, while non-steroidal anti-inflammatory drugs (NSAIDs, such as ibuprofen and naproxen) may reduce colon, breast, and prostate cancers.

Cancer Screening and Prevention in SLE

Studies show that SLE patients are less likely to keep up with their cancer screenings, such as mammograms and PAP smears, than people without SLE. It is unknown why this would occur since people with SLE see doctors often. It may be that they avoid important health maintenance visits, such as cancer screenings, because they are tired of seeing doctors.

Since SLE patients are at higher risk of cancer, they should have regular cancer screenings. Many cancers are curable when caught early. Primary care providers and gynecologists regularly recommend mammograms, pelvic exams, PAP smears, and colonoscopies (looking for colon cancer).

For men, prostate cancer can be screened for by measuring prostate-specific antigen (PSA) levels. Although high PSA levels can lead to unnecessary invasive procedures and prostate cancer overtreatment, screening can lead to lower death rates in high-risk men. PSA screening typically begins around age 50 in men who want it.

Of course, cancer prevention also includes not smoking. Obesity is also a risk factor for many cancers, such as colon cancer, so maintaining normal body weight is essential. Diets rich in omega-3 fatty acids, fruits, vegetables, and fiber may decrease the risk of some cancers. We ask all lupus patients to use daily sunscreen. Regular sunscreen use reduces skin cancers, including deadly malignant melanoma.

Cancer Treatments in SLE Patients

If chemotherapy (drugs that directly kill cancers) is used, it may help that person's lupus since chemotherapy often suppresses the immune system. At the same time, however, most chemotherapy increases infections and lowers blood counts, similar to many lupus immunosuppressants. Therefore, SLE drugs may need to be stopped during chemotherapy. However, taking anti-malarial medications, such as hydroxychloroquine (Plaquenil), is vital while on chemotherapy.

Some chemotherapy drugs can cause or worsen subacute cutaneous lupus (chapter 8). Tamoxifen (used in breast cancer) has been reported to cause lupus malar (butterfly rash), but this is rare.

LUPUS IN FOCUS

If you take hydroxychloroquine and tamoxifen, be diligent about eye exams

When tamoxifen is taken with hydroxychloroquine (HCQ), it increases the chances for anti-malarial retinopathy (damage to the retina, the back of the eye). People on tamoxifen and HCQ should get yearly eye screening tests right after starting HCQ (chapter 30).

Immune checkpoint inhibitors (ICIs) are important cancer immunotherapy drugs that use the immune system to combat cancers. In contrast to most chemotherapies, which suppress the immune system and directly attack cancer cells, ICIs increase immune system activity and cause the immune system to attack the cancer cells.

Remember that autoimmune diseases are due to the immune system being overly active. Since ICIs activate the immune system, it makes sense that they can cause some autoimmune diseases, such as lupus, to occur in the cancer patient. These types of side effects are called "immune-related adverse events" (irAEs).

Inflammatory arthritis, myositis (muscle inflammation), and vasculitis (blood vessel inflammation) are examples of irAEs. When irAEs occur, the ICI is usually stopped or switched. Steroids, such as prednisone, are generally helpful. However, other immunosuppressants, such as methotrexate and biologics (chapter 33), are needed for around 25% of irAEs. ICIs can also cause dry eyes and dry mouth, mimicking Sjögren's overlap (chapter 14), as well as scleroderma overlap (chapter 2), though rarely.

New-onset lupus from ICIs is rare. Most reported cases have been of subacute cutaneous lupus (chapter 8) and a few cases of lupus nephritis (chapter 12).

We do not know how safe ICIs are for lupus patients. Lupus patients were not allowed into the clinical trials for ICIs. However, a 2019 French study evaluated ICIs in people with autoimmune diseases. Out of 121 autoimmune disease patients, 4 had SLE, and 3 had cutaneous lupus. Only one SLE patient (who also had Sjögren's overlap) flared. It was mild and did not require treatment. It also caused problems the patient had not had before (Raynaud's and a red rash on the hands), so it may have been an irAE unrelated to the patient's SLE. Two of the three patients with cutaneous lupus developed vitiligo (an autoimmune skin disease) but not worsening of their cutaneous lupus. This suggests that ICIs may be relatively safe for lupus patients.

Radiotherapy (radiation) can sometimes worsen lupus (systemic and cutaneous). Radiotherapy has even caused SLE and cutaneous lupus (chapter 8) in people who did not previously have it. As a result, only 1 out of 10 lupus patients receive radiotherapy, even though an extensive 2019 review of the medical literature showed that only 15% of lupus patients have moderate to severe toxicity to radiotherapy. Thus, if the cancer is expected to respond well to radiotherapy, it should be offered, while also ensuring that the patient understands that there is a small risk of causing a lupus flare.

1. SLE patients have a higher risk of some cancers and a lower risk for others.

2. SLE patients tend to get some cancers at a younger age and at earlier cancer stages that are easier to treat. This may be due to their being watched so closely by their doctors.

3. SLE patients are more likely to develop non-Hodgkin's lymphoma, though it is rare.

4. Do not smoke; it dramatically increases lung cancer.

5. Cervical cancer occurs more often in SLE women due to HPV, a sexually transmitted infection.

6. Vulvovaginal, liver, kidney, and thyroid cancer happen more often in SLE.

7. Get the Gardasil HPV vaccine series if you are not in a monogamous relationship and are sexually active and between 9 and 45-years-old. It works best when given before any sexual exposure.

8. SLE women should get a pelvic exam, Pap smear, and HPV testing yearly, beginning at 21 years old. These can detect curable stages of cancer.

9. Ask your doctor when to start mammograms (for breast cancer) and colonoscopies (for colon cancer).

10. Prostate cancer screening with a PSA blood test can be done in men who understand the potential benefits and risks of the test starting around 50 years old.

11. If you have a 20-pack-year smoking history or more, get a yearly low-dose chest CT scan starting at age 50.

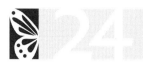

Osteoporosis

Yevgeniy Sheyn, MD, MPH, FACR, *Contributing Editor*

SLE patients are two to four times more likely (depending on the study) to get broken bones (fractures) from osteoporosis than people without SLE. These fractures reduce quality of life and shorten life span, but they are entirely preventable in most people.

Osteoporosis is a disease in which the bones become more fragile. *Osteo-* comes from the Greek word for "bone," and *-porosis* for "pore" or "passageway." Normal bones have just enough pores and passageways between the layers of hard minerals to allow blood to flow and provide nutrients and oxygen to cells that maintain the bones. Osteoporosis causes a decrease in hard bone and an overabundance of pores and passages (figure 24.1). This leads to brittle bones that are at increased risk of breaking.

The most common cause of osteoporosis is menopause, when the female hormones that are essential for keeping bones healthy decrease. Postmenopausal osteoporosis leads to broken bones, especially in the spine, hips, and wrist.

In people with osteoporosis, the spine begins to bend forward (figure 24.2) and can create a hump called kyphosis. This compresses the lungs, making it difficult to breathe. Women with multiple vertebral fractures are at increased risk of early death from lung infections due to difficulty taking full breaths. In addition, the lower rib cage is thrust down toward the pelvis, compressing the stomach and intestines, causing the abdomen to bulge. This leads to gastroesophageal reflux (heartburn), stomach upset, and constipation. People with a bent back from osteoporosis cannot stand up straight. This often causes the person to have low self-esteem.

Three years after a vertebral fracture, around half of the affected people are still alive. One year after a fracture of the pelvis, up to 25% die, and after a wrist fracture, up to 10% die.

Hip fractures also increase the risk of death. Someone with a hip fracture has about a 30% chance of dying within one year after the fracture. Around four years after a hip fracture, only one out of five survives. This is due to medical problems (such as pneumonia and blood clots) that develop from being less mobile. Hip fracture survivors have lifelong difficulties with walking and standing. Around half of survivors end up in nursing care centers due to their family's inability to care for them.

It is better to prevent these fractures in the first place by following the advice in tables 24.5 and 24.6 and by using appropriate medications.

Osteoporosis is a silent disease, meaning that the person doesn't notice it until broken bones occur. Before 1995, when the FDA approved the first effective osteoporosis

468

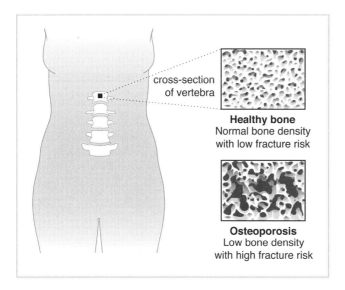

Figure 24.1 Normal bone compared to bone with osteoporosis

LUPUS IN FOCUS

Men with SLE and osteoporosis

Men with SLE are much more likely to develop broken bones from osteoporosis than men who do not have SLE. The International Society of Clinical Densitometry and the National Osteoporosis Foundation recommends that men with osteoporosis risk factors (such as SLE) begin having DXA scans at 50 years old.

---

drug (alendronate [Fosamax]), treatments were poor. Approximately half of women got hip fractures and curved spines from severe osteoporosis. It was considered a normal part of aging. Fortunately, that is not the case today.

Since medicines such as alendronate became available, we have seen a marked reduction in broken bones. We send much fewer patients to orthopedic surgeons for fracture surgeries, such as total hip replacements for hip fractures. Preventing osteoporotic fractures (broken bones due to osteoporosis) has improved the quality of life during aging.

How Osteoporosis Develops

Bones are constantly remodeled by bone cells. Some bone is removed while new bone is laid down. This can be compared to renovating a brick wall, in which some workers are removing parts of the aging and crumbling wall while others are putting in new, strong brick replacements.

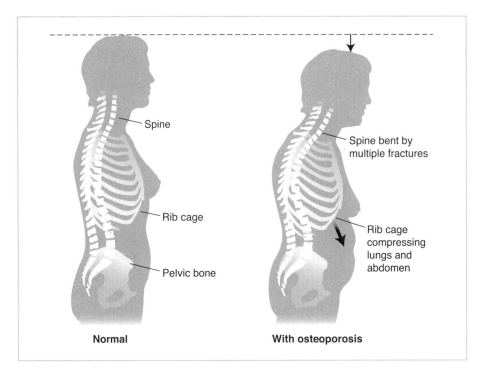

Figure 24.2 Effects of vertebral fractures from osteoporosis

The cells responsible for making new calcium-rich bone are called osteoblasts (*osteo-* is Greek for "bone," *-blast* for sprout or "germinate"). Cells that tear down old bone are called osteoclasts (*-clast* is Greek for "broken"). They continually try to improve bone architecture, ensuring that bones can support body weight and pressure during various activities.

In areas of more stress and weight, osteoblasts lay down extra mineral-enriched bony supports. This is how exercise helps strengthen bones. It is also why obese and muscular people have stronger bones than thin people and non-exercisers.

Anything that disrupts the orchestrated cycle of bone dissolving by the osteoclasts and bone-building by the osteoblasts ends up causing abnormal bone. When osteoclasts dissolve too much bone, or osteoblasts stop making more bone, there is less mineral-rich bone structure, and larger passageways and pores develop. The result is weak bones at high risk for breaking—or osteoporosis. As mentioned above, menopause, with its lack of estrogen, is the most common cause, but there are many others. Tables 24.1, 24.2, and 24.3 list osteoporosis risk factors. Go through them and mark the ones that apply to you. You have some control over some, such as drinking too much, smoking, and not exercising enough. The more risk factors people have, the more aggressively they should correct the reversible ones and use bone-strengthening drugs.

Table 24.1 Risk Factors for Osteoporosis

- **Weight ≤ 126 pounds**
- **Drinking more than 2 servings of alcohol a day (chapter 38)**
- **Vitamin D deficiency (chapters 35, 38)**
- **Lifelong low calcium intake (such as in lactose intolerance)**
- **Smoking (current and past)**
- **Taking drugs in table 24.2**
- **Balance problems, weakness, poor eyesight**, frailty, nerve or muscle problems, dementia, arthritis, dizziness: these increase risk of falling
- Menopause
- Osteoporosis in the family (especially a parent with a broken hip)
- Some diseases (table 24.3)
- History of broken bones as an adult
- Advanced age (the older you are, the higher the risk)

Note: **Bold** factors are under your control (modifiable/preventable; see also table 24.6).

How Osteoporosis Is Diagnosed

Bone biopsies are the most accurate way to diagnose osteoporosis. However, this is rarely done because it is invasive, and we have easier methods that approximate bone density well enough to be useful.

The most practical is an x-ray technique called dual-energy x-ray absorptiometry (DXA scan, for short). This type of x-ray is most often done by rheumatologists, endocrinologists, primary care doctors, gynecologists, and radiologists. The most accurate measurements are taken at the hip and spine, but the forearm is used if there is a reason that either the hip or spine measurements cannot be used. Note, though, that some diseases, such as hyperparathyroidism, affect the forearm, so in these cases, it is best to check the forearm.

DXA sends a small amount of radiation to the bone to measure its strength. Radiation exposure is minimal. A complete DXA scan uses approximately the same amount of radiation encountered while taking a round-trip flight from New York City to Los Angeles.

The DXA scan measures bone density in several different areas. It then compares it to the density expected of someone with the same height and weight at 30 years old (age of strongest bone density) and calculates the standard deviation (a statistical number). The result is reported as the T-score or the Z-score (table 24.4).

Because the DXA scan measures bone density, not bone type or bone quality, some results can be inaccurate. They can overestimate density if a person has additional bone formations, such as bone spurs from osteoarthritis (degenerative joint disease). Because of this, some people have osteoporosis and get broken bones (due to poor bone quality) even with normal DXA scans (due to bone spurs). One out of every three SLE women with osteoporotic vertebral fractures has normal DXA bone density.

Table 24.2 Drugs That Can Decrease Bone Strength

Drugs that cause bone loss (main categories followed by examples)

Steroids
- **prednisone, methylprednisolone (Medrol)**

Anti-seizure medicines (cause decreased vitamin D levels)
- **phenobarbital, phenytoin (Dilantin), carbamazepine (Tegretol)**

Blood thinners
  heparin, warfarin (Coumadin)

Thyroid hormone (when taken in excess)
  levothyroxine (Synthroid)

Hormones (non-estrogen)
  medroxyprogesterone (Depo-Provera)

Loop diuretics (fluid pills)
- furosemide (Lasix), bumetanide

Chemotherapy
- **cyclophosphamide (IV form)**, methotrexate (high doses for cancer; not the low doses used in lupus), ifosfamide (Ifex), imatinib (Gleevec)

Aromatase inhibitors (for breast cancer)
- anastrozole (Arimidex), letrozole (Femara), exemestane (Aromasin)

Thiazolidinediones (for diabetes)
- rosiglitazone (Avandia), pioglitazone (Actos)

HIV antiviral medications
  tenofovir (Viread)

Anti-androgen therapies (for prostate cancer)
- bicalutamide (Casodex), cyproterone

Drugs that may cause bone loss*

Proton pump inhibitors (decrease stomach acid)
- **esomeprazole (Nexium), lansoprazole (Prevacid), omeprazole (Prilosec), pantoprazole (Protonix), rabeprazole (AcipHex)**, and dexlansoprazole (Dexilant)

High-dose statins (cholesterol drugs)
- **> 40 mg simvastatin (Zocor)**
- **> 20 mg atorvastatin (Lipitor)**
- **> 20 mg rosuvastatin (Crestor)**

Cyclosporine (an immunosuppressant)

Antidepressants (dizziness increases risk for falling)

Vitamin A (high doses)

Note: Drugs in **bold** are commonly used in SLE. * Studies are conflicting.

Table 24.3 Disorders That Can Cause Osteoporosis

HIV

Rheumatoid arthritis

Systemic lupus erythematosus

Diabetes (type I and type II)

Hypercalciuria (high calcium leakage in the urine)

Cystic fibrosis

Hypogonadism

    Menopause in women (natural or surgical)

    Low testosterone in men (usually with testosterone levels ≤ 200 ng/dL)

Hyperthyroidism (overactive thyroid such as Graves' disease)

Kidney disease

Liver disease

Hyperparathyroidism

Malabsorption of nutrients

    Celiac disease (gluten hypersensitivity, non-tropical sprue)

    Inflammatory bowel disease (Crohn's disease and ulcerative colitis)

    Gastric bypass and similar surgeries

Table 24.4 Using DXA T-Scores and Z-Scores

T-Score	Diagnosis
–1.0 or more positive	Normal
–1.1 to –2.4	Osteopenia (also called low bone density)
–2.5 or more negative	Osteoporosis

Z-Score	Diagnosis
–2.0 or more positive	Normal
–2.1 or more negative	Low bone density for age

Another method for diagnosing osteoporosis and estimating fracture risk is the Fracture Risk Assessment Tool (FRAX). FRAX takes into account hip bone density (T-score on DXA) and other risk factors, such as smoking, excessive alcohol use, a family history of broken bones, rheumatoid arthritis, steroid use, and a personal history of broken bones. These factors are plugged them into a mathematical formula that calculates the 10-year risk for osteoporotic fractures. A person is at high risk for fractures (in other words, has osteoporosis) if the 10-year risk for a major fracture is 20% or higher or if the 10-year risk for a hip fracture is 3% or higher.

Using FRAX to estimate fracture risk in SLE

SLE patients have a higher chance for osteoporotic fractures than usual. This includes patients who have never taken steroids. Rheumatoid arthritis (RA), a systemic autoimmune disease closely related to SLE, also increases the chances of broken bones. If someone has RA, this is entered into the FRAX calculation. The FRAX score of an RA patient shows a higher risk of getting broken bones than the FRAX score of someone without RA (including SLE patients). FRAX scores for SLE patients significantly underestimate their fracture risks.

The FRAX formula is not foolproof. If someone has bone spurs around the hip joint due to osteoarthritis, the DXA can give a falsely high bone density. The FRAX calculation in this example would underestimate fracture risks. (FRAX uses the bone density of the hip but not of the spine in its measures.) Also, FRAX does not use all known risk factors for fractures.

Another way to diagnose osteoporosis is when someone has a fragility fracture, which occurs from minimal trauma that normally would not cause a broken bone. One example is when someone breaks a bone by falling from a standing height. Another would be when someone trips over their cat, sticks out their hand to catch their fall and breaks their wrist. Either would be enough evidence for osteoporosis, even with a normal DXA. If a person broke their wrist by falling down stairs, this would be considered a traumatic fracture and not an osteoporotic fragility fracture.

Another osteoporotic fragility fracture involves a vertebral fracture on x-ray not explained by previous trauma. Many vertebral fractures never cause noticeable pain and are picked up accidentally when x-rays are done for other reasons. Such a finding is enough to say the person has osteoporosis and should be treated.

Depending on the study, 15% to 50% of SLE patients have vertebral fractures, and most do not realize it. Also depending on the study, 29% to 40% of patients with vertebral fractures have normal DXA bone density. In other words, many SLE patients have osteoporotic vertebral fractures yet have no idea that they do. Once someone has a vertebral fracture, that person is at a high risk of more fractures.

Due to the high number of undiagnosed vertebral fractures, it is recommended that SLE patients who have had steroids have a vertebral fracture assessment. This is an x-ray of the entire spine by a DXA machine, which uses much less radiation than normal x-rays to find vertebral fractures.

SLE women are five times more likely to develop osteoporotic fractures than those who do not have SLE. SLE men are also at much higher risk than other men. There are multiple reasons for this. One is that the systemic inflammation from SLE decreases healthy bone production; another is that osteoporosis-causing drugs are commonly used in treating SLE (table 24.2). In addition, most SLE patients are deficient in vitamin D, which is essential for calcium absorption from the intestines and proper bone formation. Daily sunscreen use and avoiding the sun worsen vitamin D deficiency (ultraviolet light causes vitamin D production in the skin). Another reason for osteoporosis in SLE patients is inactivity. While exercise and activity are essential for the bones to stay strong and healthy, many SLE patients move around less and do not exercise much due to being ill.

Preventing Osteoporosis

Many osteoporotic risk factors can be addressed. Although you have no control over some, such as genetics and gender, you can control others (table 24.5). Below, we discuss certain preventative measures. Preventing falls is covered in table 24.6.

Get Adequate Calcium

The Food and Nutrition Board at the Institute of Medicine states that women aged 51 and older and men 71 and older should get 1,200 mg or more of calcium a day. Other adults should get 1,000 mg a day or more. Some calcium-rich foods are listed in table 24.7. If you cannot get enough calcium in your diet (such as by avoiding dairy products due to lactose intolerance), you can take calcium supplements.

Get Adequate Vitamin D

The Institute of Medicine recommends that women over 70 get 800 IU (International Units) a day or more of vitamin D; 600 IU a day or more is recommended for everyone

Table 24.5 Non-Drug Ways to Treat and Prevent Osteoporosis

- Do not smoke.
- Do not drink alcohol in excess (chapter 38).
- Exercise regularly to build strength and improve balance.
- Consume adequate calcium and vitamin D (tables 24.7 and 24.8).
- Maintain healthy body weight.
- Prevent falls (table 24.6).

LUPUS IN FOCUS

"It's impossible to get my vitamin D level normal."

It's easy to get everyone's vitamin D level to the target of around 40 ng/mL. Everyone's body absorbs and handles vitamin D differently. The optimal dose varies a lot from person to person. The way to get around this is to ask your doctor to check your level every three months. If your level is less than 40 ng/mL, simply ask your doctor to increase your dose of vitamin D. Do this every three months until your level is at this target. Some people can get away with just 400 IU a day of vitamin D3, while others may need 10,000 IU daily. Some may do well with 50,000 IU (1.25 mg) of ergocalciferol (vitamin D2) per month. Others may need it two to three times a week. Proper dosing varies between individuals.

Table 24.6 Preventing Falls

- Always use a cane or walker when walking.
- Remove throw rugs and any loose or frayed rugs.
- Remove electrical cords from areas where you walk.
- Remove all items from floors that could cause tripping.
- Have adequate lighting throughout the house, all entranceways, all outside pathways.
- Avoid wet or polished floors, and icy or slippery surfaces. Ask for help if you must walk on them.
- Avoid walking in unfamiliar places.

Table 24.7 Calcium-Rich Foods

Food Item	Serving Size	Estimated Calcium Content (in mg)
American cheese	1 ounce	175
Broccoli, cooked and drained	8 ounces (1 cup)	60
Cheddar cheese, shredded	1 ounce	205
Cottage cheese, 1% milkfat	1 cup	140
Dried figs	2 figs	55
Frozen yogurt, vanilla (soft serve)	1 cup (8 ounces)	210
Fruit juice with added calcium	6 ounces	200–345
Ice-cream, low-fat or high-fat	1 cup (8 ounces)	140–210
Kale, cooked	8 ounces (1 cup)	95
Milk, low-fat or fat-free	1 cup (8 ounces)	300
Mozzarella cheese, part-skim	1 ounce	205
Oranges	1 whole	50
Parmesan cheese, grated	1 tablespoon	70
Ricotta cheese, part-skim	4 ounces (½ cup)	335
Salmon, pink, canned with bones	3 ounces	180
Sardines, canned in oil with bones	3 ounces	325
Shrimp, canned	3 ounces	125
Soy milk with added calcium	8 ounces (1 cup)	300
Soybeans, mature, cooked, and drained	8 ounces (1 cup)	175
Swiss cheese	1 ounce	220–270
Tofu prepared with calcium	4 ounces (½ cup)	200–400
Yogurt, low-fat or fat-free (plain)	6 ounces	300

Source: National Osteoporosis Foundation and Bloomingdale Aging in Place at bloominplace.org /uploads/5/1/7/9/51791691/calcium_rich_foods.pdf

Table 24.8 Vitamin D Content of Food

Food	IUs per Serving
Cod liver oil, 1 tablespoon	1,360
Salmon (sockeye), cooked, 3 ounces	447
Mackerel, cooked, 3 ounces	388
Tuna fish, canned in water, drained, 3 ounces	154
Milk, vitamin D–fortified: nonfat, reduced fat, whole: 1 cup	115–124
Sardines (Atlantic), canned in oil, drained, 2 sardines	46
Egg, 1 large, scrambled	44

Source: National Institutes of Health at ods.od.nih.gov/factsheets/vitamind-HealthProfessional/#h3

else over 1 year of age. It is challenging for most people to get enough vitamin D through food sources alone (table 24.8).

Most SLE patients are vitamin D–deficient. Your doctor can monitor your vitamin D level through a blood test called 25-OH vitamin D. We recommend a level of around 40 ng/mL or higher to help with lupus disease activity (see chapters 3, 35, and 38).

If your level is lower than 40 ng/mL, you should take a vitamin D supplement. This can take the form of an over-the-counter vitamin D3 capsule. Your doctor may recommend taking 400 IU or more per day. The daily dose can be as high as 50,000 IU daily in patients with malabsorption (such as gastric bypass patients). Another approach is prescription vitamin D2 (ergocalciferol), most commonly 50,000 IU (or 1.25 mg) weekly.

Both vitamin D forms reliably improve blood vitamin D levels, and research studies show positive benefits from both. Neither has been proven to be better. But each has its advantages. For instance, vitamin D3 is absorbed better than vitamin D2, while the quality and dosage of vitamin D2 are more reliable. The amount of vitamin D3 in over-the-counter products varies greatly, depending on the brand, and in some cases, the actual amount of vitamin D3 in a capsule can be more or less than the bottle label states. If you take vitamin D3, we recommend taking the same brand all the time. This makes it easy to adjust the dosage based on blood level results.

After starting a vitamin D supplement, it takes about three months for blood vitamin D levels to reflect how a dose is doing, so it's best to wait about three months before checking levels. Your dose can be adjusted depending on this result.

Side effects from vitamin D supplements are rare. Although high calcium levels in the blood or urine can occur with high dosages, this happens only with 25-OH vitamin D blood levels over 88 ng/mL. In the rare person with very high calcium levels from a vitamin D overdose, symptoms can include nausea, confusion, increased thirst and urination, and kidney stones.

Be Concerned about Osteoporosis If You Are on Steroids

Taking steroids significantly increases the risk of osteoporosis. Steroids cause not only the intestines to absorb less calcium, but also the kidneys to excrete more calcium than they should. (Fortunately, taking a vitamin D supplement helps reverse these problems.) Steroids also decrease osteoblast activity and increase osteoclast activity. The result is weaker bones.

Losing bone density and breaking bones depends on steroid doses and how long they are taken. Daily doses in particular can cause bone loss within a few weeks of starting them; bone loss increases after that, especially during the first six months.

The American College of Rheumatology (ACR) recommends that everyone who takes steroids takes measures to avoid osteoporosis (table 24.5) and consume adequate amounts of calcium and vitamin D (tables 24.6 and 24.7). It also recommends that adults on steroids who are at moderate to high risk of broken bones take bisphosphonates (discussed later in the chapter). Other drugs have not been proven to be better, and bisphosphonates are less expensive.

If bisphosphonates are not tolerated or do not work, then teriparatide (Forteo) and then denosumab (Prolia) should be considered.

In postmenopausal women on steroids, raloxifene (Evista) is recommended if they cannot take the previously mentioned drugs.

Women who are capable of becoming pregnant and have an increased risk for fractures should avoid pregnancy (chapter 41) and take an oral bisphosphonate. For those who cannot take an oral bisphosphonate, teriparatide should be offered before IV bisphosphonates. There are case reports of newborn babies having problems after IV bisphosphonate treatment during pregnancy.

The ACR also recommends that everyone starting 30 mg a day or higher of prednisone take an oral bisphosphonate. High-dose steroids can cause a rapid loss of bone density soon after beginning therapy. Also, people who have taken a total of 5 grams or more of prednisone within a year should be on an oral bisphosphonate. For example, someone taking 15 mg a day of prednisone for a year would fall into this last category.

Osteoporosis and Chronic Kidney Disease

Chronic kidney disease (CKD) refers to having permanent kidney damage. CKD is divided into five stages, ranging from 1, or minimal damage, to 5, which is severe and requires dialysis. The kidneys in CKD are unable to filter the blood properly and excrete unwanted toxins into the urine beginning at stage 3.

Kidney function is measured by blood and urine tests, often by checking the glomerular filtration rate (GFR). A normal GFR should be around $100 \text{ mL/min}/1.73\text{m}^2$ and higher. When the kidney is damaged (such as from lupus nephritis, high blood pressure, or diabetes), and its ability to properly filter the blood decreases, GFR decreases.

One reliable and easy measurement is the estimated GFR (eGFR, chapter 4). People with osteoporosis and an eGFR greater than 30 mL/min (except for those with CKD-MBD, discussed below) can be treated similarly to other people. When the eGFR is less than 30 mL/min, most experts recommend not using osteoporosis drugs in patients who have not had an osteoporotic fracture.

For those with osteoporotic fractures and an eGFR less than 30 mL/min, treatment can be considered (in the absence of CKD-MDB, discussed below). The drugs of choice for patients with an eGFR lower than 30 mL/min are Prolia and Evenity. They have been used in patients with moderate to severely low kidney function. There is evidence of their decreasing broken bones and being safe. However, Prolia can cause low calcium levels, especially in those with low kidney function. Estrogen and Evista are options for postmenopausal women.

It is not broadly recommended to use bisphosphonates in people whose eGFR is less than 30 mL/min. Bisphosphonates require good kidney function to be cleared from the body properly. However, some people in bisphosphonate research studies had moderate to severely low kidney function and tolerated the drugs well. They had fewer broken bones without increased side effects. Therefore, bisphosphonates are used in low doses by some osteoporosis experts in this situation. PTH analogs (Forteo and Tymlos) should be avoided until they are studied more.

A unique situation can occur in patients with chronic kidney disease-mineral and bone disorder (CKD-MBD). This happens when the kidneys are unable to manage phosphorus (Ph), calcium (Ca), vitamin D (vit D), and parathyroid hormone (PTH). The proper balance of all of these is vital for healthy bone production. CKD-MBD occurs most commonly when the eGFR is less than 40 mL/min. It results in the production of abnormal, brittle bone called renal osteodystrophy, which is very different from osteoporosis and should be treated by a CKD-MBD expert (usually a nephrologist, or kidney expert). Clues to having CKD-MBD include having abnormal blood levels of Ph, Ca, vitamin D, or PTH.

Medications

Whether someone should take medication for osteoporosis is a complicated matter and depends on that person's risk for broken bones. In some cases, drugs may be prescribed for someone with normal bone density to prevent osteoporosis from developing in the first place (called preventative or prophylactic therapy). This section goes over the drugs used to treat and prevent osteoporosis.

After being on medication for osteoporosis, most doctors repeat the DXA scan to ensure no worsening bone density. The goal is to stabilize or increase bone density. The drugs discussed below do not just cause an increase in bone mineralization. They also improve bone structure (or architecture) and reduce the risk of broken bones.

If there is an increase in bone density, the reduction in fractures is even better. A large 2019 research study evaluated 57 osteoporosis treatment studies. A 2% improvement in total hip bone density translated into a 28% reduction in spine fractures and a 16% reduction in hip fractures. A 6% improvement resulted in a 66% and a 40% reduction, respectively.

However, DXA results can vary depending on the skill of the technician and the reviewing physician. Most physicians are not adequately trained to properly evaluate DXA results. They rely too much on the computer-calculated results rather than ensuring that the scan was done correctly. Because of this, 14% of the time, a DXA that shows worsening bone density is incorrect. This can occur due to incorrect positioning of the patient on the DXA table, which results in different bone areas being compared. This error rate tends to occur if the decrease is in one area, such as in the hip but not in the spine, and vice versa. In this case, it is probably best to repeat the DXA in a year rather than adjust therapy.

Bisphosphonates

Bisphosphonates (table 24.9) are the most prescribed osteoporosis drugs due to their ease of usage, relative safety, and proven effectiveness. They have also been used longer than most osteoporosis drugs, starting with the FDA approval of alendronate (Fosamax) in 1995.

Bisphosphonates aim to reduce osteoporotic fractures. Their effectiveness in preventing hip fractures is especially apparent. Between 1996 (soon after Fosamax first came into use) and 2006, the number of hospital admissions for broken hips decreased by 33%. A 2020 study showed that the number of hip fractures in Americans in their 80s dropped by a third to a half of what they were before osteoporosis drugs were available.

Generics available: Yes, for all except Binosto. However, generic alendronate has lower absorption, is less effective, and can have more side effects than the brand name Fosamax. This is one instance where you may want to insist on the brand name.

How bisphosphonates work: They attach directly to bone and prevent the cells that break down the bone (osteoclasts) from working. This allows the cells that produce bone (osteoblasts) to lay down more bone than what is reabsorbed.

Bisphosphonates generally take 6 to 18 months before significant bone-strengthening occurs. They work best if you consume adequate amounts of calcium and vitamin D.

Not all bisphosphonates are equally effective. Risedronate and ibandronate may not be as effective as Fosamax. Furthermore, intravenous (IV) zoledronic acid (Reclast) may be better at preventing vertebral fractures than oral forms, but experts are not sure if this is because IV zoledronic acid is a stronger drug or because doctors know 100% that patients are getting their medicine.

Do not take bisphosphonates if

- you have esophageal dysmotility, esophageal strictures, achalasia, or severe hiatal hernia. Most people with gastroesophageal reflux disease can take these safely.

- you cannot sit or stand upright for at least 30 minutes after taking the pill forms.

- you have persistently low calcium levels.

- your kidney function (eGFR or CrCl, chapter 4) is < 30 ml/min. Some studies suggest that lower doses may be safe.

Table 24.9 Bisphosphonates

Name	Medication Form, Dosage, How Often Taken
alendronate (Fosamax, Binosto)	Pill, 5 or 10 mg a day; 35 mg or 70 mg a week; Strawberry-flavored effervescent tablet (Binosto), 70 mg, dissolved in water weekly
ibandronate (Boniva)	Pill, 150 mg a month, or 3 mg IV infusion every 3 months
risedronate (Actonel, Atelvia)	Pill 5 mg a day, 35 mg a week, or 150 mg a month. Delayed-release form (Atelvia), 35 mg, with food weekly
zoledronic acid (Reclast)	5 mg IV infusion yearly

Dosage: Bisphosphonates can be administered by pills or intravenously (IV). The pills (table 24.9) have daily, weekly, and monthly types. They need to be taken first thing in the morning on an empty stomach along with water. It is important not to eat or drink anything else or take any other drugs for at least 30 to 60 minutes afterward. Even one sip of coffee prevents absorption.

One exception is Atelvia, the delayed-release form of risedronate. Atelvia can be taken with breakfast and now comes in a generic form.

Alendronate comes in a generic liquid form, as well as in a dissolvable tablet (Binosto). Binosto is the only bisphosphonate that does not come in a generic form and is, therefore, more expensive. A generic might become available in 2023.

The IV forms are preferred for people with stomach and esophagus problems. Two IV forms are FDA-approved: ibandronate (infused every three months) and zoledronic acid (infused yearly).

If your bone density worsens on an oral bisphosphonate, your doctor may recommend that you switch to one of the IV forms. You could also switch the drug type (such as to Tymlos, Forteo, Prolia, or Evenity).

If you miss a dose, take your oral (pill) form of bisphosphonate as soon as you remember (in the morning) and then take your next dose as scheduled. Do not take two doses on the same day. For the IV forms, schedule your infusion as soon as possible, then get your next injection three months (ibandronate) or one year later (zoledronic acid). Ask your doctor.

Alcohol/food interactions: Alcohol can exacerbate esophagus and stomach inflammation from the pill forms. Excess alcohol prevents your bones from getting stronger. Atelvia (but not the other oral forms) can be taken with food.

What to monitor while taking bisphosphonates:

- calcium, vitamin D, and kidney function before and while you are on the drug
- bone density via repeat DXA scan after one to three years to see if the treatment is working.

Potential side effects of bisphosphonates (table 24.10): Most people tolerate bisphosphonates with few side effects. There are exceptions.

If bisphosphonate pills are in contact with the lining of the esophagus for very long, irritation can occur, causing stomach upset, heartburn, chest pain, and potentially an ulcer. Taking the bisphosphonate with 8 ounces of water and not lying down for at least 30 minutes after taking it lowers this risk.

Zoledronic acid can cause body aches and low-grade fevers 24 to 72 hours after treatment. Taking acetaminophen (Tylenol) several times daily after the infusion usually prevents this or makes it less severe. This reaction is less likely to develop after the second infusion.

One rare potential side effect of bisphosphonates is an atypical femoral shaft fracture (or subtrochanteric fracture). "Atypical" means that these fractures (broken bones) are different from the typical fractures (called intertrochanteric fractures) that occur in the neck of the femur, which is the large leg bone that connects to the hip.

If someone breaks their hip from osteoporosis, the fracture usually occurs in the femoral neck, right next to the hip joint, and high up in the leg. In contrast, atypical hip fractures occur farther down the bone in the femur's middle section (shaft). There are usually warning signs because tiny fractures (stress fractures) occur first. Thigh discomfort during or after exercise is a common, early warning sign. An MRI can identify these early stress fractures.

Another rare side effect of bisphosphonates is osteonecrosis of the jaw (ONJ). *Osteo-* means "bone," while *-necrosis* refers to "death," so "osteonecrosis" means "death of a piece of bone." In ONJ, a small part of the jaw's bone dies, an open sore develops in the gum over the bone, and jaw pain occurs. ONJ has been seen primarily with large, frequent doses of IV bisphosphonates used in bone cancer. It is estimated that it occurs in only 1 out of every 10,000 to 50,000 people (depending on the study) who take a bisphosphonate. When someone with osteoporosis develops ONJ, it is more commonly due to some other reason (table 24.11).

Though rare, atypical femur fractures and ONJ are more likely to occur when someone has been taking bisphosphonates for a long time. For example, atypical femur frac-

Table 24.10 Potential Side Effects of Bisphosphonates

	Incidence	Side Effect Therapy
Nuisance side effects		
Low calcium and phosphate levels	Common	Supplements or mineral-rich foods.
Stomach upset, heartburn, nausea, gas, diarrhea	Common	Switch to a different drug.
Chest pain from esophagus irritation	Uncommon	Switch to a different drug.
Body aches and pains	Uncommon	Take pain relievers if bothersome. Switch to a different drug if severe.
Flu-like symptoms with IV Reclast (achiness, low-grade fever)	Common	Take acetaminophen (Tylenol) for a few days after the infusion to prevent symptoms.
Serious side effects		
Ulcers	Uncommon	Take anti-ulcer drugs. Stop the bisphosphonate.
Atypical femur fractures, subtrochanteric fractures	Rare	Stop the drug. Rest. Sometimes surgery is needed. Can avoid with a "drug holiday" after taking it for 3–10 years.
Osteonecrosis of the jaw	Rare	Avoid it by maintaining good dental health. Have major dental work done before starting these drugs. Very difficult to treat once it occurs.

Note: Side effect incidence key (these are approximations as they can vary widely from study to study): rare <1% occurrence; uncommon 1%–5% occurrence; common >5% occurrence.

Table 24.11 Causes of Osteonecrosis of the Jaw

- Sjögren's
- Dental disease (such as gingivitis, periodontitis, tooth decay)
- Smoking
- Diabetes
- Steroids
- Cancer treatments
- Dental implants
- Poor-fitting dentures

tures occur five times more often in women who take a bisphosphonate for more than eight years compared to those who take it for less than five years. The risk for these fractures rapidly decreases after the drug is stopped.

Drug holidays: Osteoporosis experts recommend a "drug holiday" from bisphosphonates for most people. This temporary cessation is like a vacation, not a retirement, and usually occurs around five years after someone has been taking an oral bisphosphonate and three years after receiving IV bisphosphonates.

Bisphosphonate drug holidays are possible because the drug remains in the bones after stopping the drug. The drug is recycled as the bones are remodeled (broken down and rebuilt by osteoclasts and osteoblasts, respectively). At the same time, the kidneys slowly get rid of (excrete) some of the recycled medicine. Over time, less of the drug is available, and fracture risk gradually increases. The best-studied drug is alendronate. One out of three patients loses bone density in the first two to three years of the drug holiday off alendronate. The risk for a broken hip at that point is about 40% higher than when the drug was stopped.

A drug holiday should be delayed for people with a high risk of broken bones or if their DXA shows worsening bone density. For example, an 80-year-old, 110-pound smoker with a high risk of falling should wait 7 to 10 years before starting a drug holiday from an oral bisphosphonate or up to 6 years on an IV form. Another option is switching to a different type of medicine, such as Forteo.

The best time to restart the bisphosphonate is unknown. Most experts agree that this should be done if a DXA worsens during the drug holiday or if new risk factors for broken bones develop. Based on research showing that the longer the drug is stopped, the more fractures occur, some experts routinely restart the medicine after three to five years of a drug holiday. Other experts base their decision on special urine tests that measure how much the bones are remodeling themselves (also called bone turnover). If these labs indicate an increase in bone loss, the doctor restarts the bisphosphonate.

While taking bisphosphonates, tell your doctor if

- you get stomach upset, nausea, vomiting, chest pain, or body pain.
- you develop an open sore on your gums, especially if the bone is exposed.
- you develop thigh or hip pain, your doctor should exclude atypical hip fracture.

Pregnancy and breastfeeding: IV bisphosphonates should not be infused during pregnancy. However, case reports of women taking oral bisphosphonates indicate that they did not show any problems. If the mother does take bisphosphonates, the newborn's calcium level should be checked after delivery.

If you are taking a bisphosphonate, wish to become pregnant, and want to stay off of it during pregnancy, it is recommended that you wait six months after stopping the bisphosphonate before becoming pregnant.

Women capable of becoming pregnant who need to take a bisphosphonate should use adequate contraception (birth control measures, chapter 41).

Safety during breastfeeding is unknown.

Geriatric use: No change in dosage required.

Bisphosphonates and surgery: Ask your rheumatologist and surgeon. However, bisphosphonates are generally safe before surgery.

PTH Analogs (Teriparatide [Forteo]) and (Abaloparatide [Tymlos])

Compared to other osteoporosis drugs, these are relatively fast-acting drugs that improve bone density within a few months. Around eight months, there is evidence for decreased broken bones.

PTH analogs (specifically Forteo) may better prevent spine fractures from steroid-induced osteoporosis than bisphosphonates.

Generic available: Yes, for teriparatide; not for Tymlos.

How PTH analogs work: PTH analogs are a form of parathyroid hormone (PTH), a natural hormone made by the parathyroid glands, which are located behind the thyroid gland, in the front of the neck just below the Adam's apple area. PTH is vital for the body's cells to correctly process calcium and vitamin D. It causes the bones to make more bone-producing cells (osteoblasts). This is very different from most other osteoporosis drugs, which work by decreasing osteoclast bone absorption.

Do not take PTH analogs if you have high calcium levels (such as in hyperparathyroidism).

Use caution if you are prone to getting calcium kidney stones.

Dosage: PTH analogs are given by injection under the skin (subcutaneously). It comes in a "pen" that contains four weeks' medication. A small new needle is attached daily. The patient inserts the needle into the skin of the stomach or thigh, then pushes a button on top to inject it.

If you miss a dose, begin your daily injections as soon as you remember. Keep track of how many pens (doses) you use. Once you get to 24, you have finished 2 years' worth. This is helpful in case you miss any doses, which is common.

Alcohol/food interactions: Excess alcohol (chapter 38) lowers the chances of your bones getting stronger. Ensure you get enough calcium and vitamin D.

What to monitor while taking PTH analogs:

- calcium and phosphate levels

- uric acid levels in people with gout (arthritis caused by uric acid)

- blood pressure if you are prone to low blood pressure

- bone density via DXA scan after one to three years.

Potential side effects of PTH analogs (table 24.12): The most reported side effects from PTH analogs are headaches, nausea, and dizziness.

Animal (rat) studies with PTH analogs showed an increase in a bone cancer called osteosarcoma. However, rat bones and human bones differ a lot. Rat bones grow throughout their lives; human bones stop growing after puberty. PTH analogs affect the active growth plates of rat bones; adult human bones lack these bone-growing sections. In addition, much higher doses of PTH analogs were used in the rat studies than prescribed for humans. Even so, the FDA recommends using PTH analogs for only two years to decrease this risk. Since 2002, when Forteo was FDA-approved, no increases in osteosarcomas have occurred.

While taking PTH analogs, tell your doctor if

- you get dizzy or light-headed.
- you get gout attacks (excruciatingly painful, red, hot swollen joints).
- you get kidney stones.

Pregnancy and breastfeeding: Not recommended during pregnancy or breastfeeding.

Table 24.12   Potential Side Effects of Teriparatide (Forteo) and Abaloparatide (Tymlos)

	Incidence	Side Effect Therapy
Nuisance side effects		
Injection site redness, tenderness	Common	Apply ice packs or cortisone cream.
Elevated blood calcium	Common	Decrease calcium intake or stop Forteo. It may be temporary and of no clinical significance.
Light-headedness, dizziness	Common	Usually goes away with regular use. Stand up slowly. If it does not get better, you may need to stop it.
Gout attacks if you have gout	Uncommon	Increase gout medicines.
Nausea, upset stomach	Common	Usually goes away with regular use. Take anti-nausea drug. May need to stop if severe.
Serious side effects		
Passing out due to dizziness	Uncommon	Call an ambulance or have someone take you immediately to a hospital. Stop the drug.

Note: Side effect incidence key (approximations, as side effects can vary widely from study to study): rare <1% occurrence; uncommon 1%–5% occurrence; common >5% occurrence.

Geriatric use: No dosage adjustments needed.

PTH analogs and surgery: Ask your rheumatologist and surgeon. It may be best to stop them a few days before surgery to avoid abnormal calcium levels.

Financial aid for PTH analogs: Teriparatide was US$2,800 monthly (according to goodrx.com in 2022); Tymlos pricing was $3,100 (per UpToDate.com). For possible aid for Tymlos call 1-866-896-5674 or go to tymlos.com/savings-support; for teriparatide go to goodrx.com or similar programs. Also, go to lupusencyclopedia.com/patient-resources

Drug helplines: Forteo, 1-866-436-7836. Tymlos, 1-866-896-5674.

Websites: www.Forteo.com, www.Tymlos.com.

Denosumab (Prolia, Xgeva)

Denosumab increases bone density and decreases broken bones.

Generic available: No.

How denosumab works: It is the only biologic for osteoporosis (biologics are discussed in chapter 33). It works by connecting to a molecule called RANKL (receptor activator of nuclear factor kappaB ligand). RANKL attaches to osteoclasts, causing them to work harder to break down and reabsorb bone. Denosumab connects to RANKL molecules, keeping them from attaching to osteoclasts. This allows the osteoclasts to work less hard and not reabsorb as much bone. Osteoblasts can then create more bone, making the bones stronger.

Denosumab also reduces joint bone destruction (called erosions) in rheumatoid arthritis. Therefore, people with rhupus (rheumatoid arthritis overlap syndrome with lupus) may benefit.

Denosumab increases bone density more than bisphosphonates do. This, however, does not necessarily mean that it is better for preventing broken bones. Comparison studies have shown that they prevent the same number of fractures.

Do not take if

- you have vitamin D deficiency, which should be normalized before starting therapy.

- you have latex allergy (packaging and needle cover may contain latex).

Use caution if you have chronic kidney disease, malabsorption, or hypoparathyroidism.

Dosage: It is given twice a year (six months apart) by an injection under the skin in the doctor's office.

If you miss a dose, schedule it as soon as possible, then every six months after that date.

Alcohol/food interactions: Excess alcohol (chapter 38) can decrease bone density. Ensure you take enough calcium and vitamin D.

What to monitor while taking denosumab:

- kidney function, calcium, magnesium, and phosphorus levels before treatment and 7 to 14 days after injection (especially if you have chronic kidney disease stage 3 or worse, have had parathyroid surgery, or have malabsorption due to gastric bypass surgery)

- bone density via DXA scan after one to three years.

LUPUS IN FOCUS

Do not be late for your denosumab (Prolia) injection

A 2020 study of over 2,500 patients showed that those who were over a month late for their Prolia injection had a 40% higher chance of vertebral fractures than those who were on time. Patients over four months late were four times more likely to fracture compared to those who were not late on their dose.

Seven to eight months after a missed Prolia injection, a high number of patients develop vertebral fractures. The bone density can even become lower than the levels before Prolia therapy. Immediately beginning a bisphosphonate after Prolia dramatically reduces this risk. A 6- to 12-month course of bisphosphonate may be sufficient in this situation.

Potential side effects of denosumab (table 24.13): Denosumab may increase some infections, although studies have found this to be unusual. If an infection occurs, it is usually a skin infection (cellulitis). Because RANKL is essential for the skin's immune system to work at its best, interfering with RANKL may decrease the skin's ability to prevent infection.

If denosumab injections are delayed past 6 months, rapid bone density loss can occur, unless it is replaced by another osteoporosis drug. Treatment delays may result in broken bones, including multiple vertebral fractures. Fractures do not typically occur unless it has been at least 6 months since the last denosumab dose. It is important to keep up with the every 6-month schedule.

While taking denosumab, call and see your doctor right away if you develop an area of red, warm, tender skin. This could be a sign of cellulitis.

Pregnancy and breastfeeding: Not recommended during pregnancy. If you become pregnant on Prolia, call the Amgen Pregnancy Surveillance Program (1-800-772-6436). Women with pregnancy potential should use adequate contraception (chapter 41).

Breastfeeding safety is unknown. Like other biologics, it is a large molecule and should not enter breastmilk very much; if any does, the baby's intestinal tract would destroy it.

Geriatric use: No changes in dosing.

Denosumab and surgery: Ask your rheumatologist and surgeon. It may be advisable not to use Prolia for several weeks before surgery to decrease the risk of infection and electrolyte abnormalities.

Financial assistance for denosumab: 1-877-776-5421 or visit amgenassist.com/copay.

Drug helpline: 1-877-4-PROLIA (877-477-6542).

Website: www.Prolia.com.

Romosozumab (Evenity)

Romosozumab is new since the first edition of this book. It was FDA-approved in 2019.

Generic available: No.

How romosozumab works: Sclerostin is a protein produced by the body that prevents bone-building cells (osteoblasts) from functioning properly and thus causes lower bone

Table 24.13 Potential Side Effects of Denosumab (Prolia)

	Incidence	Side Effect Therapy
Nuisance side effects		
Dermatitis (rash)	Common	Cortisone cream, antihistamines. Stop drug if severe.
Low calcium levels	Uncommon unless there is kidney disease	Make sure you take enough calcium and vitamin D. Stop drug if severe.
Joint, back, leg, arm pains	Common	Take Tylenol, NSAIDs. Stop taking drug if severe.
Serious side effects		
Cellulitis (skin infection) with red, hot, painful skin	Rare	Call and see doctor right away for antibiotics.
Osteonecrosis of the jaw	Rare	See main text of bisphosphonates.

Note: Side effect incidence key (approximations, as side effects can vary widely from study to study): rare <1% occurrence; uncommon 1%–5% occurrence; common >5% occurrence.

density. Romosozumab is an antibody that attaches to sclerostin, preventing sclerostin from binding to osteoblasts. This allows osteoblasts to make stronger bones.

Do not take if

- you have low calcium levels.
- you have had a heart attack or stroke in the past year or are at high risk for either one.

Dosage: Two injections are given at the same time monthly in the doctor's office for 12 months. After 12 months, it needs to be followed quickly by either a bisphosphonate or denosumab. Otherwise, bone density loss can occur rapidly.

If you miss a dose, schedule it as soon as possible, then monthly after that date.

Alcohol/food interactions: Excess alcohol (chapter 38) can decrease bone density. Ensure you take enough calcium and vitamin D.

What to monitor while taking romosozumab:

- calcium levels before and during treatment
- bone density after one to three years via DXA scan.

Potential side effects of romosozumab (table 24.14): In one study, people taking Evenity had more heart attacks and strokes than those on placebo.

Go to your closest hospital or urgent care center if you have symptoms of a stroke or heart attack (chapters 13 and 21).

Pregnancy and breastfeeding: Not recommended during pregnancy or breast feeding.

Table 24.14 Potential Side Effects of Romosozumab (Evenity)

	Incidence	Side Effect Therapy
Nuisance side effects		
Redness, tenderness at the injection site	Common	Use ice packs and cortisone cream.
Low calcium levels	Uncommon unless there is kidney disease	Make sure you are taking enough calcium and vitamin D.
Joint, muscle, and head pains	Common	Tylenol, NSAIDs. Stop taking the drug if severe.
Serious side effects		
Heart attacks, strokes	Rare	Stop Evenity.
Atypical femur fractures, subtrochanteric fractures	Rare	Stop drug; see section on bisphosphonates.
Osteonecrosis of the jaw	Rare	Stop drug ; see above section on bisphosphonates.

Note: Side effect incidence key (approximations, as side effects can vary widely from study to study): rare <1% occurrence; uncommon 1%–5% occurrence; common >5% occurrence.

Geriatric use: No changes in dosing needed.

Romosozumab and surgery: Ask your rheumatologist and surgeon.

Financial assistance for romosozumab: In 2022, the price was close to US$2,000 monthly, according to uptodate.com. Call 800-761-1558 or visit amgenassist.com/copay.

Drug helpline: 1-888-231-5663.

Website: www.evenity.com.

Raloxifene (Evista)

Raloxifene is not as good at preventing broken bones as bisphosphonates, PTH analogs, or denosumab are. If you do not have osteoporosis (such as if you have mild bone density loss or osteopenia), it can help keep you from progressing to osteoporosis.

One potential advantage of raloxifene is that it decreases the risk of breast cancer. This is particularly true for those with a strong family history of breast cancer (primarily estrogen receptor–positive invasive breast cancer). Raloxifene studies showed that breast cancers were reduced by half or more. In one study, they were reduced by 75%. The women in the research studies ranged from low to high risk for breast cancer.

Raloxifene is a good choice for women who want breast cancer prevention, have osteopenia or mild osteoporosis, and who are not at high risk for blood clots (see below).

Generic available: Yes.

How raloxifene works: Raloxifene is a selective estrogen receptor modulator. It has some estrogen (female hormone) effects in some body parts (such as bones) but not others (such as breasts and the uterus). Recall that the most common cause of osteo-porosis is the loss of estrogen after menopause. Taking raloxifene helps to provide estrogen-like bone-building effects. However, it is weaker than estrogen.

It has been shown to decrease spine fractures but not hip fractures.

Do not take raloxifene if

- you are positive for antiphospholipid antibodies.

- you smoke.

- you have had blood clots, a heart attack, or a stroke.

- you already have bothersome postmenopausal hot flashes.

- you have not gone through menopause.

- you have severe kidney function problems.

- you have had triglyceride levels greater than 500 mg/dL; it can make it worse.

- you are a man.

Dosage: Raloxifene comes in a 60 mg tablet taken daily.

If you miss a dose, take it as soon as possible, then resume daily dosing the next day.

Alcohol/food interactions: Excess alcohol (chapter 38) can decrease bone density. Raloxifene can be taken with or without food. Ensure you take enough calcium and vitamin D.

What to monitor while taking raloxifene: Bone density via DXA scan after one to three years.

Potential side effects of raloxifene (table 24.15): Raloxifene is well tolerated. The most common issues are hot flashes and muscle cramps. Hot flashes (like those in

Table 24.15 Potential Side Effects of Raloxifene (Evista)

	Incidence	Side Effect Therapy
Nuisance side effects		
Hot flashes	Common	Continue drug if mild. Stop it if severe.
Leg cramps, joint pains	Common	Continue drug if mild. Stop it if severe.
Leg swelling (edema)	Common	Wear vascular support stockings. Stop it if bothersome.
Serious side effects		
Blood clots (strokes, pulmonary embolism, deep venous thrombosis)	Uncommon	Seek medical help immediately.

Note: Side effect incidence key (approximations, as side effects can vary widely from study to study): rare <1% occurrence; uncommon 1%–5% occurrence; common >5% occurrence.

menopause) occur in 10% to 25% of women taking raloxifene and are usually mild and tolerable. But if you already have hot flashes, raloxifene may not be the right choice. Muscle cramps develop in 10% of women. These also tend to be mild and tolerable, although occasionally they can cause enough discomfort to stop the drug.

While taking raloxifene,

- Contact your doctor if you develop possible symptoms of a blood clot, heart attack, or strokes, such as a painful swollen calf, shortness of breath, chest pain, numbness or weakness, or slurred speech.

- Stop taking it at least one week before prolonged immobilization (surgery, long car or plane trips) to prevent blood clots.

Pregnancy and breastfeeding: Do not take it if you have not undergone menopause.
Geriatric use: No adjustment in dosage needed.
Raloxifene and surgery: Ask your rheumatologist and surgeon. You should not take Evista two to four weeks before surgery to prevent blood clots.
Financial assistance for raloxifene: Go to lupusencyclopedia.com/patient-resources, GoodRX.com or similar programs.

Calcitonin (Miacalcin)

Although it is one of the weakest osteoporosis drugs, calcitonin increases bone density and can reduce vertebral fracture back pain. It has not been proven to decrease hip fractures.

Generic available: Yes.
How calcitonin works: Calcitonin is a hormone produced by the thyroid gland. It attaches to osteoclasts, preventing them from breaking down bone, which allows osteoblasts to make more bone.

Do not use if you have sores in your nose.

Dosage: Although it can be prescribed as an injection, it is usually prescribed as a nasal spray. One spray in one nostril is done daily, alternating nostrils every other day. The FDA recommends using it for less than six months.

If you miss a dose, use it as soon as possible, then resume daily dosing the next day.
Alcohol/food interactions: Excess alcohol (chapter 38) can decrease bone density. Ensure you take enough calcium and vitamin D.

Potential side effects of calcitonin (table 24.16): The most common side effects of the nasal spray forms of calcitonin are nausea, nose irritation, and headaches. These quickly resolve when the drug is stopped.

While taking calcitonin nasal spray, let your doctor know if you get nose sores.
Pregnancy and breastfeeding: Calcitonin is safe during pregnancy.

Calcitonin can reduce an important breastfeeding hormone called prolactin. Therefore, it may be best to avoid during breastfeeding. However, doctors may prescribe it during breastfeeding if the benefits outweigh the risks.

Geriatric use: No dosage adjustments needed.
Calcitonin and surgery: Ask your rheumatologist and surgeon. You can use calcitonin nasal spray up to the day before surgery.

Table 24.16 Potential Side Effects of Calcitonin Nasal Spray (Miacalcin, Fortical)

	Incidence	Side Effect Therapy
Nuisance side effects		
Nose irritation and runny nose	Common	If bothersome, stop the drug.
Nasal ulceration, bloody nose	Uncommon	Stop using it.
Headache	Uncommon	Stop using it if bothersome.
Serious side effects		
Cancer	Rare	To prevent cancer, use for less than 6 months.

Note: Side effect incidence key (approximations, as side effects can vary widely from study to study): rare <1% occurrence; uncommon 1%–5% occurrence; common >5% occurrence.

Estrogen

Estrogen loss after menopause is the most common cause of osteoporosis. Estrogen is rarely prescribed for osteoporosis due to increased risks for breast cancer, strokes, blood clots, and possibly heart attacks.

In women with significant menopausal problems (such as hot flashes, vaginal dryness, aches, and pain), estrogen can decrease these symptoms while also helping with osteoporosis. It can be considered in someone who fails other postmenopausal therapies since these problems can greatly affect quality of life.

Since estrogen is most commonly prescribed by gynecologists, rather than rheumatologists, we will not discuss it in detail.

KEY POINTS TO REMEMBER

1. Osteoporosis is a disease where the bones are fragile and can fracture.

2. SLE patients are at increased risk for osteoporosis due to drugs (steroids, antiseizure medicines, blood thinners, and proton pump inhibitors) and less activity.

3. Osteoporosis is a silent disease. People do not feel poorly until their bones break.

4. Osteoporosis is treatable and preventable.

5. Osteoporosis is often diagnosed by a DXA scan.

6. If you have risk factors for osteoporosis (table 24.1), ask your doctor for a DXA scan.

7. Do the things in table 24.5 to prevent and treat osteoporosis.

8. Most SLE patients should take a vitamin D supplement. Have your vitamin D level measured regularly. We recommend a 25-OH vitamin D level of around 40 ng/mL.

9. Having a normal bone density on DXA does not mean you do not have osteoporosis. One out of three SLE patients with osteoporotic vertebral fractures has a normal bone density on DXA.

10. If you take steroids regularly, you need more calcium and vitamin D than others. You may also need to be on medicine to prevent broken bones.

11. The most effective drugs for osteoporosis are bisphosphonates, PTH analogs, Prolia, and Evenity.

12. Raloxifene can help treat osteoporosis and prevent breast cancer.

13. Do not take raloxifene if you are positive for antiphospholipid antibodies.

14. Calcitonin is no longer recommended for osteoporosis treatment. It may be useful for a short period to help vertebral fracture back pain.

15. Tymlos and Evenity are new osteoporosis drugs (since the first edition of this book). Although they may possibly work better than bisphosphonates, they are costly.

16. Evenity may increase the risk for heart attacks and strokes.

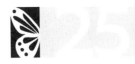

Avascular Necrosis of Bone

Hector A. Medina, MD, *Contributing Editor*

"Avascular" means "lack of blood supply," and "necrosis" means "death," so avascular necrosis of bone (AVN) is bone death due to blood supply loss. Other commonly used terms are osteonecrosis, aseptic necrosis, and ischemic bone necrosis. AVN occurs in 5% to 10% of SLE patients and is often due to high-dose steroids.

Exactly how steroids cause AVN is unknown. Steroids may reduce blood flow in the bone blood vessels, leading to bone death. The reasoning here is that since steroids can cause increased cholesterol and fat in blood, these tiny globs (called emboli) of cholesterol and fat may clog bone blood vessels. Steroids can also cause osteoporosis (chapter 24). Some experts suggest that people on steroids may first develop osteoporosis in the bone and then develop tiny, microscopic breaks or fractures in these areas of weak bone. The steroids may not allow the blood vessels to supply enough blood flow to fix these tiny fractures, causing the fractures to worsen, which in turn eventually causes the bone to die.

Although many people end up requiring surgery, such as total joint replacement, the disease process can potentially be slowed down if caught early. AVN usually occurs in the large bone of the leg (femur) connecting to the hip joint, but it also may occur in the knees and shoulders. Although it may affect just one joint, many people will develop AVN in the same joint on each side of the body.

AVN in SLE patients most commonly occurs in the femoral head at the hip. The hip joint is a ball-and-socket joint. The ball of the femur bone (called the femoral head) fits like a ball into the acetabulum of the pelvic bone (acting as the socket of the joint). This ball and socket joint allows the hips to move in many directions.

In AVN, the dead bone in the femoral head softens over time and can no longer bear weight very well. It can potentially collapse, causing the ball-shape of the femoral head to flatten out. Imagine a round orange with a soft and irregular bruised surface on one end. AVN has a similar effect on the femoral head, making movement more difficult and painful. The hip joint eventually develops arthritis (joint damage).

Since the hip joint is located in the groin area, people commonly feel discomfort in the groin when they have hip AVN. Many people find this surprising, thinking that hip arthritis would cause pain on the side of the hip. As AVN worsens, hip range of motion

Dr. Medina contributed to this article in his personal capacity. The views expressed are his own and do not necessarily represent the views of the Landstuhl Regional Medical Center, the Uniformed Services University, or the United States government.

worsens, and there may be difficulty putting on shoes, as well as trouble bearing weight, which can cause a limp when walking.

Although most SLE patients with AVN have taken high-dose steroids (often more than 20 mg a day), some develop AVN with smaller amounts. AVN can also occur in SLE patients who have taken no steroids. This suggests that there may be other causes. Some studies have considered lupus inflammation, high blood pressure, high cholesterol, Raynaud's phenomenon (where the fingers turn pale and blue with exposure to cold), vasculitis (inflammation of the blood vessels), or a history of an infected joint as factors that increase the chances of AVN, but these have not been conclusive.

Most people with AVN do not have SLE. It can be caused by problems other than steroids (table 25.1). It is essential to consider these other possible causes of AVN in SLE patients.

Diagnosing AVN

Doctors commonly diagnose AVN with x-rays. However, early in the disease process, x-rays can be normal. If the joint x-ray is normal, an MRI is the next step since MRI can diagnose AVN in its early stages. It is also a good idea to get an x-ray or MRI of the opposite joint since AVN commonly occurs on both sides of the body. AVN is often picked up on an x-ray or MRI done for other reasons.

LUPUS IN FOCUS

Hydroxychloroquine reduces the risk for AVN

As it does for many SLE problems, hydroxychloroquine (Plaquenil) reduces the chances of developing AVN.

Table 25.1 Causes of AVN

- Antiphospholipid syndrome
- Smoking, or excess alcohol drinking
- Sickle cell disease
- Trauma
- Acute lymphoblastic leukemia
- Gaucher disease (a rare genetic disorder)
- Decompression disease (when underwater divers ascend too quickly from deep water)
- Kidney transplantation
- HIV infection
- Radiation therapy for cancer
- Legg-Calvé-Perthes disease or slipped capital epiphysis (childhood developmental problems)
- Arthroscopic surgery

Once AVN is diagnosed, doctors can grade its severity on a scale of 0 to 4, with 0 being the mildest, and 4 the most severe. Stages 0 to 1 may stay the same without worsening (or even improve over time).

Stages 3 and 4 are on the opposite end of the spectrum. There is significant bone damage. Loss of joint cartilage (the smooth rubbery cushioning lining the joint bones and allowing easy movement) is present in stage 4 and commonly requires a total hip replacement.

People with stage 2 AVN have a better chance of doing well. This group has mild bone damage but no joint damage. Most people with stage 2 AVN worsen over time or remain stable. However, they are not destined to need a hip replacement as much as people with stage 3 or 4.

Symptoms (such as discomfort) may be minimal to severe, or there may be no symptoms at all. One study looked at SLE patients with AVN on MRI but with no hip pain. Over three years, 75% of these patients did not worsen, while 25% did get worse.

Preventing and Treating AVN

Since doctors do not fully understand what causes AVN, they do not know how to prevent it. Four studies have shown that blood thinners (warfarin or enoxaparin) decreased but did not eliminate the chances for AVN. Only two studies included SLE patients. More studies using blood thinners in SLE patients would be needed before doctors could use blood thinners to prevent AVN.

There are three ways to treat AVN: joint protection, conservative management (nonsurgical therapy), and surgery.

Joint Protection

Joint protection is critical no matter what stage of AVN you have. If you have stage 0 or 1, it could potentially make a big difference in preventing AVN from getting worse. Joint protection decreases stress on joint bone and cartilage. If you have knee or hip involvement, it is crucial to use an assistive device that decreases weight and stress on the joints. Examples include canes, walking sticks, walking poles, crutches, and walkers. If you use a cane, you should hold it in the hand opposite of the joint involved as this is most effective in decreasing weight on the affected joint. Also, weight loss is important if you are overweight. Also see lupusencyclopedia.com/joint-protection.

Too many people do not abide by the principles of joint protection. Instead, they rely too much on pain medications that do nothing to prevent the AVN from worsening. In addition, many people are uncomfortable with the thought of being seen in public using a cane. If that is true for you, it is vital to learn to put your health first and realize it is more important than worrying about what other people think. Also, today there are many types of stylish canes and walking sticks available, as well as Nordic sticks, which look like ski poles and are particularly popular in Europe.

Exercise is essential to maintain muscle strength, flexibility, and weight loss. Low-impact activities such as swimming or stationary bicycling are better than jogging or high-impact aerobics. You should also consider asking your doctor to refer you to a physical therapist for exercise advice.

Nonsurgical Therapies

Nonsurgical treatments for pain include using drugs such as acetaminophen (Tylenol), non-steroidal anti-inflammatory drugs (NSAIDs), and opioids. You can first try over-the-counter medicines (chapter 7) for pain. If these are ineffective, see your doctor for prescription pain relievers. Although these therapies do not prevent AVN from getting worse, they can help reduce pain, improve your ability to move, and improve the quality of your life.

Another potential therapy for AVN is bisphosphonates, a group of osteoporosis medicines (chapter 24). A couple of studies suggest that the bisphosphonate alendronate (Fosamax) may slow the progression of AVN if taken in very early stages. Using bisphosphonates for AVN is controversial since two other studies showed no improvement.

Statins, which are drugs for high cholesterol (chapter 21), may help decrease AVN damage by preventing the formation of bone fat cells, which are thought to increase pressure in the bone. While several studies have suggested they may help AVN, better studies are needed.

Iloprost (Ventavis), a pulmonary hypertension drug (chapter 11), has been shown to be helpful in some AVN patients. Iloprost may decrease the pressure inside AVN-affected bone and increase blood flow.

None of the above treatments has sufficient evidence to support its use for AVN. This does not mean they may not be helpful. We just need better research studies.

Surgery

Most stage 3 and 4 AVN, and some stage 2 AVN, eventually need total joint replacement surgery. Doctors typically recommend surgery if drugs do not control pain adequately and if the quality of life is affected. For an inactive elderly person with severe stage 4 AVN but only mild discomfort, the chances of a bad outcome from surgery may be greater than the potential benefits. So, if discomfort is tolerable and not affecting quality of life, joint replacement may not be the answer.

In contrast, a very active 30-year-old, who loves hiking, exercising, and dancing, could have enough pain from stage 2 AVN to prevent them from enjoying these activities. In that case, because quality of life is significantly affected, total joint replacement should be considered. The decision to get a joint replacement is complex, involving a detailed discussion of the potential risks and benefits with an orthopedic surgeon.

A joint replacement is performed under anesthesia. It involves removing the necrotic (dead) bone and replacing it with a new replacement part called a prosthesis. The other part of the joint may also need to be replaced. People who want a joint replacement should find an orthopedic surgeon who has done many of them. One of the best predictors for how well you do from surgery is the number of surgeries that the surgeon has done. Discuss options with your rheumatologist and primary care provider.

After choosing an orthopedist, go to the first consultation fully prepared. Bring all x-ray and MRI films plus any visit notes (called progress notes) from your recent rheumatology and primary care physician visits, as well as a list of all of your medical problems, surgeries, medications, and any recent lab results. (It is smart to bring this information to all new doctor visits.) Prepare a brief list of questions to ask the surgeon:

- Do you recommend that I have surgery? If so, what type and why?

- Approximately how many of these surgeries have you done?

- If I undergo this surgery, what are my chances of having a good outcome (decreased pain and increased ability to be more active)?

- If I undergo surgery, what are my chances for complications? How often do they occur, and how bad are they?

- If I undergo this surgery, what is rehabilitation like? How long can I expect to be out of work? Should I do the rehabilitation at home or in a rehab facility?

Core decompression is another AVN surgery in which the surgeon drills a hole into the affected bone to release built-up pressure and creates an area where new blood vessels can form. Decreasing pressure and increasing blood flow, can slow down progressive worsening of AVN. Core decompression may be effective in 50% to 77% of patients with early (stage 0, 1, or 2) AVN.

Hyperbaric oxygen is another option. It involves breathing pure oxygen in a pressurized environment. One study showed that hyperbaric oxygen therapy combined with core decompression surgery may reduce pain in early AVN. However, this therapy is not widely available, so core decompression alone is the usual treatment.

Other possible surgeries include bone grafting and osteotomy. Bone grafting places a substance in the AVN-affected bone to add support. It can come from another bone of the patient (autograft), or someone else such as a dead organ donor (allograft), an animal (xenograft), or it can be synthetic (such as ceramic). Osteotomy involves making cuts into the affected bone to redistribute weightbearing forces on the bone.

KEY POINTS TO REMEMBER

1. AVN (osteonecrosis) is a disorder in which part of the bone dies, usually in a bone next to a joint.

2. AVN occurs in 5% to 10% of SLE patients, most commonly from high-dose steroids.

3. The hip is the most commonly affected joint, causing groin pain, difficulty walking, and trouble putting on socks and shoes. The shoulders and knees can also be affected.

4. AVN is diagnosed by x-ray or MRI.

5. Doctors grade AVN severity on a scale ranging from 0 to 4.

6. If diagnosed early (stage 0 or 1) and is asymptomatic (no symptoms), there is a 75% chance of no worsening.

7. Core decompression surgery may decrease progression of early AVN (stages 0–2).

8. AVN patients should abide by joint-protection measures to slow down or prevent their AVN from progressing. See lupusencyclopedia.com/joint-protection.

9. Most patients with stages 3 and 4 (and some with stage 2) will need a total joint replacement.

Adrenal Insufficiency

Mark M. Cruz, MD, FACP, *Contributing Editor*

Anyone on steroids (such as prednisone and methylprednisolone) should understand adrenal insufficiency. It is a common and underrecognized problem.

The adrenal glands (also called suprarenal glands) sit on top of the kidneys. This is where they get their name. "Renal" is another name for "kidney"; *ad-* means "near," and *supra-* means "on top of." They produce about 50 different steroid hormones with numerous functions. Recall from chapter 17 that hormones are substances produced by endocrine glands (like the adrenal glands) that go to other body organs, instructing them to do certain functions. With steroids, this includes maintaining blood pressure, handling salts by the kidneys, responding to stress, and handling nutrients such as glucose (sugar), fats, and proteins (just to name a few). The adrenal glands also produce other hormones, such as the sex hormones DHEA (dehydroepiandrosterone) and epinephrine (called adrenaline), which is critical in keeping the blood pressure up, the heart beating, and the lung passages open.

Adrenal insufficiency occurs when the adrenal glands stop making enough of some of these hormones, especially steroids. It is helpful to know some basics about how the adrenal glands produce steroids to understand why adrenal insufficiency occurs in people taking them.

The Hypothalamic-Pituitary-Adrenal Axis

The adrenal glands work with the help of two other brain organs—the hypothalamus and the pituitary gland (figure 26.1)—in a finely orchestrated way. The medical term for these interactions is "hypothalamic-pituitary-adrenal axis."

The hypothalamus is the primary organ in charge of this whole operation (figure 26.1). The hypothalamus continuously secretes a corticotropin-releasing hormone (CRH). CRH travels to the pituitary gland to cause it to secrete another hormone called adrenocorticotropic hormone (ACTH). In turn, ACTH travels through the bloodstream to the adrenal glands, signaling them to secrete steroids (such as cortisol, which is related to cortisone, prednisone, and methylprednisolone). The body typically makes

Dr. Cruz contributed to this article in his personal capacity. The views expressed are his own and do not necessarily represent the views of the Naval Medical Center Portsmouth, the Uniformed Services University, or the United States government.

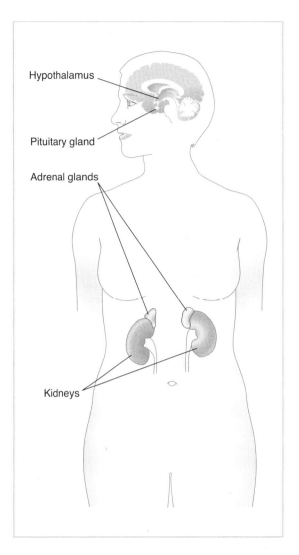

Figure 26.1 Locations of the hypothalamus, pituitary gland, and adrenal glands

the equivalent of 5 mg to 7 mg of prednisone (or 4 mg to 6 mg of methylprednisolone) daily.

More steroids are needed during periods of increased activity and stress. When the hypothalamus senses less cortisol in the bloodstream than there should be, soon after people first wake up and become active or during periods of stress (such as infections or surgery), it makes more CRH. This causes the pituitary gland to secrete more ACTH. Then the adrenal glands make more cortisol as initially demanded by the hypothalamus. After this, when the hypothalamus senses the increased cortisol in the blood, it backs off and produces less CRH. This communication system maintains proper cortisol levels. Thus, it ensures there is more cortisol during periods when needed most (stress and increased periods of activity) and less cortisol during other periods (while relaxing).

When someone takes steroids, such as prednisone and methylprednisolone, the hypothalamus senses this increase in cortisol-like steroids. When steroids are taken regularly, especially at higher doses (such as more than 7 mg of prednisone a day), the hypothalamus produces less CRH because it thinks the adrenal glands are making too much cortisol. In turn, the pituitary gland makes less ACTH, which tells the adrenal glands to stop making steroids. The adrenal glands respond to this lower amount of ACTH the way that a muscle responds to lack of exercise. Since they think they are not needed anymore to make steroids, the adrenal glands shrink. They become even smaller from higher-dose steroids or when steroids are taken over prolonged periods.

What Happens in Adrenal Insufficiency?

When someone stays on large steroid doses, they will not have physical symptoms of adrenal insufficiency since the steroid medicine replaces the steroids usually produced by the adrenal glands. The problem is not realized until one of two things happens: either a person becomes stressed while taking relatively small doses of steroids (and the body needs more steroids for the stress) or the steroid drug is decreased too quickly to small amounts or is stopped abruptly.

Stress and Adrenal Insufficiency

During stressful situations (like infections, trauma, and surgery), the hypothalamus and the pituitary order the adrenal glands to produce more cortisol. The adrenal glands can produce the equivalent of about 20 to 100 mg of prednisone a day during stress.

Let's say someone has a severe lupus flare requiring 40 mg of prednisone a day for a few weeks after which the dose is decreased gradually. This steroid amount is sufficient to cause the adrenal glands to shrink, making them less likely to respond adequately to ACTH (in other words, adrenal insufficiency). After a few weeks, the patient is down to 8 mg a day of prednisone, at which point they get the flu. The hypothalamus senses this increased stress and realizes the body needs more cortisol-like steroids during the illness. It sends an increased amount of CRH to the pituitary gland, which produces an increased ACTH amount. The smaller-than-usual adrenal glands sense this high ACTH level. Although they know they are supposed to make more cortisol in response to this elevated ACTH, they cannot. It is like telling a 90-pound weakling to lift 200-pound dumbbells. Since the adrenal glands cannot produce the proper amount of cortisol steroids, this person becomes sicker than someone who does not have adrenal insufficiency. Their fatigue becomes incapacitating, and their aches and pains become unbearable. The person is so light-headed and dizzy that they can hardly get up out of bed.

A few different scenarios could play out from this point. In one scenario, the person may try to tough it out at home. By doing so without extra steroids or cortisol, they will be more miserable. They will also probably take a lot longer to recuperate from the flu than a person with normal adrenal glands. In another scenario, the person may stay home in bed but eventually get sick enough to go to the hospital. On average, 30,000 Americans die each year from the flu. SLE patients and adrenal insufficiency patients are at high risk of this occurring. If the person is seen quickly enough, they can be treated with extra doses of steroids that can be life-saving.

The best scenario occurs when the well-educated person (like you, reading this information) calls their primary care physician at once. They know they are supposed to see the doctor ASAP with any type of fever or infection. Because they take steroids, they also realize that they may have adrenal insufficiency, so they call their rheumatologist to see if extra steroids are needed. In this case, the rheumatologist may advise increasing the prednisone dose to 20 mg a day for a few days and then tapering the dose down slowly over the next week or two. Or the person is armed with their sick-day rules (table 26.1) and increases their own steroids. Meanwhile, the internist prescribes an influenza antibiotic. Within a day or two, the person is feeling markedly better.

This temporary increase in steroid dose is called a "stress dose." If they do not take this added stress dose, they will feel much sicker for a longer time.

Whenever you have been on steroids for more than a few weeks, you should consider the possibility that you may have adrenal insufficiency. If you ever go through a period of stress, such as an infection, have significant trauma, or are preparing for surgery, always call your rheumatologist to see if you should increase your steroids or take extra steroids on your own, per the sick-day rules. Table 26.1 explains how to take increased steroids during these episodes. Talk to your doctor to discuss specific recommendations.

LUPUS IN FOCUS

Fasting and adrenal insufficiency

Fasting should be avoided by people with significant adrenal insufficiency. This can pose a problem for periods of fasting that are fundamental to religious observance (such as Ramadan for Muslims). Guidelines from the *Indian Journal of Endocrinology* published in 2012 and 2020 indicate that patients with mild adrenal insufficiency may safely practice fasting as long as they are educated about what to do if they begin to feel ill. Patients with more significant adrenal insufficiency should probably abstain from fasting. Most religions that encourage fasting, including Islam, do not encourage fasting if it harmful to the individual's health. This is important. Everyone with any degree of adrenal insufficiency should be evaluated by their physician several months before fasting and receive recommendations about proceeding.

Of course, doctors cannot prevent patients from fasting for occasions such as Ramadan. If you are someone who would fast against the advice of your physician, you must let them know. Be honest and ask for education and proper tools to use during fasting. These can include "sick day rules" and having injectable steroids at hand that can be given in the case of an emergency. It is good for those who practice Ramadan to obtain a copy of the 2012 or 2020 guidelines for reference (found at lupusencyclopedia.com/references, Siddiqui et al., or ask your endocrinologist).

Table 26.1 Sick-Day Rules for Adrenal Insufficiency

Situation	Action
Fever >100.4 or other minor illness or infections	Take 2–3 times your current steroid dose for 3 days or until illness has resolved; then return to previous dose.
Moderate illness or illness with vomiting	Take 2–3 times your current steroid dose for 2–3 days or until illness has resolved. If you vomit within 1 hour of taking your medication, repeat the dose. If you cannot do the above, use an injectable steroid and call an ambulance or immediately head to the nearest urgent care center.
Severe illness where you cannot tolerate pills or have a significant injury (broken bones, gunshot wounds, a fall from a height, etc.)	Use your injectable steroid and call an ambulance or head to the nearest urgent care center immediately.
Surgery	You may need more steroids before and after surgery. Ask your doctor.
Fasting (such as for religious and health reasons)	Strongly consider not fasting; it is better for your health. Ask your doctor.

Steroid Withdrawal

Another problem that can develop while reducing steroid doses is steroid withdrawal. This condition tends to occur when a person who has been taking steroids for a long time decreases the dose or completely stops the drug.

Usually, after a person has been on steroids for more than a few weeks, it is essential to decrease the dosage slowly (called a steroid taper). This is where the art of medicine plays a more critical role than the science of medicine. All bodies (and adrenal glands) react differently to taking steroids and to tapering them. A safe steroid taper depends greatly on the doctor's experience. After the dose is decreased to 7 mg a day and lower, the taper often needs to be done slowly enough to allow the adrenal glands to become more active, stronger, and larger. They must learn to start making their own cortisol-like steroids again. If the taper is done correctly, the patient is not likely to have any symptoms of adrenal insufficiency. If it is done too quickly, adrenal insufficiency symptoms, such as fatigue and lightheadedness, may occur (table 26.2). The affected person experiences steroid withdrawal symptoms, which are the same as adrenal insufficiency symptoms.

These symptoms can occur gradually, making it more difficult to pinpoint the steroid taper as the cause. I have seen this happen in several patients. In one situation, a patient who had been on steroids for several years for lupus nephritis (chapter 12) and whose nephritis went into remission with treatment was on a slow steroid taper. After

Table 26.2 Adrenal Insufficiency Symptoms

- Fatigue
- Weakness
- Loss of appetite
- Upset stomach, nausea, stomach pain
- Weight loss
- Body aches and pains
- Light-headedness
- Depression, confusion
- Longer recovery from mild infections such as colds

getting down to 3 mg of prednisone a day, she came in for her regular office visit. She had previously gained a lot of weight on steroids and was now happy about losing her prednisone weight. But she had absolutely no energy, had decreased appetite, was depressed and light-headed, and had headaches. It would be easy to mistake these as symptoms of depression. In her case, they were not. They were symptoms of adrenal insufficiency from taking too low a dosage of steroids. Increasing the dosage was the answer. Initially, she was very discouraged by the prospect. But after increasing her prednisone by merely 1 mg (up to 4 mg daily), she felt markedly better, like a new person. Even this tiny increase made a big difference in resolving her symptoms of adrenal insufficiency. After that, we were able to proceed with a much slower steroid taper, eventually getting her completely off steroids.

A person who has been on prednisone for a couple of months may be able to safely taper off the steroid within a few weeks. Another person on prednisone for a year or two may take a few months to a couple of years. It often takes trial and error for the patient and physician to know how quickly to taper steroids. While you are going down on your dose, if you feel adrenal insufficiency symptoms (table 26.2), it is essential to communicate this to your rheumatologist so that the steroids can be tapered a little bit more slowly. Most of our patients who have been on steroids for a while realize that if they taper their steroids and develop these symptoms, they should increase the prednisone back to the earlier dose at which they felt fine.

It can be challenging to know how quickly to taper steroids. It can be frustrating for the patient (who usually wants to get off them). The good news is that the adrenal glands work again in almost everyone, although this can occasionally take much longer than anticipated.

Steroid amounts needed to develop adrenal insufficiency vary from person to person. Doctors have some rules of thumb that help them decide which patients are at highest risk (table 26.3). These rules are not set in stone. For example, some people can develop adrenal insufficiency after taking doses lower than 10 mg a day for a few weeks. Whether or not someone develops adrenal insufficiency also varies depending on how long the steroid is taken. For example, a person who has been on just 9 mg of prednisone a day for 3 months will most likely develop adrenal insufficiency.

Table 26.3 Factors Leading to Probable Adrenal Insufficiency from Steroids

- Taking 20 mg a day of prednisone (or 16 mg a day of methylprednisolone) for 3 weeks or longer
- Taking any dose of steroids (excluding Rayos) in the evening for 3 weeks or longer
- Gaining weight or becoming puffy from steroids (called Cushingoid, chapter 31)

Taking Steroids

It is essential to take steroids (except Rayos, discussed below) in the morning, right after awakening, rather than at nighttime. When steroids are taken in the morning, they are much less likely to cause adrenal insufficiency. This is because the pituitary gland secretes the most amount of ACTH in the evening. Steroids reduce this ACTH secretion when taken at night, resulting in the adrenal glands not being activated as much by ACTH and causing subsequent adrenal gland shrinkage.

The sooner you take this medication in the morning when you get up, the better it will work, and the fewer side effects you will get. However, if you miss your steroid dose in the morning, take it later (even at nighttime). This is far better than not taking it at all. Missing a daily dose of steroids could cause problems with your lupus becoming more active or cause you to develop adrenal insufficiency symptoms that day or the following day.

If you cannot take your steroids due to nausea and vomiting, contact your doctor to get your steroids through injectable methods. If you are diagnosed with adrenal insufficiency, you should ask your doctor to prescribe injectable steroids to be used for emergencies, along with instructions on how to use the medication. The injectable steroid is commonly either 4 mg of dexamethasone or 100 mg of hydrocortisone (these two doses have similar effects). It is essential to familiarize yourself and your family with proper mixing and injecting them. It may be difficult to figure this out during an emergency.

Although steroids are usually taken in the morning, there are several situations in which doctors prescribe a nighttime dose. For example, if you have a severe SLE flare, taking steroids two to three times a day is more effective than taking them all in the morning. Thus, if you are prescribed 40 mg of prednisone, taking 20 mg twice a day is stronger and works faster than taking all 40 mg in the morning. This is because prednisone does not last long in the body.

When all 40 mg is taken in the morning, it reaches its greatest effects about two hours later. After that, it gradually decreases and is eliminated from the body. There is little to no prednisone for about seven to eight hours each night. This allows the adrenal glands to have some time to function correctly (not be suppressed by prednisone) each night. The downside is that there is little to no prednisone left to decrease inflammation starting in the late afternoon.

On the other hand, 20 mg taken twice a day produces a significant amount of prednisone within the body twenty-four hours a day. This is excellent at reducing inflammation but at the cost of more side effects. Therefore, doctors usually prescribe two daily doses for only a short period.

Another common reason for asking patients to take an evening dose of steroids is to help with morning stiffness and pain from lupus arthritis. SLE inflammation (especially of the joints) is often worse first thing in the morning after awakening. In this instance, doctors may ask patients to take a small amount (such as 1 mg to 3 mg of prednisone) at nighttime, although even this small nightly dose increases the chances of adrenal insufficiency.

A safer and more effective alternative is to take the delayed-release form of predni-sone called Rayos. When taken at night before bed, it is absorbed slowly by the intes-tines, reaching its peak effects around 6½ hours later. This helps morning pain and stiffness from SLE inflammatory arthritis (chapter 7).

If you are in one of the groups in table 26.3, consider wearing a medical alert brace-let, necklace, or card that says you take steroids or have adrenal insufficiency. These can be ordered from most pharmacies and drug stores. Ask your doctor if you are unsure. If you end up in an emergency room for any type of illness, trauma, or emergency sur-gery, the medical personnel will realize that you require extra steroids to survive the stressful event. This could potentially be lifesaving.

The bottom line is that anyone who has been on steroids for more than a few weeks is at risk of adrenal insufficiency (table 26.3). You should not decrease steroids too quickly, you should not stop them abruptly, and you should take extra steroids during stress (table 26.1). You should also consider wearing a medical alert bracelet. If you fol-low these rules, you should do very well with minimal to no problems.

KEY POINTS TO REMEMBER

1. Adrenal insufficiency occurs when someone has been on steroids for a prolonged period. The adrenal glands atrophy (shrink in size) and cannot produce enough of the body's life-sustaining steroids.

2. Those who are at greatest risk for adrenal insufficiency are noted in table 26.3. If you are unsure, ask your doctor.

3. Take steroids (except Rayos) as soon as you wake up in the morning (instead of at nighttime). This decreases the chances of adrenal insufficiency. Take steroids in the evening only if your doctor tells you to or if you missed your morning dose.

4. People with possible adrenal insufficiency must taper (decrease) their steroid dose slowly, especially when down to 7 mg of prednisone a day or less. People should never suddenly stop steroids on their own. Always follow your doctor's instructions.

5. People with adrenal insufficiency should take stress doses of steroids during stressful events, such as infections, after trauma, or during surgery (table 26.1).

6. If you develop adrenal insufficiency symptoms (table 26.2) as you decrease steroids, let your doctor know ASAP because your taper probably needs slowing down.

7. Wear a medical alert bracelet if you are in table 26.3 or if your doctor recommends it.

8. If you have adrenal insufficiency, ask your doctor for injectable steroids to keep on hand. Use this during emergencies or if too sick to take your steroids by mouth.

Fibromyalgia

Rukmini Konatalapalli, MD, *Contributing Editor*

Are you tired and achy? Have memory problems or headaches? If so, you may have fibromyalgia (FM, pronounced fy-broh-my-AL'-juh). Fibromyalgia is a painful condition related to overactive pain nerves. It is often accompanied by other problems such as headaches, insomnia, fatigue, forgetfulness, and stomach upset (table 27.1). Although it affects up to 30% of SLE patients, it is not due to lupus inflammation, so it can persist during SLE remission. This chapter describes fibromyalgia and its treatments.

Fibromyalgia Symptoms

The hallmark symptom of FM is multiple areas of pain and tenderness (termed multisite or widespread pain). For some, it begins with pain all over the body, while in others it may start in just one body part. For example, someone could be diagnosed with plantar fasciitis as a cause of their foot pain, then tennis elbow as a cause of elbow pain, and then costochondritis (breastbone cartilage inflammation) for severe chest pain. However, over time, more body parts can be affected. Eventually, it becomes clear that FM caused all these pains instead of the individual diagnoses. People with FM often say, "I hurt all over" or "I feel like I have the flu." It can cause severe fatigue, muscle and joint pains, and headaches, just like the flu.

Fatigue and difficulty sleeping are the other most common problems in FM. The sleep problems cause many FM patients to say, "No matter how much I sleep, after waking up, I feel like I was run over by a truck, and I still have no energy." This is called nonrestorative sleep because even many hours of sleep do not restore their energy.

People with fibromyalgia often have difficulty doing normal activities. Even minor activities, like light household chores, can worsen their pain and fatigue.

Each person with FM has different problems with different severities. Some have just mild achiness in their muscles and joints and do not have memory, sleep, or fatigue problems. Others have most of these symptoms to a severe, disabling degree.

FM can also cause problems commonly seen in systemic autoimmune diseases such as SLE. FM can cause Raynaud's phenomenon (where the fingers turn pale and blue with exposure to cold) and dry mouth and eyes (as in Sjögren's disease, chapter 14).

One of the most common reasons for a patient to see a rheumatologist is for a positive antinuclear antibody (ANA) test. While ANA is the most essential initial test to help diagnose SLE, FM is much more common in ANA-positive patients than SLE is. Since

Table 27.1 Common Fibromyalgia Problems

Multiple areas of pain (joints, muscles, bones, head, spine, abdomen, pelvis)

Muscle spasms

Skin and body tenderness

Tingling or numbness

Stomach upset, diarrhea, constipation (such as irritable bowel syndrome)

Fatigue

Difficulty sleeping

Non-restorative sleep

Memory and concentration problems ("fibro fog")

Ringing in the ears

Dizziness

Increased urination frequency and urination pain

Raynaud's phenomenon

Dry mouth and dry eyes

Restless legs syndrome (difficulty getting the legs comfortable in bed)

Jaw pain (as in temporomandibular joint disorder)

LUPUS IN FOCUS

Chronic fatigue syndrome and fibromyalgia

Chronic fatigue syndrome is also called myalgic encephalomyelitis/chronic fatigue syndrome (ME/CSF). The Institute of Medicine (IOM) defines ME/CSF as having severe fatigue most of the time, for at least six months. The affected person must also feel bad (malaise) after physical or mental activity, not feel refreshed after sleep, feel worse while standing upright, and/or have difficulty thinking. Like FM, ME/CFS can cause headaches, sleep problems, memory difficulties, and moodiness. Most patients with ME/CFS meet tender point criteria (described below) for FM, and 70% of FM patients meet the IOM diagnostic criteria for CFS.

both FM and SLE can cause pain, fatigue, tingling of the hands and feet, Raynaud's phenomenon, dry mouth, and eyes, figuring out if someone has FM or SLE or both can sometimes be difficult.

Since FM and SLE can cause similar symptoms, many FM patients are incorrectly diagnosed with SLE. They are even mistakenly treated with immunosuppressants and steroids because of the misdiagnosis.

One helpful clue is that lupus arthritis rarely affects the neck, back, buttocks, or sides of the hips. If these areas hurt, then FM is more likely. A blood test called the AVISE Lupus Test (chapter 4) may also be helpful. One study showed that it could help distinguish between the two.

Since FM can cause many problems, it is common to see many different specialists before a correct diagnosis is made. This includes gynecologists, nerve specialists (neurologists), heart specialists (cardiologists), lung specialists (pulmonologists), bladder specialists (urologists), dentists, and stomach doctors (gastroenterologists). These specialists may order a wide variety of tests, including ultrasounds, CT scans, magnetic resonance imaging (MRIs), upper and lower endoscopies (looking into the stomach and intestines), cystoscopy (looking into the bladder), pelvic exams, and nerve tests, including nerve conduction study/electromyogram (NCS/EMG, chapter 13) tests. Most of these end up being unhelpful.

Some FM patients undergo unnecessary joint and spine surgeries. Bulging discs are common, affecting one out of three "healthy" 35-year-olds and almost everyone 50 and over. When x-rays and MRIs show these findings in someone with severe FM back and neck pain, their pain can be mistakenly attributed to the degenerating discs. Spine surgery can be done without helping their pain.

Causes of Fibromyalgia

FM often occurs in people who have had traumatic events. It is not uncommon to develop it after a motor vehicle accident or surgery. Some people will develop it after having a severe infection such as the flu, mononucleosis, or Lyme disease.

Many people with FM have a history of profound psychological stress and abuse. Emotional, physical, and sexual abuse occur more frequently in FM patients than in those without FM. Why people suffering from trauma are more prone to FM is unknown.

Most people do not volunteer this information to their doctors, as most patients do not realize its importance. In addition, admitting abuse can be emotionally stressful and embarrassing. If a doctor discusses abuse, many people refuse to accept that their physical symptoms may be related to it. However, experts agree that people who have experienced trauma have a better chance of improving when they get psychological and psychiatric assistance. Pain rarely improves otherwise.

Although FM can cause severe pain in the body's muscles, joints, and bones, the pain is not due to damage to these structures. Our bodies are programmed to tell us there is pain when damage or injury occurs. For example, you burn your finger on the stove. Your body (via the nervous system) alerts your brain of the burn injury by way of severe pain so that you pull your hand away from the stove. This is the normal function of pain.

Most body areas have special sensory nerves that sense injury and damage. They let the brain know that an injury is happening, causing the body to respond appropriately (such as pulling back the burned finger). The spinal nerves tell the brain where the damage or injury is occurring, and in tiny fractions of a second, the brain sends neurotransmitter messages along different nerves down the spinal cord, alerting the appropriate muscles to withdraw the injured body part from the injuring source.

Suppose the injured body part (such as the burned finger) is damaged after being pulled away. In that case, the sensory nerves continue to note this injury and send pain-sensing neurotransmitters (nerve chemical messages) to the brain. If this were to continue until the body part completely healed, we would be in constant pain for a long time. However, the body protects us from sensing continuous pain by releasing other neurotransmitters in the brain and spinal cord (such as serotonin and norepinephrine).

These neurotransmitters calm down the pain messages coming up from the body's sensory nerves, so we do not feel severe, constant pain while the body part is healing.

In FM, pain nerves function abnormally. They may send these chemical messengers to each other even if there is no injury. Substance P is one of the neurotransmitters sent from one nerve to another to tell the brain that there is pain in the body. In FM, substance P levels in the spine are two to three times higher than normal.

In addition, pain messages can be persistent. While neurotransmitters, such as serotonin and norepinephrine in the brain, normally calm down pain, these helpful neurotransmitters are reduced in FM, allowing the pain nerves to stay overactive. This combination of overactive pain nerves plus a lack of inhibitory neurotransmitters to calm down the nerves is called "central pain amplification." It can be initiated by stresses such as SLE, arthritis, accidents, surgery, infections, and abuse, among others. Once started, it can be difficult to stop.

The neurotransmitter abnormalities help explain why 30% to 50% of FM patients also have depression or anxiety. People with depression and/or anxiety typically lack proper amounts of serotonin and norepinephrine, just like those who have FM. These imbalances can lead to mood problems, worrying, sleep problems, and fatigue. It is important to treat anxiety and depression as well as the FM. If you have FM, take the screening tests for depression and anxiety disorder (tables 13.3 and 13.5).

FM can run in families. If someone has FM, their parents, siblings, and children are around 10 times more likely to have it as well. Many different genes have been identified that occur more often in FM families. Most of them are involved with pain nerve pathways and neurochemical imbalances.

Medical Test Abnormalities

FM cannot be diagnosed by blood tests (except maybe the FM/a test, discussed below), x-rays, MRIs, and so on. However, abnormalities can be identified in research studies, using sophisticated tools that are too expensive for daily routine medical practices.

Some FM patients have small fiber neuropathy (see chapter 13), causing burning pain, tingling, numb feelings, and lightning-shock pains. A skin biopsy by dermatologists can show a decrease in microscopic nerves in the skin in these patients. However, FM experts do not recommend skin biopsies for small fiber neuropathy since the findings do not change the treatment. Although nerve symptoms of small fiber neuropathy can occur in FM, other nerve tests (such as NCS-EMG studies) do not show problems with larger nerves.

LUPUS IN FOCUS

Autonomic dysfunction and fibromyalgia

Just like SLE patients, people with FM can also have autonomic nervous system problems (chapter 13), which cause issues like dizziness, heart palpitations, Raynaud's phenomenon, and dry eyes and mouth.

Many people with FM do not go into the deepest parts of sleep. The brain emits different electrical signals, which can be measured by a test called an electroencephalogram (EEG). While awake, the brain exhibits much electrical activity (called alpha waves) on EEG. While sleeping, these alpha waves disappear as the person goes into deep sleep.

One of the deepest stages of sleep identified on EEG is stage IV sleep. Sleep studies show that FM patients develop alpha waves (signs of wakefulness) during this crucial deep sleep stage. These FM patients are not sleeping deeply at all. This helps explain their nonrestorative sleep. Although this is a typical finding in FM patients, EEG is not performed to help diagnose FM. This finding can be seen in other conditions, and like skin nerve biopsies, the results do not affect treatment decisions.

Other sleep problems can be associated with FM. Obstructive sleep apnea (OSA) occurs more often in FM. If you have FM, you should take the STOP questionnaire for OSA (table 6.4). If you score two or more points on the questionnaire, you should have a sleep study. OSA is treated differently than FM nonrestorative sleep problems.

Diagnosing Fibromyalgia

In 2019, the Analgesic, Anesthetic, and Addiction Clinical Trial Translations Innovations Opportunities and Networks-American Pain Society Pain Taxonomy (AAPT) developed FM criteria that can easily identify FM. Simply answer the following two questions as "yes" or "no."

1. Have you had pain in six of the following areas for three months or longer? Circle each one where you have had pain: head, left arm, right arm, left leg, right leg, upper chest, abdomen, upper back or spine, lower back or spine

2. Have you had severe sleep problems OR fatigue for three months or longer?

You probably meet FM diagnostic criteria if you answered "yes" to both 1 and 2. This does not exclude your having an additional pain-causing condition. For example, you could have numerous joints affected by osteoarthritis (OA, degenerative arthritis from aging) and meet these criteria, in which case you may have both FM and OA. If someone has both conditions, it is essential that both be treated. If only the OA is treated, the pain and other problems from FM will most likely continue.

The same is true for SLE patients who have FM. Thus, an SLE patient with FM may have their SLE go into remission on hydroxychloroquine, but have ongoing severe fatigue and pain from FM. In that case, the FM should also be treated. The ongoing symptoms of pain and fatigue are also called type 2 symptoms (chapter 5). They have non-inflammatory causes (overactive pain nerves) and do not respond to immunosuppressants.

Above, we said that you probably meet FM diagnostic criteria if you answered "yes" to both questions in the self-survey—not that you definitely have FM if you do. These diagnostic criteria are not 100% foolproof. On the other hand, some people can have FM yet not meet the criteria. If you answered "yes" to both questions, show your primary care doctor and rheumatologist the results, and see what they think. Be aware that as of February 2023, when this chapter was written, many physicians were unaware of these new criteria.

The doctor's first clue that someone may have FM is their history. They often have pain in multiple areas, fatigue, nonrestorative sleep, and/or trouble with memory and concentration. People with uncontrolled thyroid problems, infections, metabolic disorders, and other conditions can have similar symptoms. Therefore, additional testing is usually done. If one of these other conditions is diagnosed, treated, and the symptoms resolve, then it was not FM.

A physical exam is important. If the person with pain has arthritis, the physical exam usually detects it. The affected joints are typically tender, swollen, or have decreased range of motion. In FM, however, there is often tenderness in places other than the joints. This is one of the most helpful clues for diagnosing FM. A person with just arthritis will have tender joints on examination. A person with arthritis plus FM can have tenderness in and around the joints, muscles, skin, and on top of bones, ligaments, and tendons (chapter 7). People with FM and no arthritis can also have tenderness in the joints and these other places.

In 1990, the American College of Rheumatology developed FM classification criteria to ensure that doctors worldwide include similar patients in FM research studies. To diagnose FM with these criteria, the person must have had pain on both sides of the body, above and below the waist, for at least three months and at least 11 out of 18 possible tender points defined in the criteria.

However, 15% of FM patients do not fulfill these classification criteria. Tender points can fluctuate. A person with FM may have a lot of pain with many tender points on some days and few, even no tender points on good days. Not everyone with FM will have pain all over. Some will have pain mainly on the right side of the body. Others will have it on the left side or in the back, neck, and arms instead of the legs. Although they have FM, they would not meet the criteria.

While doctors look for these tender points to help diagnose FM, some people with FM can have fewer than 11 tender points. This is why FM experts established the AAPT diagnostic criteria described at the beginning of this section.

After a physical exam, a doctor will most likely do blood tests and possibly x-rays to look for other causes of widespread pain. Some medical conditions can act precisely like FM. An example is polymyalgia rheumatica (PMR), which causes severe pain in older people. However, PMR responds miraculously to small amounts of prednisone. FM, on the other hand, rarely does.

Fibromyalgia Treatments

Many therapies can help FM (table 27.2). Most patients end up needing a combination of non-drug treatments and drugs; those without depression, anxiety, or sleep problems have a better chance of responding to non-drug therapies alone.

Non-Drug Treatments

People with FM who learn about the condition are more likely to follow their doctors' recommendations and get better.

Unfortunately, FM tends to be a chronic disease, meaning that it lasts for years, if not the rest of the person's life. There is no cure. FM patients often must deal with discomfort, fatigue, and insomnia for a long time. Occasionally, though, FM can go away on its own.

FM patients should direct their efforts toward improving lifestyle habits and expectations in dealing with chronic pain. FM educational groups can help. They can also keep FM patients updated in research and treatments. One of these groups is the National Fibromyalgia Association (www.fmaware.org).

Exercise is the most important FM treatment. Exercise reconditions the muscles, reduces stress and depression, helps relaxation, improves sleep, and improves

---

Table 27.2 Fibromyalgia Treatments

Education

Exercise (chapters 7 and 38)

      Regular low-impact aerobic exercise

    Stretching exercises

      Tai chi, yoga, pilates

Mindfulness (chapter 39)

Measures to improve energy (table 6.1)

Sleep hygiene (table 6.2)

Treat conditions that worsen fibromyalgia

      Take the self-survey for depression (table 13.5).

      Take the self-survey for anxiety disorder (table 13.3).

    Take the self-survey for sleep apnea (table 6.4).

Improve memory (table 13.4)

Cognitive-behavioral therapy

Psychotherapy and counseling aimed at previous abuse

Biofeedback

Acupuncture (chapter 39)

Hydrotherapy and balneotherapy

Prescription fibromyalgia drugs

---

neurotransmitter imbalances. Exercise also works better for FM than taking the drugs noted below. If you genuinely want to get better, you must force yourself to exercise.

The resistance to exercising is understandable. How can you exercise when you are in severe pain, have muscle spasms, and fatigue? From personal experience with our patients, we know that they improve when they force themselves to exercise regularly. Many people have an "ah hah" moment when they feel better when regularly exercising. When they stop exercising, they feel worse.

You usually are not harming or injuring your joints and muscles when you exercise. Muscle pain and spasms are normal for everyone (including world-class athletes) when beginning a new exercise regimen or increasing exercise. Although it is easy to think you are injuring yourself and stop exercising when you feel pain, it is essential to remind yourself that pain will happen. If you are fearful that you are injuring yourself, ask your doctor to send you to a physical therapist. They are exercise experts. A physical therapist can evaluate your physical health (joint range of motion, strength, and so on) and design a safe and effective exercise program.

The best way to start exercising is to *start low, go up slow*. Begin with significantly easier exercises than the norm for your age, gender, and body size. Don't forget warm-up and cool-down exercises. One study found that increasing intensity by 10% every two weeks was tolerable and effective for FM patients. If you start with 10 minutes a day on the elliptical machine, increase the time to 11 minutes after 2 weeks. If you perform 10 repetitions of biceps curls with 5-pound dumbbells, increase this to 11 repetitions after 2 weeks.

Hydrotherapy, which involves physical therapy in warm water, and balneotherapy, which consists of mud and spa therapy, can be effective, according to a review (as of 2019) of 10 research studies. But these can be costly and time-consuming. They lasted an average of four hours for each session in these studies.

Several kinds of psychological therapies can help. Cognitive-behavioral therapy, for example, teaches psychological practices to reduce pain. These include using mental imagery, relaxation, self-hypnosis, breathing exercises, and stress reduction techniques.

People with FM and a history of severe abuse rarely get significantly better if they do not deal with that abuse. For these people, it is crucial to get help from an expert in abusive disorders, such as a psychiatrist, psychologist, or sociologist.

LUPUS IN FOCUS

Not ready to exercise?

A 2019 Spanish study showed that FM patients who engaged in light physical activity for 30 minutes a day daily, instead of sitting, ended up with less pain and a better quality of life. Choose 30 minutes daily to do something easy and enjoyable, such as light gardening (nothing strenuous) or slow walking. After a few weeks, slowly start to add in low-impact aerobic exercise (on an elliptical machine, or stationary bike, for example, or swimming), strengthening exercises (chapter 38), tai chi, or yoga (chapter 39).

How good are the FM treatments?

In 2019, the European League Against Rheumatism (EULAR) evaluated the research for FM therapies. They graded the quality of the treatment research results as follows:

Strong evidence to support its use: exercise

Weak evidence to support its use: mindfulness, stress reduction techniques, yoga, tai chi, qigong, acupuncture (all found in chapter 38); hydrotherapy, balneotherapy, cognitive behavioral therapy, and some drugs (duloxetine, pregabalin, tramadol, amitriptyline, and cyclobenzaprine).

Not enough evidence to recommend usage: biofeedback, capsaicin, hypnosis, massage therapy, S-adenosyl-L-methionine (SAMe, an over-the-counter supplement), NSAIDs (chapter 36), SSRIs (discussed below), and other antidepressants.

Strong evidence AGAINST its use: chiropractic therapy (safety concerns), growth hormone, sodium oxybate (Xyrem), opioids stronger than tramadol, and steroids.

Drug Treatments

The most effective FM drugs improve nerve and brain neurotransmitter imbalances. Since these are like the chemical imbalances in depression, many of these drugs are antidepressants.

Anti-seizure drugs are also used. Seizures (epilepsy) occur when the brain's nerves are overactive, causing uncontrolled body movements, loss of consciousness, behavioral changes, or hallucinations. Anti-seizure drugs work by calming down these overactive nerves. This is also how they help with FM—by calming down the brain's nerves.

Three drugs are FDA-approved for FM: pregabalin (Lyrica), DULoxetine (Cymbalta), and milnacipran (Savella). None is proven to be better than the others. The FM medicines that are not FDA-approved have cheaper generic equivalents and appear to be as effective as the FDA-approved drugs.

Most arthritis pain drugs, other than tramadol, have not been shown to help FM. Other scheduled opioid drugs (narcotics) should not be used. They disrupt the sleep cycle and decrease the usefulness of non-drug treatments. Plus, although they initially help pain, they do nothing for the disorder itself, and several studies have shown them to worsen FM symptoms over time. Also, if narcotics are taken for pain, the body becomes tolerant of them. This means that the original dose becomes less effective, and more is needed to get the same effect as previous lower doses. Many people become addicted to them.

FM can be challenging to treat. Doctors may need to try various drugs until they find an effective one. Sometimes a combination of drugs helps since they work through different mechanisms. For example, taking an antidepressant at night and an anti-seizure drug in the morning may work for one person, while using two antidepressants that work in two different ways may be better for another.

FM drugs (other than tramadol) must be taken regularly. Most are started at low doses and then increased gradually. Improving the chemical imbalances can take three to eight weeks, so it may take some time before you notice any changes. If there are no improvements after one or two months, the doctor typically increases the dose, changes the type of drug, or adds another FM drug.

The only times you should stop the drug is if your doctor asks you to or if you develop side effects. If you have side effects, contact your doctor. Withdrawal symptoms occur when you stop a drug that the body is used to too quickly. Nausea, insomnia, sweating, moodiness, stomach upset, body pain, and other side effects may occur.

The European League Against Rheumatism (EULAR) states that for severe pain, DULoxetine, pregabalin, or tramadol may be the best choices. For people with trouble sleeping, amitriptyline, cyclobenzaprine, or pregabalin may be better.

Of course, some people have tried everything and still have debilitating pain, profound fatigue, memory problems, and insomnia. There is a tremendous unmet need for better therapies. A lot of research is currently underway, and we hope that it results in better treatments.

Tricyclic Antidepressants (TCAs)

These are some of the most common drugs prescribed for FM. Amitriptyline is the most studied. They are generally given in much lower doses than those used for depression. The TCAs most used for FM include amitriptyline, nortriptyline (Pamelor), and desipramine (Norpramin).

Generic available: Yes.

How TCAs work: TCAs increase the effects of serotonin and norepinephrine, thereby decreasing brain pain nerve activity. They can take three to six weeks for the full benefit at any dose to help with pain and fatigue. Insomnia usually improves quickly.

Do not take if

- you have heart disease or seizures.

- you have closed-angle glaucoma (called angle-closure and narrow-angle glaucoma). Most people with glaucoma have open-angle glaucoma and can take TCAs.

LUPUS IN FOCUS

Other drugs studied for fibromyalgia

Drugs that have shown possible usefulness for FM in poor-quality, small studies include naltrexone (Vivitrol), memantine (Namenda), pramipexole (Mirapex), and quetiapine (SEROquel). More studies are needed.

Conflicting results have been seen with creatine and vitamin D. Some studies suggested possible benefits, while others did not.

FM research using pharmaceutical-grade cannabis and nabilone (Cesamet, a synthetic cannabinoid) had negative results.

Oxybate (Xyrem) is a controlled substance (potentially addictive) used to treat a sleep disorder called narcolepsy. It helped sleep, pain, and energy in several FM studies. The FDA and the European Medicines Agency rejected approval for FM treatment due to its numerous side effects and addictive tendencies.

Closed-angle is rare. It is usually safe if your closed-angle glaucoma has been surgically treated (ask your eye doctor).

• you take a monoamine oxidase inhibitor antidepressant; deadly side effects can occur.

Use caution when driving, climbing, or using machinery. Make sure you know how you react to the drug and that it does not make you drowsy or cause difficulty thinking.

Dosage: TCAs are best started at a low dose two to three hours before bedtime. The dose can be slowly increased over time if needed. They can cause a hungover, groggy feeling after awakening if taken too soon before bedtime.

If you miss a dose, it is usually best not to take it until the next evening. However, if you tolerate your TCA well, and it does not cause side effects, you could take one-half to a full amount right before you go to bed (instead of two hours before bed). Or take it as soon as you think about it the next day. Ask your doctor.

Alcohol/food interactions: Do not drink alcohol, which increases drowsiness, dizziness, and difficulty thinking.

Do not eat grapefruit or drink grapefruit juice, which increases TCA blood levels and side effects.

What to monitor while taking TCAs: If you are over 40, ensure that you have had an ECG to ensure your heart is OK before taking a TCA.

Potential side effects of TCAs: The most common side effects are dizziness, grogginess, and dry mouth. Others include difficulty thinking, confusion, fluid retention, weight gain, blurred vision, sweating, and problems with sexual function.

While taking TCAs, call your doctor immediately if you develop heart palpitations, fast heart rate, chest pain, or shortness of breath.

Pregnancy and breastfeeding: Some babies have withdrawal symptoms after delivery. The preferred TCAs to use during pregnancy are nortriptyline and desipramine. For insomnia, low doses of amitriptyline and imipramine are recommended. Higher doses of TCAs may be required during pregnancy due to increased metabolism.

TCAs are not recommended during breastfeeding.

Geriatric use: Older people are more sensitive to side effects. Nortriptyline is usually best tolerated.

TCAs and surgery: Ask your surgeon and anesthesiologist. Some experts recommend stopping tricyclic antidepressants 7 to 14 days before surgery to decrease the risk of heart problems.

LUPUS IN FOCUS

Drugs that interfere with sleep in fibromyalgia

Some antidepressants (doxepin, trazodone, and ramelteon) interfere with deep REM (rapid eye movement) sleep and should not be used in FM. Avoid benzodiazepines (such as lorazepam, Ativan, and Valium) for anxiety. They disrupt stage IV sleep and alter brain function the day after taken.

Financial aid for TCAs: Go to lupusencyclopedia.com/patient-resources. Also, go to www.goodrx.com or similar programs.

Selective Serotonin Reuptake Inhibitors

Selective serotonin reuptake inhibitors (SSRIs) are antidepressants. While some experts recommend them when patients fail TCAs, cyclobenzaprine, SNRIs, gabapentinoids, and tramadol, the European League Against Rheumatism FM Working Group" recommended against their use. SSRIs include fluoxetine (PROzac), paroxetine (Paxil, Brisdelle, Pexeva), fluvoxamine, and citalopram (Celexa).

Generic available: Yes.

How SSRIs work: Serotonin reduces the brain's sensation of pain. Serotonin is a neurotransmitter, meaning that it is a substance released by one nerve to send signals to other nerves. The nerve that originally produces the serotonin is also reabsorbing (or reuptaking, as the "reuptake" in the name of this drug group implies) serotonin to recycle it. SSRIs decrease the ability of the nerves to reabsorb (or reuptake) serotonin. This leads to increased brain serotonin, which calms down the brain's pain nerve signals.

FM patients have reduced brain serotonin activity, so pain messages sent to the brain are magnified and do not calm down as fast as they should. Since SSRIs increase brain serotonin, they may help some FM patients. It usually takes four to eight weeks for the full effects of improved pain, sleep, mood, and energy.

Do not to take SSRIs if

- you have severe liver or kidney disease.

- you take a monoamine oxidase inhibitor (a type of antidepressant); life-threatening side effects may occur.

- you have closed-angle glaucoma. See the TCA section above.

Use caution

- if you have bipolar mania.

- when driving, climbing, or using machinery. Make sure you know how you react to the drug and that it does not make you drowsy or cause difficulty thinking.

Dosage: This depends on the SSRI. People respond differently to different SSRIs. If an SSRI causes drowsiness, it is best taken at night. If an SSRI causes insomnia, it is best taken in the morning.

If you miss a dose, how you react to your SSRI and how often you take it determine what to do. If you take it every morning and know that it causes you insomnia (trouble sleeping) and you recall late in the day that you missed the dose, you may want to skip that day's dose. If you've missed the dose earlier in the day, you can take it as soon as you realize you did. Then resume your regular dosing the next day.

If you usually take it at nighttime because it makes you tired, take your next dosage the following evening if you miss your nighttime dose.

If you take it twice a day, and it has been just a few hours since you missed your dose, take the dose you missed as soon as you realize it and take your next dose at the regular time. If you forget your dose later in the day, just skip the dose and resume your regular schedule the next day.

Ask your prescribing doctor.

Alcohol/food interactions: Avoid alcohol; it increases side effects. They can be taken with or without food.

What to monitor while taking SSRIs: Blood tests for kidney function and liver function should be checked before starting SSRIs. Lower doses may be needed for people with decreased kidney or liver function. Blood tests are not required after starting these drugs.

Potential side effects of SSRIs: The most common side effects are drowsiness, weight gain, anxiety, dizziness, insomnia, headaches, dry mouth, blurred vision, nausea, rash, tremors, stomach upset, constipation, and problems with sexual function.

While taking SSRIs,

- inform your doctor of any side effects.

- use a slow taper if you are taken off the drug to prevent withdrawal side effects.

Pregnancy and breastfeeding: SSRIs can be taken during pregnancy if there is significant benefit. Many experts consider sertraline as the SSRI of choice in pregnancy. Some studies suggest possible heart problems, pulmonary hypertension, birth defects, and drug withdrawal problems in newborns with some SSRIs.

Use with caution or not at all during breastfeeding.

Geriatric use: Usually, lower doses are used due to increased side effects.

SSRIs and surgery: Ask your surgeon and anesthesiologist. SSRIs can increase bleeding and may react with anesthetics. They may need to be stopped several weeks before surgery.

Financial aid for SSRIs: Go to lupusencyclopedia.com/patient-resources. Also, go to www.goodrx.com or similar programs.

Dual Uptake Inhibitor Antidepressants (SNRIs)

Dual uptake inhibitors are antidepressants; they are also called serotonin-norepinephrine reuptake inhibitors (SNRIs). DULoxetine (Cymbalta) and milnacipran (Savella) are FDA-approved for FM. Venlafaxine (Effexor XR) is not, although studies suggest that it may help FM.

Generic available: Yes for all except Savella. (Savella generics could become available in 2023).

How SNRIs work: SNRIs prevent the reuptake of serotonin and norepinephrine. The way they work is similar to how SSRIs work (see above), except on norepinephrine as well as serotonin. Improved pain, sleep, and energy can take up to four to eight weeks at any particular dose.

Do not take if

- you have severe liver or kidney disease.

- you take a monoamine oxidase inhibitor antidepressant; life-threatening side effects may occur.

- you have untreated closed-angle glaucoma. See the TCA section above.

Use caution

- tell your doctor if you have a history of seizures or epilepsy.

- when driving, climbing, or using machinery, make sure you know how you react to the drug and that it does not make you drowsy or cause difficulty thinking.

Dosage: Varies depending on the SNRI. Everyone responds differently. Cymbalta is usually best taken after the evening meal. However, if it causes difficulty sleeping, it should be taken after breakfast.

If you miss a dose, see this section under SSRIs, above.

Alcohol/food interactions: Avoid alcohol; it can increase side effects. They can be taken with or without food.

What to monitor while taking SNRIs:

- blood tests for kidney function and liver function before starting. A lower dose of the SNRI might be needed in people with decreased kidney or liver function.

- blood pressure, glucose, and cholesterol should be monitored while taking SNRIs.

Potential side effects of SNRIs: Similar to SSRIs. High blood pressure, elevated glucose, and elevated cholesterol levels can also occur. SNRIs may worsen bipolar disorder.

While taking SNRIs,

- inform your doctor if any side effects occur.

- use a slow taper if you are taken off the drug to prevent withdrawal side effects.

Pregnancy and breastfeeding: SNRIs can be taken if the benefits outweigh the risks. If you get pregnant taking Savella, contact the Savella Pregnancy Registry (877-643-3010 or savellapregnancyregistry.com).

Do not use SNRIs during breastfeeding.

Geriatric use: Usually, lower doses are used due to increased side effects.

SNRIs and surgery: Ask your surgeon and anesthesiologist. SNRIs can usually be continued up to the day before surgery.

Financial aid for SNRIs: Go to lupusencyclopedia.com/patient-resources. For Savella, call 844-424-6727 or go to allergansavingscard.com/savella. Also, go to www.goodrx.com or similar programs.

Website: For Savella, go to www.savella.com.

Anti-Seizure (Antiepileptic) Medicines

Anti-seizure (antiepileptic) drugs called gabapentinoids can help FM. Pregabalin (Lyrica) is FDA-approved. Gabapentin (Neurontin) can also help FM.

Pregabalin is classified as a controlled substance in the United States. Most doctors will require you to read and sign a pain contract.

Although gabapentin is not a controlled substance per the US federal government (as of 2023), Alabama, Kentucky, Michigan, North Dakota, Tennessee, Virginia, and West Virginia consider gabapentin a controlled substance. Connecticut, the District of Columbia, Indiana, Kansas, Massachusetts, Minnesota, Nebraska, New Jersey, Ohio, Oregon, Utah, and Wyoming require pharmacies to report prescriptions in the state database. One reason is that gabapentin is often mixed with cocaine and heroin and is commonly found in the blood of narcotic death victims.

Generic available: Yes.

How pregabalin and gabapentin work: They decrease over-activity of pain nerves that send too many pain messages to the brain.

Use caution

- if you have a history of drug or alcohol abuse, there is an increased risk of drug dependency with pregabalin.

- if you have decreased kidney function, lower doses may be needed.

- when driving, climbing, or using machinery, make sure you know how you react to the drug and that it does not make you drowsy or cause difficulty thinking.

Dosage: They are taken one to three times a day. Both are often started at a low dose and increased slowly. Gabapentin also comes in a once-daily, slow-release form, Gralise, taken with the evening meal.

If you miss a dose, see SSRIs.

Alcohol/food interactions: Avoid alcohol; it increases side effects.

Gabapentin can be taken with or without food. Pregabalin and Gralise are best taken with food (Gralise with the evening meal).

What to monitor while taking pregabalin or gabapentin: Regular urine or blood drug tests are needed to ensure that you are not taking other controlled substances and that you are taking your medicine.

Potential side effects of pregabalin and gabapentin: The most common side effects are edema (ankle swelling), weight gain, dizziness, drowsiness, dry mouth, concentration problems, increased appetite, and blurred vision.

While taking pregabalin or gabapentin,

- alert your doctor of any side effects.

- do not abruptly stop the drug. It is best to decrease the dose gradually.

Pregnancy and breastfeeding: Both drugs can be used in pregnancy if the risks outweigh the benefits. They are probably best to avoid while breastfeeding.

Geriatric use: Lower doses are usually used due to increased side effects.

Pregabalin and gabapentin and surgery: Ask your surgeon and anesthesiologist. These can usually be continued up to the day before surgery.

Financial aid for pregabalin and gabapentin: Go to lupusencyclopedia.com/patient-resources. Also, go to www.goodrx.com or similar programs.

Cyclobenzaprine (Flexeril, Amrix, Fexmid)

Cyclobenzaprine is a muscle relaxant. Some of its effects are like those of tricyclic antidepressants, so much of the information in this section is like that of the TCA section.

Generic available: Yes.

How cyclobenzaprine works: See section on TCAs.

In people with FM, 20% have less pain, but it can take up to four weeks to work. Most people sleep better immediately.

Do not take if

- you have heart disease.
- you have difficulty urinating (as in benign prostatic hypertrophy).
- See also this section under TCAs.

Use caution if you have an overactive thyroid (hyperthyroidism). Inform your doctor.

Dosage: The immediate-release forms (generic cyclobenzaprine and Fexmid) are usually taken two to three hours before bed to prevent a morning hangover feeling. Sometimes, a low dose can be taken in the morning if it does not cause drowsiness. Extended-release Amrix is taken once daily. Never crush or bite Amrix because it would be absorbed too quickly and cause side effects.

If you miss a dose, see TCAs.

Alcohol/food interactions: Avoid alcohol to prevent increased side effects.

The immediate-release forms (generic cyclobenzaprine and Fexmid) can be taken with or without food. The extended-release form (Amrix) has increased absorption when taken with food. If you usually take it on an empty stomach, you should continue to do so. If you were to take it with food, you could have unexpected side effects such as drowsiness.

What to monitor while taking cyclobenzaprine: No blood work needed.

Potential side effects of cyclobenzaprine: The most common side effects include drowsiness, feeling hungover after waking, dizziness, dry mouth, and constipation.

While taking cyclobenzaprine, contact your doctor if you have any side effects.

Pregnancy and breastfeeding: Use caution during pregnancy. Probably safe while breastfeeding.

Geriatric use: Generally avoided in older people or used in smaller doses due to increased side effects.

Cyclobenzaprine and surgery: Ask your surgeon and anesthesiologist. Cyclobenzaprine can usually be continued up to the day before surgery.

Financial aid for cyclobenzaprine: Go to lupusencyclopedia.com/patient-resources. Also, go to www.goodrx.com or similar programs.

Tramadol (Ultracet, Ultram, Ultram ER, Ryzolt, Rybix, ConZip)

Tramadol is an opioid pain reliever and, therefore, can cause physical dependency (chapter 36). However, its opioid effects are weak, and it is rarely addictive. From 1995 to 2014 it was not a controlled substance in the United States. In 2014, it was made a controlled substance after addiction cases were reported in people with previous addiction (psychological dependence, chapter 36) problems. Most doctors require patients to read and sign pain contracts before starting it.

Generic available: Yes.

How tramadol works: In addition to being a weak opioid (chapter 36), it also blocks serotonin and norepinephrine reuptake, decreasing pain (see the section on dual uptake inhibitors).

Most people can get 50% or more pain reduction.

Do not take if

- you have a history of drug or alcohol abuse. Let your doctor know; you may have an increased risk for addiction.

- you have ever had seizures or epilepsy.

Use caution if

- you have decreased kidney or liver function; lower doses are generally needed.

- you have been diagnosed with increased intracranial pressure (such as pseudo-tumor cerebri, see chapter 13) or have had a brain injury. Inform your doctor.

Dosage: Immediate-release forms (generic tramadol, Ultracet, Ultram) are generally taken three to four times a day. Extended-release forms (tramadol ER, Ultram ER, ConZip) are typically taken once a day. Do not crush or bite extended-release forms: they would be absorbed too quickly and cause side effects.

Immediate release forms can disrupt sleep if taken later in the day. Some people should not take any after 5:00 P.M. or so.

If you miss a dose of immediate-release tramadol, take that dose as soon as you realize you missed it. Usually, immediate-release tramadol is taken a similar number of hours apart while awake, such as one or two tablets every six to eight hours (for example, 8:00 A.M., 2:00 P.M., and 8:00 P.M.). If you realize at 10:00 A.M. that you missed your morning dose, go ahead and take the morning dose, then take your next dose six hours later at 4:00 P.M., and then the last dose of the day six hours later at 10:00 P.M. If it is too late in the day and past your bedtime, just skip the last dose and resume your regular dosing schedule the next day.

If you miss a dose of extended-release tramadol, take that dose as soon as you remember you missed it that day, then resume your usual schedule the next day. If you do not realize you forgot your dose until the following day, you have two choices, depending on how you tolerate it: you can take one dose when you wake up the next day, then a second dose in the evening, or you can take just one dose that day. Ask your physician.

Alcohol/food interactions: Avoid alcohol; it increases side effects.

Extended-release forms (tramadol ER, ConZip, and Ultram ER) are absorbed faster when taken with fatty foods. Therefore, it is usually best to take them on an empty stomach to prevent side effects. Immediate-release forms are not affected by food.

What to monitor when taking tramadol: Regular urine or blood drug tests are needed to ensure you are not taking other controlled substances and that you are taking your medicine.

Potential side effects of tramadol: The most common side effects are drowsiness, nausea, itchiness, constipation, dizziness, and headaches. If stopped too quickly, withdrawal symptoms (anxiety, agitation, memory problems, sweating, feeling hot, high heart rate, stomach upset, muscle spasms) can occur.

While taking tramadol,

- let your doctor know if you develop side effects.

- do not stop abruptly to avoid withdrawal symptoms.

LUPUS IN FOCUS

Poor long-term effectiveness of FM drugs

A 2017 Israeli study showed that only 9% of FM patients taking TCAs (such as amitriptyline) continued their drug after one year due to it not working or having side effects. A 2020 Taiwanese study showed that only 12% of FM patients taking pregabalin stayed on it after one year. Another 2020 study of close to 30,000 FM patients showed that no drug produced long-term improvements in pain or quality of life.

Pregnancy and breastfeeding: Do not take it during pregnancy or breastfeeding.
Geriatric use: Lower doses are used to prevent side effects.
Tramadol and surgery: Ask your surgeon and anesthesiologist. When tramadol is stopped, there is a risk of withdrawal symptoms. Your surgical team may need to give you an alternative around the time of surgery to prevent withdrawal symptoms and pain.
Financial aid for tramadol: Go to lupusencyclopedia.com/patient-resources. Also, go to www.goodrx.com or similar programs.
Drug helpline for tramadol: 800-222-1222 for mild overdose; 911 for a life-threatening overdose.

KEY POINTS TO REMEMBER

1. FM is a problem in which overactive pain nerves cause pain and many other issues (table 27.1).

2. FM occurs in up to 30% of SLE patients.

3. Take the self-survey at the beginning of the "Diagnosing Fibromyalgia" section to see if you might have FM. If you score positive, show the results to your doctor.

4. FM pain is not treated with immunosuppressants.

5. The most important treatment for FM is exercise.

6. FM can be treated with drugs that improve pain nerve chemical imbalances.

7. Treatment usually includes a combination of therapies, including exercise, as outlined in table 27.2. Drugs alone are not very effective.

8. Antidepressants and anti-seizure medicines are commonly used FM drugs.

9. There are three FDA-approved FM drugs (Cymbalta, Savella, and Lyrica). There is no evidence that they work any better than other FM drugs.

10. FM drugs (other than tramadol) need to be taken on a regular schedule and take three to eight weeks to work. Often a low dose is started and gradually increased.

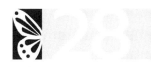

Gastroesophageal Reflux Disease and Peptic Ulcer Disease

Rodger Stitt, MD, *Contributing Editor*

Gastroesophageal reflux disease (GERD) and stomach ulcers are usually not caused by lupus directly (except when esophageal dysmotility causes GERD, chapter 15). Nonetheless, they are common in SLE patients and are often related to drug side effects.

Gastroesophageal Reflux Disease

GERD is commonly called acid reflux and is often recognized by feeling heartburn. A tight, circular muscle called the lower esophageal sphincter normally prevents acidic stomach contents from backing up into the esophagus (figure 28.1). It relaxes when swallowed food travels down the esophagus into the stomach and then tightens after the food contents enter the stomach. This closes the entrance to the stomach, allowing the food to remain there and be digested. GERD develops when the stomach's acidic contents back up, or reflux, through this barrier and up into the esophagus.

GERD occurs in SLE for many reasons (table 28.1). Some drugs commonly used for SLE, such as calcium channel blockers (used for Raynaud's), can cause the sphincter to relax too much. So can other substances such as tobacco, caffeine, chocolate, peppermint, alcohol, and fatty foods. Patients who feel heartburn or have GERD should avoid them.

A hiatal hernia can also cause this sphincter muscle to work improperly and not keep acidic contents in the stomach. "Hiatal," which comes from the Latin word for "opening," refers to the opening between the esophagus and the stomach. A hiatal hernia is when part of the stomach protrudes through this opening (figure 28.2) up into the chest cavity, where the lungs are. While mild hiatal hernias are usually not problematic, worse ones can make it difficult for food to go down into the stomach, leading to heartburn, chest pain, trouble swallowing, and even regurgitation of food up into the mouth.

Obesity is a common cause of GERD. Excess abdominal fat puts pressure on the stomach, causing it to push acidic contents up through the lower esophageal sphincter and into the esophagus. Other causes of increased abdominal pressure that worsen GERD include coughing, bending over, and wearing a tight belt.

About 30% to 50% of people with SLE have decreased saliva formation due to Sjögren's overlap (chapter 14). Saliva normally flows down from the mouth and through the esophagus, keeping fluids moving down into the stomach. When there is less saliva, stomach contents can back up. Decreased saliva (and worse GERD) can also occur from drugs that cause dry mouth (chapter 14).

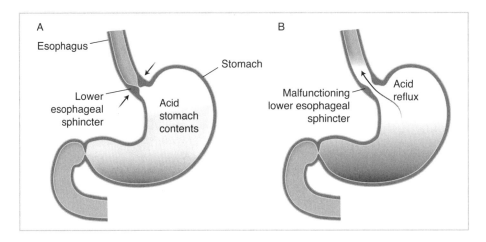

Figure 28.1 The lower esophageal sphincter keeping stomach contents away from the esophagus (A) compared to an abnormal sphincter causing GERD (B)

GERD symptoms are due to the stomach's acidic contents irritating the esophagus. These include heartburn, difficulty swallowing, feeling a lump in the throat, increased salivation, nausea, and even stomach contents coming up into the mouth. Heartburn can even cause chest pain that feels like a heart attack. It is not uncommon for someone to develop a sensation of severe chest pressure radiating into the arm, go to the emergency room, and find out it was due to GERD and not a heart attack. However, never assume this on your own. Heart attacks and strokes are the number one cause of death in SLE, and a doctor should always evaluate these symptoms.

GERD's less typical symptoms include hoarseness if acid drips on the vocal cords (laryngopharyngeal reflux) and cough (from acid contents going down the windpipe into the lungs). Cough or hoarseness can sometimes be the only GERD symptoms.

If left untreated, GERD can cause problems (table 28.2) from repetitive irritation of acid exposure in the esophagus, vocal cords, and lungs. While the stomach has a protective lining that prevents acid damage, these other tissues do not. The esophagus can develop inflammation (called esophagitis). If the inflammation becomes severe, it can damage the esophagus (an esophageal ulcer), causing pain and trouble swallowing. Scar tissue can form in the esophagus, causing an esophageal stricture (narrowing). This can cause swallowing problems. In addition, repeated exposure of the esophagus cells to acid can cause a precancerous condition called Barrett's esophagitis, which can develop into esophageal cancer if not treated appropriately.

Another complication occurs when acid contents drip down the trachea (windpipe), causing inflammation of the larynx (voice box, laryngitis) and hoarseness. As in the esophagus, scar tissue can form in the trachea, creating a stricture, and cancer can also develop. If acidic contents drip into the lungs, they can cause a persistent cough or even asthma. Worsening lung damage from GERD contents is common in SLE (chapter 10). People with lupus inflammatory lung disease need both the lung problem and GERD treated.

Table 28.1 Causes of GERD

Drugs that relax the lower esophageal sphincter (LES)

    calcium channel blockers (such as nifedipine, amlodipine, etc.) for blood pressure and Raynaud's

    pain relievers (such as tramadol and opioids)

    antidepressants and anti-anxiety drugs

    beta-blockers (for high blood pressure)

    antihistamines (for allergies)

    sedatives (sleeping pills)

    Parkinson's disease drugs

    theophylline and other asthma drugs

    drugs for urinary incontinence

    some glaucoma drugs

    progestin female hormones (for birth control, menopause, and to decrease uterine blood flow)

Other substances that relax the LES

    tobacco, cigarettes

    alcohol

    caffeine

    chocolate

    peppermint

    fatty foods

Drugs that worsen GERD by other means

    NSAIDs (table 36.1)

    steroids (such as prednisone)

    bisphosphonates for osteoporosis (table 24.9)

    tetracyclines (such as doxycycline and minocycline)

    potassium and iron supplements

Conditions that worsen GERD

    esophageal dysmotility

    decreased saliva flow (Sjögren's and some medicines that cause dry mouth)

    hiatal hernia

    obesity

    tight clothes and belts

    pregnancy

Note: Terms in **bold** are common causes of GERD in SLE patients.

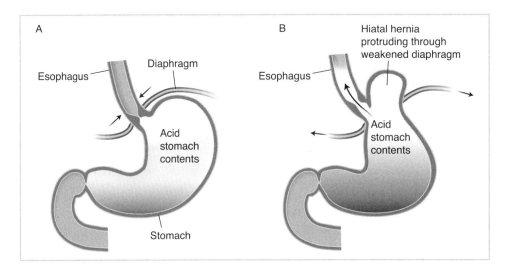

Figure 28.2 Hiatal hernia

Table 28.2 Potential GERD Complications

Esophagitis (esophagus inflammation)

Esophageal ulcer

Esophageal stricture (narrowing from scarring)

Barrett's esophagitis (a precancerous condition)

Esophageal cancer

Laryngitis and hoarseness

Tracheal stricture (narrowing of the windpipe)

Throat cancer

Asthma

Cough

Worsening of lupus lung disease

Doctors usually diagnose GERD from symptoms alone. Someone with heartburn, which may worsen with eating or lying down, can be diagnosed and treated for GERD without further testing. The first step in treating GERD is to change lifestyle habits that worsen it (table 15.2). These measures can address many GERD causes without the need for medications (table 28.3). Relying on anti-acid drugs alone can lead to more problems. Anti-acid drugs reduce stomach acidity but do not reduce the amount of stomach contents refluxed up the esophagus.

Anti-GERD drugs should be considered if changing lifestyle habits or offending medications does not stop the symptoms. If symptoms are mild and intermittent, then over-the-counter preparations can be tried. These include Tums, Alka-Seltzer, Pepto Bismol, Mylanta, Rolaids, Prilosec, Pepcid Complete, and cimetidine (Tagamet). Check

Table 28.3 Proton Pump Inhibitors (PPIs)

dexlansoprazole (Dexilant)

esomeprazole (Nexium, Esomep-EZS)

omeprazole (Prilosec, Zegerid, OmePPi)

lansoprazole (Prevacid)

pantoprazole (Protonix)

rabeprazole (Aciphex)

with your doctor before taking these. Some interact with other drugs or should not be used with some medical problems.

Your doctor may put you on anti-acid prescription medicine, which can help you feel better and prevent some GERD complications. For example, aluminum sucrose sulfate (Sucralfate), which coats and protects the esophagus and stomach lining, can help people with mild GERD, especially when problems occur after eating.

Other anti-GERD drugs typically lower stomach content acidity. Those that are prescription-strength drugs are divided into two main groups: proton pump inhibitors (PPIs) (table 28.3) and histamine type 2 (H2) blockers.

H2 blockers include cimetidine (Tagamet), famotidine (Pepcid), and nizatidine. While PPIs usually work better than H2 blockers, H2 blockers tend to be less expensive than PPIs, so some insurance companies require people to take an H2 blocker before taking a PPI.

PPIs are not all the same, though. One PPI may work better than another. Therefore, trials of different PPIs at different doses are sometimes needed. It is important to take the PPI on an empty stomach one hour before eating a meal with protein. Some people also do better if they take a PPI in the morning and an H2 blocker in the evening. They work in two different complementary ways. It is not recommended to take both at the same time.

PPIs are generally safe. However, they can decrease magnesium and vitamin B12 absorption. We check vitamin B12 and magnesium levels regularly in patients taking PPIs.

Prolonged PPI use can potentially cause other problems. These include osteoporotic fractures (chapter 24), *C. difficile* infection (an intestinal bacterial infection), microscopic colitis (inflammation in the large intestine), and atrophic gastritis (an abnormality of the stomach lining). Doctors recommend limiting PPI use to avoid these. A common approach is to use a PPI daily for eight weeks and then cut it down to an "as needed" basis.

Another reason for cutting down on PPIs is that studies suggest that they cause chronic kidney disease, dementia, or pneumonia. However, we do not know if these are real side effects or not—the studies suggesting that PPIs may cause these are not well-designed and do not prove that these are problems.

Suppose that the GERD symptoms do not improve with treatment. Or, say that someone has symptoms suggesting a significant complication, such as trouble swallowing. Then, it is appropriate to do more testing. One test is an upper endoscopy, also called an esophagogastroduodenoscopy (EGD), which is usually done under sedation. A doctor

PPIs can lower mycophenolate blood drug levels

PPIs can lower mycophenolate mofetil (CellCept) drug levels by around 35%, making it less effective for treating lupus. PPIs reduce the conversion of mycophenolate to its active substance, mycophenolic acid, in the body. It is probably better to take mycophenolic acid (Myfortic) if you need a PPI. Ask your doctor; this is not a well-known interaction.

inserts a thin, fiberoptic tube (or scope) down the esophagus (*esophago-*) and into the stomach (*-gastro-*), and the duodenum (*-duodeno-*); see figure 28.3. The doctor can see inflammation, ulcers, cancers, or other problems, and biopsies can be done if needed.

A barium swallow is another test performed by having the patient swallow a substance that coats the esophagus and stomach and shows up on an x-ray. It can show if stomach contents are refluxing up into the esophagus (GERD). It can also show problems such as hiatal hernias, strictures, tumors, or ulcers (if large enough to be seen on x-ray). However, a barium swallow can miss mild GERD, small ulcers, and cancers. Therefore, a normal result does not mean nothing is wrong. An EGD is usually needed. Other studies for diagnosing GERD include manometry and pH monitoring. However, they are performed less often and will not be discussed.

Surgery (such as a Nissen fundoplication) can be performed for a severe hiatal hernia to eliminate it. This is reserved for severe cases that do not respond to other treatments.

KEY POINTS TO REMEMBER

1. GERD and esophageal irritation are common in SLE for multiple reasons (table 28.1).

2. The most common GERD symptoms are heartburn, chest pain (which can even feel like a heart attack), and difficulty swallowing.

3. If chest pain occurs, do not assume it is GERD. Chest pain requires a doctor's evaluation.

4. Unusual GERD symptoms include hoarseness (from laryngopharyngeal reflux), cough, and asthma-like symptoms. These can happen without any heartburn.

5. To treat GERD, follow the advice in table 15.2. Anti-GERD drugs mainly cover up symptoms. They do not decrease the contents that reflux up from the stomach.

6. For mild or intermittent GERD, try over-the-counter (OTC) heartburn drugs.

7. If OTC drugs do not work, then your doctor may prescribe Sucralfate, a prescription-strength PPI, or an H2 blocker.

8. If you take a PPI long-term, try to cut down to an as-needed basis. Ask to have your vitamin B-12 and magnesium levels checked regularly.

Peptic Ulcer Disease

"Peptic" refers to stomach's digestive juices, and an ulcer is a hole on the surface of a part of the body. Peptic ulcer disease is a condition in which ulcers occur in the stomach or small intestine due to stomach acid (figure 28.3). If a peptic ulcer is mild, it is called an erosion. Although SLE itself does not generally cause peptic ulcer disease, it can occur from drugs used in SLE, such as NSAIDs (table 36.1), steroids (such as prednisone), and bisphosphonates (table 24.9). Other causes include stress, aspirin, cigarette smoking, and alcohol.

Ulcers and erosions can produce many possible symptoms, depending on where they occur. The classic stomach ulcer (and erosion) pain is a discomfort in the upper part of the abdomen with a burning, gnawing, cramping, or "hunger-like" quality. Bloating, heartburn, nausea, or an early feeling of fullness after eating are other possible symptoms. Eating food or taking an antacid often helps. Symptoms do not always follow this classic description. Some people have right or left upper abdominal discomfort, and eating makes some people's symptoms worse instead of better.

Duodenal ulcers behave differently. Usually there are no symptoms right after eating. Digesting food decreases acidity of stomach contents entering the duodenum. Typically, symptoms develop three to five hours after eating, when the food is gone from the stomach. The stomach contents become more acidic again and enter the duodenum, irritating the ulcer and causing pain. Stomach acid is at a maximum between 11:00 P.M. to 2:00 A.M., so this is a typical time for duodenal ulcer pain.

Some people have severe ulcer complications. One complication is a bleeding ulcer. If a stomach ulcer bleeds and the person throws up, the coagulated blood in the vomit looks like coffee grounds (called coffee ground emesis). If the blood goes through the intestines and is excreted, it creates black and tarry stool (melena), which is thick and sticky with a strong, foul, hard-to-forget smell. A bleeding ulcer can potentially be deadly, so if you have coffee ground emesis or melena, seek medical attention (such as an emergency room) at once.

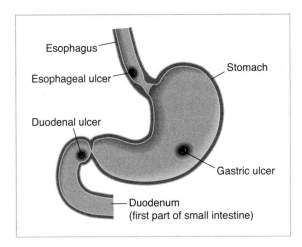

Figure 28.3 Possible locations of peptic ulcers

531

Barium swallows and EGD (both discussed in the GERD section) are used for diagnosing peptic ulcer disease. EGD is usually the better test. It can visualize smaller ulcers and obtain biopsies if needed.

NSAIDs (chapter 36) are a leading cause of peptic ulcers. NSAIDs reduce the production of prostaglandins, which have many crucial body functions. One of these is sensing pain. Prostaglandins are necessary for helping send pain messages from spinal nerves to the brain. Decreased prostaglandins due to NSAIDs can cause the spinal nerves to send fewer pain signals. Prostaglandins are also crucial for producing inflammation. NSAIDs can decrease inflammation and the pain it causes, but they can also cause fewer prostaglandins to be made. That is a problem because prostaglandins help produce the stomach's protective mucous layer (protecting itself from stomach acid). Taking NSAIDs can thus lead to less protective mucus, thus allowing stomach acid to damage the stomach lining and leading to inflammation (gastritis), erosions, or ulcers.

Yet, most patients do not get ulcers when they take NSAIDs. Sometimes there is no rhyme or reason why one person gets an ulcer and another does not. Still, it is possible to predict who is at highest risk. They include people who take steroids, blood thinners, or an SSRI (chapter 27) along with an NSAID. The American College of Gastroenterology (ACG) has created guidelines suggesting the highest risks (table 28.4).

Most of the time (70% or higher), NSAID-induced ulcers do not cause pain. This may be because NSAIDs reduce body pain. Most people with an ulcer from NSAIDs realize they have it after they develop complications. These include anemia from slow bleeding or having coffee ground emesis or melena from a large bleed. Some will not have any warning signs. They may pass out from massive blood loss, develop severe abdominal pain or vomiting due to perforation (a catastrophic hole through the stomach wall), or develop an intestinal blockage. We bring this up because people are often reluctant to take additional medication (such as a PPI or misoprostol, table 28.5) to prevent ulcers while on NSAIDs. They may say, "The medicine never bothers me; I never get belly pain, so I don't need a medicine to prevent ulcers." You should realize that most people who take NSAIDs do not get any warning of having an ulcer at all, so do not let this keep you from taking a PPI or misoprostol if your doctor recommends it.

Table 28.4 Ulcer Risk Levels from NSAIDs

High risk (having either of the following):

    History of a complicated ulcer (such as one that bled)

    Three or more moderate risk factors below

Moderate risk (having one or more of these risk factors):

    Age > 65

    High-dose prescription NSAID (table 36.2)

    History of an uncomplicated ulcer

    Aspirin (even low-dose), steroids, or blood thinners

Low risk:

    None of the risk factors listed

If you need an NSAID and fall into the medium- or high-risk category for ulcers, you should consider taking a preventative drug (table 28.5). Ask your doctor.

If an EGD or barium swallow shows a peptic ulcer, it needs treatment. The doctor will usually test for *Helicobacter pylori*, a stomach bacterial infection that can cause ulcers and stomach cancer. *H. pylori* can be diagnosed by biopsy during the EGD. A breath test to diagnose *H. pylori*, called the urea breath test (UBT), can also be done separately from the EGD. The UBT is most often done by a gastroenterologist (the same doctor who most commonly does EGDs). The stool antigen test is a simpler and less expensive diagnostic method. It accurately shows if there is an active infection, and it can be used to see if the infection goes away after treatment. While *H. pylori* can also be detected through a blood test, this test is not as reliable. It can either miss the infection in someone who has it or show a positive result for someone who doesn't. *H. pylori* is treated with a combination of antibiotics plus a PPI.

If an ulcer is active, NSAIDs should be stopped. A big question is whether the NSAID can be added after the ulcer heals. If the ulcer occurred during an *H. pylori* infection or if the person was not taking misoprostol or a PPI at the time, it may be possible to resume the NSAID. However, it is prudent to take one of the drugs in table 28.5. This is especially important if the person has significant arthritis pains and quality of life issues become problematic off the NSAID.

Ulcers are treated with a PPI for various amounts of time, depending on how large the ulcer is, its location, whether the person was on an NSAID, and if there is an *H. pylori* infection. It is also essential to stop smoking and decrease alcohol intake. Avoiding certain foods does not speed up healing, but if some foods bother you (such as acidic or fatty food), not eating them can help. Although stress, depression, and anxiety appear to increase the risk of ulcers, there is no medical evidence that resolving these issues makes the ulcers heal more quickly. At the same time, though, having these problems increases the risk of ulcers recurring after healing. Therefore, it is vital to decrease stress (chapter 38) and treat depression and anxiety.

Table 28.5 Drugs to Prevent NSAID Ulcers

Misoprostol (Cytotec) as an add-on drug

Diclofenac plus misoprostol combo pill

PPI as an add-on drug (table 28.3)

    naproxen plus esomeprazole (Vimovo)

Non-acetylated salicylate (less likely to cause ulcers but are weak pain drugs)

    diflunisal

    salsalate

COX-2 inhibitor (only if not taking aspirin)

    celecoxib (Celebrex)

    meloxicam (Mobic) at 7.5 mg a day

Duexis (ibuprofen plus H2 blocker famotidine combo pill)

---

1. Peptic ulcers occur from stomach acid eroding the lining of the stomach or duodenum.

2. Peptic ulcers commonly occur in people with SLE because they have *H. pylori* infection or they take NSAIDs.

3. If you are at increased risk of ulcers from NSAIDs (table 28.4), ask your doctor for one of the treatments in table 28.5.

4. Most ulcers due to NSAIDs have no warning signs (like abdominal pain) until they get complications such as bleeding.

5. Coffee ground emesis or melena can mean peptic ulcer bleeding. Seek immediate medical attention.

6. EGD and barium swallow x-rays can diagnose peptic ulcers. An EGD often is required to obtain a biopsy to rule out *H. pylori* infection, cancer, or other problems.

7. If *H. pylori* infection is found (by EGD biopsy, breath test, blood test, or stool test), then a PPI plus combination antibiotics are used.

8. Doctors prescribe a PPI to treat ulcers.

9. If you are on an NSAID and get an ulcer, you need to stop taking it.

10. Stopping smoking and decreasing alcohol help ulcers heal.

11. If you take mycophenolate mofetil (MMF) and a PPI, it is probably better to change MMF to mycophenolic sodium (Myfortic). PPIs reduce MMF effectiveness.

PART IV

Treating Lupus

Medications and Lupus

George Stojan, MD, *Contributing Editor*

Lupus treatment is complex. Since lupus is an autoimmune disease in which the immune system is overactive and attacks the person's body, the primary treatment is to use drugs that calm down the immune system. This chapter details doctors' thought processes when prescribing medicines while also giving you insight into how best to take them. Later chapters go into more detail about individual therapies.

There are many different ways to treat lupus. It is possible to treat the same person in different ways successfully. Doctors choose therapies based on their own personal training and experience. Not all treatments work the same for everyone. Often a trial-and-error approach to different drugs may be needed before the best combination is found.

Since the first edition of this book came out, major rheumatology organizations have published lupus treatment guidelines—a significant advancement in itself. This chapter will include many of these recommendations, which are listed in table 29.1.

When doctors evaluate SLE patients, they note the different problems it is causing and identify the most severe ones. This helps categorize whether the SLE is mild, moderate, or severe. They also figure out if any of the problems require different therapies.

Research tools such as the Systemic Lupus Erythematosus Disease Activity Index (SLEDAI, table 29.2) provide formal definitions for mild, moderate, and severe SLE. Most rheumatologists do not use these tools, nor do they always write down "mild," "moderate," or "severe" in patients' records. But they are thinking along these lines when choosing treatments.

In most cases, doctors would likely agree on what makes for a mild, moderate, or severe case of lupus. For example, if an SLE patient has slightly decreased blood cell counts, minor skin problems, or mild Raynaud's (chapter 11), doctors would likely agree that the condition is mild.

If there is significant major organ involvement (of, say, nerves, brain, heart, lung, liver, or kidney) doctors would agree that it is severe. This is especially true if there is a chance for organ failure or death if the disease is not treated aggressively.

SLE problems that are not mild or severe fall into the moderate category. For example, according to table 29.2, someone with discoid lupus on the face and lupus arthritis would have a score of 6 points, which is moderate.

It is a good idea to get a sense of how severe your SLE is. Some patients resist added treatment when we recommend it. They think their lupus is not bad enough to call for additional drugs or higher doses. Nevertheless their SLEDAI score may show otherwise.

Table 29.1 SLE Treatment Recommendations

- An anti-malarial drug (hydroxychloroquine, chloroquine: HCQ, CQ) should be considered in all patients.
- Check for antiphospholipid antibodies (aPLAs).
- See patients regularly (usually every 3 months) for a history, physical exam, and labs, including a complete blood count, liver enzymes, chemistry panel, kidney function, anti-ds DNA, C3, C4, ESR, CRP, urinalysis, and a random protein/creatinine ratio. (I also recommend EC4d and anti-C1q if positive for these, chapter 4).
- If the urine protein/creatinine is greater than 0.5 (or >500 mg protein in a 24-hour urine sample), a kidney biopsy should be done (if safe to do so).
- Ensure patients get proper vaccinations, including for influenza, pneumonia, shingles, human papillomavirus, hepatitis, and COVID-19 (details in chapter 22).
- Cardiovascular risk factors including hypertension, diabetes, hyperlipidemia, obesity, should be aggressively treated.
- Screening should be done for avascular necrosis (chapter 25), thyroid disease, osteoporosis, and cancer.
- Labs should be done regularly for patients on immunosuppressants to ensure no side effects.
- Eye exams (preferably VF 10-2 and an SD-OCT) are needed at baseline, then annually after 5 years on HCQ and CQ. Asians also need a VF 24-2 or 30-2.
- Pregnancy and contraception should be addressed with all child-bearing aged women. Anti-Ro/anti-La and aPLAs need to be checked before pregnancy.
- Suggest non-drug interventions: sunscreen, ultraviolet light avoidance, vitamin D, exercise, stress reduction, adequate sleep, and proper diet.
- Get patients off steroids or on the lowest dose possible.
- Consider topical steroids or tacrolimus for skin lupus.
- Use immunosuppressants or biologics to help reduce steroids.
- Address type-2 symptoms (widespread pain, fatigue, insomnia, memory issues, depression, anxiety)
- Treatment should be adjusted and aimed at stopping lupus flares, even mild flares, if possible.
- Treatment goal is remission. If remission is not possible, aim for low disease activity.

Rheumatologists can also underestimate disease severity. This is where the usefulness of the SLEDAI tool comes in. Consider the following scenario.

A week ago, you had your typical monthly lupus flare during your menstrual cycle. You were fatigued, and arthritis pains in multiple joints kept you from doing some of your customary activities. As usual, the flare resolved after a few days. Now, when you're at your rheumatologist's, you explain that you've been feeling fine except for those few days. A physical exam finds three mildly tender joints and a few small sores on the roof of your mouth that you didn't notice. Labs show an elevated anti-dsDNA and a low C4 complement level. Many doctors would think this was a mild flare.

Table 29.2 SLE Disease Activity Index (SLEDAI)

Add up the points for each active problem present during the past 10 days. Follow definitions exactly. Non-lupus causes must be excluded. Lupus headache is rare; do not count unless told to do so by a doctor. Terms are highly technical; this is the actual SLEDAI used in research.

Score interpretation: 1–5 points (low disease activity), 6–10 points (moderate), 11+ points (high disease activity).

Points	Lupus Problem	Definition
8	Seizure	Active seizure
8	Psychosis	Hallucinations, incoherent, bizarre behavior, catatonia
8	Organic brain syndrome	New onset memory loss, not oriented, reduced consciousness, plus 2 of the following: imperception incoherence insomnia or daytime drowsiness abnormal psychomotor activity
8	Lupus retinopathy	Retinal bleeding, cytoid bodies, choroiditis, or optic neuritis disease
8	Cranial neuropathy	New
8	Lupus headache	Severe, constant, narcotics don't help
8	Stroke	New
8	Vasculitis	tender finger nodules, nail fold infarcts (purple spots on the cuticle around the nail), splinter hemorrhages, vasculitis ulcer or gangrene, biopsy or angiogram showing vasculitis
4	Arthritis	Inflammatory arthritis in 3 or more joints (prolonged morning stiffness, tender joints, non-bony joint swelling)
4	Myositis	Shoulders or hip/thigh muscle pain or weakness and high CPK/aldolase or positive muscle biopsy
4	Urine casts	Red blood cell, heme, or granular casts
4	Hematuria	6 or more red blood cells per high power field in urine
4	Pyuria	6 or more white blood cells per high power field in urine

(*continued*)

Table 29.2 (*continued*)

4	Proteinuria	New or recent increase of urine protein >.5 gm/24hrs or protein/creatinine >0.5
2	Lupus rash	Active inflammatory lupus rash
2	Alopecia	Abnormal patchy or diffuse hair loss not from other causes
2	Mucosal ulcers	Mouth or nose ulcers or erosions from lupus
2	Pleurisy	Chest pain with deep breathing, with imaging showing pleural fluid or scarring or a "rub" is heard on physical exam
2	Pericarditis	Chest pain with deep breathing with rub on physical exam, pericardial fluid on echo, or pericarditis on ECG
2	Low complement	Low CH50, C3, or C4
2	High anti-ds DNA	High anti-ds DNA antibody
1	Fever	>100.4° F oral temperature with no infection or other cause present
1	Low platelets	<100,000 platelets/mm^3 (or <100 × 10^9/L)
1	Leukopenia	<3,000 white blood cells/mm^3 (or <3.0 × 10^9/L) not due to drugs

But suppose your rheumatologist measures your SLEDAI score. In that case, you would have had a total of 10 points (arthritis, mouth sores, increased anti-dsDNA, and low complement). This would qualify as moderate disease activity, bordering high disease activity. Research shows that even mild flares increase ongoing organ damage over time. Your rheumatologist should consider adjusting your treatment to better control your SLE.

The goal of lupus treatment is remission (chapter 5). Low (mild) disease activity is the second-best goal. Many of our patients with active SLE have gone into remission merely by being better about taking their medicines. The following sections discuss medications commonly prescribed for lupus

Immunomodulators

Immunomodulators, or immunomodulating drugs, affect the immune system to varying degrees. A drug that suppresses the immune system in an individual is called an immunosuppressant (table 22.1).

Antimalarial drugs are immunomodulators. They do not suppress the immune system—they calm it down. They also decrease the risk of infections, in contrast to immunosuppressants, which increase the risk.

SLE treatments continue to improve

One sign of improvement is shown by the pattern of lupus disease activity. In 1999, approximately 50% of SLE patients had persistently active disease (called a chronic-active pattern in a Johns Hopkins study). Around 30% had periods of remission interspersed with periods of flares (called a relapsing-remitting pattern).

Twenty years later (2019), a large lupus center in Toronto, Canada, showed that only 10% of their SLE patients had persistently active SLE; 70% had a relapsing-remitting pattern. Today, more patients have periods of no disease activity compared to the past. SLE patients also do not need hospitalizations nearly as often (chapter 19) and live significantly longer.

Antimalarials

Most lupus experts treat SLE patients with an antimalarial such as hydroxychloroquine (HCQ, Plaquenil) or chloroquine (chapter 30). These are the safest drugs for calming the lupus immune system. HCQ is the most commonly used and the most studied antimalarial in SLE. When discussing antimalarial therapy, this chapter refers primarily to HCQ. The benefits of HCQ are many and are listed in table 30.1. HCQ is the only drug proven to increase life spans in SLE patients and is one of two drugs to be classified as a disease-modifying agent, proven to reduce SLE organ damage. Belimumab is the other as of December 2022 (chapter 34).

One problem with HCQ is that it can take a long time to work. In some, it can start helping after a month, but it can take up to a year for full effectiveness. For mild lupus, HCQ may be the only drug needed. If there are other problems that cannot wait a month or so to resolve, such as severe joint pain, severe pleurisy (chapter 10), disfiguring rash, profound fatigue, or others, it is important to use something in addition to HCQ—often a steroid such as prednisone. Steroids (discussed below) work much faster than other lupus drugs, often within hours of taking them. The next-fastest is anifrolumab (Saphnelo, chapter 34), which can start working after the first infusion in some patients.

Some SLE patients need an immunosuppressant in addition to HCQ. Immunosuppressants are stronger than HCQ.

Corticosteroids

The only lupus drugs that work immediately are corticosteroids (steroids, chapter 31). SLE patients who feel quite sick and those who have any significant internal organ involvement (such as the kidneys, lungs, brain, or heart) usually need steroids right away. Some doctors consider steroid use a bridge therapy, in which the steroid quickly controls SLE while waiting for the slower-working drugs to work.

Lupus inflammation can cause permanent organ damage. The faster doctors stop this inflammation, the better the chances of preventing permanent damage. Although some people resist taking steroids because of their side effects, it is worth dealing with

LUPUS IN FOCUS

Hydroxychloroquine drug levels

The ability to measure hydroxychloroquine (HCQ, Plaquenil) drug levels (chapter 4) has revolutionized our SLE patients' treatments. When we first began measuring levels, we were surprised at the number of patients who were not regularly taking their Plaquenil. We even had patients who told us they rarely missed doses of their Plaquenil, only to have their levels come back as zero. We would show our nonadherent patients their results and educate them about how vital Plaquenil is for treating SLE. The vast majority of patients eventually became very good at taking their medication regularly. As a result, most of them had less SLE inflammation, and many went into remission.

We aim to have our patients' HCQ levels between approximately 1,000 ng/mL to 1,200 ng/mL. However, the best target is not entirely understood at the time of this writing. The science of HCQ drug levels is in its infancy, and much research on this topic continues to change our understanding of how to best use this blood test. At this moment, if a patient's level is too high (generally > 1,500), we lower the dose in the hopes of preventing side effects such as eye damage (retinopathy). Although the American Academy of Ophthalmology (AAO) recommends dosing Plaquenil at less than 5 mg/kg of body weight per day, there are differences in the ways that people handle (metabolize) the drug. To have an optimal level, some require higher doses than the 400 mg daily that the AAO recommends to have an optimal level. I have three patients with malabsorption from gastric bypass surgery who require 500 mg to 600 mg a day to maintain the proper drug levels. I would not have realized this without the ability to measure HCQ drug levels.

those side effects rather than risking permanent damage to a vital organ by undertreating lupus. Once the steroids calm disease activity, doctors lower (taper) the dose.

Steroids can cause many side effects, so it is important to use safer therapies (HCQ, sunscreen, vitamin D, and so on) to control SLE so that steroids can be stopped, or at least tapered down to the lowest possible doses.

Even low-dose steroids are of concern. Several studies have shown a small association between low-dose steroids (such as doses lower than 5 mg daily or the use of higher doses for 2 weeks or less) with side effects such as infections (though they occur rarely with these low doses).

Using steroids initially for moderate to severe lupus problems can help decrease organ damage and even be lifesaving by immediately reducing inflammation. At the opposite extreme, steroids can cause damage when taken for extended periods (this amount varies from person to person). These problems include cataracts, skin damage, osteoporotic fractures (chapter 24), avascular necrosis (chapter 25), diabetes, hardening of the arteries (chapter 21), heart attacks, and strokes. A 2017 Canadian study showed that SLE patients who had taken any steroids at all were twice as likely to develop damage compared to patients who never did. Therefore, the decision to use steroids is not to be taken lightly.

LUPUS IN FOCUS

The hierarchy of steroid use and safety

Steroids can be listed in order of their ability to cause side effects. This parallels their use for the severity of SLE. Life-threatening problems (such as severe lung or kidney inflammation) require the highest doses. These carry the most side effects, but they may be needed for their life-saving qualities. Mild inflammation (such as minor pleurisy or arthritis) may do well with steroids at the safer side of the spectrum. Here is a list of steroids, ranging from the safest (but also weakest) at the top to the strongest (with the most side effects) at the bottom:

- Topical steroid creams, ointments, and gels
- Intramuscular injections(triamcinolone, dexamethasone, or Depo-Medrol)
- Short course of oral steroids (such as 6 days of methylprednisolone: Medrol Dose Pack)
- Every-other-day low-dose steroids (such as 7 mg every other day)
- Daily low-dose steroids (less than 6 mg daily prednisone)
- Higher daily doses of steroids
- Pulse IV steroids (1–3 days of 250 mg to 1,000 mg methylprednisolone) followed by daily steroids. Note, though, that pulse steroids can be safer than daily steroids in certain regimens. For example, 500 mg IV methylprednisolone followed by 20 mg a day of prednisone with a taper is safer than 60 mg a day oral taken for a lengthy period without IV steroids.
- Split dosing of high-dose steroids (such as 20 mg prednisone three times daily, which is stronger than 60 mg taken each morning)

Other Medications

Sometimes different individual problems caused by lupus must be treated with specific drugs. And sometimes additional medications are needed to prevent or treat the side effects of some lupus drugs. Understanding why you need so many drugs can make it easier to accept the treatment plan and take the drugs as prescribed.

Some lupus problems are not due to active inflammation. These problems require other therapies (table 29.3) along with immunomodulating medicines that treat lupus inflammation.

One example of a non-inflammatory problem is Raynaud's phenomenon (chapter 11). This occurs when the arteries of the hands and feet become smaller than usual during periods of stress and in cold temperatures. As a result, blood supply to those extremities decreases, and they become painful. In these situations, drugs may be needed to open the blood vessels and increase blood flow. Immunomodulating drugs (such as HCQ and prednisone) usually do not help Raynaud's attacks (chapter 11).

Some SLE patients have blood clots because of antiphospholipid syndrome (APS) due to antiphospholipid antibodies. Blood thinners such as warfarin (Coumadin) are used for APS. For someone who is positive for the antibodies but has never had a blood clot, aspirin may be prescribed for blood clot prevention.

Table 29.3 Non-Immunomodulatory Drugs for SLE Problems

Drugs to dilate arteries in Raynaud's phenomenon (chapter 11)

Blood thinners for antiphospholipid syndrome (chapters 9 and 11)

Drugs for dryness in Sjögren's (chapter 14)

Pain relievers (chapters 7 and 36)

Table 29.4 Treatments for SLE Drug Side Effects

Side Effect	Treatment
Prevent methotrexate side effects	folic acid or folinic acid (leucovorin)
For stomach upset or GERD due to drugs and to prevent ulcers in high risk patients	anti-acid drugs (such as PPIs, table 28.3)
Prevent and treat osteoporosis from steroids	bisphosphonates (table 24.9)
	calcium supplement with vitamin D
Prevent infections from immunosuppressants	dapsone or atovaquone (prevent pneumocystis pneumonia)
	isoniazid, rifampin, or rifapentine (prevent active TB)

Between 30% and 50% of SLE patients have Sjögren's disease, which causes dryness, especially in the mouth and eyes. Sometimes drugs to increase fluid production are needed. Most immunomodulating drugs do not help Sjögren's dryness.

Some people need pain medicine. Non-steroidal anti-inflammatory drugs (NSAIDs) such as ibuprofen (Motrin) and naproxen (Naprosyn) are commonly used.

Other medications are needed to treat or prevent lupus drug side effects (table 29.4). Although adding them to a patient's regimen may make the overall treatment more costly and complicated, it ensures that lupus drugs are used safely. For example, for someone taking methotrexate, it is vital to take a vitamin called folic acid or folinic acid (leucovorin) to lower the risk for low blood counts, liver inflammation, and other side effects. For side effects from NSAIDs and steroids, such as stomach upset, heartburn, or ulcers, your doctor may prescribe a drug to reduce stomach acidity. An acid-reducing drug could be prescribed in the absence of stomach upset if you are at increased risk for ulcers (table 28.4).

One of the worst side effects from steroids is osteoporosis, in which the bones become brittle and can break. To counter these side effects, doctors prescribe calcium supplements, vitamin D, and a drug to keep the bones healthy (such as a bisphosphonate).

Immunosuppressants can greatly increase the risk of infections in some scenarios. It may be important to take antibiotics with them. This includes taking pneumocystis pneumonia antibiotics when high-dose steroids are used with cyclophosphamide or mycophenolate and taking anti-TB drugs by people with a positive tuberculosis test (chapter 22).

Weighing Drug Benefits and Risks

Anything taken internally for a medical purpose can have side effects. This is true for something as harmless-seeming as a multiple vitamin, which can cause stomach upset.

Prescribed drugs usually include a list of possible side effects. While most are nuisance side effects, some can be hazardous or even life-threatening.

With any drug, it is important to weigh the risk of potential side effects against the drug's benefits. For example, penicillin, an antibiotic prescribed for infections (such as pneumonia) comes with warnings about severe allergic reactions and even death. These are real possibilities—close to 400 Americans die every year from penicillin— but they are rare. Many more lives are saved by penicillin than are lost. The chances of dying or having permanent body damage from untreated infection is far greater than the chances of life-threatening side effects from the antibiotic. People rarely refuse to take antibiotics because this logic is easy to understand.

This is what we mean by weighing benefits and risks (figure 29.1). Medications should always have more proven benefits than possible risks.

How do we know whether a medication is safe?

In the United States, the Food and Drug Administration (FDA) is the agency responsible for ensuring drug safety. The approval process begins after a drug has undergone rigorous research (called clinical trials) on humans. Then panels of experts at the FDA review the research results and determine whether the drug does what it is supposed to do for a disorder (efficacy) and whether it is safe before approving it for use.

This decision for FDA approval involves weighing benefits and risks. For example, a drug used to treat a mild skin rash with hardly any side effects will likely be approved. But what about a medicine used to treat a rapidly deadly disease (such as some forms of cancer)? It could have some major side effects, but if no other therapies are available, it could be approved because it could be lifesaving.

You should always report side effects to your doctor, even if they are mild. In some cases, they may be more of a nuisance than a danger, but even then the doctor may decrease the dosage or switch you to a different medication. Note, too, that the severity of side effects can vary a lot from medicine to medicine. For example, while mild stomach upset on an antibiotic may be considered worth putting up with to get rid of an infection, mild stomach upset on an NSAID (for example, Motrin) can be a warning sign of a stomach ulcer. Your doctor may want you to either stop the medicine entirely or take an anti-ulcer medicine along with Motrin.

It is best not to decide how mild a side effect of a medicine is on your own. It is always better to contact your doctor's office for advice instead. In this book, medications used to treat lupus are accompanied by charts with lists of possible side effects. We list only those definitely known to occur with the drug (removing the guesswork) and indicate whether they are mild or severe, how often they occur, and what you should do if

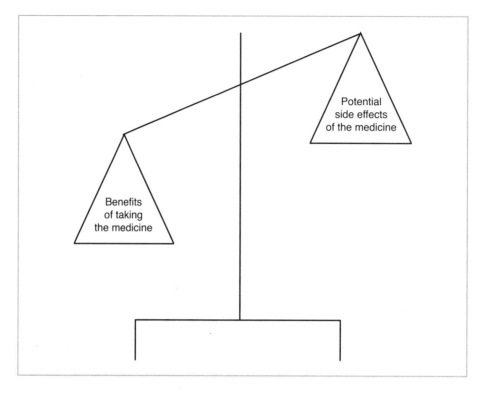

Figure 29.1 Weighing the risks versus the benefits of a medicine

you get the side effect. Even with these charts, you should contact your doctor if you get a drug side effect.

Be careful about what you hear on the news. The purpose of the news is not just to provide information. Media outlets also need to gain people's interest. Thus, it can be advantageous for the media to take the results of a medical study, report them as soon as possible, and even sensationalize them. Unfortunately, this can sometimes lead to people worrying too much about something that may not be true at all or may be blown out of proportion.

The same goes for drug advertisements (called direct-to-consumer advertising). Realize that they are required to list dangerous side effects as listed by the FDA on the drug package insert, even if that side effect is not truly a side effect. One example is the TNF inhibitors (chapter 33). Their ads usually state that they can cause a white blood cell cancer called lymphoma. In the clinical trials, people taking TNF inhibitors developed more lymphoma than expected in the general population. Therefore, it was listed as a possible side effect. However, the studies were done in patients at increased risk of lymphoma because of their disease (severe rheumatoid arthritis, RA). We expected to see more lymphomas in those patients because of their RA. These drugs have now been out for around 25 years, and numerous studies have been done looking at lymphoma occurrence. We have not seen any more lymphoma in patients with RA taking TNF inhibitors compared to RA patients not on TNF inhibitors. In other words, the lymphoma occurred because of the disease, not because of the drug. Yet, lymphoma remains a potential side effect listed on the package insert (and in advertisements).

A list of side effects from the pharmacy often includes side effects that are very rarely seen and even side effects that are not seen. For example, many of the side effects listed for methotrexate refer to those seen when high-dose methotrexate is used intravenously (IV) for cancer. We use markedly lower doses in SLE, and we never see many of those side effects.

Doctors prescribe so many drugs daily that they have a better feel for how often side effects actually occur and how severe they can be. In their practices, they find that most side effects from most drugs are nuisance side effects, which are tolerable and quickly resolve after the drug is stopped or its dose decreased. We also monitor for side effects closely (such as following blood cell count, liver function, and kidney function blood tests). When we catch a drug side effect, it is usually mild and reversible by simply adjusting the drug dose. If you are afraid of side effects you read about with a prescribed drug, ask your doctor what the realities are regarding how often and severe they are, how to prevent them, and what to do if they occur.

We have also taken steps in this book to ensure that we provide comprehensive and accurate information about lupus drug side effects, including which ones can occur, how often, and what to do if you get any. Methotrexate (chapter 32) is an example of where we provide more accurate information than available from most sources. Methotrexate side effects and drug interactions listed on pharmacy-provided patient information are not accurate. They include those that are seen with high-dose IV methotrexate, and they do not apply to low-dose methotrexate used for lupus. We also give advice on how to prevent the side effects of many drugs.

Learn as much about your medicine as you can using the information in this book.

Managing Your Medications

Managing your medications means adhering to—or sticking to—the plan your doctor prescribes. You should regularly see your doctor and get the necessary tests to ensure that any medicine does not cause side effects. It is crucial to take most lupus drugs

How often should you see your rheumatologist?

We believe that most SLE patients should see their rheumatologist at least every three months. The primary reason is to ensure there is no active SLE that should be treated differently. For example, lupus nephritis (kidney inflammation), which develops in close to half of people with SLE, causes no symptoms until it becomes severe. If we catch it early, before symptoms occur, by collecting a urine sample every three months, we have a better chance of treating it quickly and getting it into remission. People with active SLE may need to be seen more often, even as often as every one or two weeks. At the other end of the spectrum, some rheumatologists feel comfortable seeing very stable patients who are in complete remission and at a low-flare risk every 6–12 months. Monitoring for drug side effects also dictates office visit frequency. For example, if you are in remission and your mycophenolate mofetil (CellCept) is changed to azathioprine (Imuran) in preparation for pregnancy, you may need to be seen every two to four weeks at first.

regularly. Most of them must build up in the body to reach steady blood levels to exert their beneficial effects.

As Dr. C. Everett Koop, former surgeon general of the United States, said, "Drugs don't work if people don't take them." If you frequently forget to take your medicine, it won't help your condition. When your doctor sees you and notes that your lupus is not doing well, it is essential to let them know if forget to take your medicine. Otherwise, your doctor will assume that the drug is not working and may incorrectly add something to your drug regimen or switch to another drug. It is better to admit to not taking a drug as prescribed so that you and your doctor can figure out a plan to help you take it regularly.

Studies show that drugs for chronic diseases (such as lupus) are taken only about 50% (and less) of the time. Many studies focusing on lupus find similar results for patients on HCQ. This is worrisome because HCQ is by far the safest drug to treat lupus, and it has numerous benefits (table 30.1). People who regularly take it are much less likely to get severe internal organ involvement or even die from lupus. Patients who do not regularly take their HCQ are playing with fire. They are inviting their lupus to become more active. If this occurs, they may need high doses of steroids and other strong immunosuppressants with many more side effects than HCQ.

A 2019 Italian study showed that people with SLE who did not take HCQ regularly were five times more likely to have flares than those who took their HCQ. Another way of saying this is that the HCQ-taking patients were 75% less likely to flare than those who did not. That is a huge difference.

Another example of the importance of sticking to a drug regimen comes from a 2019 Brazilian study, which looked at HCQ adherence in SLE patients with kidney inflammation (lupus nephritis). Those who missed HCQ doses were almost six times more likely to have a nephritis flare than those who regularly took their HCQ. The problems this can cause cannot be overstated. Each lupus nephritis flare dramatically increases the risk of going into complete kidney failure, which would require dialysis and a kidney transplant. One bad flare of lupus nephritis can permanently destroy as much as one-third of the kidneys' filtering units. Once they are permanently damaged, they can never be replaced.

It can be challenging to remember to take your medications regularly, especially if they need to be taken at different times of the day or on different days of the week. Strategies to help you take medication regularly are listed in table 29.5. An essential first step is to recognize what a serious disease SLE is, that you truly have the disorder (don't be in denial) and that you need to take your medications regularly to do well.

Some people (especially younger people who were previously very healthy) can go into denial about their illness, which contributes to their not taking their drugs as prescribed. Others can have conditions such as depression, which make them less likely to stick to their treatment regimen. If you have any depression symptoms (such as feeling blue, not being motivated to do things, feeling tired, or having difficulty sleeping), take the self-test on depression in table 13.5. If you score high on this test, see your doctor about evaluating you for possible depression.

Table 29.5 Strategies for Help with Taking Medications Regularly

- Convince yourself of the importance of taking your medicines.
- If you are depressed (table 13.5), ask your doctor for help.
- Educate yourself about how the medicine works, how long it takes to work, and what lupus can do to you if you do not take it regularly. Look it up in the index to find it in this book.
- Ask your doctor if there is a drug that is easier to take, such as a once-a-day drug.
- If a drug is too expensive, ask for a cheaper alternative. Use a pharmacy that packages pills in dated/timed packets (such as PillPack). This makes it easy to see if you miss doses.
- If you miss a dose: look your drugs up in this book's index.
- Keep your medicines in easy-to-remember places (such as your work desk or next to your toothbrush).
- Fill up a large pill organizer once a month.
- Set cell phone, smartphone, or smart device (such as Amazon's Alexa or Google's Assistant) alarms to remind you.
- Ask a family member to remind you.
- Stick to a regimen that will get you into the habit of taking your medicine (e.g., taking it after breakfast or after you brush your teeth).
- If you miss doses due to side effects, ask your doctor for an alternative.
- If your drug regimen is complicated, ask your doctor to simplify it or write it down in easy-to-understand language.
- Plan for refills to make sure you do not run out.
- If you can get a 90-day supply with your prescriptions, do so. It saves time and money.

Educating yourself about how your medicines work can also help you take them regularly—and realize what can happen to you if you don't. Some drugs can take a while to take effect. People who don't understand this can stop taking their medicine after just a few doses, thinking that it is not working. In contrast, people who know that a drug takes, say, three months to work, will not stop taking it prematurely.

It is also much easier to take a drug once a day than two or three times a day, and you're much more likely not to forget a dose. If you find yourself missing the second or third dose of a medicine on some days, ask your doctor if there are once-a-day alternatives.

Drug affordability is important. Doctors usually prescribe what they feel is best for their patient's conditions. They want to give the safest treatments that are most likely to be taken regularly. A doctor is more likely to prescribe a new drug that is taken once a day than a cheaper, generic medicine taken four times a day. They know the four-times-a-day generic drug is rarely going to be taken properly. Doctors may also have samples of a new drug available. If they do, they may want to give patients some samples first to ensure that a particular medicine works and is tolerable before committing them to a full medication prescription. What doctors can't do is keep track of all the different insurance plans their patients have and the drugs they cover. If you are prescribed medicine that is not covered or unaffordable, you're probably not going to take it, or you will take it only some of the time. Either way, that particular drug is not going to work for you. You should let your doctor know that you cannot afford it and ask for an alternative. Most of the time (but not always), more affordable drugs are available. The cheaper generic drugs are usually just as good as the more expensive ones, as long as they are taken regularly and properly. Referring to the example at the beginning of this paragraph, you will do better taking an affordable four-times-a-day drug most of the time, than an expensive, new once-a-day drug that you can't afford and rarely end up taking.

There are many types of pill organizers that can help remind you to take your medicine. One of the most helpful can hold an entire month's worth, having sections for four

LUPUS IN FOCUS

Special pharmacies can make it easier to take medicines

An example is PillPack (www.pillpack.com or call 855-745-5725), which prepackages pills in small packets that are dated, timed, and conveniently placed in a roll dispenser. All the packets are attached with serrated edges that pull apart easily. The evening doses are next on the roll after the morning doses. If you miss an evening dose, the next morning the next packet reminds me because it says "take at 8:00 P.M." You may be able to make up for the missed dose. What to do in case of missed doses varies from drug to drug. You can look up your drugs in this book to figure out what to do.

Other pharmacies (such as CVS) are now following PillPack's example and offering this convenient packaging system. If your insurance plan allows for this type of specialty pharmacy, I cannot recommend using this highly enough.

separate weeks divided by days of the week. If you spend time filling it once a month, it can help make a big difference in ensuring that you do not miss any doses during the month.

Cell phones, smartphones, and smart devices (such as the Echo Alexa and Google's Assistant) can help remind you when to take medication. Every day at 6:00 P.M., my Alexa announces, "This is a reminder. Take your medicine." I rarely miss taking my medicine thanks to this. Drug-timer apps that you can download onto your phone are also available. Of course, there is also the old-fashioned way of asking a family member for help. This can be especially important if you have difficulties with memory. If you do ask for help, remind yourself that you give that person permission to prompt you. That way, you won't feel that you are being nagged and get annoyed at them.

Make taking your medicines habit-forming. Pick a particular time of day or regularly performed activity that will remind you to always take your medicine and stick to that schedule. For example, if you choose to take your medicine every time you brush your teeth in the morning or after you eat your breakfast, you will be more likely to stick to your regimen. Keep your drugs in locations that will remind you to take them, such as next to your toothbrush and at your work desk.

Sometimes people do not take their medicines regularly because they have side effects such as stomach upset. This is considered a mild, nuisance side effect in most cases, but if it ends up making you miss doses, it is not a good idea to continue the drug. Let your doctor know about this so they can see if there are alternatives. The same goes for difficulty taking medicine for other reasons. For example, if a pill is large and you have trouble swallowing it, ask your doctor if it comes in a different size or in an easier-to-consume alternative such as a liquid or topical patch.

Unfortunately, the medication regimens taken by SLE patients can be complicated. If your doctor changes your treatment regimen, and you are not 100% clear on how to take your medicine, make sure to ask them to write down the instructions in easy-to-understand terms. Sometimes doctors forget that what sounds simple to them may not be simple to others, so never be afraid to tell your doctor that you do not understand something. Doctors would rather have patients understand how to take their medicines instead of leaving the office with unanswered questions.

Ensuring that you do not run out of your prescriptions is essential. This means planning ahead to keep up with your refills. When you pick up your medicine, make sure to note how many refills remain. This will be noted on the bottle. If it says, "0 refills," then it is vital that you know when and how to get it refilled so that you do not run out. Some doctors want you to ask your pharmacist to fax them or send a computer request for refills (called electronic prescribing or e-prescribing). Some doctors want to see you personally for an appointment to give you the refill. And still others may want you to call their office to get your refill. Either way, do not wait until the last minute. Make sure that you request refills a week or so before needed. If your pills are gone on Saturday, don't think you can call your doctor late Friday afternoon to get it filled.

Also, find out if your prescription plan allows 90 days' worth at a time. It's a lot easier to pick up such a prescription than one that you have to get every 30 days. In addition, mail-order pharmacies that handle 90-day prescriptions can save you time. Getting 90 days' worth is also usually cheaper in the end. Plus, many prescription plans have made cost-saving deals with certain pharmacies to save their members more money. Just make sure to ask your doctor to prepare your prescription for 90 days at a time.

An essential part of taking medications is knowing how to take them correctly. For example, some medicines are best taken without food; some are better taken with food for better absorption. Some medicines should not be taken at the same time as other medicines. These instructions will be on your pill bottle or on a printout given to you by your pharmacist. We discuss the most commonly used drugs for lupus in this book and supply much of this advice in the following chapters.

If you forget to take a dose of your medicine, find out what you should do from your pharmacist or doctor. Specific instructions on how to deal with missed doses of lupus drugs are also included in the following chapters.

Sometimes crushing or cutting tablets can make it easier to take them. A large tablet can go down more easily when crushed and added to applesauce, for example. Note, though, that some medicines should never be chewed, crushed, or split in two, especially not drugs designed for slow release. These medicines will often have the letters CR (controlled release), DR (delayed-release), XR (extended-release), SR (slow release), or XL (extended life) in their names. If these are cut or crushed, the medicine is absorbed too quickly and can cause dangerous side effects.

Some pills have a protective coating to make them easier on the stomach or so that they can be absorbed later in the intestines. These will often be followed by the letters EC (enteric-coated). Some pills have two different drugs or substances designed to be released at different times in the intestinal system (such as diclofenac-misoprostol, Arthrotec).

Make sure your medications have not expired. All prescription packages should have an expiration date on them. The medicine should always be stored in the original bottle with the original identification information on it.

The FDA recommends not storing drugs in the bathroom because heat and moisture can cause them to expire prematurely. Also, do not keep them with dangerous materials (such as cleaners) to avoid inadvertently opening the wrong container.

Other Practicalities

Medicine Lists

One of the most important things we recommend for patients is to maintain an updated medication list that includes their drug intolerances (such as sulfa antibiotics) and

---

LUPUS IN FOCUS

What to do if you have difficulty swallowing pills

Difficulty swallowing pills is common. Many people with SLE have less saliva formation, making it difficult to swallow. Others have an esophagus (tube between the mouth and stomach) that does not move pills down to the stomach as it should. Page 314 includes practical advice on measures you can take to swallow medication more easily.

always keep it with them. This can be helpful, even life-saving, for many reasons. For example, if you have a list like this and you end up in an emergency room, the medical personnel will not give you any drugs that you do not tolerate, that could interact dangerously with yours, or that could flare your lupus. This way, you will receive the best medical care possible.

A medication list like the one in table 29.6 is useful. It can be handwritten or kept on your computer or smartphone. Whenever there is a change in any drug, you should immediately update your list and throw away the old one. Put a new copy in your pocketbook or wallet right away. Keeping it on a computer simplifies this process; a new one can be printed out each time a change is made. It is easy to find medication list forms that you can download off the internet.

At a minimum, you want the list to include the name of the drug, what dose each tablet, capsule, or liquid has, how many you take at a time, and how often you take it. However, to be complete and if you have enough room, you should consider adding the other information as well. The dose section should have the dose per pill or tablet. This is usually labeled in milligrams (mg) on the bottle. Other measurement units are sometimes used, such as micrograms (mcg) or international units (IU). If your medicine is a liquid, make sure you note the concentration (for example, 25 mg/mL or 50mg/2mL for liquid methotrexate). You should also include over-the-counter drugs, vitamins, and herbal supplements.

Also, write down what you are actually taking, which may not be the same as what you should be taking. For example, if your doctor wants you to be taking a drug twice a day, but you have been taking it only once a day most of the time, be honest and write down once a day on your list. When your doctor notes this discrepancy, it can lead to a discussion about why you are taking it only once a day, whether this may negatively affect your health, and if a better alternative is available.

When a nurse or medical assistant asks what you are taking, do not answer "yes" and "no" to their list of drug questions. Mistakes are easily made when done this way. Instead, hand them your current medicine list. They can double-check your list against what is in your chart. I for one always take an updated medicine list to my doctors' appointments. Even though I know my medicines inside and out, I realize it is easy to accidentally say "yes" when you mean "no," or vice versa. Handing the nurse or medical assistant my list prevents potential mistakes.

Table 29.6 Medication List Form (Example)

Drug Name	Dose	How Much Taken at a Time	How Often Taken	Why Taken (for what purpose)	Prescribing Doctor

It is not uncommon for patients to tell my medical assistant, "You should know what I'm taking. You have the list of medicines in your records." Doctors agree that most medication lists in our patients' charts are not 100% correct. Computerized electronic health records (EHRs) are complicated. Changing medications in them involves many steps of removing items, altering items, and adding items in specific spots. If any one step is incorrect, the list becomes incorrect.

In our EHR, when a drug gets down to zero refills, the computer automatically drops that medication down into the inactive drug list. This could be disastrous when this happens with a vital lupus medication, such as mycophenolate. For example, suppose the patient sees one of my partners, who does not realize that this occurred and so does not renew the prescription for this essential drug. However, if the patient shows an up-to-date medicine list, this mistake can be easily figured out and corrected.

A medication list kept by the patient and double-checked by the doctor during each visit ensures everyone is on the same page. It can also help catch any mistakes made by the pharmacy.

Some people find keeping a list of their medicines too bothersome. In that case, they should bring all of their drugs and vitamins in a bag to every doctor's visit. Another option is to photograph each drug label with your smartphone and show these at your appointment. Doctors would rather have their patients do this than possibly have an incorrect drug list in their charts.

Pharmacies

If you can, always go to the same pharmacy, especially if you take drugs prescribed by different doctors. That way the pharmacist will know all of your medications and alert your doctors if there are any critical interactions. If you go to several different pharmacies, you will miss having this safety net.

Going to one pharmacy also helps build a good relationship with the pharmacist, which can help you get high-quality service. In addition, if you take a medicine that is difficult to obtain or requires special ordering, you can more easily contact that pharmacist a week or so before you need your refill and ask them to ensure you don't run out.

When you pick up your medications at the pharmacy, always open the bottles before leaving and inspect them. If they are generic, they may come in different shapes, sizes, and colors each time. Pharmacies often buy the least expensive generic drugs to minimize costs. If your medicine looks different, you want to ensure that it is the correct drug and that a mistake was not made in filling the prescription. Ask the pharmacist to confirm that it is the right drug before leaving. If you are at home before you notice the difference, you can find out whether it is the correct medicine at Drugs.com (www .drugs.com/imprints.php) or WebMD (www.webmd.com/pill-identification/default .htm).

Another reason for checking your pills before you leave the pharmacy is to ensure that you have the correct number of tablets. If you are shortchanged (given too few) by mistake, you could run out of your medicine too soon and possibly develop withdrawal side effects. If you don't realize this until you get home, it's too late to do anything. Checking your pills at the pharmacy is especially important with substances controlled by the Drug Enforcement Administration (DEA), commonly called narcotics. These drugs are sometimes used for recreational purposes, otherwise abused, or sold on the street. Someone in the pharmacy could potentially have an ulterior motive for taking some of your pills. Although highly illegal, this does occur. You want to figure this out while you are standing at the counter in full view of the pharmacy clerk and pharmacist.

Disposing of Medicines

If you must stop a drug and have some left over, it is crucial to know how to dispose of them (table 29.7). Some will have disposal instructions printed on the prescription. You can also go to fda.gov/drugs/safe-disposal-medicines/disposal-unused-medicines-what-you-should-know. The best method is to drop them off at a local Drug Take Back Site (see table 29.7). If it is a controlled substance, you can take it to one of those sites, but even better, take it to a DEA-recommended site (table 29.7).

These sites are not convenient for everyone, so there are alternative methods. Most drugs (but not controlled substances) can be thrown into the trash, but you should take precautions, starting with checking with your pharmacist whether doing so is legal. If it is, scratch out your personal information on the container to reduce the chances of someone else using it to get refills of the medicine. Then, take out the drugs and mix them with something unappealing, such as coffee grounds or kitty litter, place the mix in a sealable container, and put it in the trash. Mixing them in kitty litter or coffee grounds reduces the chances for pets or children from consuming them.

Never give your medicine to friends or relatives. You cannot be sure it is safe for them.

Most drugs should not be flushed down the toilet; otherwise, they could up in drinking water, streams, and lakes. There are some exceptions, though. The FDA recommends that drugs that people seek to abuse and drugs that can potentially kill someone if one dose is taken should be flushed. These include many opioid pain relievers (narcotics), such as oxycodone, hydrocodone, morphine, fentanyl patches, and OxyCONTIN. Flushing them is considered safe for the environment. By getting rid of them immediately, they will be less likely to be swallowed by children or pets or stolen by others for inappropriate usage. To see the FDA "Flush List," go to fda.gov/media/85219/download.

Table 29.7 Disposing of Drugs

- Remove personal information from prescriptions.
- Take controlled substances (such as opioids) to a Controlled Substance Public Disposal Location: apps.deadiversion.usdoj.gov/pubdispsearch/spring/main
- Drop off any drug off at your local Take Back Site: go to www.safe.pharmacy
- Many drugs can be thrown out in the trash in many communities.
- Contact your local government and pharmacist for details.
- Mix drugs in kitty litter or coffee grounds, seal in a container, place in the trash.
- Some drugs *should* be flushed down the toilet (e.g., Percocet, morphine, fentanyl patches, OxyCONTIN).
- Most others *should not* be flushed down the toilet.

Dispose of drugs your doctor asks you to stop taking

People often keep discontinued drugs, thinking they could be useful in the future. However, it is safer to dispose of them at once. There are several reasons. First, when pill bottles pile up, you can easily make a mistake such as retaking an old drug instead of the correct one. Also, if you become ill and a family member must care for you, figuring out what medicine to give you can turn into a nightmare for them. Still another is that you do not want your drugs to get into the wrong hands. It is not uncommon for prescription drugs to be stolen, even by those who are closest to us.

However, do not dispose of drugs that you may need in the future. For example, the dose of some medications (like steroids) may be increased and decreased over time. Ask your doctor.

Handling of Sharps

Many drugs must be given by injection instead of pill form. These include the biologics discussed in chapters 33, 34, and 37. Some osteoporosis drugs, such as Forteo and Tymlos (chapter 24), also involve needles. Learning how to properly handle needles and other sharp devices is essential. You want to prevent others from injury, exposure to your drug, or possibly contracting a blood-borne disease (such as viral hepatitis or HIV). Each state has its own laws on the proper disposal of needles and other sharps. To learn more, go to safeneedledisposal.org. If you do not have internet access, contact your pharmacy or physician for guidance. Also, many pharmaceutical companies help with needle disposal. Contact the pharmaceutical company directly, either by calling—the number in the drug information that most patients receive—or by going to the drug's website (usually www.[fill in the drug name].com). You can also ask them for disposal containers. This is usually a free service.

1. Sometimes, it is necessary to take many drugs for SLE. Some calm down the immune system. Others treat symptoms (such as pain); others reduce side effects.

2. Learn the reason for taking each drug. This can help you stay adherent to your regimen.

3. The benefits of a drug should outweigh potential side effects. Ask your doctor for their advice.

4. Always contact your doctor's office when you develop a side effect to determine how you should respond. You can also look up your drug in this book.

5. The most common reason for drugs not working is not taking them regularly or taking them incorrectly.

6. Use the strategies in table 29.5 to ensure you take your medications regularly.

7. Keep an updated medicine list that includes drug intolerances (such as sulfon-amide antibiotics) with you at all times (table 29.6).

8. Use one pharmacy to fill all prescriptions, if possible.

9. Check your prescription for accuracy when you pick it up at the pharmacy.

10. Dispose of drugs properly (table 29.7).

11. If you use injectable medicines, go to safeneedledisposal.org/ for disposal information. You can also contact the drug company to see if it can provide you with sharps disposal equipment.

Antimalarials

Yashaar Chaichian, MD, and Ziv Paz, MD, *Contributing Editors*

Patients sometimes ask, "Why do drugs used to treat malaria also work for autoimmune diseases like lupus?" First, understanding how the immune system works helps explain the answer. One key immune system activity is antigen presentation (figure 30.1A). Antigens are substances that cause the immune system to make antibodies directed toward those specific antigens to protect the body (chapters 1 and 3). For example, suppose you are infected with a virus called parvovirus, which can cause a cold-like illness and sometimes rash, joint pain, and other lupus-like symptoms. The immune system recognizes the virus substances (which function as antigens), realizes they do not belong to the body, and launches an all-out war against the virus. It does this by making antibodies that attach to the parvovirus antigens. Your immune system develops "memory" via antibodies that recognize parvovirus for the rest of your life. Thus, if you are infected by parvovirus in the future, you most likely will not get sick from it again.

So now, let us go a little deeper into how the body makes these antibodies, focusing on a concept called antigen processing (figure 30.1A). Although this is a technical discussion, it can be interesting for someone who wants to know more about how antimalarial drugs (antimalarials for short) work. White blood cells known as macrophages and plasmacytoid dendritic cells (pDCs) are key to finding foreign antigens. You can think of these cells, also known as antigen-presenting cells (APCs), as frontline soldiers who identify unusual antigen substances such as viruses, bacteria, and cancer cells. In the figures, you can replace the macrophage-engulfing damaged body cells mentioned there with viruses, bacteria, and cancer cells as well. The same process occurs.

In SLE, the immune system attacks parts of the body itself, the antigens it thinks are foreign are actually substances that naturally occur in the body. When macrophages and other antigen-presenting cells see these substances (antigens), they engulf them in tiny bubbles called vacuoles (figure 30.1A). The vacuoles digest these antigens into smaller components, reassemble them, then attach these reassembled structures to their outer surface. These APCs can then show the antigens (or present them) to other white blood cells (especially T-cells). The T-cells think that these substances normally found in the body are dangerous. The T-cells then cause B-cells (white blood cells that makes antibodies) to make antibodies directed against the body's own substances (antigens). The antibodies produced to attack the body's own antigens are called auto-antibodies. Examples of these auto-antibodies are anti-dsDNA, anti-Smith, and anti-SSA (chapter 4).

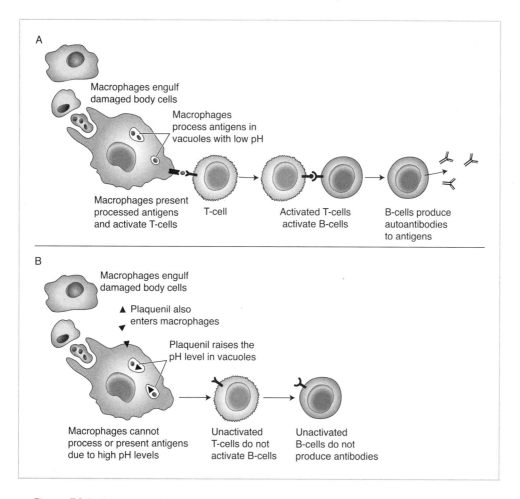

Figure 30.1 Skin antigen processing to T-cell causes lupus rash (A); Plaquenil interferes with skin antigen presentation to T-cell (B).

A well-known example of this occurring in SLE is when ultraviolet (UV) light damages skin cells. Damaged skin cells release their inner contents, such as the nucleus and DNA, into the surrounding tissues. Thinking that the DNA is a foreign invader, the macrophages and other APCs engulf the damaged cells' contents, such as its DNA. In this case, the DNA is being dealt with as if it were a foreign substance or antigen. The rearranged DNA molecules are then presented by the APCs to T-cells that then tell the B-cells to make anti-DNA antibodies. The anti-DNA autoantibodies can then attach to the person's own DNA anywhere in the body. This combination of the body's own DNA bound to the anti-DNA antibody is called an immune complex. Such immune complexes can then travel throughout the body, depositing in other tissues where the lupus immune system can cause inflammation and damage. One of the most concerning places is the kidneys, where these DNA immune complexes can cause lupus nephritis (chapter 12). In short, UV light exposure can cause not only a lupus rash in the area of exposure

LUPUS IN FOCUS

HCQ calms down the immune system, but does not suppress it

Although HCQ decreases autoantibody formation, it does not control lupus completely in all patients. This is because other parts of the immune system still function abnormally in SLE.

In addition, HCQ doesn't completely stop antigen processing and auto-antibody formation; it merely decreases the amount of processing. And thank goodness for that. We need antigen processing so that our immune system fights off infections, cancers, and more. We call HCQ an immunomodulator and not an immunosuppressant. It calms down the immune system (or modulates it) without suppressing it.

but also inflammation in distant body parts such as the kidneys. This is why we ask all SLE patients to use sunscreen all the time. They can develop problems such as lupus nephritis from UV light without getting a rash.

The APCs' vacuoles must have a low pH (be acidic) for antigen presentation to occur. When antimalarials (hydroxychloroquine, chloroquine, and quinacrine) enter the APCs, they concentrate inside the vacuoles and create higher pH levels (figure 30.1B). The APCs' digesting enzymes are unable to function in this higher pH and cannot break down the antigens to present to T-cells. The T-cells cannot "see" these antigens and, thus, do not signal B-cells to make lupus autoantibodies. Therefore, antimalarial medications calm down the immune system.

However, antimalarials do not actually cause immunosuppression. In other words, the immune system still functions normally in different areas, continuing to protect the person from infections and cancer.

Increasing vacuoles' pH levels to reduce antigen processing and antibody formation is not the only way antimalarials work. In lupus, toll-like receptors (a part of the immune system) become overactive and work abnormally, causing inflammation and damage. Antimalarials stop these toll-like receptors from working abnormally, resulting in less lupus inflammation. Delving deeper into this topic is beyond the scope of this book.

"Hydroxychloroquine Is Lupus Life Insurance"

This is a common saying among rheumatologists. As Dr. Michelle Petri, the director of the Lupus Center at Johns Hopkins, Baltimore, Maryland, observes, "Hydroxychloroquine is the only drug proven to prolong survival in lupus." Although we suspect that other treatments (such as belimumab) will join this list in the future, hydroxychloroquine (HCQ) is the only drug proven by large research studies to prolong life expectancy in SLE (as of 2023).

Doctors always try to find effective therapies that cause the fewest side effects. That is truly the case for HCQ. It has numerous benefits for lupus patients (table 30.1). When you compare the long list of benefits to its low risk of side effects, it is one of the best drugs available.

Table 30.1 Benefits of Antimalarial Drugs

- Help arthritis, rashes, serositis, fatigue, fevers, and low blood counts
- Reduce lupus flares while increasing remission and low-disease activity
- Reduce skin UV sensitivity
- Reduce the amount of internal organ involvement
- Reduce the need for higher steroid doses
- Reduce long-term organ damage
- Reduce blood clots from antiphospholipid antibodies
- Lower total cholesterol and bad cholesterol (LDL) levels
- Reduce the risk of developing diabetes
- Lower the risk of heart attacks (when used with low-dose aspirin)
- Increase successful pregnancy outcomes
- Help prevent congenital heart block from anti-SSA antibodies
- Help prevent other types of neonatal lupus from anti-SSA antibodies
- Improve quality of life and increase life expectancy in SLE patients
- Reduce infections and some cancers
- Have less chance of significant side effects compared to other lupus drugs

In this chapter, we talk mainly about HCQ because it is the best-studied antimalarial in lupus. However, chloroquine (CQ) and quinacrine have their place, and we discuss them further toward the end of the chapter.

HCQ is especially useful for milder lupus problems. It can help reduce lupus arthritis joint pain and skin inflammation. It also reduces skin UV sensitivity, though taking HCQ does not negate using sunscreen and avoiding the sun. In addition, HCQ can increase blood cell counts in lupus patients with low blood counts. In someone with SLE fatigue, HCQ can increase energy levels, as well.

Quinacrine in particular appears to help with energy and can even improve memory and concentration, as it works as a central nervous system stimulant. However, you must be careful not to over-interpret antimalarials' effect on fatigue. As discussed in chapter 6, fatigue is more commonly due to other problems such as depression, fibromyalgia, or lack of sleep. Antimalarials do not help with these causes of fatigue.

Antimalarials decrease the number and severity of lupus flares. A study by the Canadian Rheumatology Group showed that 73% of patients who did not take an antimalarial medicine developed flares of their lupus. In comparison, only 36% of those who took an antimalarial had a flare. Their flares were also milder overall compared to the patients who did not take an antimalarial.

Some people have symptoms suggestive of SLE but do not have full-blown SLE. They are often diagnosed with undifferentiated connective tissue disease (UCTD), incomplete lupus, or lupus-like disease (chapter 2). Treating UCTD with HCQ can decrease the chances of it developing into severe SLE. As of early 2023, a large research study is being done to see if HCQ can prevent SLE in these individuals—The Study of anti-Malarials in Incomplete Lupus Erythematosus (SMILE). We hope the results will be available in a year or so.

While HCQ helps with milder SLE problems, it is not strong enough for inflammation of the brain, nerves, kidneys, heart, and lungs. If you have significant inflammation of any major organs, your rheumatologist needs to use stronger immunosuppressants (table 22.1) along with HCQ. Patients with major organ involvement, such as the kidneys, do much better when they take HCQ with their immunosuppressants. HCQ increases the chances for remission when used with an immunosuppressant for severe SLE problems. This means that patients can be in a state in which they have no symptoms, signs, or lab abnormalities related to the previously affected organ. Taking HCQ can also help decrease the doses needed of the other stronger drugs. This can lead to fewer side effects.

Some people with mild lupus may not feel sick and may say, "Why should I take anything when I feel so good?" The reason is that over time, anyone with SLE can develop more severe lupus. Between 40% and 50% of SLE patients develop lupus nephritis (kidney inflammation). It can occur at any time and usually does so without warning. Someone with mild SLE who takes HCQ regularly is less likely to (a) develop lupus nephritis and (b) have it be as severe if it does develop, compared to someone who does not take HCQ.

Steroids can be lifesaving when used right away for severe SLE. However, virtually 100% of people who take steroids for any significant time develop side effects, such as infections, congestive heart failure, bleeding ulcers, and organ damage. Studies show that staying at 7.5 mg/day of prednisone or less, or ideally less than 6 mg/day, reduces steroid-related organ damage. Nevertheless, no "safe" steroid dose is universally agreed upon. The goal is to limit the amount to the lowest necessary and to take it for the shortest duration. Therefore, doctors use other medicines (such as HCQ) to decrease the use of steroids ("steroid-sparing effect").

Antimalarials also decrease the amount of permanent damage within organs affected by lupus. The damage from lupus occurs in two stages. The first is the inflammatory stage, in which the immune system attacks an organ (for example, the kidneys). The second is when the inflammation heals, leaving permanent scar tissue that prevents that part of an organ to function properly. This is what we are referring to when we talk about long-term organ damage from lupus.

When doctors treat lupus patients, they have two goals in mind. First, they want the treatment to help them feel better right away (such as relieving them of their rashes, pain, fever, and so on). Second, they also want to decrease the amount of inflammation as quickly as possible so that permanent damage does not occur in the body's organs. Regular HCQ usage reduces long-term organ damage.

Between 30% and 50% of SLE patients are positive for antiphospholipid antibodies (aPLAs) such as anticardiolipin antibodies, lupus anticoagulant, and beta-2 glycoprotein I antibodies. Over time, approximately 50% of aPLA-positive patients develop problems, such as blood clots in the legs or lungs, heart attacks, and strokes (all discussed in chapter 9). Regularly taking HCQ decreases the chances of these blood clots. A 2010 Canadian study showed that lupus patients who took antimalarials were 68% less likely to develop blood clots than patients who did not.

The Johns Hopkins Lupus Center found a similar result in 2021 when they looked at SLE patients who were aPLA-negative. Their study showed that patients who took

HCQ regularly with an HCQ drug level of at least 1068 ng/mL were 68% less likely to develop blood clots than those with levels less than 648 ng/mL. It is thought that fewer blood clots form because HCQ prevents platelets from clumping together and reduces aPLA blood levels.

Heart attacks and strokes are among the most common causes of death in SLE. One risk factor for heart attacks and strokes is high cholesterol. Regularly taking HCQ reduces cholesterol levels (both total cholesterol and LDL, or "bad" cholesterol). A study also showed that people with lupus who took HCQ were less likely to develop diabetes (another risk factor for heart disease) compared to those who did not take it. A 2023 study showed that HCQ reduced heart attacks and strokes, while a 2017 Italian study suggested that taking low-dose aspirin with HCQ reduced heart attacks by even more.

HCQ also increases life expectancy in SLE. Numerous studies have shown that HCQ reduces the risk of dying by more than half. Some have shown even better results. For example, in a 2021 Canadian study that followed over 3,000 patients with SLE over an average of 6 years, those who did not take HCQ were 4 times more likely to die than those who took HCQ.

A 2011 study from China even went so far as to say, "Our analyses show that antimalarials are the only class of drugs that exerted a clear protective effect on survival." This study looked at about 2,000 patients hospitalized with SLE and all the medications they were taking. Those taking antimalarials at the start of their hospitalization were much less likely to die.

Much of the credit for antimalarials increasing life expectancy is due to the way that they help control lupus. In addition, people who take HCQ regularly are less likely to need stronger immunosuppressants and steroids, which increase the risk of infections. Recall from chapters 19 and 22 that infections are among the leading causes of death in SLE.

With HCQ having so many good effects, it is impressive that it rarely causes severe side effects. While 10%–20% of people who take it may experience mild side effects like stomach upset, difficulty sleeping, rash, or headaches, these are typically mild and tolerable or go away when the dose of the medicine is decreased. Severe side effects are unusual.

The two primary downsides of HCQ are that it is slow to work (see specific drug information in the HCQ section below) and that patients need eye exams regularly while taking it.

Eye Problems and Antimalarials

The most significant potential side effect of HCQ and CQ is antimalarial retinopathy (also called antimalarial maculopathy). The retina (chapter 16), which is the back part of the eye, is responsible for capturing light that enters the eye and allows your brain to see the world you live in. Over time, these drugs can accumulate in the retina, causing damage. Retinopathy refers to a disease of the retina. The macula, which is the central part of the retina, is responsible for high-definition vision. This is the retina area most often affected by antimalarials and is called maculopathy when it occurs here.

Antimalarial retinopathy can lead to blurred vision, difficulty reading, light intolerance (photophobia), and sometimes seeing flashing lights. In severe cases, antimalarial retinopathy causes concentric rings of pigmentation (looking like the bull's eye of a dartboard) on the retina—hence the term "bull's eye retinopathy" or "bull's eye macu-lopathy." This is what the eye doctor can see when examining the retina on physical exam.

Note the dark round area above and to the right of the pointer in figure 30.2. This is the bull's eye. It is surrounded by a clear area and then another ring of dark pigment. Though this example is not perfect, its shape is like that of a dartboard with the bulls-eye in the middle.

This should never occur anymore because the newer eye exams can diagnose early stages of antimalarial retinopathy before a "bull's eye" can be seen on physical exam. However, if someone does not keep up with their eye exams and develops the bull's eye, it can cause vision problems.

Another rare eye problem with antimalarials is that the drugs can deposit in the clear, front part of the eye (called corneal deposits). This can lead to seeing halos around lights and having difficulty tolerating light. These side effects tend to occur from two weeks to a few months after starting the drug. Usually, they are mild and transient; most people do not need to stop their medicine. If significant vision problems occur, the con-dition resolves on lower doses or stopping the drug.

Do not let the very small chances of antimalarials affecting your eyes scare you. Most people taking them never develop retinopathy. Specifically, only an estimated 2% of

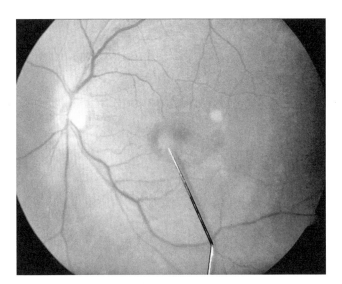

Figure 30.2 Bull's eye maculopathy due to HCQ. The tip of the metal pointer shows the center of the bull's eye maculopa-thy in the photo. This woman was on HCQ for SLE. Fortu-nately, her vision was not impaired (most patients with this have some vision loss). This was picked up by her ophthalmol-ogist during an eye examination before the better tests (like SD-OCT) became available. Photo courtesy of retinologist Omar Ahmad, MD

patients taking HCQ for 10 years have retinopathy. While the risk increases for patients on HCQ for more than 10 years, most never develop retinopathy.

When vision problems occur in patients taking HCQ, it is almost always due to other problems. For example, dry eye from Sjögren's disease (chapter 14) is one of the most common causes of blurred vision in SLE. Cataracts (clouding of the lens, chapter 16) is also a common cause. So is the need for a new eyeglass prescription. It is essential to see your eye doctor so that any eye issue is properly diagnosed, and the right treatment is given. Do not jump to the conclusion that HCQ is causing your problems. It very rarely is.

Furthermore, vision loss related to retinopathy from antimalarials, particularly in the case of HCQ, should no longer occur if current screening recommendations are followed. The next section describes the dosing of CQ and HCQ and the eye tests needed.

Hydroxychloroquine and Chloroquine Dosing

In 2016, the American Academy of Ophthalmology (AAO) released new dosing guidelines for HCQ and CQ. These recommendations were based on a 2014 research study using a large health care organization database (Kaiser Permanente).

The 2016 AAO recommendations state that patients should not take more than 5 mg of HCQ per kg of actual body weight per day. *Actual* body weight needs to be emphasized. The AAO's earlier recommendations (as described in this book's first edition) were based on ideal body weight, which was calculated using height, sex, and actual body weight. Using actual body weight makes dosage calculations much easier (table 30.2).

Regarding CQ, no more than 2.3 mg/kg daily is recommended. A shortcut in the United States, where pounds are used, is to not take a higher number of milligrams of CQ than your body weight in pounds. For example, a 170-pound person should not take more than 170 mg of CQ daily.

These doses were recommended because abnormal eye exams were seen in some patients on higher doses in the Kaiser Permanente study. However, there were questions over what doses of antimalarials patients were actually taking and whether the abnormal eye exams were truly due to antimalarial retinopathy or other eye problems unrelated to the drugs. Study results are therefore problematic.

In addition, the recommended doses were designed to minimize the possibility of retinopathy; the AAO did not assess the effectiveness of these doses for SLE. It is important to base drug dosing on safety balanced with efficacy.

Therefore, many lupus experts do not agree with these dosing recommendations. Since HCQ is the most crucial drug for SLE and is much safer than immunosuppressants

Table 30.2 Hydroxychloroquine Dosing

Body Weight Pounds (kilograms)	Maximum Daily HCQ Dose
Greater than 175 pounds (>80 kg)	400 mg
132–174 pounds (60 kg–79 kg)	300 mg–395 mg
Less than 132 pounds (<60 kg)	295 mg or less

Note: These recommendations are based on taking 5 mg/kg actual body weight or less daily.

(table 22.1), we should use it to reach its full effectiveness while also lowering the risk of side effects such as retinopathy. The FDA-approved package insert for HCQ (as of 2023) recommends a dose of 200 mg to 400 mg daily to treat lupus. It recommends yearly eye exams if more than 5 mg/kg/day is used.

My strategy for HCQ dosing is a hybrid of the two versions mentioned above. When I first put a patient on HCQ, I usually begin with a maximum dose of 5 mg/kg per day (per the AAO recommendation), with one exception.

If someone has moderate to severe disease, I start them on 600 mg a day (200 mg 3 times a day). I reduce the dose to 5 mg/kg per day one to three months later. This is because HCQ begins working very slowly at a dose of 400 mg daily or less.

A rheumatoid arthritis (RA) study showed that patients starting on doses higher than 400 mg a day responded faster. That has been the case in my experience with SLE patients. The FDA-approved package insert says that 600 mg a day can be used as a loading dose in RA, an autoimmune disease closely related to SLE. In addition, UpTo-Date (an online medical management site for doctors) states that a loading dose of up to 600 mg per day can be used for up to 3 months if needed to achieve lupus disease control.

But we don't need to rely only on these recommendations. One of the most important advances in managing lupus is the ability to measure whole blood HCQ drug levels (or HCQ drug levels for the sake of simplicity), which is now widely available in the United States and is covered by most insurance plans. The Johns Hopkins Lupus Center showed that patients with HCQ levels above 1,752 ng/mL had an increased risk for retinopathy, while those with levels less than 1,183 ng/mL had the lowest risk. Another study in France showed that similarly high levels predicted other side effects such as stomach problems and skin discoloration.

At the same time, other studies have shown that patients with HCQ blood levels lower than 1,000 ng/mL have high rates of lupus flares and worse disease activity. Therefore, my ideal HCQ drug level is 1,000 ng/mL or above for better disease control, yet below 1,200 for the lowest retinopathy risk.

A 2022 US study showed that 23% of patients taking the AAO-recommended HCQ (doses 5 mg/kg per day or less) had moderate to severe disease flares during a 6-month period. In addition, patients taking the AAO-recommended dose had more flares compared to patients on higher doses. This suggests that this recommended dose is not effective for many of our patients.

In my practice, I (Don Thomas, MD) use HCQ drug levels to adjust dosing. I aim for 1,000 to 1,200 ng/mL. For some patients, it can be difficult to fine-tune the dose to such a narrow target, so I'll allow up to 1,500 ng/mL in them. In patients with hard-to-control disease, allowing a level up to 1,700 ng/mL may be optimal (it is close to the 1,752 level in the Johns Hopkins study mentioned above).

I have had quite a few patients on the AAO-recommended dose who had active SLE with flares and low HCQ drug levels. Using their drug levels as a guide, I've had many of these patients take higher than the AAO-recommended dose, which resulted in better disease control.

The correct time to check an HCQ drug level is right before a scheduled dose (called a trough level). After someone takes HCQ, levels rise as much as 30%, with the maximum level reached around 4 hours later and gradually decreasing after that.

A low drug level at any time is good evidence for poor adherence. However, a higher HCQ drug level does not necessarily mean that the patient is taking HCQ regularly, especially if the level is measured three to four hours after their dose. For example, someone who misses HCQ doses and who would normally have a trough level of 770 ng/mL (not at our target of 1,000) could have a level of 1,001 ng/mL if measured 4 hours after they took their dose. This can make it falsely appear that they are taking their drug regularly and that they have an ideal drug level. In other words, it is essential to insist on a trough level for accurate dose adjustments and identification of poor adherence.

HCQ drug levels can be checked one and a half months after initiating HCQ therapy or one month after changing a dose, per the French Plaquenil LUpus Systemic (PLUS) study.

Eye Screening Tests

In 2016 the AAO updated eye exam recommendations to ensure that patients do not develop antimalarial retinopathy. In 2021, the AAO (in collaboration with rheumatology and dermatology medical societies) recommended that the first retinal exam occurs within a few months of starting HCQ. This evaluation and later exams need to include two eye tests sensitive to retina problems: a spectral-domain optical coherence tomography (SD-OCT, figure 30.3) and a visual field (VF) 10-2 test. If you are Asian, you also need a third eye test each time: either a VF 24-2 or a VF 30-2. Many Asians have a different part of the retina involved from antimalarials than other ethnicities, requiring this additional visual field exam (see chapter 19 for an in-depth discussion).

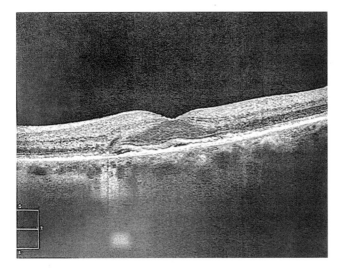

Figure 30.3 HCQ retinopathy on an SD-OCT. In the center of the picture, just above the horizontal white line, is a dark area that looks a bit like an alien spaceship from old-sci-fi movies. This is called the "flying saucer sign" and is a classic finding with HCQ retinopathy. Photo courtesy of Doctors Grant Hom, Thais Conti, and Rishi Singh, Cleveland Clinic

The machinery necessary to perform these tests is not found in all eye doctors' offices (especially the SD-OCT and VF 10-2). Alternatives tests include either a fundus autofluorescence (FAF) or the more accurate multifocal electroretinogram (mfERG). If your eye doctor can do the VF 10-2 test, ask if they can do a VF 10-2 using a white target (figure 30.4) to ensure a more reliable result than you can get with a simple red target. If not, ask for a referral to an eye specialist closest to you who can do the correct tests.

After their first eye exam, many patients can wait five years before the next test. It is rare to develop antimalarial retinopathy before five years. After that, though, you should have two of the tests mentioned above (three if you are Asian) performed yearly. Preferably, these tests would be a VF 10-2 and an SD-OCT (along with a VF 24-2 or a VF 30-2 if Asian). If, however, you are at increased risk for eye problems, you should have annual exams beginning the first year. These earlier yearly exams are recommended for people with decreased kidney function, people who already have a retina problem, people taking tamoxifen (a breast cancer drug that causes retinopathy), and people on antimalarial doses higher than the 2016 AAO recommendations.

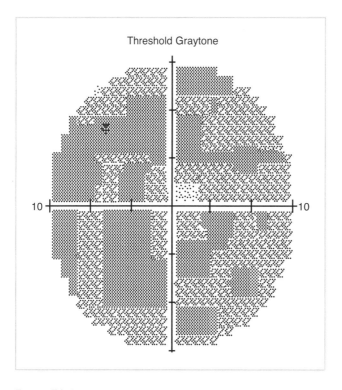

Figure 30.4 HCQ retinopathy on a VF 10-2 test. Note the darker gray areas. Those are areas of vision loss in the patient with HCQ retinopathy in figure 30.3. The gray and white areas are normal vision. Photo courtesy of Doctors Grant Hom, Thais Conti, and Rishi Singh Cleveland Clinic

ANTIMALARIALS

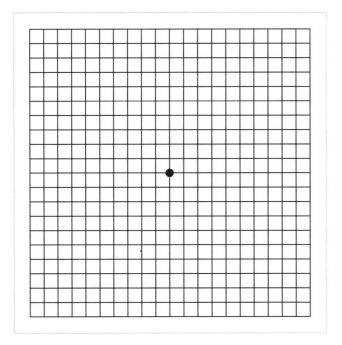

Figure 30.5 Amsler grid

When the eye testing outlined above is followed closely, your eye doctor can detect problems before you would ever notice any visual changes, thus, making antimalarials incredibly safe.

If you are still nervous about retinopathy after reading this chapter, you can comfort yourself by taking an Amsler grid test, which you can easily do at home (figure 30.5). It was developed in 1945 by Dr. Marc Amsler (a Swiss ophthalmologist) to help identify retina problems.

How to Use an Amsler Grid

- If you wear reading glasses, wear them when looking at the grid.

- Hold the grid out at a comfortable reading distance where it is in good focus.

- Cover one eye and look at the central dot. You should be able to see all lines clearly. They should all be straight and connect at 90-degree angles. You should also see all four outer sides plus the corners. If any lines appear blurred, wavy, or distorted, or parts are missing, see your eye doctor.

- Cover your other eye and repeat the above.

If you do have difficulty seeing parts of this grid, it is almost always due to problems other than HCQ retinopathy. These include diabetic retinopathy, hypertensive retinopathy, vitreomacular traction, epiretinal membrane, posterior vitreous detachment, and macular degeneration. The latter three problems are very common in older people and are often identified by an abnormal Amsler grid. If the test is abnormal,

Table 30.3 Preventing Antimalarial Retinopathy

- Make sure your dose is based on table 30.2, or ask your rheumatologist to measure your whole blood HCQ drug level to help adjust dosing.

- Have your first eye exams within a few months of starting an antimalarial.

- Before making an appointment with an eye doctor, call them and ask if they specifically do VF 10-2 and SD-OCT tests. If not, find an office that does (if possible, in your area).

- Make sure you get a visual field (VF) 10-2 and an SD-OCT eye test.

  - If these tests are not available, other options are a FAF or mfERG test.

  - If Asian, you also need a VF 24-2 or a VF 30-2 test (a total of 3 eye tests)

- After initial exams, begin having annual exams starting in the fifth year of treatment.

- If you are at increased risk for eye problems (e.g., decreased kidney function, have other retina disorders, or take tamoxifen), begin annual exams immediately.

- Do an Amsler grid exam at home monthly. If results are abnormal (see main text), see your eye doctor.

---

make an appointment with your ophthalmologist as soon as possible. Conditions such as early macular degeneration are treatable.

Note that the Amsler grid does not replace the need to have the visual field 10-2, SD-OCT, or other screening tests. If you take the proper precautions (table 30.3), vision problems from antimalarials should not occur.

Everyone with SLE should be taking antimalarials if they are not truly allergic. The medicine's many advantages (table 30.1) far outweigh any risk of significant side effects, including eye problems. The rest of this chapter goes into more detail about the three antimalarials used to treat lupus.

Hydroxychloroquine (HCQ, Plaquenil)

HCQ is most helpful for lupus arthritis, rashes, mouth sores, fatigue, fevers, and low blood counts. It is not adequate by itself for severe lupus problems such as kidney, nerve, brain, heart, and lung involvement. However, it increases remission rates when used with immunosuppressants.

Generic available: Yes.

How HCQ works: HCQ is a slow-working drug. It takes about a month before its effects are noticed, and it takes three to six months before its full effects occur in most people. It can even take up to a year for some. Starting with a dose of 600 mg daily for 1–3 months helps it work faster. Also, see table 30.1.

Do not take if

- you are allergic to it.

- you have a severe eye problem that makes it impossible to screen for retinopathy (the ophthalmologist would make this determination).

- you develop retinopathy from HCQ.

- you have congenital long QT syndrome, continuous QT measurements > 500 milliseconds on ECG, dangerous low heart rate disorders, certain heart arrhythmias (ask your cardiologist), uncorrected low magnesium or potassium levels, a recent heart attack, or severe congestive heart failure (ask your cardiologist).

Dosage: See table 30.2 for the doses recommended by the American Academy of Ophthalmology. We can calculate the total amount of HCQ that can be taken weekly (based on actual body weight and no more than 5 mg/kg/d), then divide it by 7 days to figure out the daily dose. Read the section on Hydroxychloroquine and Chloroquine Dosing above.

HCQ comes in 100 mg, 200 mg, 300 mg, and 400 mg tablets. As of 2023, the costs of the 100 mg, 300 mg, and 400 mg tablets were significantly higher than the 200 mg tablets and are usually not covered by insurance plans.

If you are on 400 mg a day, try taking both 200 mg pills once a day to decrease your chances of missing doses. If it bothers your stomach by taking both together, split up the amount by taking one pill twice a day instead. If you take it in the morning or daytime and it causes nausea, take it before bed. It is less likely to cause nausea at bedtime. Taking it with food also avoids stomach upset.

If you are prescribed 300 mg a day (1½ daily of the 200 mg tablets), an alternative is to take one tablet one day (200 mg), alternating with 2 tablets (400 mg) the next. Taking one pill on odd-numbered days of the month and two tablets on even-numbered days is an easy way to remember.

Your pharmacist may tell you that you should not cut your pills. That is the formal recommendation by the manufacturer because the tablets are not scored (and are difficult to cut exactly in half), and the cut pills have an unpleasant taste. However, an inexact cut is not a problem. Due to the way HCQ is absorbed and handled in the body, slightly different doses on each day do not make a difference. Do the "alternate 1 tablet with 2 tablets every other day" dosing if the taste is too unpleasant.

Some rheumatologists will initially prescribe 600 mg a day for the first 1–3 months then lower it to the doses in table 30.2. HCQ works faster when dosed in this manner.

Tests for whole blood HCQ drug levels can be used to help adjust dosage. HCQ drug-level blood tests are best done just before a dose. The optimal level is 1,000 ng/mL to 1,200 ng/mL (with exceptions as discussed in the main text earlier).

Patients with malabsorption problems (such as after gastric bypass surgery) may need higher doses, and those with decreased kidney function may need lower doses than what is recommended in table 30.2.

A lower dosage should be used in people with severely low kidney function. As of 2022, lupus expert Dr. Daniel Wallace used 200 mg daily of HCQ in end-stage kidney disease. Dr. Michelle Petri (Johns Hopkins Lupus Center, Baltimore, MD) used one 200 mg dose after each dialysis treatment. I (Don Thomas, MD) use HCQ drug levels to determine the optimal dose in patients with kidney failure.

If you miss a dose, take your next amount on the same day as soon as you realize you forgot it.

If you do not remember until the following day that you forgot your previous dose, take a double amount on the day you remember. For example, if you remember at 8:00 A.M. that you forgot the previous day's 11:00 A.M. dose, take your full dose right away,

LUPUS IN FOCUS

Drugs that prolong the QT interval when used with antimalarials

In 2020, due to flawed research, there was a surge of HCQ use for COVID patients. Subsequently numerous research studies showed that HCQ was ineffective for COVID. In those studies there was an increase in ECG abnormalities called QT-interval prolongation (abbreviated "QTc"; see chapter 11 for details), which can potentially cause heart rhythm problems. However, the doses of HCQ used in these research studies varied from 600 mg to 1,200 mg daily, much higher than we use in SLE.

A 2020 study found no association between HCQ use and QTc prolongation among patients with SLE or RA. Only when HCQ was combined with an antipsychotic did they observe QTc prolongation. An even larger 2022 Canadian study of over 23,000 SLE and RA patients taking HCQ showed no increase in heart rhythm problems.

Another study from 2021 limited to patients with lupus found no association between HCQ use and QTc prolongation, regardless of blood level, dose prescribed, chronic kidney disease, or known heart issues. Mild QTc prolongation was seen among those on other potential QTc-prolonging drugs.

Nevertheless, it would not be unreasonable to check the ECG in patients at high risk of QTc-interval prolongation. This could include patients with rhythm problems (arrhythmias) and those with preexisting QT prolongation, although even in these patients, the risk is low.

In high-risk patients, precautions could be taken in prescribing other drugs that can increase QTc-intervals. For example, if there is an alternative drug, let's say an antibiotic other than azithromycin (which can increase QTc), it could be used instead. Another choice for drugs used for a short period (such as antibiotics) would be to stop HCQ or CQ during that short time. This rarely causes problems with lupus since the effects of HCQ and CQ last a long time.

If a drug that prolongs the QT interval must be used for a long time (such as an antipsychotic), and if there are no alternatives, an ECG could be done before adding the drug, and you could consult with a cardiologist. ECGs could be checked while on both medications. Another alternative for high-risk SLE patients who are in remission is to decrease the dose of HCQ. QT prolongation is less likely to occur on lower doses.

The bottom line for most HCQ and CQ patients is that there is no need to worry about QT prolongation.

then repeat the same amount at 8:00 P.M. that night. Resume your regular schedule the next day.

Ask your doctor.

Alcohol/food interactions: Avoid alcohol if you get stomach upset. HCQ can be taken with or without food. Taking it with food helps reduce stomach upset.

HCQ may decrease atrial fibrillation in SLE

Atrial fibrillation (Afib, chapter 11) is a heart rhythm problem that increases heart failure and stroke risks. SLE patients are at increased risk of AFib compared to the general population. A 2020 study of 1,647 patients with SLE showed that HCQ decreased the chances of AFib by 88%.

What to monitor when taking HCQ: See table 30.3.

Potential side effects of HCQ (table 30.4): Most people get no side effects. Stomach upset is the most common and easily goes away with lower HCQ doses. However, it is better to try taking it with food or with Pepto Bismol or taking smaller doses at a time spread out over the day to see if you can tolerate your full daily dose. It is uncommon to have significant side effects from HCQ. Do not be afraid to take it because of the rare possibility of developing eye problems. Read the section on retinopathy in this chapter for more information and follow the recommendations in table 30.3.

Although the old package insert for HCQ recommended caution in patients with a deficiency in an enzyme called G6PD, this has been shown not to be a problem. G6PD testing is not needed.

Some people taking HCQ develop dark areas of skin (hyperpigmentation) on the nails, forearms, shins, and inside the mouth while taking HCQ. This happens most often in people on blood thinners (such as aspirin) and people with high HCQ drug levels. The discoloration can become lower after reducing the dose or stopping the drug but is usually permanent.

While taking HCQ, see your ophthalmologist if you experience blurred vision or light sensitivity, or see halos around lights, see your ophthalmologist. These problems are usually due to something other than HCQ.

Vaccines and HCQ: You can get all vaccines (including live virus vaccinations) while taking HCQ. You do not need to stop taking it.

Pregnancy and breastfeeding: Never stop taking HCQ during pregnancy. HCQ reduces lupus flares, preeclampsia, stillbirth, miscarriage, congenital heart block, and neonatal lupus. HCQ significantly increases live birth rates in lupus patients.

HCQ is safe during breastfeeding.

Geriatric use: People with retina disease or severe kidney disease may need annual (or more frequent) eye exams as soon as they start HCQ. Otherwise, doses do not vary with age.

HCQ and surgery: Ask your rheumatologist. However, it is generally safe to take up to the time you are told to stop taking medications by mouth before surgery, and it can be started soon after surgery.

Financial aid for HCQ: Go to lupusencyclopedia.com/patient-resources, GoodRX .com, or similar programs.

Website: lupusencyclopedia.com/top-tips-on-taking-hydroxychloroquine-for-lupus

Table 30.4 Potential Side Effects of Hydroxychloroquine

	Incidence	Side Effect Therapy
Nuisance side effects		
Stomach upset, nausea, diarrhea, weight loss, appetite loss	Most common	Take with food or Pepto Bismol. Take in smaller amounts spread out over the day. Or decrease the dose.
Rash	Common	Contact doctor. Resolves when the drug is stopped. If mild, may be able to start back at a lower dose or use a desensitization protocol.
Blue, black, gray pigmentation of the skin and gums	Common	Decreases on lower doses or when stopped. Can be permanent.
Insomnia, nervousness, anxiety	Uncommon	Take in the morning if insomnia. Usually resolves at lower doses.
Headaches, lightheadedness	Uncommon	Usually resolves with continued use. Can reduce the dose.
Seeing halos around lights, light sensitivity due to corneal crystals	Rare	Usually of minimal consequence, not requiring intervention. Resolves if stopped or dose is lowered.
Low white blood count, anemia	Rare	Improves on lower doses or if drug is stopped.
Serious side effects		
Retinopathy (maculopathy). No symptoms when picked up early. Causes blurred vision if diagnosis is delayed.	Uncommon when ≤ 5–10 years of use	Preventable; see table 30.3
Muscle, nerve, heart (hypertrophic, restrictive cardiomyopathy) damage	Very rare	Diagnosed by biopsy. Stop HCQ.

Note: Side effect incidence key (approximations, as side effects can vary widely from study to study): rare <1% occurrence; uncommon 1%–5% occurrence; common >5% occurrence.

Chloroquine (CQ, Aralen)

CQ is sometimes used instead of HCQ. While HCQ can take 3 to 6 months (and, on occasion, up to 12 months) to achieve complete efficacy, CQ's full effects are reached at around 2 to 3 months. Therefore, it is sometimes used for severe skin (cutaneous) lupus, especially a type called discoid lupus (chapter 8), or when other SLE flares require a more rapid response. In some countries, CQ is more readily available or cheaper than HCQ.

Generic available: Yes.

How CQ works: CQ may start to work within a couple of weeks, and the full impact occurs in two to three months. It is most helpful for arthritis, rashes, mouth sores, fatigue, fevers, and low blood counts from SLE. It is not adequate by itself for severe lupus problems such as kidney, nerve, brain, heart, and lung involvement.

Do not to take CQ if

- you are allergic to it.

- you have a severe eye problem that makes it impossible to screen for retinopathy.

- you develop CQ retinopathy.

- you have congenital long QT syndrome, continuous QT measurements > 500 milliseconds on ECG, persistent low heart rate disorders (ask cardiologist), history of heart arrhythmia, uncorrected low magnesium or potassium levels, a recent heart attack, or severe congestive heart failure (ask cardiologist).

Dosage: CQ comes in 250 mg and 500 mg tablets. Do not take more than 1 mg of CQ per pound (or no more than 2.3 mg per kg) of actual body weight daily. We are unable to measure CQ drug levels.

If you miss a dose, follow the instructions given in the HCQ section.

Alcohol/food interactions: Alcohol should be avoided if stomach upset occurs. CQ can be taken with or without food; taking it with food reduces stomach upset.

What to monitor while taking CQ: See table 30.3.

Potential side effects of CQ (table 30.5): The risk of developing retina damage (retinopathy) with long-term use may be greater with CQ than with HCQ. See the main text above and table 30.3 for the recommended eye exams.

Table 30.5 Potential Side Effects of Chloroquine

	Incidence	Side Effect Therapy
Nuisance side effects		
Rash, itchy skin	Common	Contact doctor. Itchy skin can sometimes go away while staying on the drug. Rash resolves when the medicine is stopped. May be able to start back at a lower dose.
Stomach upset, nausea, weight loss, loss of appetite	Common	Take with food or Pepto Bismol. Take in smaller amounts spread out over the day. Or decrease the dose.
Insomnia, nervousness	Common	Take in the morning if insomnia. Usually resolves at lower doses.
Blue-black pigment changes of skin and gums	Common	Decreases on lower doses or when stopped. But it can be permanent.
Low white blood count, anemia	Uncommon	Resolves on lower doses or when stopped.
Seeing halos around lights, light sensitivity due to corneal crystals	Uncommon	Usually of minimal consequence, not requiring intervention. Resolves if medicine stopped.
Serious side effects		
Retinopathy (maculopathy). No symptoms when picked up early. It can cause blurred vision if the diagnosis is delayed.	Uncommon	See table 30.3 to prevent.
Muscle, nerve, heart (hypertrophic, restrictive cardiomyopathy) damage	Very rare	Diagnosed by biopsy. Stop CQ.

Note: Side effect incidence key (approximations, as side effects can vary widely from study to study): rare <1% occurrence; uncommon 1%–5% occurrence; common >5% occurrence.

As with HCQ, some people will develop dark areas of skin due to CQ. This happens most often in people taking blood thinners (such as aspirin). It usually occurs on the nails, forearms, shins, and inside the mouth, especially in areas of bruising. These dark areas can become lighter after lowering the dose or stopping the drug, but the discoloration is permanent.

While taking CQ, see your ophthalmologist if you have blurred vision or light sensitivity, or see halos around lights.

Vaccines and CQ: You can get all vaccines (including live virus vaccines) while taking CQ. You do not need to stop taking it.

Pregnancy and breastfeeding: CQ is safe during pregnancy and breastfeeding.

Geriatric use: People with retina disease or severe kidney disease may need annual (or more frequent) eye exams as soon as they start CQ. Otherwise, doses do not vary with age.

CQ and surgery: Ask your rheumatologist. However, CQ is generally safe to take up to the time you are told to stop taking medications by mouth before surgery and can be started soon after surgery.

Financial aid for CQ: Go to lupusencyclopedia.com/patient-resources, GoodRX.com, or similar programs.

Quinacrine

Quinacrine, which was discussed in the first edition, is omitted here and placed online at lupusencyclopedia.com/quinacrine. Quinacrine was unavailable for a few years. As of 2022, it is again available from some compounding pharmacists who can prepare pills and medicines that are unavailable from pharmaceutical companies and most pharmacies.

KEY THINGS TO REMEMBER

1. All SLE patients should take an antimalarial unless they are intolerant.

2. SLE patients who take HCQ regularly have less severe disease and live longer than people who do not take it. There are many other benefits (table 30.1).

3. Antimalarial retinopathy is very uncommon. It can be easily detected early before it should ever cause vision problems (see table 30.3).

4. QTc prolongation and heart problem concerns were exaggerated during COVID research that used much higher doses of HCQ than used in SLE. Discuss with your rheumatologist and cardiologist.

Steroids

Jess D. Edison, MD, *Contributing Editor*

Steroids (also called glucocorticosteroids and corticosteroids) are important in treating SLE. Chapter 26 explains how steroids are normally made by the body and their vital role in everyday functioning. It is a good idea to read that chapter before this one.

There are several reasons why doctors use steroids (table 31.1). They are the fastest-working drugs for lupus. Other immunosuppressants (table 22.1) can take several months to work. When someone has life-threatening lupus or major organ involvement, several months is not an option: waiting that long would mean irreversible organ damage. Steroids can provide rapid improvement, save lives, and decrease permanent damage.

Uses and Doses

High doses are needed for life-threatening SLE or when it attacks major internal organs. Prednisone for severe lupus is often dosed at around 1 mg per kilogram of body weight per day. For a 130-pound person, this would amount to 60 mg per day. In the most severe cases, up to 2 mg per kilogram may be used.

However, sometimes this is not enough, and we use intravenous (IV) pulse steroids. In the past, this typically meant giving 1,000 mg of IV methylprednisolone (SOLU-Medrol) a day, three days in a row, followed by around 60 mg of prednisone daily. Today, many of us tend to use much lower doses of IV steroids followed by lower prednisone doses, such as 20 mg to 40 mg daily.

Using these lower doses was confirmed as being effective when the Lupkynis (chapter 34) research studies used IV pulses of just 250 to 500 mg a day of methylprednisolone followed by just 20 to 25 mg of prednisone daily. This effectively treated severe lupus nephritis.

Moderate lupus (such as serositis, arthritis, severe discoid lupus, and high fevers) may require doses of 10 mg to 20 mg per day because other immunosuppressants take too long to work. Doctors call this "bridge therapy." Thus, if an SLE patient taking hydroxychloroquine (HCQ, Plaquenil) has severe joint pain, prednisone can function as a "bridge" to quickly calm the inflammation and pain while waiting for HCQ to work.

Dr. Edison contributed to this article in his personal capacity. The views expressed are his own and do not necessarily represent the views of the Walter Reed National Military Medical Center, the Uniformed Services University, or the United States government.

Table 31.1 Reasons to Use Steroids

Treat SLE that affects major organs or is life-threatening

Rapidly improve quality of life by reducing pain and fatigue

As a "bridge therapy" while waiting for slower-working drugs to work

As a topical treatment for cutaneous lupus

As joint cortisone injections for arthritis

As intramuscular cortisone injections for flares

LUPUS IN FOCUS

Why the weird spelling of drugs such as "Solu-MEDROL"?

The Institute for Safe Medication Practices (ISMP) developed a "tall man" (mixed case) naming system for drugs. This uses upper-case (capital) letters and lower-case letters in drug names to decrease prescription errors.

For example, the lupus arthritis drug Celebrex looks similar to the anti-depressant Celexa. A busy pharmacist could reach for the wrong drug. They are used for different things, and the doses are very different. It would be dangerous to get Celexa 200 mg instead of the prescribed Celebrex 200 mg. The typical dose for Celexa is up to 40 mg daily. The tall man names of CeleBREX and CeleXA can prevent this mistake.

The prednisone dose can be reduced once the HCQ works. (See chapters 26 and 29 about steroid tapering.)

Steroids taken by mouth or IV are classified as systemic steroids. The steroid enters the bloodstream to exert its effects on all organ systems (systemic). This way, the steroid calms the immune system, which is present throughout the body. Since all organs are affected, the steroid can cause unwanted side effects (table 31.3) in multiple areas.

This contrasts with topical steroids applied to and meant to work in one area, resulting in minimal to no side effects elsewhere. Examples of topical steroids include steroid eye drops for lupus eye inflammation, joint cortisone injections for lupus arthritis, steroid ear drops for itchy ear canals from Sjögren's dryness (chapter 14), nasal cortisone spray for lupus nose sores, inhaled steroids for asthma, and topical steroids for the skin.

Topical skin steroids are used for cutaneous lupus (chapter 8). If cutaneous lupus is one of the main problems and does not cover a large body area, this is a safer approach than steroid pills. Examples include creams, gels, lotions, foams, pastes, or ointment, often used two to three times daily for a couple of weeks at a time.

Steroids can also be injected into the muscles (intramuscular, IM). A Johns Hopkins study showed that an intramuscular injection of steroids in the buttock helps lupus flares. Compared to prednisone pills, the IM steroids worked faster and with no side effects other than discomfort at the injection site and sometimes a localized decrease in fat (lipodystrophy). Lipodystrophy is an unwanted loss of fat, leaving a dimple at the injection area. This occurred because triamcinolone was used in the study, and triamcinolone easily dissolves in fat. Instead of triamcinolone, my office uses a combination of methylprednisolone and dexamethasone, which dissolve in water and do not often cause lipoatrophy.

Steroids can also be injected into the joints or around tendons for lupus arthritis or tendonitis (chapter 7).

Many different steroids are used in SLE (table 31.2). Prednisone is the most common, but prednisolone or methylprednisolone can be used if patients have difficulty tolerating prednisone.

Table 31.2 Systemic Steroids Commonly Used in SLE

Steroid Name	Prednisone Equivalent Dose	Usage
Triamcinolone (Kenalog, Zilretta)	1.3 mg	Injections, especially in the joints and IM. Zilretta is only for knee joints.
prednisone (Rayos)	1 mg	Pills and liquid. Rayos is taken at night for morning lupus arthritis symptoms.
prednisolone	1 mg	Pills and liquid. More tolerable in some people. Often used in patients with severe liver damage.
methylprednisolone (Medrol, DEPO-Medrol, Solu-Medrol)	1.3 mg	Pills and IV. Often used for "pulse" IV steroids.
dexamethasone	6.7 mg	Liquid, pills, and injections. May help prevent fetal heart block (chapters 18 and 41).
betamethasone	8.3 mg	Injections. May help prevent fetal heart block (chapters 18 and 41).

Note: Prednisone Equivalent Dose: 1 mg of the steroid is equal to this amount of prednisone.

LUPUS IN FOCUS

Converting prednisone dosing to methylprednisolone dosing

Equivalent doses of different steroids are in table 31.2. For example, a 5 mg tablet of prednisone is equivalent to a 4 mg tablet of methylprednisolone, while 20 mg of prednisone is equal to 16 mg of methylprednisolone.

Side Effects: Preventing Them and Treating Them

It is vital to learn the potential side effects (table 31.3) of steroids, how to prevent them (table 31.4), and how they are treated. Steroid side effects are best dealt with by going through each organ system. While other drug side effects in this book are usually labeled as occurring "commonly," "uncommonly," or "rarely," we do not use this system with steroids. The potential side effects vary greatly, depending on the steroid dose, how long and how often it is used, and how the individual person reacts. Some people are sensitive to steroids and get many side effects at relatively low doses. Others can take high doses and have relatively few.

Take steroids immediately when waking up in the morning and take the entire daily dose at once (unless directed otherwise). This reduces side effects, especially adrenal insufficiency (chapter 26).

Steroids remain in the blood system for only a few hours, so if the full dose is 60 mg per day, taking one 20 mg tablet every 8 hours is more effective than taking 3 of them in the morning. The body ends up seeing a high dose of steroids for a longer amount of time throughout the day. Splitting up the quantity is especially useful in treating severe problems, such as severe brain, heart, and lung inflammation, but it also causes more side effects than taking the entire daily dose in the morning. So while doctors may prescribe several doses a day to treat severe lupus, as soon as things improve, they tend to combine the dose to be taken once each morning. If you are prescribed more than one tablet of steroids a day, make sure to ask if you are to spread out the dose or take it all in the morning. If you are told to spread out the quantity, find out when you should combine the amount in the morning to decrease side effects.

If you miss a dose, make sure to take it as soon as you remember that you forgot your dose. This is so that you do not develop adrenal insufficiency problems (chapter 26). Then take your next amount at the usual scheduled time.

Do not reduce the steroid dose or stop the drug without your doctor's instructions. If you have been on steroids for a short time, they can be safely stopped without slowly lowering the dose (or what we call steroid tapering). If you have been on high doses or

---

LUPUS IN FOCUS

Rayos for lupus arthritis

Most SLE patients have joint pains or inflammatory arthritis (chapter 7). This inflammation is often worse in the morning when the person wakes up. Generic prednisone taken in the mornings does not reach its full effects until a few hours later. By this time, the person has already had their worst symptoms.

Rayos is an alternative. It is taken with food before bed. The intestines start to absorb it 4 hours later, reaching its maximum blood levels 6 to 6½ hours after taken. When waking up 8 hours after going to bed, Rayos is at its full effect.

However, it is costly; a month's supply of 5 mg Rayos was US$3,600.00 (per GoodRX.com, December 2022) while generic prednisone was as low as $8.00.

Table 31.3 Potential Side Effects of Systemic Steroids

Organ System Affected	Steroid Side Effects
Bones	Osteoporosis (chapter 24)
	Avascular necrosis (chapter 25)
	Stunted growth in children
Muscles	Steroid myopathy (weak and smaller muscles)
	Muscle spasms and pain
Joints	Joint pains while reducing steroid doses
Skin	Skin thinning
	Stretch marks
	Bruising
	Acne
	Scalp hair loss
	Unwanted hair on the face
	Poor wound healing
	Increased blood vessels under the skin (telangiectasias)
Endocrine (hormone) and metabolic systems	Hunger and craving for sweets, carbohydrates, and fats
	Weight gain
	Increased fat in central body areas
	Moon-shaped face
	"Buffalo hump" on the upper back
	Fluid retention and swelling from sodium (salt) retention
	Decreased potassium
	Elevated cholesterol and triglycerides
	Elevated glucose and diabetes
	Adrenal insufficiency (chapter 26)
	Irregular menstrual cycles
	Decreased fertility
Heart and blood vessels	High blood pressure
	Hardening of the arteries, heart attacks, strokes, peripheral vascular disease
Brain and nerves	Depression, anxiety, moodiness
	Restlessness, tremors, heart palpitations, increased energy
	Trouble sleeping
	Hallucinations, bizarre thinking and behavior
	Decreased memory
Eyes	Cataracts
	Glaucoma
Gastrointestinal system	Nausea
	Peptic ulcer disease when used with NSAIDs
	Bowel perforation from ulcers or diverticulitis
Immune system	Increased infections

Table 31.4 Preventing Steroid Side Effects

- Take dose first thing in the morning as soon as you wake up unless directed otherwise. (Rayos is taken before bed.)
- If prescribed more than one tablet daily, take them all in the morning unless directed otherwise.
- Never miss a dose.
- If you forget a dose, see "Uses and Doses" section.
- If lupus is under good control, ask your doctor every visit if you can reduce your dose.
- Do not reduce steroid doses or stop them on your own.
- Do not smoke.
- Do not drink alcohol.
- Take a vitamin D supplement regularly if you have a low vitamin D level. Your 25-OH vitamin D level goal is around 40 ng/mL or higher.
- If your vitamin D level is normal, take at least an 800 IU vitamin D3 supplement daily.
- Do weight-bearing exercise 5 days a week, 30 minutes at a time to keep bones strong.
- Do strength-training exercises 3 days a week.
- Do aerobic exercise 5 days a week, trying to get to 30 minutes each time.
- Get adequate calcium (table 24.6).
- Take a drug to prevent osteoporosis (like a bisphosphonate, table 24.9).
- Take potassium or drink tonic water for muscle spasms.
- Use acne medicines if needed.
- Use steroid creams only as directed; work closely with a dermatologist.
- Eat a low-sodium diet; eat lots of fresh fruits, vegetables, and fiber; eat only low-fat meats.
- Use potassium salt substitutes in food (if approved by doctor).
- See a dietician or go to a group such as Weight Watchers to learn proper eating habits.
- If you have high cholesterol, diabetes, prediabetes, or high blood pressure, see your doctor regularly. You may need higher doses of your medicines to control these problems.
- Wear a medical alert bracelet if you use steroids more than a month.
- Alert your surgeon that you take steroids prior to any surgeries.
- If you are under increased stress (such as from trauma or infection), you may temporarily need more steroids (table 26.1).
- Inform family members of potential steroid side effects such as moodiness, depression, or anger.
- Ask your family to let you know immediately if they observe symptoms of moodiness or depression: discuss them with your doctor.
- Avoid caffeine.
- Use good sleep hygiene techniques, as described in table 6.2.
- If you get heartburn, nausea, or an upset stomach, consider taking Tums or Prilosec, with doctor's permission.
- If you take an NSAID and steroids, consider taking a daily PPI (table 28.3) to prevent peptic ulcer disease.
- Avoid infections (table 22.4).
- Tell your doctor if you have been positive for TB in the past or have been exposed to TB.

have been taking steroids for a longer period, you could have adrenal insufficiency. It can be dangerous to lower the dose too quickly or abruptly stop the drug. Steroid tapering is needed. Usually, the longer you have been on steroids and the higher the dose, the slower the steroid taper needs to be. For example, someone taking 5–10 mg of prednisone for 3 weeks may be able to taper off over a week's time. However, someone taking 5 mg daily for several years may need to go down by just 1 mg a day every 3 months, or even just ½ mg at a time.

Bones

Osteoporosis and avascular necrosis are discussed in chapters 24 and 25.

Prolonged use of steroids in children, especially at high doses, can cause the bones' growth plates to weaken, and the limbs (arms and legs) can end up being shorter (chapter 20). This can lead to a shorter height than their peers.

Muscles

Most everyone has heard about steroids used by athletes to make their muscles larger and stronger. Those are anabolic steroids, which break down fat and produce more muscle. Steroids for lupus are catabolic steroids and do the opposite: they break down muscle and make more fat.

When taken for long periods and at high doses, catabolic steroids cause the body's muscles to shrink and weaken (muscle atrophy).

In severe cases, they can cause steroid myopathy (*myo-* comes from the Greek word for "muscle," and *-opathy* means "accident" or "suffering" and can refer to an abnormality). In steroid myopathy, the individual microscopic muscle cells become smaller (atrophy). This usually occurs in the muscles of the neck, shoulders, upper arms, thighs, buttocks, and upper legs. It usually begins in the hip region muscles, followed by the shoulders and neck. It can be difficult standing up from a chair without using the hands, as well as raising the arms to brush hair or teeth. Most patients first notice symptoms several months after beginning steroids, but they can begin as fast as three weeks in some. It is treated by decreasing the steroid dose, although this could cause lupus to become more active if the steroids are essential in controlling it.

Muscle enzymes (such as CPK, chapter 4) are normal in steroid myopathy while electromyogram (EMG, chapter 13) can show muscle abnormalities or can be normal. Diagnosis is usually made by the classic symptoms above. The diagnosis is confirmed if muscle strength improves a few weeks after steroid dose reduction. Muscle biopsies are usually not needed, but if done to exclude other causes, they show muscle cell atrophy and no inflammation (as would be seen in lupus myositis, chapter 7).

The best way to prevent the possibility of muscle atrophy or steroid myopathy is to perform strengthening exercises regularly. This is best done as soon as you begin taking the steroids to maintain or build up muscle mass instead of waiting until you notice the muscles getting weaker. Consider doing muscle-strengthening exercises three days a week with a day of rest between each session, allowing the muscles to recuperate.

If you have never performed muscle-strengthening exercises before, you can join a gym and get help from a certified personal trainer. You can also ask your doctor to send you to a physical therapist (PT). The advantage of PT is that they will be more knowledgeable about your medical condition and design a program based on your health.

Some inexpensive dumbbells may be all the equipment you need after seeing a PT. Trainers and PT can be quite expensive, so another option is to learn on YouTube, where many experts, such as physical therapists, provide excellent exercise instructions. Make sure that you watch an instructor who has proper technique.

Fortunately, steroid myopathy resolves in almost everyone after steroids are stopped.

Other common side effects are muscle spasms, cramps, and pain. These can occur at high doses of steroids or when the steroid dose is lowered. Pain and spasms are not due to steroid myopathy. Muscle spasms may occur from electrolyte (mineral) abnormalities, such as potassium. Taking a potassium supplement may help. It should not be taken by people with kidney problems or who take an ACE inhibitor or angiotensin receptor blocker (blood pressure pills, table 12.4) without asking your doctor.

Volume depletion (the medical term for dehydration) can worsen muscle cramps. This occurs from not drinking enough water daily or from some medications (such as diuretics or fluid pills). Reduced body water from dehydration causes abnormalities of minerals such as calcium, potassium, and sodium and leads to the muscles not working properly. Therefore, it is good to drink at least nine glasses of water daily when on steroids (unless your doctor says otherwise) and avoid dehydrating substances such as alcohol and caffeine.

Exercising regularly, including stretching, strengthening, and aerobic exercises, help reduce muscle spasms and pain.

Joints

Steroids can cause avascular necrosis (chapter 25).

Steroids can also cause joint pains (arthralgia, chapter 7) without causing actual arthritis. Sometimes, especially when high doses are reduced, people can develop pain in the joints and muscles (myalgia), which can feel like a lupus flare. Your doctor would need to figure out what is causing the pain. If the pains are due to a lupus flare, your doctor may find joint swelling on physical exam, active inflammation on ultrasound, or other indicators of increased SLE, such as low complements and high anti-dsDNA levels (chapters 5 and 7). In this case, the steroid dose may need to be increased and your medications may need adjusting (such as higher doses of immunosuppressants).

If it is due to steroid withdrawal (instead of lupus arthritis), the dose won't be changed, but the pain will gradually decrease over several weeks. Your doctor may slow down your steroid taper. Treatment includes exercising and taking pain drugs (chapters 7 and 36).

Skin

Steroids can cause the skin to become thin, wrinkle, and bruise easily. Bruises can occur anywhere (but not commonly on the face) without preceding injury. Stretch marks (striae) can also occur. The delicate skin can become fragile and tear easily with minimal trauma. Unfortunately, stretch marks tend to be permanent. Skin thinning can improve once you are off steroids but can also be permanent.

Acne can occur, especially on the face, upper back, and chest. Using acne treatments can help, and the acne resolves after steroids are stopped.

Steroids can also cause an increase in tiny blood vessels under the skin (telangiectasia, chapter 8), especially on the face. Unfortunately, these can be permanent.

Rosacea from steroids can look like the SLE butterfly rash

Steroid-induced rosacea commonly causes telangiectasia with red splotches on the cheeks, similarly to the lupus malar (butterfly) rash. It is important to distinguish between them with the help of a dermatologist. Active SLE with a malar rash may need increased steroids, while steroid-induced rosacea needs decreased steroids. See example at lupusencyclopedia.com/book-photos.

High doses or long-term use of smaller doses can cause hair loss similar to what is seen in men (male pattern baldness). Fortunately, this is reversible, and hair growth resumes after the steroids are stopped. The opposite can also happen: increased hair growth (hypertrichosis) may occur anywhere. Facial hair from hypertrichosis can be especially upsetting for women. This usually improves when steroids are stopped.

Skin wounds, scratches, and cuts can take longer to heal, especially after taking steroids for a long time and at higher doses. This is one reason why surgeons like patients to be on the lowest possible doses of steroids before surgery. However, never lower your steroid dose on your own without consulting your rheumatologist or doctor who treats your lupus. Many people need more steroids around surgery for adrenal insufficiency.

Endocrine (Hormone) and Metabolic Systems

Steroids often cause hunger, especially cravings for sweets, carbohydrates, and fatty foods. The only way to decrease this urge is to reduce the steroid dose but only with your doctor's help.

Weight gain is one of the most dreaded side effects. As mentioned, steroids break down muscle and produce fat. Smaller muscles, often accompanied by less physical activity from lupus fatigue and pain, results in fewer calories being used. Increased fat production from steroids with increased calorie intake from steroid-induced hunger results in unwanted weight gain.

The fat typically forms in the face, back, chest, shoulders, and abdomen (central body areas), while steroid muscle atrophy causes thinner arms and legs. The face can become round and puffy, like a moon (called a moon facies). Fat can accumulate above the collarbones or on the upper back (the latter is known as a buffalo hump). This fat accumulation and weight gain produce what is known as a Cushingoid appearance (Cushing's syndrome from steroids).

The best way to minimize weight gain is to try to prevent it before it happens. Once it occurs, it is very hard to get rid of (except by reducing the steroids). Eat a healthy diet and exercise regularly as soon as you start taking steroids. Muscle-strengthening exercises several days a week improves muscle mass, strength, and calorie usage (larger muscles use up more calories).

Aerobic exercises burn extra calories. Aerobic exercise includes activities where you are moving large muscle groups continuously for a significant time. It can be done on stationary bicycles, treadmills, or elliptical machines. Swimming and brisk walking are also good (chapters 7 and 38). Since most SLE patients are ill when placed on steroids, seeing a physical therapist to design a safe and effective exercise regimen should be considered.

If you have gained weight and accumulated extra fat you are presumed to have adrenal insufficiency. Read chapter 26 and follow its recommendations closely.

Steroids can cause the kidneys to retain sodium and lose potassium. Excess sodium retains more water, causing swelling, especially in the legs and ankles. The person will often say they feel bloated or swollen all over. Leg swelling typically worsens after sitting or standing throughout the day and gets better after lying down. Therefore, it is usually less noticeable when getting out of bed and is more evident after being upright. This leg swelling is called edema.

Eating less salt and drinking more water reduce edema. The increased water intake helps the kidneys get rid of the extra sodium. Do not add salt to food and learn to avoid hidden sodium. Most pre-prepared foods are high in sodium. This includes anything in a can, fast food, food prepared by most restaurants or convenience stores, pizza, many bagged snacks, such as chips and pretzels, and soda pop. It is much better to cook your own food using fresh ingredients and spices (other than salt). The largest single source of sodium in the U.S. diet is bread, so it is important to limit bread intake. It can be beneficial to see a dietician.

Fluid retention is especially problematic in people with congestive heart failure, kidney disease, or liver cirrhosis. More fluid can build up, especially in the lungs, causing breathing and heart problems.

Potassium loss may cause muscle spasms and pain. Taking a salt substitute with potassium salts instead of sodium can help. Check with your doctor first because people with kidney problems or who take certain blood pressure drugs should avoid too much potassium. They should have potassium blood levels monitored.

Steroids can increase total cholesterol, bad LDL cholesterol, and triglycerides (chapter 21). Steroids increase the risk of heart attacks and strokes. See your primary care doctor or cardiologist (heart doctor) regularly to watch your cholesterol. Exercising and eating right help reduce this complication. However, if these levels are elevated, it is usually best to take medication, especially a statin (table 21.5). It may be important for you to remind your primary care provider and cardiologist that lupus patients get heart attacks and strokes younger than other people.

Glucose (sugar) levels can increase (hyperglycemia), especially in those with diabetes, metabolic syndrome (chapter 21), prediabetes, and obesity, as well as in those with a family history of diabetes. Proper diet and exercise help prevent this. If they do not, then diabetes drugs may be needed. Interestingly, the diabetic drug most used in this situation, metformin, may help reduce lupus inflammation (chapter 35). Hyperglycemia increases the chances of heart attacks and strokes. If you have pre-existing diabetes, it is important to follow up more often with the doctor who treats your diabetes. You may need higher doses of your diabetic medicine.

Steroids can also cause irregular menstrual cycles. High doses can reduce fertility rates in both men and women. This is believed to be due to sex hormone production problems. These problems resolve with lower doses.

Heart and Blood Vessels

Steroids can increase blood pressure. Sodium retention is one of the reasons. It is crucial to exercise regularly and eat a diet low in sodium to prevent this. If you have high blood pressure, you should see the doctor who treats your blood pressure more often.

SLE patients develop heart attacks, strokes, and peripheral vascular disease (hardening of the arteries) at a younger age than the general population (chapter 21). Unfortunately, steroids increase this risk, especially in those with lupus nephritis.

Brain and Nerves

Steroids may cause moodiness. Even people not predisposed to depression or anxiety may feel very nervous on steroids, cry for no apparent reason, and get angry easily. Inform your loved ones that you are taking steroids early on and that these are possible side effects. This is important because you may not notice this yourself. You may lash out at your loved ones without realizing it. They need to understand that it is probably not their fault or your fault, but it is due to the steroids. If they tell you it is occurring, discuss this with your doctor. Reducing the steroid dose may help, but sometimes a mood stabilizer or antidepressant may be needed.

Learning how to minimize stress can also help (table 38.9).

It is often difficult to sleep on steroids, which can make the mind race. Do everything in tables 6.2 and 6.3.

Steroids can cause nerve overactivity, creating anxiety, tremors, restlessness, and heart palpitations (feeling the heart pounding in the chest). Caffeine and tobacco worsen these problems, so avoid using them.

A rare side effect is steroid psychosis. Psychosis is a brain problem that causes bizarre thoughts, behavior, or hallucinations. The person may lose touch with reality, have delusions, or become paranoid. If steroid psychosis develops, it usually does so on higher doses. It is more common in patients with a family history of depression or alcoholism, which suggests a genetic cause.

Steroid psychosis is treated by reducing the steroid dose. If it can't be, antipsychotic drugs (used to treat conditions such as schizophrenia and bipolar disorder) may be needed.

Another complicating issue is that severe SLE can cause brain inflammation and lupus psychosis (chapter 13). As a result, it can be tough for doctors to figure out if the psychosis is from steroids or from SLE. If it is from SLE, more steroids are needed (just the opposite of what doctors do for steroid psychosis).

Memory problems can develop after using steroids, usually at prednisone doses greater than 5 mg a day for three months or longer. This is most common in older patients.

Eyes

Steroids may cause cataracts. Cataracts (chapter 16) occur when the eye's clear lens (the part of the eye that focuses light on the retina) becomes clouded. They are more common in people on higher doses of steroids taken for a long time, but they can also occur on low doses (less than 5 mg a day) or even with every-other-day steroid regimens. The

Drug-induced organ damage

An important research tool called the SDI (SLICC/ACR Damage Index) measures organ damage in SLE. In addition to measuring organ damage from SLE, the SDI includes organ damage from the drugs used to treat SLE. Steroid-induced organ damage in the SDI includes cataracts, muscle atrophy, osteoporotic fractures, skin damage, avascular necrosis, and diabetes. Steroids can also contribute to other damage in the SDI, such as strokes, heart attacks, hardening of the arteries, and blood clots. Other SLE drugs that can cause organ damage in the SDI include cyclophosphamide and some of the other immunosuppressants.

It is very important that we try to use drugs that help SLE but do not cause problems such as organ damage. Thus far (as of January 2023), the only two drugs proven to reduce organ damage in SLE are hydroxychloroquine and belimumab (Benlysta, chapter 34).

only way to prevent cataracts is by working with your doctor to decrease your steroid dose as much as possible. Cataracts can cause blurred vision, seeing halos around lights at night, and nighttime blurred vision. You should regularly see an ophthalmologist to follow the use of your anti-malarial (such as hydroxychloroquine). During these visits, your eye doctor should check for cataracts. If they develop and become severe enough, cataract surgery may be needed. Eating a diet high in fruits and vegetables may decrease cataract formation due to aging.

Steroids can also increase pressure inside the eyeball (intraocular hypertension or glaucoma, chapter 16). If you have a family history of glaucoma, already have glaucoma, or have been labeled a "glaucoma suspect" by your eye doctor, see your eye doctor more often while taking steroids.

Gastrointestinal System

Gastrointestinal system problems can occur early on from steroids. Nausea, heartburn, and upset stomach are the most common. Tums or over-the-counter stomach acid reducers (such as Prilosec) can help. If unhelpful, alert your doctor; PPIs may help (table 28.3).

If you take an NSAID (table 36.1) in addition to steroids, you have an increased chance for peptic ulcer disease (chapter 28). To prevent ulcers, ask your doctor about the drugs in table 28.5.

People with active ulcers when they are put on steroids or who have diverticulosis (small pockets sticking out of the large colon) are at increased risk of bowel perforation. A perforation is a hole in the stomach or intestine lining that can allow stomach or intestinal contents to leak into the abdomen. This is potentially life-threatening. It is important to regularly take an anti-ulcer medicine if you have peptic ulcer disease while on steroids. If you develop severe abdominal pain, seek medical attention at once.

Immune System

Steroids are immunosuppressants. The higher the dose of steroids, the greater the risk of infection. Out of all the immunosuppressants (table 22.1), steroids are the most common cause of infections. If you have any infection symptoms (chapters 22 and 40), see a health care provider right away. If it is an evening or a weekend, go to your closest urgent care center. Steroids can decrease the body's ability to mount a fever, so do not make the mistake of thinking that you do not have an infection if you do not have a fever.

You should stop taking other immunosuppressants during infections, but do not stop your steroid. The body makes more steroids during infections (to help during the stressful event), so your rheumatologist may need to have you take a higher dose during infections. When you get an infection, in addition to seeing your primary care provider for treatment of the infection, you should contact your rheumatologist to see if you need a higher dose of steroids. See table 26.1 for sick-day instructions for people with adrenal insufficiency.

Do everything possible to prevent infections (table 22.4). Let your doctor know if you have ever been exposed to tuberculosis (TB) or have had a positive skin or blood test for TB. Most people infected with TB do not get very sick from the infection, but the infection can live in their bodies for life. If a TB-infected person is put on high-dose steroids, severe TB can occur. This can be prevented with antibiotics.

Potential Side Effects in Special Uses of Steroids

Because IV steroids are a much larger dose, the chances of diabetics developing much higher glucose levels are present. Work closely with your diabetic doctor while getting IV pulse steroids. Blood pressure can also become elevated and heart rate can change during and soon after IV steroids. The nurse giving the medicine will check these closely. After the infusion, mood changes and insomnia may occur.

Topical steroids for cutaneous lupus can cause skin side effects, such as skin thinning and telangiectasia. Use topical steroids only on the skin areas with active lupus inflammation. This may be difficult to figure out on your own. A common mistake is to use them on skin areas with permanent damage (such as on red sites due to telangiectasia). See a dermatologist to ensure that you are using these drugs correctly.

Joint steroid (cortisone) injections are one of the safest ways to use steroids. Most of their effects occur at the joint. However, some of the drug is absorbed into the bloodstream and affects other parts of the body. The most common side effect is skin flushing, especially in the face, which can become warm and pinkish in color. This is a natural reaction due to the blood vessels dilating (getting larger). It is not an allergic reaction. It typically comes on during the first 24 hours after the injection and can last for a few days.

Some diabetics can have high glucose (sugar) levels after joint cortisone injections, so it is important to know what to do ahead of time from your diabetes doctor. In patients whose diabetes worsens after cortisone injections, lower doses of cortisone or Zilretta can be used. Zilretta is a brand of steroid that is bound inside microscopic balls, which release the drug slowly into the joint over three months. Zilretta is FDA-approved for knee injections only.

In rare cases, a steroid joint injection can cause joint swelling, pain, and redness. If this occurs, it is usually within the first few days after the injection and resolves on its own or with using ice packs. Always contact your doctor to ensure it is not a joint infection. The best way to prevent this is to use an ice pack on the joint for 5–10 minutes as soon as you get home after the injection and repeat this hourly for the rest of the day. Then do not use the joint very much during the first few days.

Infection from a joint injection is rare. If you get a red, hot, swollen joint that is very painful to move after the first few days, see your rheumatologist at once. A joint infection is dangerous. It needs to be identified and treated immediately to prevent permanent joint destruction. If your rheumatologist is not immediately available, go to an emergency room.

One question that comes up is how often intra-articular steroid injections (joint cortisone injections) can safely be given. This has never been studied in SLE. Rheumatologists generally give no more than four injections a year into any joint.

Steroid Drug Facts

Steroids are the fastest-working lupus drugs. Decreased joint pain, fever reduction, and an overall feeling of well-being can be seen within 3 to 24 hours.

Generic available: Yes, except for Rayos, a delayed-release form of prednisone.

How steroids work: They suppress the immune system and decrease inflammation.

There are no absolute contraindications for steroids (reasons not to take them) for life-threatening lupus or lupus affecting the major internal organs.

If someone is allergic to a specific steroid preparation (such as prednisone), another can be used (such as methylprednisolone).

Let your doctor know if you have ever been positive for a TB skin or blood test or have ever been exposed to someone with TB.

Dosage: See the "Uses and Doses" section above.

If you miss a dose, see the section on "Uses and Doses" above.

Alcohol/food interactions: Alcohol can increase stomach upset. For Rayos (taken before bed), have a light snack when you take it if it has been more than two and a half hours since your last meal.

Taking steroids with food reduces stomach upset. Try not to take calcium supplements at the same time as steroids. Steroids can decrease calcium absorption. Limit caffeine (or stop it); caffeine increases tremors, moodiness, heart palpitations, and difficulty sleeping. See the "Endocrine (Hormone) and Metabolic Systems" section above for more advice.

You may need extra calcium (taken at least a couple of hours away from your steroid dosing), potassium, vitamin D, and other vitamins such as vitamin B6, folate, and vitamin C. Ask your doctor.

What to monitor when taking steroids:

- your lupus. See your doctor regularly to ensure you are not getting any side effects and check how your lupus is responding. If it is in good control, always ask your doctor if you can decrease your steroid dose.

- blood pressure, as well as hemoglobin, glucose, vitamin D, cholesterol, and potassium levels

- TSH levels and thyroid drugs. These may, or may not, need adjusting. Consider seeing a thyroid expert (endocrinologist).

- bone density via DXA scan (chapter 24)

- eyes, regularly, by an eye doctor, to ensure you don't develop glaucoma or cataracts.

Potential side effects of steroids: See the "Side Effects: Preventing Them and Treating Them" section above.

While taking steroids,

- if you have poorly controlled diabetes, high blood pressure, congestive heart failure, or severe cirrhosis, see the doctors who treat these conditions more often.

- do everything in tables 22.4 and 31.4.

Pregnancy and breast-feeding: Steroids can be used during pregnancy, at the lowest possible dose. There are cases of babies having cleft lip and cleft palate when steroids are taken during the first trimester, but this risk is low.

Steroids are safe while breast-feeding. If you take more than 40 mg a day of prednisone, wait at least 4 hours after each dose before breast-feeding (chapter 41).

Geriatric use: Dosing is no different. However, side effects are more likely.

Steroids and surgery: Ask your rheumatologist because it can be complicated. If you have been on them briefly and are not at risk of your lupus flaring, then they can be stopped before surgery. This is an optimal situation since steroids delay surgical wound healing and increase the risk of infections.

However, most of the time, they should be continued during surgery to prevent lupus flares and in case there is adrenal insufficiency (chapter 26). For major surgeries, your rheumatologist may recommend higher doses of steroids around the time of surgery (stress doses, discussed in chapter 26).

Financial aid for steroids: Go to lupusencyclopedia.com/patient-resources, GoodRX.com, or similar programs.

Website: rheumatology.org/patients/prednisone-deltasone

Corticotropin (Adrenocorticotropic Hormone, ACTH)

Corticotropin (also called adrenocorticotropic hormone or ACTH) is not a steroid, but it increases body steroid production (see chapter 26).

For many decades, ACTH has been used for inflammatory diseases, such as gout, lupus, and rheumatoid arthritis. ACTH therapy can cause similar effects as prednisone and other steroids. The treatment results and side effects of steroids also apply to ACTH treatment.

ACTH may also help inflammatory diseases by binding to special receptors (called melanocortin receptors) on the surfaces of some cells. They are found on many body cells, including most immune system white blood cells. When ACTH attaches to these receptors, it can directly lower inflammation. Steroids do not work in this way.

ACTH has not been proven safer or more effective than steroids and is markedly more expensive. It does have a role in treatment, though. When necessary—as when a patient does poorly on steroids or in someone who is unable to take oral steroids—I have used it with excellent results.

The brand names for ACTH are Acthar and Cortrophin. The information in this chapter also applies to these drugs.

Go to www.acthar.com to learn more about Acthar and www.cortrophin.com for Cortrophin.

KEY POINTS TO REMEMBER

1. Steroids are one of the most important drugs to treat moderate to severe lupus. They can be lifesaving.

2. However, they cause side effects and organ damage if taken at high doses or for extended periods. Read the "Side Effects: Preventing Them and Treating Them" section above.

3. Corticotrophin gel injections (Acthar and Cortrophin) are expensive alternatives for steroids. Whether they are safer or more effective than steroids has not been proven.

4. If you take steroids or use corticotrophin gel, do everything in table 31.4 to decrease your risk of side effects.

Other Immunosuppressants

George Bertsias, MD, PhD, *Contributing Editor*

Antimalarial drugs (such as hydroxychloroquine) calm down the immune system but do not actually suppress it to the point of causing infections. They are safer than immunosuppressants (table 22.1), which can increase infection risk. While doctors always hope that antimalarials alone can be used to treat lupus, stronger immunosuppressants are needed in moderate to severe lupus.

Steroids (chapter 31) are one way to suppress the immune system and treat lupus. They are fast-acting and can be lifesaving. But almost everyone who takes them will get side effects eventually.

It is better to supplement steroids with an antimalarial and one of the other immunosuppressants described in this and chapters 33, 34, and 37 to help get people on lower steroid doses or hopefully off steroids. While steroids are based on cortisone-like steroid hormones produced in the body, these other immunosuppressants are synthetic drugs unrelated to steroids. The immunosuppressants discussed in this chapter and in chapters 33 and 37 were all developed and FDA-approved for diseases other than lupus. However, they have been shown to help lupus patients in research studies. Since they are not FDA-approved for lupus, they are used off-label to treat lupus. This does not mean they don't work as well as the FDA-approved immunosuppressants (chapter 34).

Azathioprine (AZA, Imuran, Azasan)

AZA is used for moderate to severe SLE. One of its significant strengths is that it is safe to take during pregnancy.

Generic available: Yes.

How AZA works:

It is a slow-working drug that suppresses the immune system. It takes about six weeks to begin working and usually takes about three to six months to achieve the full effects of reducing or stopping lupus inflammation.

Do not take if

- you are completely deficient in TPMT.

- you have an infection.

Vaccination against COVID-19

Several vaccines against COVID-19 were available in the United States as of January 2023. Since they do not contain live virus, patients taking immunosuppressants can (and should) get the COVID-19 vaccinations.

Some drugs (for example, methotrexate, mycophenolate, prednisone, rituximab, Janus kinase inhibitors, and abatacept) may decrease the effectiveness of some vaccines. The American College of Rheumatology published recommendations on what to do with these drugs when getting COVID vaccines, and these recommendations are updated as new research emerges. You can find them at lupusencyclopedia.com/4th-covid-vaccines and at rheumatology.org/covid-19 -guidance.

Let your doctor know if you have been exposed to TB in the past. If you have ever had a positive TB skin test (PPD) or blood test (QuantiFERON or T-SPOT.TB), also let your doctor know.

Dosage: AZA is taken in pill form (50 mg, 75 mg, and 100 mg tablets). Dose is based on body weight (up to 3 mg per kilogram of body weight per day). Most doctors start with a low dose and go up gradually. This slow increase helps reduce nausea and upset stomach.

Let your doctor know if you are taking allopurinol or febuxostat (Uloric) for gout, kidney stones, or high uric acid levels. These two drugs can cause AZA blood levels to become dangerously high. Much lower doses of AZA must be used with these drugs.

Your doctor may measure a thiopurine methyltransferase (TPMT) blood level before starting AZA. If your level is low, you may be at higher risk for side effects, and you may be started at a lower than the usual dose and monitoring labs (see below) may be done more often.

If you miss a dose, if it is the same day as your missed dose, take your missed dose as soon as possible with food, then resume your usual schedule after that. If it is the next day that you remember, skip the missed dose, and resume your normal schedule. Ask your doctor.

Alcohol/food interactions with AZA: Alcohol may increase stomach upset. Best taken after eating.

What to monitor while taking AZA:

• complete blood cell count and liver enzymes (chapter 4) every two to four weeks, then every two to three months (as determined by your doctor).

Potential side effects of AZA (table 32.1): The most concerning are low blood counts and infections. Infection risk is higher with low white blood cell counts.

While taking AZA, see your primary care provider or go to an emergency room immediately if you have infection symptoms (table 22.3). Practice all measures to prevent infections (table 22.4).

Table 32.1 Potential Side Effects of Azathioprine

	Incidence	Side Effect Therapy
Nuisance side effects		
Nausea, vomiting, loss of appetite, diarrhea	Common	Take an anti-nausea or anti-diarrhea drug. Take it after eating. Divide up or reduce the dose.
Mouth sores	Rare	Reduce dosage. Use mouth rinses and creams prescribed by your doctor.
Hair loss	Rare	Stop the drug or reduce the dose. Hair grows back after drug is stopped.
Rash	Uncommon	Reduce dosage or stop the drug.
Serious side effects		
Low white blood cell counts	Common; severe on rare occasions	Reduce dosage or stop the drug. Can be treated with Neupogen (with caution, chapter 9).
Low platelet counts	Uncommon; severe on rare occasions	Reduce dosage or stop the drug. Platelet transfusions can be used if severe.
Anemia (low red blood cells)	Common; severe on rare occasions	Reduce dosage or stop the drug if severe. Can be treated with erythropoietin (such as Epogen or Procrit).
Infection	Common	Seek medical attention immediately for any fever or infection symptoms. Do not take during infection.
Lung inflammation (pneumonitis)	Rare	Stop the drug.
Liver inflammation (hepatitis)	Uncommon	Stop the drug.
Pancreas inflammation (pancreatitis)	Rare	Stop the drug.

Note: Side effect incidence key: rare <1% occurrence; uncommon 1%–5% occurrence; common >5% occurrence.

Vaccines and AZA: Although it is a live vaccine, it is safe to get a Zostavax (shingles vaccine) when taking AZA. Stopping the drug for one to two weeks after vaccines (if your lupus is under excellent control) may help the vaccine work better. Ask your doctor.

For in-depth information, go to lupusencyclopedia.com/4th-covid-vaccines and lupusencyclopedia.com/2022-vaccine-recommendations.

Pregnancy and breast-feeding: It is one of the lupus drugs of choice during pregnancy and breast-feeding.

Geriatric use: Lower doses are often used initially due to possible increased side effects in older people.

AZA and surgery: Ask your rheumatologist and surgeon. AZA can be continued during surgery. In people with mild SLE in remission, it can be stopped one week before surgery, then resumed after they have healed well after surgery, and if there is no infection.

Financial aid for AZA: Go to lupusencyclopedia.com/patient-resources, goodrx.com, and similar programs.

Drug helpline: Call 1-888-825-5249 (for brand name Imuran only)

More information: Go to https://rheumatology.org/patients/azathioprine-imuran.

Baricitinib (Olumiant), Tofacitinib (Xeljanz), and Upadacitinib (Rinvoq)

These drugs are in a class called Janus kinase inhibitors (JAKi). Chapter 3 discussed how the immune system's white blood cells communicate by sending chemical messages called cytokines. Some cytokine messages decrease inflammation, while others increase inflammation. When inflammation-producing cytokines attach to a white blood cell's surface, many rely on an enzyme (a type of chemical or molecule) inside the cell called Janus kinase. If Janus kinase does not work correctly, the cytokine cannot cause the white blood cell to become more active, resulting in less inflammation and immune system activity. JAKi prevent some types of Janus kinases from working, resulting in better disease control.

Although FDA-approved for other diseases, like rheumatoid arthritis, JAKi have been found to help lupus in some studies. I (Don Thomas, MD) had some SLE patients participate in phase 1 and phase 2 clinical trials (see chapter 37) for tofacitinib use in SLE. One of them had severe, difficult-to-control SLE arthritis (she did not have RA or rhupus). A few weeks after treatment, she had a fantastic response with the complete disappearance of arthritis. After the research ended and she had to stop the study drug, she again had a severe arthritis flare. She went into remission after I prescribed tofacitinib (Xeljanz) and remains in remission today. Therefore, I use JAKi in some SLE patients with excellent results and good tolerability.

Generic available: No.

How JAKi work: See above.

Patients can usually tell within the first couple of weeks if it is helping. The longest they take is around four to five weeks.

Do not take if

- you have an active infection.

- your blood counts are too low, liver enzymes are too high, or kidney function decreases by too much.

- you have severe anemia or severely low white blood cell counts.

- you have cancer. If you had cancer in the past, discuss it with your doctor.

Use caution if

- you have had a blood clot, stroke, or heart attack in the past.

- you have diverticulitis (a large intestine infection).

- you have had squamous cell or basal cell carcinoma of the skin.

Let your doctor know if you have been exposed to TB, hepatitis B, hepatitis C, or HIV in the past. If you have ever had a positive TB skin test (PPD) or blood test (QuantiFERON or T-SPOT.TB), also let your doctor know.

Dosage: For RA, the approved dose for baricitinib is a 2 mg pill once daily; tofacitinib is 5 mg twice daily or 11 mg once daily; upadacitinib is 15 mg a day. The SLE clinical trial for baricitinib showed that 4 mg a day worked better than 2 mg a day.

As of January 2023, baricitinib has an "emergency use authorization" by the FDA in treating very sick, hospitalized patients infected with COVID-19 using 4 mg daily, and tofacitinib at 10 mg twice daily.

If you miss a dose, take your next dose on the same day as soon as you remember that you forgot it. For example, if you usually take it at 11:00 A.M. every day and realize at 8:00 P.M. that you forgot to take your medicine, go ahead and take your tablet for that day. Resume taking your next dose at 11:00 A.M. the next day. However, if you do not remember until the next morning you forgot your previous day's dose, just wait until 11:00 A.M. and take your usual dose for that day, totally missing the previous day's dose. Ask your doctor.

Alcohol/food interactions: There are no alcohol or food interactions; can be taken with or without food.

What to monitor while taking a JAKi:

- blood counts, liver function tests, and kidney function

- lipid profile (cholesterol panel)

- skin cancer screenings from a dermatologist.

Potential side effects of JAKi (table 32.2): The increased risk of infection is the most significant potential side effect, especially if used with steroids. JAKi also increase the risk of shingles. Tell your doctor if you develop an uncomfortable, burning, or painful rash, which can be a sign of shingles. But it's better to make sure you have your shingles shot before you start a JAKi. The Shingrix shot (chapter 22) is preferable (it works best and is not a live vaccine). If you get the live vaccine (Zostavax), make sure you get it at least 30 days before starting a JAKi. If you are already on a JAKi, you can go ahead and get the Shingrix vaccine but not Zostavax.

JAKi may increase the risk of blood clots. They have occurred mainly in obese patients and in those with a history of blood clots. The problem has been seen most commonly with doses higher than those FDA-approved for RA. A phase 1/2 clinical trial of tofacitinib for SLE did not note any increase in blood clots using the standard dose (5 mg twice daily). This included patients who were positive for antiphospholipid antibodies. However, there were more blood clots in the group taking high-dose 10 mg twice daily.

If you develop abdominal pain, let your doctor know, because intestinal perforations (chapter 15) have been noted but are rare.

Table 32.2 Potential Side Effects of JAK Inhibitors

	Incidence	Side Effect Therapy
Nuisance side effects		
Diarrhea, nausea	Common	Take with food, lower the dose, or stop it.
Elevated cholesterol	Common	Unsure if this is an important issue.
Increased CPK level	Common	Probably not an important issue.
Headaches	Uncommon	See your doctor, lower the dose, or stop it.
Mild anemia (defined by doctor)	Uncommon	Monitor if very mild or reduce dosage.
Rash	Uncommon	Lower the dose or stop the drug.
Elevated liver enzymes	Uncommon	No intervention if mild; stop the drug if severe.
Serious side effects		
Infections, especially shingles	Common	Seek medical attention immediately for fever or infection. symptoms. A painful blistering rash could be shingles.
Severe anemia (defined by doctor)	Uncommon	Reduce dosage. It can be treated with erythropoietin (Epogen or Procrit). Or stop the drug.
Low white blood cells	Uncommon	Reduce dosage or stop it. Can be treated with Neupogen (with caution, chapter 9).
Blood clots	Rare	Immediately go to emergency room and stop the drug.
Heart attacks, strokes	Rare	Immediately go to emergency room and stop the drug.
Gastrointestinal perforation	Rare	Immediately go to emergency room and stop the drug.
Cancer	Rare	Treat the cancer and stop the drug.

Note: Side effect incidence key: rare <1% occurrence; uncommon 1%–5% occurrence; common >5% occurrence.

While taking a JAKi, see your primary care provider or go to an emergency room immediately if you have infection symptoms (table 22.3). Practice all measures to prevent infections (table 22.4).

Vaccines and JAKi: Do not get live vaccines (chapter 22). If your lupus is under excellent control, stopping the drug for one to two weeks after vaccines may help vaccines work better. Ask your doctor.

JAK inhibitors are labeled "small-molecule drugs"

The JAK inhibitors (JAKi) are as effective as biologics in treating rheumatoid arthritis (RA). While biologic drugs are very large molecules, JAKi are much smaller. We use the term "disease-modifying agents for rheumatic diseases" (DMARDs) for the older small-molecule drugs, such as methotrexate and azathioprine.

However, JAKi tend to work better and faster in RA than the older DMARDs. Therefore, to differentiate JAKi from biologics and DMARDs, we group them under "small-molecule drugs." This term will become handier in the future. Other non-JAKi small-molecule drugs that are being tested in SLE patients would be included in this group.

For in-depth information, go to lupusencyclopedia.com/4th-covid-vaccines and lupusencyclopedia.com/2022-vaccine-recommendations.

Pregnancy and breast-feeding: Use good birth control (chapter 41). Do not take a JAKi while pregnant. A JAKi should be switched to a pregnancy-safe drug (such as AZA) before getting pregnant.

Do not take while breast-feeding.

Geriatric use: A lower dose may be needed.

JAKi and surgery: Ask your rheumatologist and surgeon regarding specific instructions. If someone's lupus is at high risk of flaring, it may be continued during surgery. If not, it may be stopped four days before surgery and restarted once the wound is healing well without infection.

Financial aid for JAKi: Go to lupusencyclopedia.com/patient-resources, olumiant .com, xeljanz.com, and rinvoq.com.

Websites: olumiant.com, xeljanz.com, and rinvoq.com

Cyclophosphamide (CYC)

CYC is one of the strongest immunosuppressants. It is the drug of choice for severe or life-threatening SLE, such as severe vasculitis, kidney, brain, heart, or lung inflammation.

Generic available: Yes.

How CYC works: CYC is an alkylating agent chemotherapy drug; it adds a molecule called an alkyl group to the DNA of reproducing cells. This results in the destruction of actively dividing cells. Since it does this to all body cells, it strongly suppresses the entire immune system. It can begin to work as quickly as a couple of weeks after the first dose.

Do not take if

- you have an infection. Wait until it is gone.

- your blood counts are too low. Wait until they improve.

Let your doctor know if you have been exposed to TB in the past. If you have ever had a positive TB skin test (PPD) or blood test (QuantiFERON or T-SPOT.TB), also let your doctor know.

Dosage: CYC is most used in intravenous (IV) form in SLE. There are two common dosing regimens: the high-dose National Institutes of Health (NIH) regimen and the low-dose Euro-Lupus regimen.

The high-dose NIH regimen of 750 mg to 2,000 mg at a time is usually given monthly for six months by IV. A white blood cell count is typically measured 10 days after each dose to help with dosage adjustments. After six months, many patients are switched to a different longer-term treatment (called maintenance therapy), such as mycophenolate mofetil (MMF, CellCept). Others may continue getting CYC every three months for up to a total of two years before maintenance therapy. For membranous lupus nephritis (WHO Class V), it is sometimes given every other month for a year.

The Euro-Lupus regimen uses lower doses of IV CYC (500 mg) every two weeks for six doses, followed a week or two later with maintenance therapy (such as with MMF or AZA). It was as effective as, and safer than, the NIH regimen when tested in European patients. There were fewer infections and low blood cell count problems, and it did not cause infertility as the NIH regimen does.

Another study done in the US and Mexico (the Abatacept and CYC Combination Efficacy and Safety Study) used the Euro-Lupus regimen in Black and Hispanic patients. Those patients did well in the short term without high rates of side effects.

Due to the Euro-Lupus regimen's superior safety, we now primarily use this regimen in most of our SLE patients who need CYC.

Since the high-dose NIH regimen has been studied more in severe lupus nephritis (such as rapidly progressive glomerulonephritis, chapter 12) and non-Europeans (African and Hispanic descent), some doctors prefer the NIH regimen in these groups.

CYC can also be taken orally (pills), but it is rarely used this way in the United States since it causes more side effects than the IV form. Oral CYC is used more often in some countries due to its low cost.

If you miss a dose, set up your CYC infusion as soon as possible (if there is no reason you should not get it, such as having very low blood counts or infection). Then reset your schedule accordingly. For example, if your monthly infusion was scheduled on January 10 and for some reason, you had to reschedule it for January 21, get your next infusion scheduled as close to February 21 as you can and resume monthly dosing after that. Ask your doctor.

Alcohol/food interactions: No alcohol or food interactions occur with the IV form.

What to monitor while taking CYC on the high-dose NIH regimen:

- a complete blood cell (CBC) count 8–12 days after each infusion
- a regular chemistry panel (to check liver and kidney function) and urinalysis.

What to monitor while taking CYC on the Euro-Lupus regimen: monthly CBC, urinalysis, and chemistry panels.

Potential side effects of CYC (table 32.3): If hair loss occurs, it begins to grow back 3–12 weeks after the last infusion, sometimes in a different color or texture. Nausea and vomiting typically occur 6 to 10 hours after the infusion. You should be armed with an anti-nausea medicine, which should be provided to you by your doctor. Take it at any hint of nausea. Do not wait until you really start to feel sick because it can be harder to get nausea under control. If your anti-nausea medicine does not work sufficiently, make sure to let your doctor know so they can try a different one or give you a larger dose.

Generally, we talk about drug side effects in this book as being "potential"—that is, they usually do not occur in most people. However, a low white blood cell count is expected in almost everyone taking CYC. The lowest levels occur around the tenth day after the infusion and then improve over time. Your doctor will use blood count results to determine the best dose when using the NIH regimen.

Infections are one of the most serious side effects. Infection risk correlates with how low the white blood cell count gets and how much steroids are used. The lower the white blood cell count is, the higher the chances of infection. Also, the higher the dose of steroids, the greater chance for infection. Try to get all vaccines (such as COVID-19, pneumococcal, flu shot, Gardasil, and Shingrix) before CYC.

Some doctors give an antibiotic to prevent a lung infection due to *Pneumocystis jirovecii* bacteria. The two most used antibiotics in SLE are dapsone and atovaquone. We recommend avoiding trimethoprim-sulfamethoxazole (Bactrim) due to the increased risk of lupus flares and other reactions in SLE patients to sulfonamide antibiotics (chapter 5).

The high-dose NIH regimen can cause infertility. The EuroLupus regimen does not. The chances of infertility are higher in older women (that is, women in their thirties and forties, rather than in their teens and twenties). Infertility can be reduced by taking hormone drugs (such as Lupron) while on CYC. Freezing your eggs (chapter 41) is another option. If you wish to have children in the future, discuss this with your doctor before starting the NIH regimen.

It can also cause infertility in men. If you are a man and want to ensure that you can have children in the future, you can investigate the possibility of receiving testosterone or storing your sperm in a sperm bank before treatment.

However, since CYC is used for severe lupus, which often occurs without warning, it is often impractical to store sperm or freeze eggs.

CYC increases some cancer risks (chapter 22), primarily in people who have received multiple rounds of high-dose CYC. The more CYC you receive in your lifetime, the greater the chance. It increases cancers associated with human papillomavirus (such as cervical and anal cancer) and blood cancers (leukemia and lymphoma). These usually occur many years after treatment. The risk of getting one of these cancers is around double that of the general public. Fortunately, CYC does not cause cancer in most patients.

IV CYC, or any dose of oral CYC, can occasionally concentrate in the urinary bladder and cause inflammation, leading to visible blood in the urine (called hemorrhagic cystitis). This increases the risk for bladder cancer. It is less likely to occur with lower doses (as in the EuroLupus regimen) and when lower total overall doses are given (as in the EuroLupus regimen, rather than the NIH regimen). However, it can occur at any dose. Some genes can greatly increase this risk, but we do not have a way to measure them outside of a research setting. Drink lots of water the day before and after your IV infusions to minimize this possibility. Also, frequently empty your bladder, especially before bed. This reduces the toxic chemicals in the bladder. Using a drug called Mesna can help prevent this complication.

While taking CYC, see your primary care provider or go to an emergency room immediately if you have infection symptoms (table 22.3). Practice all measures to prevent infections (table 22.4).

- Drink lots of fluids, as discussed above.

- Take an antibiotic to prevent pneumocystis pneumonia if you have very low lymphocyte counts and are on prednisone greater than 20 mg daily.

Vaccines and CYC: Do not get live vaccines unless it is at least 30 days before the first infusion. If your lupus is under excellent control, stopping the drug for one to two weeks after vaccines may help the vaccine work better. Time your intravenous CYC to be given one week after vaccines, if possible.

For in-depth information, go to lupusencyclopedia.com/4th-covid-vaccines and lupusencyclopedia.com/2022-vaccine-recommendations.

Pregnancy and breast-feeding: Men and women on CYC need strict birth control (chapter 41). Life-threatening SLE during the second or third trimester may be treated with CYC. If you decide to become pregnant after stopping CYC, wait at least three months before trying to have a baby. If you get pregnant on CYC and live in the United States or Canada, contact MotherToBaby at mothertobaby.org or 866-626-6847 to learn more.

Do not breast-feed while taking CYC.

Geriatric use: Lower doses are typically used; older people usually have reduced kidney function, which can increase side effects.

CYC and surgery: Ask your rheumatologist and surgeon. Elective surgeries should not be done on CYC. For emergency surgeries, do not resume CYC treatments until surgical wounds heal and there is no infection.

Financial aid or CYC pills: Go to lupusencyclopedia.com/patient-resources, goodrx.com, or similar programs.

More information: See https://rheumatology.org/patients/cyclophosphamide-cytoxan.

CyclosporineA (CsA, SandIMMUNE, Neoral, and Gengraf)

Cyclosporin (also spelled ciclosporin and cyclosporine) is usually used for lupus nephritis. Occasionally, it is also used for other lupus problems, such as cutaneous (skin) lupus and severely low blood counts.

Generic available: Yes. Because the body absorbs each type of CsA differently, it is crucial to stick with the same brand or generic producer.

How CsA works: CsA suppresses the immune system, especially a subset of immune cells known as T cells, and improves podocyte function (chapter 12).

A decrease in urine protein can be seen as quickly as a few weeks after starting therapy for lupus nephritis.

Do not take if

- you are allergic to it or your blood pressure is poorly controlled.

- you have significant fibrosis (scarring) on kidney biopsy.

- use caution if you have had squamous cell or basal cell carcinoma of the skin.

Table 32.3 Potential Side Effects of Cyclophosphamide

	Incidence	Side Effect Therapy
Nuisance side effects		
Nausea, vomiting, loss of appetite, diarrhea	Common	Take an anti-nausea or anti-diarrhea drug.
Mouth sores	Common	Reduce dosage. Use mouth rinses and creams prescribed by your doctor.
Hair loss	Common	Hair grows back after treatment is stopped.
Rash	Uncommon	Reduce dosage.
Runny nose, congestion, watery eyes, sneezing immediately after infusion	Uncommon	Slow down the rate of infusion during later treatments.
Serious side effects		
Low white blood cell counts	Common	Reduce dosage or stop it. Can be treated with Neupogen (with caution, chapter 9).
Low platelet counts	Uncommon	Reduce dosage. It can be treated with platelet transfusions if severe.
Anemia (low red blood cells)	Common	Reduce dosage if severe. It can be treated with erythropoietin (Epogen or Procrit).
Infection	Common	Seek medical attention immediately for any fever or infection symptoms. Do not get infusion during infection. Take prophylactic antibiotics during treatment to prevent lung infections.
Cancer, usually years later	Uncommon	Treat the cancer.
Lung inflammation (pneumonitis)	Rare	Stop the drug.
Liver inflammation (hepatitis)	Rare	Stop the drug.
Infertility	Common with high doses	It may be mitigated by hormone treatments (women) or sperm donation before treatment (men).

Note: Side effect incidence key: rare <1% occurrence; uncommon 1%–5% occurrence; common >5% occurrence.

Let your doctor know if you have been exposed to TB in the past. If you have ever had a positive TB skin test (PPD) or blood test (QuantiFERON or T-SPOT.TB), also let your doctor know.

Dosage: CsA is available in both tablet and liquid form. It is usually taken twice a day.

If you miss a dose, take your next dose at the usual time, and do not try to squeeze in an extra dose unless it has been just a few hours or less since the missed dose. Ask your doctor.

Alcohol/food interactions: No known interactions with alcohol.

Do not drink grapefruit juice or eat grapefruit; they increase CsA blood levels and thus side effects. It can be taken with or without food, but it is best taken at the same time each day and with the same pattern regarding meals. This helps your doctor adjust your drug dose accurately.

What to monitor while taking CsA:

- blood test for kidney function (serum creatinine and estimated glomerular filtration rate [eGFR]) and blood pressure, every one to two weeks for the first few months after starting or after dose increases, then every one to three months if doing well

  - a cholesterol panel (including triglycerides)

  - blood pressure at home; alert your doctor if it increases above your baseline.

Potential side effects of CsA (table 32.4): See the tacrolimus section below regarding calcineurin-inhibitor-induced pain syndrome.

While taking CsA,

- contact your doctor if you develop any side effects.

- *see your primary care provider or go to an emergency room immediately if you have infection symptoms (table 22.3).* Practice all measures to prevent infections (table 22.4).

Vaccines and CsA: Do not get live vaccines (chapter 22). If your lupus is under excellent control, stopping the drug for one to two weeks after vaccines may help the vaccine work better. Ask your doctor.

For in-depth information, go to lupusencyclopedia.com/4th-covid-vaccines and lupusencyclopedia.com/2022-vaccine-recommendations.

Pregnancy and breast-feeding: CsA is safe during pregnancy.

CsA is considered safe during breast-feeding.

Geriatric use: Usually, the doses are the same as those used in younger adults, but there may be an increased risk for side effects, especially high blood pressure and decreased kidney function.

CsA and surgery: Ask your rheumatologist and surgeon. If someone's lupus is at high risk of flaring, it may be continued during surgery. If not, it may be stopped one week before surgery and restarted once the wound is healing well without infection.

Financial aid for CsA: For SandIMMUNE and Neoral contact 800-245-5356 and novartis.com/us-en/patients-and-caregivers/patient-assistance. Go to lupusencyclopedia.com/patient-resources

Medication use in patients after weight loss surgery

Some patients who have undergone gastric bypass surgery (GBS, Roux-en-Y surgery) may have trouble absorbing pills and capsules due to having a smaller stomach and small intestine. Less stomach acidity and less bile result in lower absorption of fat-absorbed drugs. Two small GBS studies suggest that higher hydroxychloroquine and higher cyclosporine doses may be required for some patients, based on HCQ and cyclosporine drug levels. Health care providers should consider using drug levels to monitor certain oral drugs.

While we do not know which drugs are not absorbed well after GBS, we can get a good idea about a particular oral medication if it does not achieve a satisfactory response. If an inadequate response occurs, options include crushing pills, opening capsules and sprinkling them on food, changing pills to liquid form, using nonoral forms (such as injections), and using immediate-release instead of extended-release forms. Liquid medications containing nonabsorbable sugars (mannose, sucrose) can worsen a dumping syndrome GBS problem and may need to be avoided. An example is liquid acetaminophen (Tylenol).

Another type of weight loss surgery, gastric sleeve, may increase tacrolimus and mycophenolate mofetil absorption. Lower doses and drug level monitoring should be considered.

Some drugs can increase the risk of ulcers at the stomach surgical site after GBS and gastric sleeve surgery. Nonsteroidal anti-inflammatory drugs (NSAIDs), such as ibuprofen and naproxen, and oral bisphosphonates (such as alendronate) should be avoided. Steroids should be used in the lowest doses needed.

More information: https://rheumatology.org/patients/cyclosporine-neoral-sand immune-gengraf.

Leflunomide (LEF, Arava)

Arava was FDA-approved for rheumatoid arthritis (RA) in 1998 but has been shown to help some patients with SLE.

Generic available: Yes.

How LEF works: LEF suppresses the immune system. It is a slow-working drug. In RA, it tends to start working several weeks after starting it, and it takes about three months before the full effects of reducing or stopping joint inflammation. Taking a higher loading dose at first (see below) helps it work faster.

Do not take if you have an active infection or liver disease.

Use caution if you have had hepatitis or a history of excessive alcohol use; let your doctor know.

Dosage: LEF comes in 10 mg and 20 mg tablets. Some people may be started on 10 mg a day, especially if used with MTX. Sometimes, 100 mg daily for the first three days is prescribed, so it will work faster.

Table 32.4 Potential Side Effects of Systemic Cyclosporine and Tacrolimus (TAC)

	Incidence	Side Effect Therapy
Nuisance side effects		
Nausea, vomiting, loss of appetite, diarrhea	Common	Take with food. Decrease dosage or stop the drug.
Headache	Common	Reduce dosage or stop the drug.
Increase in body hair	Common	Reduce dosage or stop the drug.
Weight loss and weight gain	Common	Change diet and exercise regimens. Reduce dosage or stop the drug.
Rash	Common	Reduce dosage or stop the drug.
Leg cramps	Common	Reduce dosage or stop the drug.
Tremors	Common	Reduce dosage or stop the drug.
Tingling in hands and feet	Common	Reduce dosage or stop the drug.
Dizziness	Common	Reduce dosage or stop the drug.
Fluid retention, swelling of ankles (edema)	Common	Reduce dosage or stop the drug.
Swelling of the gums	Common	Reduce dosage or stop the drug.
Serious side effects		
High blood pressure	Common	Reduce dosage or stop taking the drug.
Decreased kidney function	Common	Reduce dosage if the kidney function is more than 25% below baseline.
Elevated triglycerides (chapter 21)	Common	Reduce dosage or stop the drug.
Infection	Common	Seek medical attention immediately for any fever or infection symptoms. Do not take during infections.
Diabetes mellitus (new-onset or worsening of existing diabetes)	Uncommon with CsA, common with TAC	Reduce dosage or stop the drug
Cancer (lymphoma)	Rare	Treat the cancer.

Note: Side effect incidence key: rare <1% occurrence; uncommon 1%–5% occurrence; common >5% occurrence.

If you miss a dose, if it is the same day as your missed dose, take your missed dose as soon as possible with food, then resume your usual schedule after that. If it is the next day that you remember, skip the missed dose and resume your normal schedule. Ask your doctor.

Alcohol/food interactions: Limit alcohol intake to minimize liver inflammation. See chapter 38 for safe alcohol amounts. Discuss with your doctor.

LEF may be taken with or without food. Taking it with food may decrease stomach upset.

What to monitor while taking LEF:

- CBC, liver enzymes, and chemistry panel blood tests, every two to four weeks for the first three to six months, then every two to three months

- blood pressure.

Potential side effects of LEF (table 32.5): If dangerous side effects occur, cholestyramine can be prescribed to absorb the LEF and rid it from your body (called cholestyramine elimination). Cholestyramine is usually taken 3 times a day for 11 days, after which the LEF blood levels are checked. Medicinal charcoal can also be used instead of cholestyramine.

While taking LEF,

- *see your primary care provider or go to an emergency room immediately if you have infection symptoms (table 22.3).* Practice all measures to prevent infections (table 22.4).

- contact your doctor if you develop yellow-colored skin and eyes, which may be a sign of jaundice from liver inflammation.

Vaccines and LEF: Do not get most live vaccines. It is OK to get Zostavax. If your lupus is under excellent control, stopping the drug for one to two weeks after vaccines may help the vaccine work better. Ask your doctor.

For in-depth information, go to lupusencyclopedia.com/4th-covid-vaccines and lupusencyclopedia.com/2022-vaccine-recommendations

Pregnancy and breast-feeding: The 2020 American College of Rheumatology (ACR) Guideline for Reproductive Health recommends against taking it during pregnancy and to do a cholestyramine elimination program (see above) before pregnancy or if pregnancy occurs while taking LEF. They recommend getting two negative LEF blood test results before getting pregnant. Cholestyramine may need to be used again if the blood level is not zero.

However, it is possible that LEF may be safer than we thought. A 2020 research study, published after the ACR Guidelines were published, evaluated 222 LEF pregnancies. No more birth defects than expected occurred. Those that did were different from each other, which led the authors to conclude that LEF most likely does not cause birth defects. (If a drug causes birth defects, they usually are the same types.) Ask your doctor.

LEF is probably safe for men to take while trying to father a child.

If you get pregnant on LEF and live in the United States or Canada, contact MotherToBaby at mothertobaby.org or 866-626-6847 to learn more.

It is not recommended to take LEF while breast-feeding.

Geriatric use: Same dosing as younger adults.

Table 32.5 Potential Side Effects of Leflunomide

	Incidence	Side Effect Therapy
Nuisance side effects		
Diarrhea	Common	Usually resolves while taking LEF. Try Imodium (OTC). If intolerable, decrease the dosage or stop the drug.
Nausea, vomiting, loss of appetite	Common	Take with food. Take anti-nausea medicine; or reduce dosage or stop the drug.
Hair loss	Common	Reduce dosage or stop the drug. The hair grows back.
Rash or itchy skin	Common	Reduce dosage or stop the drug.
Serious side effects		
High blood pressure	Common	Reduce dosage or stop the drug.
Liver inflammation (hepatitis)	Common	If liver enzymes are mildly elevated, the drug can be continued. The dose may need to be reduced for higher levels, or the drug may need to be stopped. For very high levels, cholestyramine elimination is needed.
Nerve damage (peripheral neuropathy)	Uncommon	Stop LEF. Cholestyramine elimination procedure may be needed.
Infection	Rare	Seek medical attention immediately for any fever or infection symptoms.

Note: Side effect incidence key (these are approximations as they can vary widely from study to study): rare <1% occurrence; uncommon 1%–5% occurrence; common >5% occurrence.

LEF and surgery: Ask your rheumatologist and surgeon. LEF does not need to be stopped for surgery as per the "2022 Perioperative Management of Antirheumatic Medication in Patients with Rheumatic Diseases Undergoing Elective Total Hip or Total Knee Arthroplasty."

Financial aid: Go to lupusencyclopedia.com/patient-resources, goodrx.com, or similar programs.

More information: https://rheumatology.org/patients/leflunomide-arava

Methotrexate (MTX, Otrexup, Rasuvo, RediTrex, Xatmep, Trexall)

Methotrexate is one of the most commonly used drugs for SLE. It is considered a weak immunosuppressant at the doses used in SLE.

Generic available: Yes for all except Xatmep and Trexall.

How MTX works: MTX suppresses the immune system. It is slow-working, but faster than AZA. It can begin working in a few weeks after starting but can take up to three months for the full effects of reducing or stopping lupus inflammation.

Do not take if

- you have an active infection or liver disease.

- you are on dialysis.

Use caution if

- you have a history of alcoholism or hepatitis.

- have decreased kidney function.

- you have had squamous cell or basal cell carcinoma of the skin before.

Let your doctor know if you have been exposed to TB in the past. If you have ever had a positive TB skin test (PPD) or blood test (QuantiFERON or T-SPOT.TB), also let your doctor know.

Dosage: MTX (MTX) is taken orally or by subcutaneous (SQ, SC, under the skin) injection once a week. The maximum dose of pills is generally 25 mg a week, 30 mg for SQ.

Generic MTX pills come in 2.5 mg tablets, while the brand name version Trexall comes in 5, 7.5, 10, and 15 mg tablets. Trexall is scored, so pills are easy to split if your doctor asks you to.

In people who have trouble swallowing pills, there is brand name Xatmep liquid solution. A cheaper alternative is to mix injectable MTX in water or juice (but not milk or caffeinated drinks).

To use generic injectable MTX, you must be able to draw it up out of the MTX vial with a needle and syringe and be able to handle the smaller syringe for injecting. This can be difficult for people with bad hand arthritis or nerve weakness problems. If you have trouble using the generic form, ask your doctor to prescribe Rasuvo, Otrexup, or Redi-Trex, which are brand name forms. They come in convenient pre-filled clickable pens.

Take tablets all at the same time weekly; this minimizes side effects. A higher percentage of MTX is absorbed at lower doses (7.5 mg to 15 mg) than at higher doses. For example, there can be a 30% less absorption of a 20 mg dose than a 10 mg dose. A 10 mg dose may achieve a MTX polyglutamate blood level (chapter 4) of 35 nmol/L (nanomoles per Liter). If the doctor increases the dose to 20 mg weekly, the measured blood drug

---

LUPUS IN FOCUS

MTX may increase skin cancer risks

A single study suggested that MTX may increase skin squamous cell carcinoma risk. People at higher risk for skin cancer (fair-skinned, a history of high amounts of sun exposure, and a family history of skin cancer) may want to regularly see a dermatologist for a skin examination. Methotrexate should also not be used in patients undergoing cancer radiation therapy.

level may be 60 nmol/L, instead of an anticipated level of 70 nmol/L if it were absorbed as well as the 10 mg dose. Much MTX is excreted in the feces, especially at the higher doses.

If your lupus is still active while taking all your pills once a week, your doctor may ask you to split your dose up over 12 to 24 hours. When this is done, a higher percentage of each dose is absorbed (compared to taking it all at once), resulting in more effective drug levels. Splitting up the dose can also reduce some side effects, such as stomach upset.

Never split up MTX by more than 24 hours. Taking one tablet seven days a week is dangerous compared to taking all seven tablets at the same time once a week. A higher proportion of medicine is absorbed from a single tablet than from seven taken all at once. We have seen severely low blood counts after patients accidentally took one tablet daily. After taking all the tablets weekly at once, their blood counts were better.

When MTX is injected, 100% of the drug enters the body. Up to 30 mg a week can be taken SQ. Rasuvo brand SQ MTX comes in doses up to 30 mg. Generic injectable MTX comes in 25 mg/mL concentration (often labeled as 50 mg/2 mL on the bottle). If generic is used, 30 mg would be 1.2 mL (the same as 1.2 cc).

You should take either folic acid or folinic acid (leucovorin) while taking MTX. Folic acid is taken 1 mg to 5 mg daily, while leucovorin is best taken once a week, 10 mg to 25 mg, 8 to 12 hours after your MTX dose.

If you miss a dose, take the dose you missed right away. For example, if you miss your Monday dose and do not realize you missed it until Wednesday, take it on Wednesday. Then do not take your next dose until the following Wednesday and proceed with weekly dosing on Wednesdays instead of Mondays.

An alternative would be to take the dose on Wednesday, then take your usually scheduled dose the following Monday and continue Monday doses. This latter method may be preferred if your SLE is not in remission. Ask your doctor.

If you take leucovorin (folinic acid), which is usually taken once a week, similarly reset your leucovorin schedule. If you take folic acid, continue taking it every day.

Alcohol/food interactions: It can be safe to drink alcohol in moderation or small amounts (if you do not have a reason not to drink, such as alcoholism or have liver problems). This decision is made on a case-by-case basis. Ask your doctor. Read chapter 38 to learn what a safe amount of alcohol is.

LUPUS IN FOCUS

MTX polyglutamate drug level testing

Some doctors check MTX drug levels (MTX polyglutamates). This should be done at least 36 hours after the previous dose and three months after a previous dose change. It can help ensure treatment adherence, especially in those not in remission. In rheumatoid arthritis, patients with levels above 60 nmol/L (nanomoles of MTX polyglutamates per liter of blood) tend to have less inflammation and better disease control. I check levels in my patients who are reluctant to increase their MTX dose when their SLE is not in full remission. Many are more willing to increase their dose or switch their pills to injections if their level is low.

MTX is best taken on an empty stomach. However, if you get stomach upset, taking it with food can reduce stomach issues but result in reduced amounts of MTX in your system. Milk products reduce absorption even more.

Caffeine may interfere with how well MTX works. If you take MTX and your SLE is hard to control, consider stopping caffeine for a few months to see if it helps.

What to monitor while taking MTX:

- complete blood cell counts and liver function tests, every 2–12 weeks
- a baseline chest x-ray before or soon after starting MTX.

Potential side effects of MTX (table 32.6): As with the other immunosuppressants, the biggest concern is low blood counts and infections. The risk for infections is especially high if the white blood cell count decreases or when taking steroids, such as prednisone.

One of the most common side effects of MTX is liver enzyme elevations (AST and ALT, chapter 4). Although this occurs in half of patients taking MTX, it rarely indicates any liver problems. Real liver damage with MTX is more common in people with a history of heavy alcohol drinking, people who have had hepatitis or fatty liver, obese patients, and people with diabetes. In a 2020 study, only 5 out of 2,391 MTX users developed severe liver problems (cirrhosis). All but one were obese, and all were diabetic. This emphasizes the importance of maintaining normal body weight and ensuring excellent glucose (sugar) control.

Do not be alarmed if you get a call from your doctor asking you to lower your MTX dose because your liver enzymes are elevated. If the levels are followed closely and proper dose adjustments are made, MTX should not cause an actual problem. But if your liver enzymes are elevated five times or more in a year, your doctor may want to get a liver biopsy or order additional blood tests to make sure that everything is OK. Because there are so many other effective SLE drugs, liver biopsies are rarely done these days. Most doctors switch patients to a different drug instead.

It is not uncommon for the blood counts to go down on MTX. This problem is usually mild and resolves when the dosage is decreased. Taking MTX can cause an enlargement of the red blood cells, identified as an elevated mean corpuscular volume (MCV) (chapter 4) on the complete blood cell counts. This is common and rarely problematic.

Hair thinning occurs in less than 10% of MTX users and is reversible. The hair slowly grows back after the dose is decreased or after MTX is stopped. If you are taking folic acid and notice some thinning of your hair, ask your doctor if you can switch to leucovorin (folinic acid), which may work better. Decreasing the dose of MTX can also help. Note that it may take 4–12 months after these changes to notice increased hair growth again.

Another potential side effect is lung inflammation due to hypersensitivity (allergic reaction) pneumonitis. It is rare and most commonly occurs within the first year of treatment. The symptoms are similar to those of pneumonia, including cough (often coughing up sputum), fever, and shortness of breath. The chest x-ray can look identical to pneumonia due to infection. It may be impossible to tell if someone who has pneumonia while on MTX has it due to infection or from MTX-induced hypersensitivity pneumonitis. Therefore, both possibilities may need treatment using a combination of antibiotics, high doses of steroids, and stopping MTX. Pneumonitis is more common in smokers and in those with preexisting lung problems. Both infectious pneumonia and MTX-induced hypersensitivity pneumonitis are dangerous. If you develop these symptoms, it is important to stop MTX and seek medical attention immediately.

Although MTX can cause lung inflammation, it is generally safe to use in patients with preexisting interstitial lung disease (ILD) (chapter 10).

If you get headaches, dizziness, feel out of sorts, confused, or have "the blahs" after taking MTX, take one tablet of Mucinex DM with your methotrexate, then take another tablet eight hours later along with leucovorin. Dextromethorphan (the active ingredient) can reduce these side effects.

MTX can cause sun sensitivity (already a problem in lupus). You should already be taking adequate precautions (tables 38.2, 38.3, and 38.4). If you ever get a sunburn, some experts recommend not taking the next dose of MTX (skip one week).

Folic acid and leucovorin help prevent and treat MTX side effects. Folinic acid (leucovorin) is probably more effective than folic acid. See the "How MTX is taken" section above.

While taking MTX, see your primary care provider or go to an emergency room immediately if you have infection symptoms (table 22.3). Practice all measures to prevent infections (table 22.4).

Vaccines and MTX: Do not get most live vaccines while using MTX. It is OK to get Zostavax when taking low-dose MTX (as is used in SLE). If your lupus is under excellent control, stopping the drug for one to two weeks after vaccines may help the vaccine work better. Ask your doctor.

For in-depth information, go to lupusencyclopedia.com/4th-covid-vaccines and lupusencyclopedia.com/2022-vaccine-recommendations.

Pregnancy and breast-feeding: MTX has a high chance of causing miscarriage or congenital abnormalities. Strict birth control must be used to prevent pregnancy (chapter 41). If a woman on MTX wishes to become pregnant, she should stop taking MTX. After the next menstrual cycle, she can then try to become pregnant. After stopping MTX, a woman should take a folic acid supplement every day and then continue taking it throughout pregnancy to increase the chances for a successful, safe conception and pregnancy.

Men should continue MTX while attempting pregnancy with their female partners. Even though the FDA-approved drug label warns against this, subsequent research showed it is no problem.

If you get pregnant on MTX and live in the United States or Canada, contact MotherToBaby at mothertobaby.org or 866-626-6847 to learn more.

MTX is not recommended during breast-feeding.

Geriatric use: Lower doses may decrease the potential of side effects.

MTX and surgery: Ask your rheumatologist and surgeon. Many experts recommend that MTX be continued during surgery because it has not been shown to increase infections after surgery. Some rheumatologists like to be extra cautious. If SLE is in remission and the person is at low risk for flaring, MTX can be stopped one week before surgery, then resumed after the surgical wound is healing well, and if there is no infection.

For people with significantly decreased kidney function (ask your doctor) who undergo major surgery (like heart surgery), it may be wise to stop MTX the week before surgery and readd when the surgical wound is healing. If kidney function decreases even more (related to the surgery and anesthetics), the MTX drug level could increase, potentially causing side effects.

Should you stop MTX after vaccines?

MTX can decrease the response to vaccines. A 2019 study showed that patients with rheumatoid arthritis who were in remission and skipped their MTX for two doses (two weeks) after the flu shot (influenza vaccine) responded to the vaccine better. They also did not have many arthritis flares.

Because of this, I have lupus patients who are in remission and who are not at high risk for a lupus flare stop their methotrexate for one to two weeks after all vaccines. A 2022 study showed that when MTX was stopped after COVID vaccines for one to two weeks, patients had better responses to the vaccines with few flares, thus supporting this approach.

Always consult with your physician.

Financial aid for MTX: Go to lupusencyclopedia.com/patient-resources, goodrx.com, or similar programs.

More information: https://rheumatology.org/patients/methotrexate-rheumatrex-trexall-otrexup-rasuvo

Mycophenolate mofetil (CellCept) and mycophenolate sodium (Myfortic)

Mycophenolate is the most popular drug (other than steroids) for lupus nephritis. Studies show it is helpful for other SLE problems as well. It is as effective as cyclophosphamide (CYC) for many cases and may be safer. MMF is superior to azathioprine when used as maintenance (long-term) therapy for lupus nephritis. A 2017 Spanish study showed that the related drug, mycophenolate sodium (Myfortic), was superior to azathioprine in treating non-kidney SLE in 240 SLE patients.

MMF works better for lupus nephritis in Hispanic and Black patients than CYC. Another advantage over CYC is that it does not cause sterility (infertility) in women.

Generic available: Yes.

How mycophenolic acid works: It is usually used for moderate to severe SLE. However, it is a slow-working drug, usually taking several months (up to six) to work.

Proton pump inhibitors (table 28.3) used for decreasing stomach acidity can reduce the conversion of mycophenolate mofetil (CellCept) to the active molecule, mycophenolic acid, by as much as 35%. Therefore, patients taking a PPI may be better off taking mycophenolate sodium (Myfortic) than CellCept.

Do not take if

- you are allergic to it.

- you have an active infection.

- you have an active ulcer in the gastrointestinal system.

- you are allergic to polysorbate 80, an ingredient in some brands.

Table 32.6 Potential Side Effects of Methotrexate

	Incidence	Side Effect Therapy
Nuisance side effects		
Elevated liver enzymes	Common	Lower the dose. Change folic acid to leucovorin or increase leucovorin dose. Stop MTX if the condition persists.
Nausea, vomiting, loss of appetite, diarrhea	Common	Spread the dose over 24 hours. Take with meals. Change folic acid to leucovorin or increase the leucovorin dose. Reduce MTX dose. Take an anti-nausea drug.
Mouth sores	Common	Spread the dose over 24 hours. Change folic acid to leucovorin or increase the leucovorin dose. Reduce MTX dose. Use mouth rinses and creams prescribed by your doctor.
Hair loss	Common	Change folic acid to leucovorin or increase the leucovorin dose. Reduce MTX dose or stop the drug. Hair returns after MTX is stopped or dose is reduced.
Headache, dizzy, feeling out of sorts, confused, "the blahs."	Common	Take dextromethorphan as indicated in the text. Spread the dose over 24 hours. Change folic acid to leucovorin or increase the leucovorin dose. Reduce MTX dose or stop the drug.
Rash, often sun sensitive	Uncommon	Follow advice in tables 38.2, 38.3, and 38.4. Reduce dosage or stop MTX.
Serious side effects		
Low white blood cell counts	Common; rarely severe	Reduce dosage or stop MTX. Can be treated with Neupogen (with caution, chapter 9).
Low platelet counts	Uncommon; rarely severe	Reduce dosage or stop MTX. It can be treated with platelet transfusions.
Anemia (low red blood cells)	Common; rarely severe	Reduce dosage or stop MTX. It can be treated with erythropoietin.
Infection	Uncommon	Seek medical attention immediately for any fever or infection symptoms. Stop MTX during infections.
Skin cancer (not melanoma)	Uncommon	Treat the cancer. Get regular skin cancer screenings if you are fair-skinned or have had much sun exposure in the past.
Lung inflammation (pneumonitis)	Uncommon	Stop MTX and seek medical attention immediately.
Cirrhosis of the liver	Very rare	Stop MTX.

Note: Side effect incidence key (these are approximations as they can vary widely from study to study): rare <1% occurrence; uncommon 1%–5% occurrence; common >5% occurrence.

Let your doctor know if you have been exposed to TB in the past. If you have ever had a positive TB skin test (PPD) or blood test (QuantiFERON or T-SPOT.TB), also let your doctor know.

Dosage: Mycophenolate mofetil (MMF, CellCept) comes in 250 mg and 500 mg tablets or capsules. It also comes in a liquid preparation for people with difficulty swallowing pills. The extended-release form (Myfortic as mycophenolate sodium) comes in 180 mg and 360 mg tablets. MMF is commonly prescribed at 500 mg to 1,500 mg (180 mg to 1,080 mg for Myfortic) twice a day. Because people with African ancestry tend to metabolize it (break it down inside the body) or absorb it from the intestinal system differently than other ethnicities, they are usually prescribed 1,500 mg twice a day. White patients are often started at 1,000 mg twice daily at first then increased to 1,500 mg twice daily after a month, if not significantly better by that time. However, Asians can be more sensitive to mycophenolate, and lower doses are often used.

It is often initiated at a small dose (such as 500 mg twice a day) and then gradually increased to the maximum prescribed dosage. This "start low, go up slow" technique minimizes gastrointestinal side effects, like nausea, diarrhea, or stomach upset. The enteric-coated delayed-release tablet (Myfortic) may have less of these side effects compared to MMF.

If you miss a dose, take your next dose at the usual time. Do not try to squeeze in an extra dose unless it has been just a few hours or less since the missed dose. Ask your doctor.

Alcohol/food interactions: There are no known interactions with alcohol.

Mycophenolate is absorbed best on an empty stomach. But if stomach upset or diarrhea occurs, it can be easier to tolerate when taken with food. In the long run, it is just as effective when taken with or without food.

What to monitor while taking mycophenolic acid:

- blood counts, liver function, and kidney function, done anywhere from once a week up to every three months

- skin cancer screening if you are at high risk (fair-skinned, strong family history, or have had excessive sun exposure).

Potential side effects of mycophenolic acid: See table 32.7

While taking mycophenolic acid see your primary care doctor or immediately go to an urgent care center if you develop any infection symptoms (table 22.3). Practice all measures to prevent infections (table 22.4).

The FDA requires that the pharmaceutical companies producing mycophenolate offer health care professionals and patients an opportunity to participate in a risk evaluation and mitigation study (REMS). Women who are capable of getting pregnant and take mycophenolate should go to mycophenolateREMS.com or call 800-617-8191 to enroll.

Vaccines and mycophenolic acid: Do not get live vaccines. If your lupus is under excellent control, stopping the drug for one to two weeks after vaccines may help the vaccine work better. Ask your doctor.

For in-depth information, go to lupusencyclopedia.com/4th-covid-vaccines and lupusencyclopedia.com/2022-vaccine-recommendations.

Pregnancy and breast-feeding: Mycophenolate can cause birth defects. Do not take while pregnant and use strict birth control (read chapter 41).

If you get pregnant on mycophenolate and live in the United States or Canada, contact MotherToBaby at mothertobaby.org or 866-626-6847 to learn more.

Do not use while breast-feeding due to unknown safety.

Geriatric use: It is usually the same as in younger adults, although older people tend to have more stomach upset and infections.

Mycophenolic acid and surgery: Ask your rheumatologist and surgeon. A common recommendation is to stop it one week before surgery, then start taking it again after the surgical wound is healing well and there is no evidence of infection. The drug may be continued during surgery for SLE patients who are at risk for lupus flares.

Financial aid: Go to lupusencyclopedia.com/patient-resources, goodrx.com, or similar programs.

More information: https://rheumatology.org/patients/mycophenolate-mofetil-cellcept-and-mycophenolate-sodium-myfortic

Table 32.7 Potential Side Effects of Mycophenolic Acid

	Incidence	Side Effect Therapy
Nuisance side effects		
Nausea, vomiting, appetite loss, diarrhea, weight loss	Common	Take with food. Reduce the dosage or stop the drug. Antinausea drugs; Imodium for diarrhea.
Tremors or anxiety	Uncommon	Reduce dosage or stop the drug.
Rash	Uncommon	Reduce dosage or stop the drug. Cortisone cream, oral steroids, antihistamines.
Serious side effects		
Low white blood cell counts	Uncommon	Reduce dosage or stop the drug. Can be treated with Neupogen (with caution, chapter 9).
Low platelet counts	Uncommon	Reduce dosage or stop the drug. It can be treated with platelet transfusions.
Anemia (low red blood cells)	Uncommon	Reduce dosage or stop the drug if severe. It can be treated with erythropoietin, such as Epogen or Procrit.
Infection	Common	Seek medical attention immediately for any fever or infection symptoms. Do not take it during infections.
Cancer (skin cancer)	Rare	Treat the cancer.

Note: Side effect incidence key (these are approximations as they can vary widely from study to study): rare <1% occurrence; uncommon 1%–5% occurrence; common >5% occurrence.

Tacrolimus (TAC, Astagraf XL, Envarsus XR, and Prograf) and Topical Ointment (Protopic)

TAC is related to CsA and voclosporin (chapter 34) within a drug class called calcineurin inhibitors. TAC is considered an improved form of a calcineurin inhibitor compared to CsA and is referred to as a second-generation drug. Its improvements include more predictable results with more reliable dosing and fewer side effects than CsA.

Generic available: Yes

How TAC works: TAC suppresses the immune system, especially a subset of immune cells known as T cells, and improves podocyte function (chapter 12).

When used for lupus nephritis, TAC can significantly lower urine protein levels and improve serologies (anti-dsDNA, C3, and C4, chapter 4) within weeks.

The ointment is used for cutaneous lupus and works within six weeks.

Do not take oral TAC if

- you are allergic to tacrolimus.

- you have significant fibrosis (scarring) on kidney biopsy.

- use caution if you have had skin squamous cell or basal cell carcinoma.

- you have prolonged QTc (chapters 11 and 30). Although hydroxychloroquine and TAC can potentially increase QTc intervals, this problem has not been reported on the low doses of these drugs used for lupus.

Let your doctor know if you have been exposed to TB in the past. If you have ever had a positive TB skin test (PPD) or blood test (QuantiFERON or T-SPOT.TB), also let your doctor know.

Dosage: For the oral form, the more commonly used immediate-release form is taken twice daily. The extended-release is once a day. The two types are not interchangeable.

TAC tablets and pills are FDA-approved to prevent organ transplant rejection (such as after getting a kidney transplant). They are generally used in much lower doses for lupus nephritis. We usually begin at 0.5 to 1 mg twice daily. If needed, we slowly increase the dose. In lupus nephritis research studies, doses as high as 0.15 mg/kg daily were used.

Some doctors measure TAC drug blood levels to help guide dosing. Drug levels are measured 30 minutes before a dose (called a trough level when blood levels are at their lowest); 4 to 6 ng/mL concentrations have been suggested as a safe and effective target. The doctor increases or decreases the dose based on the result, then repeats the drug level measurements to see if further adjustments are needed.

The ointment comes in a 0.03% and a stronger 0.1% version. It should be rubbed in completely on active inflammation areas twice a day regularly (not just as needed).

If you miss a dose, take your next dose at the usual time; do not try to squeeze in an extra dose unless it has been just a few hours or less since the missed dose. Ask your doctor.

Alcohol/food interactions: Avoid alcohol with extended-release TAC since it can increase the drug's absorption. There is no alcohol restriction with the immediate-release form. Alcohol may cause increased flushing and redness at the application site of the ointment. This is not a dangerous reaction but something to be aware of.

Food (especially fatty foods) can decrease absorption by as much as 75%, so it is best to take TAC on an empty stomach (such as first thing in the morning and right before bed).

Do not consume grapefruit since it can increase drug levels.

What to monitor while taking oral TAC:

- drug levels 30 minutes before a planned dose of 2 mg twice daily or more (not needed with just 1 mg twice daily)

- blood pressure at home (alert your doctor if it increases above your baseline)

- blood cell counts, liver function enzymes, chemistry panel (electrolytes, glucose, and kidney function), and HbA1c.

Potential side effects of TAC (table 32.4): An uncommon side effect of TAC and CsA is calcineurin-inhibitor-induced pain syndrome. If it occurs, it is usually within six months of starting treatment. It causes severe and sometimes disabling pain in the legs (especially the feet, ankles, and knees), as well as in the back. Blood work will often show a high alkaline phosphatase level. Gabapentin may help the pain.

The primary side effects of TAC ointment are irritation, redness, swelling, pain, or rash at the application area. Report it to your doctor if this occurs.

While taking oral TAC,

- contact your doctor if you develop any of the side effects mentioned above.

- *see your primary care provider or go to an emergency room immediately if you have infection symptoms (table 22.3)*. Practice all measures to prevent infections (table 22.4).

Vaccines and oral TAC: Do not get live vaccines. If your lupus is under excellent control, stopping the drug for one to two weeks after vaccines may help the vaccine work better. Ask your doctor.

For in-depth information, go to lupusencyclopedia.com/4th-covid-vaccines and lupusencyclopedia.com/2022-vaccine-recommendations.

Pregnancy and breast-feeding: TAC can be used safely during pregnancy and while breast-feeding.

Geriatric use: There are no special considerations.

TAC and surgery: Check with your rheumatologist and surgeon. A common recommendation is to stop taking it one week before surgery, then resume taking it after the surgical wound is healing well and there is no infection. For SLE patients at risk of flaring, it is usually continued during surgery.

Topical TAC can be used up to surgery time unless you use it directly at the surgical site. If the surgery involves the skin where you are using tacrolimus, consult your prescribing doctor when you should stop using it.

Financial aid: Go to lupusencyclopedia.com/patient-resources, goodrx.com, and similar programs.

Websites: astagrafxl.com, envarsusxr.com

KEY POINTS TO REMEMBER

1. Immunosuppressants are used for moderate to severe lupus.

2. Because immunosuppressants usually take a while to work (weeks to months), steroids are typically used as bridge therapy. When the immunosuppressant begins to work, the steroid dose is gradually reduced (chapter 31).

3. Immunosuppressants are considered steroid-sparing drugs: they help decrease the dose of steroids needed.

4. All immunosuppressants increase infection risks. If you get infection symptoms (table 22.3), stop the immunosuppressant, immediately contact your primary care provider or go to the emergency room.

5. Do everything to prevent infections when taking immunosuppressants (table 22.4).

6. Do not get live vaccines while using these medicines (although you can get a Zostavax to prevent shingles if you take MTX, LEF, or AZA).

7. All of these drugs (except tacrolimus ointment) need labs done regularly.

8. Some of these drugs have strict rules on how they are used or not used in people who may want a baby. Make sure that you are aware of these recommendations.

Biologic Agents

Andrea Fava, MD, *Contributing Editor*

Biologic agents are also called biologic drugs or biologics. They are produced in any living (hence, biologic) system, including microscopic organisms (such as bacteria), animal cells, or plant cells. This contrasts with other drugs produced in a laboratory by mixing chemicals together (called chemical agents). Immunosuppressants (chapter 32), steroids (chapter 31), and antimalarials (chapter 30) are all chemical agents.

Rituximab (Rituxan) is a commonly used biologic in SLE and is included in this chapter. Belimumab (Benlysta) and anifrolumab (Saphnelo) are biologics FDA-approved for SLE, and they will be discussed in the next chapter. Some others can be used in SLE, but not as often, and are discussed in chapter 37.

This chapter discusses biologics in much greater detail, but first, it explains some important immunology concepts that make the biologic section easier to understand.

Cytokines: How White Blood Cells Talk to Each Other

Among their many functions, cells can release molecules to send messages to other cells. These communication particles are called cytokines. *Cyto-* comes from the Greek word for cell, while *-kine* comes from the Greek word meaning "to move" or "to stir up."

Here is an example of how they work. When macrophages (chapter 30) of the immune system recognize an invading army of microbes (such as viruses or bacteria), they release large amounts of a cytokine called lymphocyte-activating factor (now renamed interleukin-1, or IL-1 for short). As the name implies, this cytokine activates lymphocytes (a type of white blood cell). These cytokines tell the lymphocytes and other members of the immune system to become activated, or "stirred up," and to reproduce and move to the area of invasion to destroy the viruses or bacteria and protect the body (figure 33.1). This IL-1 (or lymphocyte-activating factor) also causes fever, a common symptom during infections.

In autoimmune diseases such as SLE and rheumatoid arthritis (RA), many of the cytokines that cause inflammation are produced in excess (figure 33.2), while the cytokines that calm down inflammation are not being made as much as they should.

Could doctors control these diseases by decreasing cytokines that cause inflammation or by increasing cytokines that reduce inflammation? Could it be possible to design drugs that target what is going wrong with specific parts of the immune system instead of suppressing the entire immune system (the way that immunosuppressant

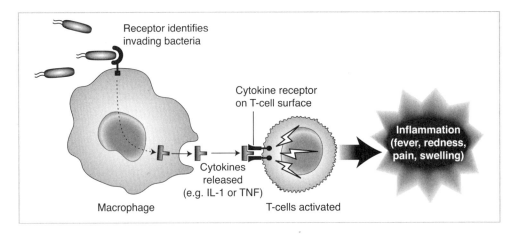

Figure 33.1 Cytokines causing normal immune response with inflammation

medications do)? Along came an essential technique called recombinant DNA technology that would allow the production of large amounts of cytokines for research.

In 1975, a cytokine that was produced by macrophages and could kill mouse cancer cells was identified. It was named tumor necrosis factor (TNF; figure 33.3). TNF increases body inflammation, including increased white blood cells, fever, loss of appetite, and weight loss. In the mid-1980s, it was discovered that RA patients had excessive TNF activity (especially one called TNF alpha).

The Birth of Biologic Drugs: Miracle Drugs for Rheumatic Diseases

The next logical step was to develop a way to decrease this TNF alpha (also written as TNF-α) activity. Recall from chapter 1 that an antibody is a molecule of the immune system that attaches to an antigen molecule to remove it from the body. In the early 1990s, antibodies were developed that could attach to TNF-α. This antibody was made into a drug called etanercept (Enbrel) and was the first in a new class of drugs called TNF inhibitors. In 1998, the FDA approved its use for RA. Within a few years, TNF inhibitors were shown to dramatically reduce RA joint damage and deformities. This was truly miraculous. Since then, biologics such as TNF inhibitors have become some of the most important drugs for rheumatic diseases like SLE. (We discuss "biologics" below.)

Since the immune systems of lupus patients produce too many inflammation-producing cytokines (including TNF-α), doctors tried these TNF inhibitors in SLE patients (see figure 33.3) who failed other treatments. The first studies, published in 2002 and 2003, showed that TNF inhibitors helped SLE patients. Infliximab (Remicade, a TNF inhibitor) helped some patients with lupus nephritis (kidney inflammation) and arthritis. After that, many lupus experts began recommending TNF inhibitors for SLE patients who failed other therapies.

TNF inhibitors are produced using bacteria or mouse cells. Compared to the laboratory techniques used in the production of chemical medications, the biological processes used to produce biologic agents are complex (table 33.1).

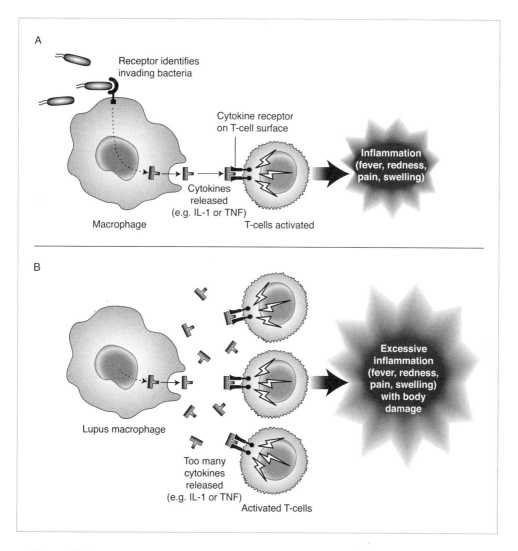

Figure 33.2 Normal immune response (A) versus inflammation from an overproduction of inflammatory cytokines (B) in SLE

Biologics are produced in living systems, including microscopic organisms (such as bacteria), animal cells, or plant cells. These drug molecules are much larger than those produced by chemical processes. They also tend to be more fragile. Due to their large size and complexity, stomach acid would destroy the drugs before they could be absorbed. Therefore, they cannot be taken orally in pill form. They are administered by injection through an IV into a vein or a needle injecting it into a muscle or under the skin (called subcutaneous, SC, or SQ).

Biologics are costly, ranging from tens of thousands of US dollars per year to over US$100,000 for just one patient. One reason for their being so expensive is that the

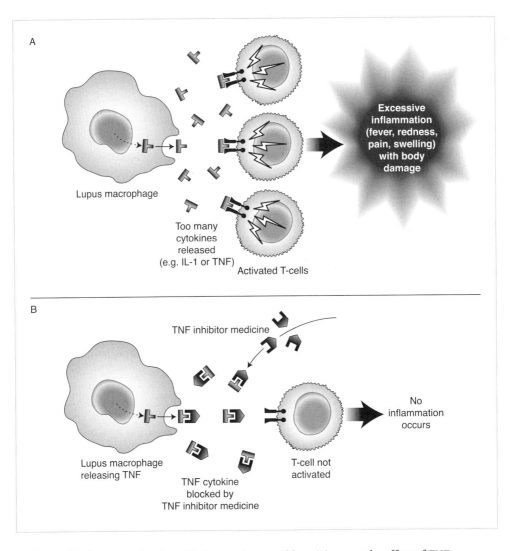

Figure 33.3 Overproduction of inflammatory cytokines (A) versus the effect of TNF inhibitor treatment (B)

Table 33.1 Biologic Agents versus Chemical Agents

Biologics (examples: rituximab, belimumab, anifrolumab)	Chemical Drugs (examples: prednisone, hydroxychloroquine)
Made by complex biological processes	Made by simpler chemical processes
Very expensive	Less expensive
Very large, complex molecules	Smaller, "simpler" molecules
Usually given by injection	Many can be taken by mouth

factories producing biologics must be completely sterile at every step to keep the bacteria, or other organisms producing the biologic, safe and pure. Not even one tiny contamination can occur. Everyone who enters the facility must put on a sterile suit. In addition, each batch of the biologic must be evaluated using expensive biologic systems instead of simpler chemical systems.

Other biologics used for SLE include rituximab (Rituxan), belimumab (Benlysta), and anifrolumab (Saphnelo). Not all biologics attack cytokines. Some of them interfere with the immune system in other ways.

This chapter discusses the TNF inhibitors and rituximab (Rituxan), while chapter 34 covers belimumab (Benlysta) and anifrolumab (Saphnelo). Other biologics, like tocilizumab (Actemra), abatacept (Orencia), and ustekinumab (Stelara) are not used as often and are in chapter 37.

Biosimilars: Generic Equivalents for Biologics

When a new drug is made, the pharmaceutical company that makes it has legal patents that protect against other companies manufacturing the same drug. These patents typically last for at least seven years and can be much longer for complicated drugs. When the patent expires, other companies can produce the drug, usually at a lower cost than the original brand (trade) medicine. An example for lupus is mycophenolate mofetil, the generic equivalent of the brand-named CellCept. Reasons for the initial brand-name drug being so expensive have to do with the incredibly high price for research and development that went into discovering and developing the original drug, producing it, and then educating health care providers and patients about its use. An additional unseen cost comes from the fact that for every drug that becomes FDA-approved, many others fail. The research costs of these failed drugs are made up in the price of new drugs produced. A pharmaceutical company needs to recoup all these costs and make a profit that motivates investors to continue investing in the search for better treatments.

Biosimilars are the generic equivalents for biologics. They are what drug companies develop after the patent for the original biologic has expired. In 2016, Infliximab-dyyb (Inflectra) became the first biosimilar rheumatic drug. It is similar to infliximab (Remicade), which was FDA-approved 18 years earlier.

Biologics and their biosimilars are made by biological systems (such as bacteria) that are not 100% controllable and predictable. This is unlike chemical drug processing methods, which are predictable. Since the resulting drug molecules are similar to the original biologic but not exactly like the original, the term "biosimilar" is used instead of "generic." While we expect generic molecular structures to be precisely like the original, the FDA states that a biosimilar is "highly similar to, and has no clinically meaningful differences from another biologic that's already approved by the FDA."

TNF Inhibitors (adalimumab/Humira, certolizumab/Cimzia, etanercept/Enbrel, golimumab/Simponi, infliximab/Remicade)

Although TNF inhibitors were recommended to treat SLE in the early 2000s, they are rarely used for SLE today. Better drugs are now available. There is also concern that this group of drugs could worsen lupus in some patients, though this has not been proven. SLE patients on TNF inhibitors today usually fall into one of two categories. Either they were placed on them in the early 2000s or they have RA overlapping with lupus (rhupus, chapter 2), and the TNF inhibitor is being used for their RA.

Biosimilars available: Yes, except for golimumab and certolizumab as of February 2023.

How TNF inhibitors work: Each of them works in a slightly different way to prevent the cytokine TNF-α from attaching to and activating white blood cells so that the TNF-α molecules cannot create as much inflammation.

Inflammatory arthritis may respond as quickly as a week (but can take up to several months), resulting in decreased pain, swelling, and stiffness.

Do not take if

- you have uncontrolled congestive heart failure (chapter 11); seen mainly with infliximab.

- you have bladder cancer treated with Bacillus Calmette-Guerin (BCG), a bacteria related to TB, which can become active and spread through the body if the treated person uses a TNF inhibitor.

- multiple sclerosis, Guillain-Barré syndrome, chronic inflammatory demyelinating polyneuropathy, or optic neuritis.

- you are allergic to latex: then avoid adalimumab (Humira), etanercept (Enbrel), certolizumab (Cimzia), and golimumab (Simponi) pre-filled syringes, which have latex in the rubber parts of the syringes.

Before starting treatment, everyone should be tested for hepatitis B (a blood test) and TB (a skin test and/or blood test). If you have been infected with TB in the past, you should be treated for TB with antibiotics before starting a TNF inhibitor. You can often begin taking the TNF inhibitor soon after starting the antibiotic (ask your doctor). Do not use a TNF inhibitor if you have an untreated, active infection.

Some also recommend testing for HIV before use.

Dosage: Some are given intravenously (IV) while others are SQ (subcutaneous) forms injected in the doctor's office or by patients themselves at home. Dose and frequency vary between the different brands.

If you miss a dose, give yourself an SQ injection, or have your infusion scheduled as soon as you realize that you missed a dose. Then you need to reset your schedule from that date.

For example, if you inject yourself with adalimumab every two weeks on Mondays, and you realize on Saturday that you forgot your Monday dose, give yourself your SQ injection on that Saturday and resume your next injections every two weeks on Saturdays. However, it is possible to do the injections sooner than this and catch up on your missed doses. If you are not in remission, your doctor may advise you to give yourself the injection on that first Saturday, then proceed with your every other week schedule on the normally scheduled Monday, nine days later. Always ask your doctor.

Alcohol/food interactions: None known.

What to monitor while taking TNF inhibitors:

- your lupus labs

- skin for cancer if you have had skin cancer.

Potential side effects of TNF inhibitors (table 33.2): While the package insert states that cancers, including lymphoma (cancer of the lymph nodes and white blood cells), may occur with TNF inhibitors, these drugs have been available for over 24 years, and many detailed studies have shown no increase in any cancers, except for the possibility of some skin cancers (basal cell and squamous cell carcinoma, but not melanoma). Therefore, it is most likely safe for you to take these drugs if you have had cancer. However, since drugs that suppress the immune system can theoretically increase cancer risk, this warning will remain on the package label, even if no cancer is proven to occur.

Some studies have shown no increased risk of skin cancer, while others have suggested an increased risk for basal cell and squamous cell carcinoma. Consider having your skin checked periodically by your primary care doctor or a dermatologist. Do everything in tables 38.3 and 38.4 to reduce this possibility.

There have been case reports of TNF inhibitors causing drug-induced lupus (discussed in chapter 1) in patients who did not previously have SLE. However, they have not been shown to worsen SLE in lupus patients.

Infusion reactions are common with the IV (intravenous) forms, but they are usually mild and temporary. Most doctors treat their patients with an antihistamine (such as Benadryl), Tylenol, and steroids before the infusion to prevent these reactions. The most common infusion reaction symptoms include headaches, chills, body aches, nausea, upset stomach, and itchy skin. Infusions may also cause a more severe, life-threatening reaction (anaphylaxis), but this is rare.

While taking TNF inhibitors, contact your primary care provider or go to an urgent care center immediately if you develop infection symptoms (table 22.3). Practice all measures to prevent infections (table 22.4).

Vaccines and TNF inhibitors: Do not get live vaccines. You do not need to stop the drug for flu shots, pneumonia shots, Shingrix, Gardasil, or the COVID-19 vaccine. These recommendations are based on the latest medical evidence as of January 2023. However, your situation may dictate otherwise, or newer research studies may recommend otherwise. Ask your doctor.

The reason not to get a live vaccine while taking a biologic such as a TNF inhibitor is that the patient could potentially get an infection from it. However, in a 2019 research study that evaluated the live vaccine Zostavax (for shingles) in over 300 TNF inhibitor

Table 33.2 Potential Side Effects of TNF Inhibitors

	Incidence	Side Effect Therapy
Nuisance side effects		
Injection site reaction	Common	Usually mild and tolerable. Can use ice compresses or cortisone cream on the site.
Infusion reaction with IV forms	Common	It can be prevented or made less severe by taking Benadryl, Tylenol, and steroids before and during the infusion. The rate of the infusion can also be slowed down.
Headache	Common	Take Tylenol or NSAIDs (ask your doctor if it is OK). If severe, go down on the dose or stop the drug.
Nausea, stomach upset	Common	Usually mild. Take anti-nausea drugs for nausea. If severe, may need to reduce the dose or stop the drug.
Rash	Common	Usually mild. Use cortisone cream or antihistamines such as Benadryl. If severe, reduce the dose or stop the drug.
Psoriasis rash	Uncommon	Stop the drug and treat psoriasis with cortisone creams. Sometimes the drug can be continued if mild.
Temporary joint pain	Uncommon	Usually mild. Can treat with Tylenol or use steroids.
Serious side effects		
Infection	Common	See your primary care doctor or go to the emergency room immediately. Do not take the drug during infections.
Severe infusion reaction	Uncommon	Stop the drug.
Drug-induced lupus	Rare	Stop the drug. May need steroids or other immunosuppressant.
Skin cancer	Rare (unknown if truly a side effect or not)	Get skin examined annually by a dermatologist.
Congestive heart failure (CHF), primarily infliximab	Rare	Avoid in patients with uncontrolled CHF; treat CHF and stop the drug.

Note: Side effect incidence key (these are approximations as they can vary widely from study to study): rare <1% occurrence; uncommon 1%–5% occurrence; common >5% occurrence.

Store and travel with biologic drugs properly

Biologics need to be stored correctly to ensure that they remain stable and effective. It is recommended to keep them at 35°F to 46°F. Avoid the lower crisper portion of the fridge where meats and produce are usually stored; it could be too cold. When placed at room temperature (for example, before giving yourself an injection), keep the biologic at less than 77°F.

Etanercept and adalimumab can be safely kept up to 14 days at a temperature up to 77°F (out of sunlight). Certolizumab may be kept up to a week.

If your biologic is improperly stored, discard it (chapter 29) and contact the pharmaceutical company for a replacement.

patients, none became infected with shingles after receiving the vaccine. This challenges the idea of live vaccines being forbidden, but more research is needed.

For in-depth information, go to lupusencyclopedia.com/4th-covid-vaccines and lupusencyclopedia.com/2022-vaccine-recommendations.

Pregnancy and breast-feeding: Safe during pregnancy (mainly the first two trimesters) and breast-feeding (see chapter 41).

Geriatric use: No differences in dosing.

TNF inhibitors and surgery: Check with your rheumatologist and surgeon. A standard recommendation is to schedule your surgery on the date of your usual TNF inhibitor dose. Then resume your TNF inhibitor on your usual schedule once the wound is healing well without infection (typically two weeks later). In SLE patients who may flare if there is a delay in treatment, no changes in TNF inhibitor scheduling may be recommended.

Studies have shown no increased risk for infections after surgery, so some rheumatologists do not stop these drugs for surgery.

Financial aid: Each TNF inhibitor has its own website. Just type in the name of the brand followed by .com—for example, remicade.com and enbrel.com.

Drug helpline: Each has its own website. See above.

More information: rheumatology.org/patients/tumor-necrosis-factor-tnf-inhibitors. Also, each drug has its own website. See above.

Rituximab (Rituxan)

Rituximab is a biological agent that decreases B-cell lymphocyte production (see figure 30.1 and chapter 30). It was initially FDA-approved in 1997 to treat B-cell lymphoma, but since autoimmune diseases such as RA and SLE have been noted to have overactive B-cells, rituximab was studied in these disorders. The FDA approved it for RA patients in 2006. Since then, it has been shown to be helpful in other rheumatologic conditions, including SLE.

Biosimilars available: Yes.

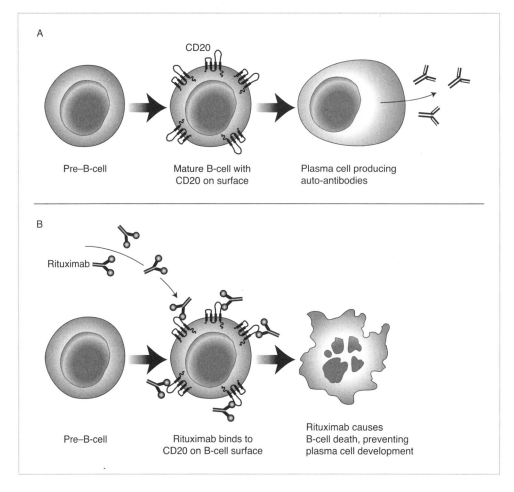

A

CD20

Pre–B-cell   Mature B-cell with   Plasma cell producing
                    CD20 on surface   auto-antibodies

B

Rituximab

Pre–B-cell   Rituximab binds to   Rituximab causes
                CD20 on B-cell surface   B-cell death, preventing
                                    plasma cell development

Figure 33.4 B-cell maturation and involvement of CD20 in SLE (A); Rituximab attaches to B-cells causing them to die and not produce SLE autoantibodies (B).

How rituximab works: Rituximab binds to the outer surface of B-cells on a receptor (attachment) called CD20 and causes the CD20 B-cells to become inactive or die (figure 33.4A). CD20 is an identification badge worn by several types of B-cells.

One of the primary problems seen in lupus is that the immune system makes too many antibodies that attack the body itself (called autoantibodies, chapter 1). Specialized B-cells (called plasma cells) make these autoantibodies. Rituximab attaches to the CD20 labels on the maturing B-cells and prevents them from producing the autoantibody-producing plasma cells. Since fewer lupus autoantibodies are made, less inflammation and damage may occur (figure 33.4B).

Low blood counts from SLE (low platelets and autoimmune hemolytic anemia, chapter 9) can improve within a few weeks, while lupus arthritis may take a few months to begin to improve. It may help some patients with Sjögren's (chapter 14) and in patients with RA and SLE overlap (rhupus). It is also used for severe lupus problems such as lupus nephritis (kidney inflammation) after other drugs fail.

Do not take if

- you have chronic hepatitis B infection.

- you have an active infection.

- you have uncontrolled congestive heart failure or have severe heart arrhythmia; ask your doctors.

You should have hepatitis B and TB tests before starting rituximab (chapter 22).

Dosage: Rituximab is given as an IV infusion over about six to eight hours. A typical dosing schedule is to get 1,000 mg, followed by a similar infusion two weeks later. This is often repeated every six months (in other words, four infusions a year). It is sometimes given as often as every four months. Other dosing schedules are used as well. IV steroids are usually given before rituximab to decrease the chances of an allergic-type reaction.

If you miss a dose, schedule your infusion as soon as possible. Then reset your schedule from that date. For example, let's say that you did not get your biweekly rituximab as scheduled (maybe it had to be canceled for some reason or you forgot). You should reschedule that dose as soon as possible and then schedule your next dose to occur two weeks later. Consult your prescribing doctor to double-check these instructions, but these guidelines will be enough for most people.

Alcohol/food interactions: None noted.

What to monitor while taking rituximab: Your doctor will want to check a blood cell count, immunoglobulin levels (chapter 4), and a chemistry panel periodically

Potential side effects of rituximab (table 33.3): The most significant is increased infections. Infections are more likely to occur in patients with low neutrophil counts (a type of white blood cell) and those with low IgG immunoglobulin levels (hypogammaglobulinemia, chapter 22). As with other immunosuppressants, if you have any infection symptoms (table 22.3), you should see your primary care provider or go to an urgent care center immediately. Also, you should not take your medicine during infections.

One infection needs special mention: progressive multifocal leukoencephalopathy (PML). We discuss PML here in detail because the FDA requires the pharmaceutical company to include it as a potential side effect in its package insert and advertise it to the public. PML is a brain infection caused by the JC (John Cunningham) virus. Close to 90% of all people have been infected with the JC virus, most commonly as children. It usually does not make you sick. The virus can live inside our bodies for the rest of our lives, and our immune systems keep it under control. If the immune system is suppressed, JC virus can multiply and damage the central nervous system, a condition called PML. PML can cause confusion, memory and coordination problems, muscle weakness, difficulty speaking, and double vision.

Unfortunately, PML is usually deadly. PML occurs in approximately 1 out of every 25,000 RA patients who receive rituximab, so it is very rare. How often it occurs in SLE is unknown. There have been only a few case reports of its occurring in SLE patients taking rituximab.

PML has occurred in SLE patients while taking almost any lupus drug. More than 40% of those patients received very little immunosuppression, suggesting SLE itself may increase the risk for PML.

In a New York City study that followed 7,455 SLE patients from 1986 to 2013, there was only 1 case of PML. The individual had been treated with cyclophosphamide and high doses of prednisone (not rituximab). None of the rituximab patients developed PML.

If you develop any neurologic symptoms seen with PML, listed above, you should seek immediate medical attention. Since most of these same symptoms also occur in people with strokes, it is best to go to an emergency room.

Infusion reactions are common, but they are usually mild and temporary. Most doctors treat their patients with an antihistamine, Tylenol, and steroids before and during the infusion to prevent these reactions. The most common infusion reaction symptoms include headaches, chills, body aches, nausea, upset stomach, and itchy skin. They typically occur with the first infusion in about one-third of people with RA and become less common after that. More severe allergic infusion reactions (anaphylaxis), which can cause shortness of breath, swelling in the throat, hives, vomiting, and blood pressure changes, are much less common. Your infusion center will be prepared to treat any of these.

Since intravenous steroids are usually given along with rituximab, some of the side effects can be from the steroid rather than Rituxan. These include ankle swelling, elevated glucose levels, flushing, and high blood pressure.

While taking rituximab, contact your primary care provider or go to an urgent care center immediately if you develop infection symptoms (table 22.3). Practice all measures to prevent infections (table 22.4).

Vaccines and rituximab: Your B cells are necessary to respond well to vaccines. For example, when you get a shingles vaccine, the vaccine instructs your B-cells to produce the antibodies that can fight off shingles. With fewer B cells after rituximab treatment, the response to the vaccine will be weaker.

Since rituximab gets rid of large numbers of your B-cells, it is best to get any non-live vaccination two to five weeks before each cycle's first rituximab treatment. If you get a vaccine soon after your rituximab, your body would not respond well to the vaccine.

It is best to get your flu vaccine in September or October each year (in the Northern Hemisphere). Some patients should consider adjusting their rituximab schedule (with the help of their prescribing doctor) if needed. Suppose you were to get your rituximab the first two weeks of September, you had not had your flu shot yet, and your next rituximab was scheduled in March. In that case the best time to get your flu shot would be two to five weeks before the March rituximab. Flu season is almost over by then. It is better to reschedule your September rituximab a few weeks later, ideally in October (if this won't jeopardize your lupus), and get the flu shot in early September, two to five weeks before rituximab.

COVID-19 vaccines are equally tricky. If you are just starting the initial vaccine shots (called the primary series), get the first vaccine four to five weeks before your first rituximab and the booster shot one to two weeks before the second rituximab. If you need a one-shot booster, get it two to four weeks before rituximab. Since we most commonly give rituximab cycles every four to six months, this means waiting four to six months between each booster shot, longer than recommended for people not on rituximab.

Many of us try to delay rituximab treatments in the hope that the vaccines will work better. For example, if a patient who is in remission or low disease activity is scheduled for rituximab in six months and also needs a COVID booster, they could try to wait eight months before getting rituximab. Those extra two months help the B cells increase in number so that the patient could respond better to the vaccine. The decision process is complicated. Ask your doctor well ahead of your scheduled infusions (prepare months, not weeks, ahead).

As of January 2023, rituximab patients may need as many as six total COVID vaccines. For more information, go to lupusencyclopedia.com/4th-covid-vaccines and lupusencyclopedia.com/2022-vaccine-recommendations.

Do not get live vaccines while on rituximab.

Pregnancy and breast-feeding: Rituximab is usually avoided during pregnancy. However, it can be used for severe SLE flares. Rituximab can be used during breast-feeding.

Geriatric use: Older people are at increased risk for infections, lung problems, and heart problems while using rituximab.

Rituximab and surgery: Ask your rheumatologist and surgeon. A standard recommendation is to schedule your surgery on the date of your usual rituximab dose (and skip the rituximab). Then resume your rituximab once the wound is healing well without infection (typically two weeks later). In SLE patients who may flare if there is a treatment delay, no changes in rituximab scheduling may be recommended.

Financial aid: Call 877-436-3683.

Drug helpline: 888-835-2555.

More information: rituxan.com and rheumatology.org/patients/rituximab-rituxan-and-mabthera

LUPUS IN FOCUS

How well does rituximab work in SLE?

A 2019 Italian study of 80 patients treated with repetitive rituximab courses showed that 1 out of 3 patients went into remission after the first treatment and stayed in remission for an average of 2 years. After the study was over and rituximab was stopped, the researchers watched 75% of those patients. Half of them were still in remission after an additional 18 months of no rituximab treatment (the treatment study had ended). SLE patients who were most likely to go into remission were those who had severe disease, had not failed numerous previous treatments, and did not have lupus arthritis.

Table 33.3 Potential Side Effects of Rituximab (Rituxan)

	Incidence	Side Effect Therapy
Nuisance side effects		
Flushing, rash, sweats, itchiness	Common	Usually mild; stop the drug if significant.
Ankle swelling (edema)	Common	Usually resolves on its own. Avoid salt and salty foods the day before, day of, and day after your infusion. Can use diuretics (fluid pills) if severe.
Infusion reactions	Common	Taking Benadryl, Tylenol, and steroids before and during the infusion can help prevent this. The rate of the infusion can be slowed down in the future to help prevent this. They are treated with the same drugs used to prevent it.
Elevated liver enzymes	Common	Usually mild requiring no treatment. Stop the drug if severe.
Stomach upset, nausea, diarrhea	Common	Usually mild and temporary; can take anti-nausea or anti-diarrhea drugs; stop rituximab if severe.
Serious side effects		
Infections	Common	Treat infections; don't get rituximab during infections.
Elevated blood pressure	Common	Usually mild and temporary. May not require treatment. Blood pressure medicines can be used.
Severe infusion reaction	Uncommon	Treated by the infusion center. Rituxan treatments most likely would be stopped.
Low white blood cell counts and hypogammaglobu-linemia	Common	Usually requires no treatment. Your treatment may be delayed if it persists. If infections occur with hypogammaglobulinemia, IVIG can be given (chapter 35)
Low red blood cells (anemia) or platelets (thrombocytopenia)	Uncommon	Usually mild, requiring no treatment. Your treatment may be delayed if the condition persists.
Bowel perforation/ obstruction	Rare	Go to the emergency room if you develop abdominal pain, especially if it is severe or occurs with fever.
Severe rash	Rare	Requires treatment by your doctor. Stop rituximab.

Note: Side effect incidence key (these are approximations as they can vary widely from study to study): rare <1% occurrence; uncommon 1%–5% occurrence; common >5% occurrence.

1. Biologics are produced by biological processes (such as bacteria or mouse cells) instead of simple chemical processes.

2. Due to production complexities, biologics are very expensive.

3. Due to the large size and fragility of the molecules, biologics are usually given by injection (SQ or IV); otherwise, stomach acid would destroy them.

4. The most commonly used biologics for SLE are rituximab (Rituxan), anifrolumab (Saphnelo), and Benlysta (belimumab).

5. Just as with other immunosuppressants, there is an increased risk of infections with biologics.

6. Make sure not to use biologics during active infection.

7. Contact your primary care provider or go to the emergency room immediately if you have infection symptoms.

8. Do everything in table 22.4 to prevent infections.

9. Do not get live vaccines (including a Zostavax for shingles) if you are on a biologic.

Newest FDA-Approved Drugs for SLE

Timothy Niewold, MD, *Contributing Editor*

On March 9, 2011, belimumab (Benlysta) became the first drug that the FDA approved for lupus since April 18, 1955, when it approved hydroxychloroquine. Back then, color television sets were popping up in US homes for the first time, and Dwight D. Eisenhower was president. All new drugs used to treat SLE from 1956 to 2010 (over five decades) were borrowed from other diseases.

Currently, the only drugs that are FDA-approved for treating lupus are steroids, hydroxychloroquine, aspirin, anifrolumab, belimumab, and voclosporin. FDA approval requires meeting such a high bar that these drugs deserve their own chapters. HCQ and steroids were discussed in chapters 30 and 31, respectively. Anifrolumab, belimumab, and voclosporin are discussed in this chapter.

Anifrolumab (Saphnelo)

Anifrolumab was FDA-approved in 2021 on the basis of two phase 3 clinical trials called the Treatment of Uncontrolled Lupus via the IFN Pathway (TULIP) trials. Phase 3 clinical trials are the final research studies performed before a pharmaceutical company asks the FDA to approve its drug as a safe and effective therapy. An advantage of anifrolumab over many other lupus drugs is that it appears to work faster in some patients, often as soon as after one infusion.

Biosimilar available: No.

How anifrolumab works: Around 70% of SLE patients have high type I interferon levels. Interferon is an immune system molecule, a type of cytokine (chapters 3 and 33). These high levels cause increased lupus inflammation. Anifrolumab binds to the cell surface receptor (attachment) for type I interferon and keeps interferon from working, which results in less lupus inflammation and better disease control in many patients.

Some patients see improvements during the first month of treatment. By the third month, most patients who are going to respond to it already have improvements.

It appears to be especially useful in decreasing active inflammation, redness, tenderness, and itching in moderate to severe cutaneous lupus. In the clinical trials, 49% of those with at least moderately severe cutaneous lupus had at least a 50% disappearance of skin inflammation by three months compared to 25% of those receiving the usual lupus treatments (called standard of care in the studies). That is a remarkable difference.

636

Aspirin is FDA-approved for SLE, but we do not use it in that way

Aspirin is. FDA-approved for lupus pleurisy and lupus arthritis. However, when prescribed for these conditions, very high doses are used, which cause significant side effects in most patients. Therefore, we do not use aspirin anymore for its FDA-approved indications. Instead, we use it for three other reasons.

First, we use low-dose (LD) aspirin to help prevent heart attacks and strokes. We use LD-aspirin to help prevent blood clots from antiphospholipid antibodies. Lastly, we use LD-aspirin to improve pregnancy outcomes (chapters 9, 21, and 41).

Anifrolumab can significantly reduce lupus inflammatory arthritis pain and swelling. It also improves low blood cell counts due to SLE. Immune system activity markers of lupus (anti-dsDNA, C3, and C4) tend to improve as well. In addition, it can decrease the number and frequency of lupus flares and help reduce the need for steroids.

Patients with severe kidney inflammation (lupus nephritis) and severe neuropsychiatric lupus (chapter 13) were excluded from the research studies. Therefore, we do not know how they will do on anifrolumab. Studies are underway for lupus nephritis.

Interferon levels are high in other related disorders such as scleroderma, dermatomyositis, RA, and Sjögren's. Experts hope that it may be beneficial in these. As of January 2023, research studies are being conducted using anifrolumab in scleroderma, RA and Sjögren's patients.

Do not take if

• you have an active infection.

• you have an immune deficiency disorder (chapter 22), HIV, viral hepatitis B or C, or a history of severe herpes infections.

Before starting treatment, patients should be checked for HIV, hepatitis B, and hepatitis C infection.

Dosage: 300 mg of anifrolumab is given by IV monthly.

If you miss a dose, get your infusion ASAP. If this infusion is more than 14 days before your next scheduled anifrolumab, you can stick to your usual schedule and resume every-4-week dosing after that. Anifrolumab doses need to be at least 14 days apart.

For example, if you miss your January 1 anifrolumab and get it on January 10 instead, you can get your next anifrolumab on January 29 (4 weeks after the missed dose date) and resume every-4-week dosing after that. However, if you get your infusion on January 20 (instead of January 1), you must wait until at least February 12 (14 days later) before your next infusion and resume every-4-week dosing after that.

Alcohol/food interactions: No known food or alcohol interactions.

What to monitor while taking anifrolumab: only the usual lupus labs.

Potential side effects of anifrolumab (table 34.1): Severe infections (including opportunistic infections such as tuberculosis and pneumocystis pneumonia, see chapter 22) were not seen more frequently with anifrolumab than in patients treated with

Table 34.1 Potential Side Effects of Anifrolumab (Saphnelo)

	Incidence	Side Effect Therapy
Nuisance side effects		
Infection, especially shingles, pharyngitis, bronchitis, URI	Common	Treat as needed. Do not use during infections. Keep up on all vaccines, especially Shingrix and flu shots.
Allergic reactions	Uncommon	Treat the reaction. Stop the drug if severe.
Serious side effects		
Severe allergic reaction (anaphylaxis)	Rare	Treat anaphylaxis and stop the drug.

Note: Side effect incidence key (these are approximations as they can vary widely from study to study): rare <1% occurrence; uncommon 1%–5% occurrence; common >5% occurrence.

placebo (fake infusions). However, we do need to exercise some caution. Interferon is essential to fighting viral infections. Patients taking anifrolumab were three times more likely to develop shingles than those in the placebo group, although no severe shingles attacks occurred. Patients should get the Shingrix (shingles) shot before they start anifrolumab or soon thereafter.

More patients had influenza, upper respiratory tract infections (URI, like the common cold), bronchitis, and pharyngitis (throat infection) compared to those on placebo. Anifrolumab patients should keep up with their flu shots every September and October (in the Northern Hemisphere).

As of February 2023, research results for patients who had taken anifrolumab for three years showed no increase in side effects over that time. During the period when COVID vaccines were available, there were no alarms for any more COVID problems in the anifrolumab group compared to the placebo group.

Although infusion reactions may occur, they are usually mild and temporary. The most common infusion reactions include headaches, chills, body aches, nausea, upset stomach, and itchy skin. Antihistamines, acetaminophen (Tylenol), and steroids can be given before infusions to prevent these. However, most patients in the clinical trials were not treated with these drugs and the vast majority did not have infusion reactions.

While taking anifrolumab, contact your primary care provider or go to an urgent care center immediately f you develop infection symptoms (table 22.3). Practice all measures to prevent infections (table 22.4).

Vaccines and anifrolumab: Try to get at least one Shingrix shot (for shingles, chapter 22), two weeks or more before your first infusion. Anifrolumab increases the risk of shingles. If you are on anifrolumab and have not had your Shingrix, get it as soon as possible.

Do not get live vaccines. You do not need to stop anifrolumab for flu shots, pneumonia shots, Gardasil, Shingrix, or the COVID-19 vaccine. However, your situation may dictate otherwise, or newer research studies may recommend essential changes. Ask your doctor.

For in-depth information, go to lupusencyclopedia.com/4th-covid-vaccines and lupusencyclopedia.com/2022-vaccine-recommendations.

As of February 2023, a research study assessing how anifrolumab patients do after getting flu shots is being conducted in the United States.

Pregnancy and breast-feeding: Do not use anifrolumab while pregnant or breast-feeding; neither has been studied. Since anifrolumab is a large molecule, very little of it probably gets into breast milk. Even if it did, the baby's stomach acid would most likely destroy it. Ask your doctor.

Geriatric use: Anifrolumab has not been studied in many older people.

Anifrolumab and surgery: Check with your rheumatologist and surgeon. A standard recommendation is to schedule your surgery on the date of your usual anifrolumab dose. Then resume your anifrolumab on your usual schedule once the surgical wound is healing well without infection (typically two weeks later). In SLE patients who may flare if there is a delay in treatment, no changes in anifrolumab scheduling could be recommended.

Financial aid: Go to Saphnelo.com or call 844-275-2360.

Drug helpline: Go to saphnelo.com/patient/support/support-way or call 866-727-4635.

Website: lupusencyclopedia.com/saphnelo-vs-benlysta

Belimumab (Benlysta)

Belimumab was FDA-approved for SLE in 2011. Thereafter, it became the first FDA-approved drug to treat pediatric SLE patients as young as five years old (2019) and then the first drug ever to be FDA-approved for lupus nephritis in children and adults.

In 2022, belimumab was shown to be a disease-modifying drug in lupus (shown to reduce organ damage, including kidney damage, over time). It and hydroxychloroquine are the only drugs proven to be lupus disease-modifying drugs.

Biosimilar available: No.

How belimumab works: Belimumab works by combining with a particular immune system molecule (cytokine) called B lymphocyte stimulator (BLyS for short, pronounced like "bliss"). BLyS is also called B-cell activating factor. BLyS keeps antibody-producing B cells alive. Typically, when B-cells (and mature B-cells called plasma cells) produce antibodies, they die after a short time, unless kept alive by BLyS. Think of BLyS as "B-cell fertilizer." The immune system makes BLyS during active infections to keep the important B-cells alive. When the infection is gone, it stops making BLyS, and the un-needed B-cells can retire and die (a process called apoptosis).

Most SLE patients' immune systems make too much BLyS. Lupus B cells that make autoantibodies (such as antinuclear antibody, anti-SSA, and anti-DNA antibodies) that attack body organs stay alive and continuously produce these dangerous antibodies. Belimumab works by attaching to BLyS in the bloodstream and removing it. The dangerous autoantibody-producing B-cells can finally die since the "B-cell fertilizer" is no longer around. While there are no longer as many autoantibodies to attack the person's body, the immune system can still produce B-cells to fight infections and other foreign invaders. Therefore, belimumab tries to restore a more normal balance to the immune system instead of suppressing it. This is very different from rituximab, which depletes B-cells (chapter 33).

Belimumab can take 3 to 6 months to work. However, some people notice benefits within one to two months. Patients with severe neuropsychiatric lupus (chapter 13) were not included in the research studies. Therefore, we do not know how these patients would do on belimumab.

It appears to work especially well for patients with cutaneous lupus, lupus arthritis, fatigue, and lupus nephritis. Patients with high anti-dsDNA levels, low C3 complement, or low C4 complement levels have a better chance of responding to the drug. Patients with more severe SLE are more likely to respond than those with mild lupus problems.

In the phase 3 clinical trials, twice as many patients treated with belimumab went into low disease activity (chapters 5, 19, 29) as those treated with standard of care plus placebo.

If you ever read that belimumab does not work in people of African ancestry, this is simply not true. The phase 3 clinical trials had too few Black patients in them to draw any accurate conclusions. Since then, two extensive studies (the OBSErve and the EMBRACE trials) showed that Black patients responded well to belimumab, had better disease control, and could lower their prednisone dose.

Do not take if you have an active infection.

Dosage: The intravenous (IV) infusion is dosed at 10 mg per kilogram of body weight infused into a vein. Three infusions are given during the first month at two-week intervals. This is followed by one IV infusion every four weeks. It takes about one hour to infuse the drug, and IV dosing is the same for SLE and lupus nephritis.

The self-injectable subcutaneous (SC, SQ) form is FDA-approved for adults 18 years old and older who have SLE or lupus nephritis. It comes in a prefilled syringe as well as an autoinjector. The dose for SLE without nephritis is 200 mg weekly. For lupus nephritis, the amount is two 200 mg injections (total of 400 mg) each of the first four weeks, then just one 200 mg injection weekly after that.

Take the self-injectable SC form out of the fridge 30 minutes before the injection. If you leave it out for more than 12 hours, discard it and contact the manufacturer at benlysta.com.

If you miss a dose, have your infusion scheduled as soon as possible. Then you reset your schedule from that date. For example, let's say that you did not get your monthly infusion on January 10, as scheduled, and you reschedule that dose on, say, January 20. In that case, you should schedule your next infusion to occur four weeks after January 20.

LUPUS IN FOCUS

Belimumab reduces long-term organ damage

In 2020, a study showed that patients taking belimumab for seven years were 61% less likely to get organ damage each year of treatment than patients taking other lupus drugs. There were no unexpected side effect problems, and some side effects decreased over time.

If someone has to miss a few months of belimumab infusions for some reason, we will often "reload" it with one infusion every other week for the first few doses (similar to what we give a new patient).

For self-injectable belimumab, take your missed dose as soon as you can. Resume your next dose on the date it is normally scheduled, but do not take two doses on the same day. Ask your doctor.

Alcohol/food interactions: No known alcohol or drug interactions.

What to monitor while taking belimumab: the usual lupus labs.

Potential side effects of belimumab (table 34.2): Slightly more infections and allergic reactions occurred in patients who received belimumab than those who did not, but the difference was not statistically significant.

After more than 12 years of study, we are not seeing any more cancers in the belimumab group than expected in the general population.

Another area of possible concern is depression and psychiatric problems. Most people in both the placebo group and the belimumab group who developed depression already had preexisting depression. We cannot say that belimumab worsens depression from these data, but this should be watched. Although 2 two out of 1,458 patients who took belimumab committed suicide, this number is far too small to draw any conclusions. Both of these patients had significant depression before the study. These

Table 34.2 Potential Side Effects of Belimumab (Benlysta)

	Incidence	Side Effect Therapy
Nuisance side effects		
Nausea/diarrhea	Uncommon	Consider anti-nausea drugs and Imodium for diarrhea. Ask your doctor.
Difficulty sleeping	Uncommon	Consider a sleeping aid. Avoid steroids as a premedication for infusions.
Pain in the arms and legs	Uncommon	Take Tylenol or NSAIDs (if OK with your doctor).
Serious side effects		
Infection	Uncommon	Treat infection. Do not use the drug during infections.
Depression or anxiety	Uncommon	Treat depression or stop the drug.
Allergic reaction (usually mild), anaphylaxis	Uncommon	Treat allergic reaction. May need to stop the drug if severe.
Low white blood cell count	Uncommon	No intervention if mild. Decrease dose or stop the drug if severe.

Note: Side effect incidence key (these are approximations as they can vary widely from study to study): rare <1% occurrence; uncommon 1%–5% occurrence; common >5% occurrence.

major depression problems were seen only in the intravenous (IV) research studies. They were not seen in the self-injectable subcutaneous (SC) belimumab studies, which did not allow patients with severe psychiatric issues to participate in the research study.

While taking belimumab,

• *if you develop infection symptoms (table 22.3), contact your primary care provider or go to an urgent care center immediately.* Practice all measures to prevent infections (table 22.4).

• *if you feel more depressed than usual while taking belimumab, and especially if you develop any suicidal thoughts, let your doctor know ASAP.*

Vaccines and belimumab: Do not get live vaccines. You do not need to stop it for flu shots, pneumonia shots, Gardasil, Shingrix, or the COVID-19 vaccine. It is recommended to stop SC belimumab for one to two weeks after COVID-19 vaccines (if not at high risk of lupus flares).

For in-depth information, go to lupusencyclopedia.com/4th-covid-vaccines and lupusencyclopedia.com/2022-vaccine-recommendations.

A 2017 study showed that belimumab did not decrease the effectiveness of Pneumovax vaccines in SLE patients. This is reassuring.

Pregnancy and breast-feeding: The 2019 American College of Rheumatology pregnancy guidelines recommend against using belimumab while pregnant (unless approved by your doctor). However, after over 12 years of study, it appears that belimumab may not cause problems with the fetus during pregnancy. Ask your doctor.

If you get pregnant on belimumab, contact the Belimumab Pregnancy Registry at 877-681-6296 or go to https://pregnancyregistry.gsk.com/belimumab.html.

LUPUS IN FOCUS

Belimumab and rituximab combination therapy?

Autoantibody-producing B-cells are bad. They produce autoantibodies, like anti-dsDNA, that attack the body.

Although rituximab reduces B-cells in the bloodstream, it is not as effective at depleting lymph node B-cells. In addition, after rituximab treatment, some patients have a surge of extra BLyS (B-cell fertilizer), creating long-living autoantibody-producing B-cells—just what we do not want in SLE.

Belimumab causes autoantibody-producing B-cells to die more quickly. Then B-cells hiding in the lymph nodes go out into the bloodstream more quickly (where rituximab can get rid of them).

Giving a patient belimumab followed by rituximab, or vice versa, could potentially have better results than using just one of these drugs. However, this needs to be proven to be safe and more effective. Combination studies are now (2023) being done in SLE, Sjögren's, immune thrombocytopenic purpura (ITP), scleroderma, membranous nephropathy, and vasculitis.

Belimumab is safe during breast-feeding.

Geriatric use: No dosing adjustments are needed.

Belimumab and surgery: Ask your rheumatologist and surgeon. A standard recommendation is to schedule your surgery on the date of your usual belimumab dose. Then resume your belimumab on your usual schedule once the wound is healing well without infection (typically two weeks later). In SLE patients who may flare if there is a delay in treatment, no changes in belimumab scheduling may be recommended.

Financial aid: Call 877-423-6597 or go to benlysta.com.

Drug helpline: 877-423-6597.

Website: lupusencyclopedia.com/saphnelo-vs-benlysta.

Voclosporin (Lupkynis)

Voclosporin (Lupkynis) was approved to treat lupus nephritis (kidney inflammation) classes III, IV, and V on January 22, 2021. It is a third-generation calcineurin inhibitor (same family as cyclosporine, first generation, and tacrolimus, second generation, chapter 32). It does not require drug-level monitoring. It is also stronger, more dependable, and safer. Diabetes and cholesterol problems, which can occur with the other drugs, are not seen with voclosporin.

In the research studies, voclosporin was used with mycophenolate mofetil and steroids (the most common lupus nephritis drugs). Most patients were also taking hydroxychloroquine.

Generic available: No.

How voclosporin works: It suppresses the immune system. It also improves how podocytes work (chapter 12).

A decrease in urine protein can be seen as quickly as two weeks after starting therapy. Almost twice as many patients go into remission compared to those receiving MMF without voclosporin. Patients on voclosporin had marked protein reductions in their urine twice as fast as those on MMF without voclosporin. Patients on voclosporin and MMF can reduce their steroids more than patients not on voclosporin.

Do not take if

- you are allergic to it.

- you have severely decreased kidney or liver function.

- if you take ketoconazole, itraconazole, or clarithromycin.

Caution:

- pravastatin, fluvastatin, or rosuvastatin are preferred over simvastatin, lovastatin, or atorvastatin for cholesterol control.

Dosage: It is taken orally: three 7.9 mg capsules, two times a day (23.7 mg twice daily). Try to take it every 12 hours and at least 8 hours apart.

Lower doses should be used in patients with decreased liver or kidney function (ask your doctor).

Lower doses (half dosage) also need to be prescribed if someone is taking certain drugs such as verapamil, diltiazem, fluconazole, miconazole, and erythromycin.

If you miss a dose, take your next dose if it has been less than four hours since the missed dose. If it has been more than four hours, wait until your next dose's scheduled time before taking your voclosporin and skip the dose you missed.

For example, suppose you usually take voclosporin at 8:00 A.M. and 8:00 P.M., and realize you forgot to take your morning dose at 11:00 A.M. Since this is less than four hours since your scheduled dose, you can take your missed dose at 11:00 A.M. and take the next dose at your regularly scheduled time of 8:00 P.M. Then resume your usual schedule the next day.

Alcohol/food/herbal interactions: No known interactions with alcohol.

Take on an empty stomach. Do not drink grapefruit juice or eat grapefruit, which can increase the absorption and blood levels of voclosporin.

Avoid cat's claw, Echinacea, wild cherry, chamomile, and black licorice, which can increase voclosporin drug levels. Avoid St. John's wort, which interferes with voclosporin drug levels. Do not take higher than recommended curcumin (turmeric) doses, which could increase voclosporin levels.

What to monitor when taking voclosporin:

- blood pressure every two weeks during the first month. The manufacturer recommends not taking voclosporin if the blood pressure is higher than 165/105 mmHg. Monitor your blood pressure at home. If you get a high reading, contact your prescribing doctor ASAP.

- blood cell counts, random urine protein to creatinine ratio, and potassium levels

- kidney function every other week the first month of treatment, then every month after that

- routine ECGs if you are at increased risk of QT prolongation (chapter 11).

Potential side effects of voclosporin (table 34.3): Voclosporin is a calcineurin inhibitor. This class of drugs is expected to cause elevated blood pressure and decreased kidney function. In the clinical trials, high blood pressure elevations were seen primarily in the first few months but responded well to blood pressure medications. In patients followed over three years, those on voclosporin had similar blood pressure as those on placebo.

Calcineurin inhibitors cause decreased blood flow through the microscopic filters of the kidneys, resulting in decreased kidney function. In clinical trials, this was seen in the first few months. It is reversible with lower doses. The dose of voclosporin is decreased (or stopped) if kidney function declines too much. With appropriate dose changes, there were no differences in kidney function in patients on voclosporin compared to placebo at the 24-week and the 52-week marks. In patients who were followed over three years, there was overall less loss of kidney function over time than in patients on placebo.

While taking voclosporin, contact your primary care provider or go to an urgent care center immediately if you develop infection symptoms (table 22.3). Practice all measures to prevent infections (table 22.4).

Vaccines and voclosporin: Do not get live vaccines. You do not need to stop it for flu shots, pneumonia shots, Gardasil, Shingrix, or the COVID-19 vaccine.

Why voclosporin is not recommended during pregnancy

One capsule of voclosporin contains 21 mg of alcohol. To put this into perspective, one 5-ounce serving of red wine contains around 4,000 mg of alcohol. The Centers for Disease Control states that there is no known safe amount of alcohol during pregnancy.

Table 34.3 Potential Side Effects of Voclosporin (Lupkynis)

	Incidence	Side Effect Therapy
Nuisance side effects		
High blood pressure (rarely severe)	Common	Treat with blood pressure drugs. See main text.
Decreased kidney function	Common	See main text
Cough	Common	Treat as needed. May need to lower dose or stop the drug.
Hair thinning	Common	Use Rogaine if OK by doctor. May need to lower dose or stop the drug.
Headache	Common	Treat as needed. May need to lower dose or stop the drug.
Nausea/diarrhea/stomach upset/decreased appetite	Common	Treat as needed. May need to lower dose or stop the drug.
Mouth soreness or ulcers	Common	Treat as needed. May need to lower dose or stop the drug.
Tremor	Uncommon	No treatment needed if mild. May need to lower dose or stop the drug. Beta-blocker blood pressure drugs may help.
Serious side effects		
Infection	Common	Treat infection. Do not use the drug during infections.

Note: Side effect incidence key (these are approximations as they can vary widely from study to study): rare <1% occurrence; uncommon 1%–5% occurrence; common >5% occurrence.

For in-depth information, go to lupusencyclopedia.com/4th-covid-vaccines and lupusencyclopedia.com/2022-vaccine-recommendations.

Pregnancy and breast-feeding: Not recommended during pregnancy or when breast-feeding.

Geriatric use: Older individuals who have a higher chance of decreased kidney function may need a lower dose.

Voclosporin and surgery: Ask your rheumatologist and surgeon. If your lupus nephritis could flare if there is a delay in treatment, no changes in voclosporin may be recommended.

Financial aid: Call Aurinia Alliance at 833-287-4642, go to lupkynis.com, fax to 833-213-1001, or email Aurinia Alliance at support@AuriniaAlliance.com

Website: lupkynis.com and lupusencyclopedia.com/lupkynis-phase-3-data-for-lupus-nephritis.

KEY POINTS TO REMEMBER

1. Anifrolumab, belimumab, and voclosporin are the first drugs approved by the FDA for lupus since Eisenhower was president.

2. They are the only drugs specifically developed for lupus. All other drugs came from use in other diseases.

3. IV belimumab is the only FDA-approved drug for SLE and lupus nephritis patients as young as five years old.

4. Belimumab and voclosporin are the only FDA-approved drugs to treat lupus nephritis.

5. Anifrolumab was not evaluated in patients with severe lupus nephritis. Belimumab and anifrolumab were not studied in patients with severe CNS lupus.

6. Do everything listed in table 22.4 to prevent infections.

7. Do not get any live vaccines if you are being treated with these drugs.

8. See your primary care provider or go to the urgent care center immediately if you have any infection symptoms, increased depression, or suicidal thoughts.

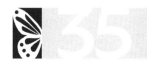

Other Medical Therapies for Lupus

Ian Ward, MD, FACP, FACR, *Contributing Editor*

While antimalarials, steroids, immunosuppressants, and biologics are the most commonly used drugs for SLE, other lupus therapies do not fall into one of these categories. Some were accidentally found to help lupus, while others were tried based on their known immune system effects. This chapter discusses these other medical therapies. It is not intended to be exhaustive and does not discuss rarely used drugs (such as gold and sulfasalazine).

Thalidomide (Thalomid)

Thalidomide is FDA-approved for multiple myeloma (a white blood cell cancer) and erythema nodosum leprosum (a skin complication of leprosy, an infection). It is also used for severe cutaneous lupus (chapter 8) that fails other therapies.

Generic available: No.

How thalidomide works: Thalidomide decreases immune system inflammation.

It works well in up to 98% of people with severe discoid lupus (chapter 8), with up to 85% of patients achieving complete remission. It begins working within two weeks and reaches full effectiveness by eight weeks. An added benefit is that it can significantly slow down lupus hair loss from scarring alopecia and increase hair growth in lupus nonscarring alopecia (chapter 8).

Do not take if you have preexisting nerve disease, seizures, heart disease, or a history of blood clots.

Dosage: Thalidomide comes in 50 mg to 200 mg capsules. It is best taken before bedtime, at least one hour after eating.

If you miss a dose, do not take an extra dose if you forgot to take it the preceding day. Ask your doctor.

Alcohol/food interactions: Avoid alcohol; it increases drowsiness. Take at least one hour after eating.

Dr. Ward contributed to this article in his personal capacity. The views expressed are his own and do not necessarily represent the views of the Dwight D. Eisenhower Army Medical Center, the Uniformed Services University, or the United States government.

What to monitor while taking thalidomide: You must be active in the Thalomid Risk Evaluation and Mitigation Strategies (THALOMID REMS) program. You can enroll by calling 888-423-5436 or by going to thalomidrems.com/patient.html.

Potential side effects of thalidomide (table 35.1): Thalidomide has a high rate of side effects. Most people get drowsy, and 25% of people can get nerve damage (peripheral neuropathy), causing numbness in the feet and hands.

While taking thalidomide, you must be active in the THALOMID REMS program. You can enroll by calling 888-423-5436 or by going to thalomidrems.com/patient.html. Let your doctor know at once if you are pregnant, miss a period, get numbness or burning sensations in the feet or hands, dizziness, shortness of breath, chest pain, weakness in an arm or leg, slurred speech, a rash, or a red, swollen, painful leg.

Vaccines and thalidomide: No need to stop it for vaccines.

Table 35.1 Potential Side Effects of Thalidomide

	Incidence	Side Effect Therapy
Nuisance side effects		
Drowsiness	Common	Take the drug at bedtime.
Erectile dysfunction	Common	Decrease dose or stop the drug.
Headache	Common	Treat the symptoms. Decrease dose or stop the drug.
Weight gain, edema, fluid retention	Common	Decrease dose or stop the drug.
Fatigue, malaise (feeling poorly)	Common	Decrease dose or stop the drug.
Dizziness, vertigo	Common	Decrease dose or stop the drug.
Constipation, diarrhea, stomach upset, nausea	Common	Treat the symptoms; decrease dose or stop the drug.
Serious side effects		
Blood clots	Common	Seek medical attention immediately and stop the drug.
Severe fetal malformations	Very common	Must use two forms of contraception simultaneously.
Nerve damage	Common	Decrease dose or stop the drug.
Rash, itchiness (sometimes severe)	Common	Treat the symptoms; Decrease dose or stop the drug.
Low red blood cell and white blood cell counts	Common	Decrease dose or stop the drug.

Note: Side effect incidence key (these are approximations as they can vary widely from study to study): rare <1% occurrence; uncommon 1%–5% occurrence; common >5% occurrence.

Pregnancy and breast-feeding: Thalidomide can cause severe birth defects of the arms and legs. Never take it during pregnancy. If you are a woman taking thalidomide or the female partner of a man taking thalidomide, you must use at least two forms of effective contraception (chapter 41) and enroll in an FDA-required program called Thalomid REMS at thalomidrems.com/patient.html. Using an IUD (intrauterine device) plus another form of birth control is most effective in lupus patients. Women must have periodic pregnancy tests.

Do not use while breast-feeding.

Geriatric use: Drowsiness and other side effects may be more common in older patients.

Thalidomide and surgery: Ask your rheumatologist and surgeon. To prevent blood clot side effects, stop thalidomide at least a few days before surgery, then resume it when you can walk normally again.

Financial aid: Call 800-931-8691.

Drug helpline: Call 888-423-5436.

Website: thalomidrems.com/patient.html

Dapsone (Diamino-Diphenyl Sulfone)

Dapsone is an antibiotic used to treat leprosy, as well as various forms of cutaneous lupus, lupus panniculitis, cutaneous vasculitis, and bullous lupus) in patients who have not been helped by antimalarials, or topical drugs (like steroids and tacrolimus). It is often the preferred and most effective drug for bullous forms of lupus (chapter 8).

Generic available: Yes.

How dapsone works: Dapsone decreases immune system inflammation. It works fast for bullous lupus erythematosus. Blisters often stop forming within one to two days of starting it, and existing blisters start healing soon thereafter.

Dapsone can also prevent pneumocystis pneumonia (a severe lung infection), primarily in those taking high-dose steroids with mycophenolate or cyclophosphamide.

Do not take if you are deficient in an enzyme called glucose-6-phosphate dehydrogenase (G6PD). G6PD needs to be checked before treatment. G6PD deficiency can cause severe anemia from dapsone.

Dosage: Dapsone comes in 25 mg and 100 mg tablets. A typical dosing regimen is 100 mg a day.

If you miss a dose, take your dapsone dose on the same day you forgot it, then resume your regular schedule the next day. Do not take extra doses in a day if you forgot to take it the preceding day. Ask your doctor.

Alcohol/food/herbal interactions: No interactions with alcohol or food. Avoid St. John's wort, which can decrease dapsone levels.

What to monitor while taking dapsone: A complete blood cell count (CBC) and chemistry panel should be checked regularly (consider a CBC every one to two weeks initially).

Potential side effects of dapsone (table 35.2): Hemolytic anemia may occur with dapsone. It can be severe in G6PD-deficient patients. Taking vitamin E daily may reduce anemia and headache risks.

Table 35.2 Potential Side Effects of Dapsone

	Incidence	Side Effect Therapy
Nuisance side effects		
Stomach upset, nausea	Common	Decrease dose or stop the drug.
Fever, headaches, insomnia, dizziness	Uncommon	Treat the symptoms. Decrease dose or stop the drug. Taking vitamin E can prevent headaches.
Elevated liver enzymes	Uncommon	If mild, no changes needed. If severe, decrease dose or stop the drug.
Rash	Common	Decrease dose or stop the drug. Cortisone cream can help.
Serious side effects		
Anemia	Common	Decrease dose or stop the drug. Taking vitamin E may prevent anemia.
Male infertility	Uncommon	Reversible by stopping the drug.
Low white blood cell count	Uncommon	Stop drug since severely low counts can occur. Consider Neupogen (with caution, chapter 9).
Hepatitis (liver inflammation)	Uncommon	Stop the drug.
Nerve damage	Uncommon	Stop the drug.

Note: Side effect incidence key (approximations, as side effects can vary widely from study to study): rare <; uncommon 1%–5% occurrence; common >5% occurrence.

While taking dapsone, let your doctor know if you become short of breath, fatigued, develop a rash, have numb feet, or develop yellow eyes (jaundice).

Vaccines and dapsone: No need to stop it for vaccines.

Pregnancy and breast-feeding: It can be taken during pregnancy, but alert your obstetrician because anemia can occur in the newborn. Men may have fertility difficulties.

Do not use it while breast-feeding G6PD-deficient babies.

A CBC should be followed in newborn and breast-fed babies to ensure no anemia, especially in infants less than one month old.

Geriatric use: No special considerations.

Dapsone and surgery: Ask your rheumatologist and surgeon. Dapsone is probably safe to take up to the time of surgery.

Danazol

Danazol is a hormone related to male testosterone. It is typically used for the treatment of endometriosis or hereditary angioedema.

Generic available: Yes.

How danazol works: How it works in SLE is not understood. Danazol increases platelet counts in two out of three SLE patients with low platelets (thrombocytopenia, chapter 9). It may help some lupus patients who flare around their menstrual cycle. In addition, it can help with discoid lupus, mouth sores, and hemolytic anemia. It can start working as fast as two weeks but takes at least six months for its full effects.

Do not to take danazol if

- you have severe kidney, liver, or heart disease.

- you have a condition called porphyria.

- you have abnormal vaginal bleeding.

Dosage: Danazol comes in 50 mg, 100 mg, and 200 mg capsules. Doses as high as 800 mg daily are used, divided up over two to three times a day.

If you miss a dose, skip the dose you missed and resume at your next regularly scheduled dose. Do not take extra doses if you missed a dose. Ask your doctor.

Alcohol/food interactions: No interactions with alcohol. Can be taken with or without food. However, meals can delay absorption speed, while fatty foods increase the total amount absorbed. Try to keep a similar daily pattern regarding how you take danazol (with or without food) so your doctor can reliably change dosing if needed.

What to monitor while taking danazol: Liver enzymes and a cholesterol panel should be checked periodically.

Potential side effects of danazol (table 35.3): The majority of side effects are related to its male sex hormone effects. These include developing extra body hair, deepening of the voice, smaller breasts, a larger clitoris, and abnormal menstrual cycles.

While taking danazol, let your doctor know if you develop side effects due to the male hormone influence.

Vaccines and danazol: No need to stop it for vaccines.

Pregnancy and breast-feeding: Do not take while pregnant. When on danazol, you must use effective birth control.

Do not use while breast-feeding.

Geriatric use: No changes.

Danazol and surgery: Ask your rheumatologist and surgeon. To help prevent blood clots, it may be best to stop it five days before surgery. Resume after surgery once able to walk around.

Dehydroepiandrosterone (DHEA, prasterone)

DHEA is a type of steroid produced by the adrenal glands and converted into male androgen sex hormones. DHEA levels are generally lower in SLE patients.

Generic available: DHEA (chapter 6) is available in two forms (prescription and over the counter, OTC). Most OTC brands are of low quality; some even have no DHEA at all.

Table 35.3 Potential Side Effects of Danazol

	Incidence	Side Effect Therapy
Nuisance side effects		
Irregular menstrual cycles	Common	No intervention if mild; otherwise reduce dose or stop the drug.
Weight gain, feet swelling (edema)	Common	Can take fluid pills or use compression stockings for edema. Reduce dose or stop the drug.
Depression, moodiness, nervousness, headaches, insomnia	Not noted	Treat symptoms; reduce dose or stop the drug.
Low sex desire	Not noted	Reduce the dose or stop the drug.
Rash (especially with sun exposure)	Not noted	Abide by UV protection (tables 38.3, 38.4). Treat symptoms; reduce drug dose or stop it.
Stomach upset	Not noted	Treat symptoms; reduce drug dose or stop the drug.
Elevated liver enzyme blood tests	Not noted	Reduce dose or stop the drug.
Acne, oily skin	Not noted	Reduce dose or stop the drug.
Elevated cholesterol levels	Not noted	Reduce dose or stop the drug.
Serious side effects		
Decreased breast size	Common	Stop the drug.
Male and female infertility	Not noted	Stop the drug.
Worsening of SLE	Not noted	Stop the drug.
Loss of menstrual cycles	Not noted	Stop the drug.
Enlargement of the clitoris	Rare	Stop the drug.
Deepening of the voice	Rare	Stop the drug.
Male pattern hair growth	Rare	Stop the drug.
Decreased testicle size	Rare	Stop the drug.

Note: Side effect incidence key (approximations, as side effects can vary widely from study to study): rare <; uncommon 1%–5% occurrence; common >5% occurrence.

If you decide to take DHEA, it is best to get a doctor's prescription and fill it with a compounding pharmacist to ensure you get a pure product.

How DHEA works: DHEA may improve mild lupus symptoms and fatigue. Some people may be able to reduce their steroids. Some may see an increase in bone density.

Do not take if you have polycystic ovarian syndrome.

Table 35.4 Potential Side Effects of DHEA

	Incidence	Side Effect Therapy
Nuisance side effects		
Acne	Common	Reduce dose or stop the drug.
Increased hair growth on the face and other body areas	Common	Reduce dose or stop the drug.
Decrease in HDL (good) cholesterol	Uncommon	Reduce dose or stop the drug.
Elevated liver enzymes	Uncommon	Reduce dose or stop the drug.
Serious side effects		
Elevated blood pressure	Uncommon	Reduce dose or stop the drug.
Increased psychiatric problems	Rare	Reduce dose or stop the drug.

Note: Side effect incidence key (these are approximations as they can vary widely from study to study): rare <1% occurrence; uncommon 1%–5% occurrence; common >5% occurrence.

Use caution if you have significant liver disease.

Dosage: Most SLE studies used 200 mg a day, but it may be beneficial at lower doses as well.

If you miss a dose on a given day, you can take it later that day. Do not take extra doses the next day. Ask your doctor.

Alcohol/food/herbal interactions: Do not drink alcohol. It may be taken with or without food.

What to monitor while taking DHEA: blood pressure, cholesterol levels, and liver function.

Potential side effects of DHEA: See table 35.4.

While taking DHEA,

- your insulin dose may need to be adjusted if you have insulin-requiring diabetes.

- inform your doctor if you develop increased hair growth or acne.

Vaccines and DHEA: No need to stop it for vaccines.

Pregnancy and breast-feeding: Avoid during pregnancy and breast-feeding.

Geriatric use: No dose adjustments required.

DHEA and surgery: It may be safe to take it up to the time of surgery. Ask your rheumatologist.

Intravenous Immune Globulin (IVIG)

Immunoglobulins (or immune globulins, IG) are antibodies. Intravenous (IV) infusions of immunoglobulins (IVIG) are useful in people with recurrent infections and a deficiency in IgG immune globulins (hypogammaglobulinemia, chapter 22). It can also help some SLE problems.

Generic available: No.

How IVIG works: IVIG can decrease immune system overactivity. IVIG can help cutaneous lupus (chapter 8), lupus nephritis, muscle inflammation (myositis), low blood cell counts (including myelofibrosis, chapter 9), lung inflammation, myocarditis (chapter 11), arthritis, severe antiphospholipid syndrome, and neuropsychiatric lupus (chapter 13). A small 2012 study also suggested that it may help prevent congenital heart block in the babies of anti-SSA-positive women. IVIG has been used successfully to treat lupus flares during co-existent infections when other treatment options were not safe. It works rapidly, even within days after treatment.

Do not receive IVIG if you are allergic to IVIG or any of its ingredients (ask your doctor).

Use caution if you have preexisting heart disease, kidney disease, and a history of blood clots. Having these conditions increases the chances of developing them on IVIG.

IVIG brands containing IgA can cause severe allergic reactions (anaphylaxis) in patients with severe IgA deficiency (chapter 22). Gammagard S/D brand of IVIG is generally safe in IgA deficiency.

Dosage: The infusion is usually given once or twice a month and takes several hours to complete. A self-injectable form is available.

If you miss a dose, reschedule as soon as you realize you missed your dose, then reset your schedule from that point. Ask your doctor.

Alcohol/food interactions: None noted.

What to monitor while receiving IVIG: periodic blood cell counts and kidney function tests.

Potential side effects of IVIG: See table 35.5.

While receiving IVIG seek medical attention at once if you develop a red, painful, swollen leg, shortness of breath, chest pain, slurred speech, or arm or leg weakness.

Vaccines and IVIG: No need to stop it for non-live vaccines (like Shingrix, Gardasil, influenza, pneumonia, and COVID-19). IVIG may decrease the response to some live vaccines. Ask your doctor about the timing with live vaccines (table 22.5).

Pregnancy and breast-feeding: Can be used during pregnancy and breast-feeding.

Geriatric use: There may be an increased risk for side effects such as kidney problems, heart problems, and blood clots.

IVIG and surgery: IVIG can potentially increase the risk of blood clots and probably should not be used close to surgery. Ask your doctor.

More information: Go to https://www.lupusencyclopedia.com/intravenous-immuno globulin-ivig-for-lupus.

Plasmapheresis (Therapeutic Plasma Exchange)

Plasmapheresis is a medical treatment in which blood is removed from a person's vein and is put through sterile tubing into a machine that filters out the largest substances, including autoantibodies (chapter 34). Since lupus makes autoantibodies that attack the body, this can be helpful in SLE.

In plasma exchange (a type of plasmapheresis), when the blood is filtered, you receive donated blood products or an IV fluid called albumin.

Table 35.5 Potential Side Effects of IVIG

	Incidence	Side Effect Therapy
Nuisance side effects		
High blood pressure	Common	Treat the high blood pressure.
Mild infusion reactions (headache, body aches, fever, hives, chills, stomach upset, nausea, abdominal pain)	Common	Nurse will slow down the rate of infusion.
Headaches	Common	Treat symptoms; or reduce dose or stop the drug.
Fatigue	Common	No treatment needed. Dose can be reduced next time if needed.
Elevated liver enzymes	Common	Usually, no intervention; or reduce dose or stop the drug.
Anemia or low white blood cell counts	Common	Usually, no intervention; or reduce dose or stop the drug.
Rash, skin vasculitis	Common	Treat symptoms; or reduce dose or stop the drug.
Serious side effects		
Severe allergic reaction (anaphylaxis, low blood pressure, wheezing)	Uncommon	Stop the drug.
Severe headache, aseptic meningitis	Uncommon	It may be prevented with antihistamines, steroids, and pain drugs. May need to reduce dose or stop the drug if severe.
Kidney failure	Rare	Stop the drug.
Increase in lupus flares	Rare	Stop the drug.
Blood clots	Uncommon	Seek immediate medical attention. Stop IVIG.

Note: Side effect incidence key (these are approximations as they can vary widely from study to study): rare <1% occurrence; uncommon 1%–5% occurrence; common >5% occurrence.

Generic available: Not applicable.

How plasmapheresis works: Plasmapheresis can be lifesaving for hospitalized SLE patients with diffuse alveolar hemorrhage (lung bleeding, chapter 10), neuropsychiatric lupus (chapter 13), thrombotic thrombocytopenic purpura (chapter 9), catastrophic antiphospholipid syndrome (chapter 9), myocarditis (heart inflammation, chapter 11),

What to do during plasma exchange if you do not want blood products

Plasma exchange removes some of your plasma (one part of your blood), so it is standard to receive donated blood products or albumin (a protein found in humans) to replace it. If you have religious or other objections to receiving blood products, plasma exchange can be performed using a fluid mixed with starch instead.

kidney inflammation (lupus nephritis), cryoglobulinemic vasculitis (chapters 8 and 11), and severe disease in pregnancy.

Do not receive plasmapheresis if your blood pressure is low.

Dosage: Usually, multiple sessions of plasmapheresis are done over a couple of weeks.

Alcohol/food/herbal interactions: Not applicable.

What to monitor while getting plasmapheresis: Blood pressure and a chemistry panel.

Potential side effects of plasmapheresis (table 35.6): Plasmapheresis is given to very sick, hospitalized patients. Medical personnel closely watch the patient for possible side effects and deal with them if they occur (table 35.6). Because plasmapheresis removes many drugs from the body (like azathioprine, cyclophosphamide, and rituximab), these should be given to the patient again after the procedure. Steroids (which are smaller molecules) are not affected.

Pregnancy and breast-feeding: Can be used for severe SLE during pregnancy. Although it may increase the risk for premature delivery and other complications, severe SLE is more dangerous than plasmapheresis. Breastfeeding is no problem.

Geriatric use: No different from other age groups.

Cholecalciferol (Vitamin D3) and Ergocalciferol (Vitamin D2)

White blood cells have receptors (attachment areas) for vitamin D inside their cytoplasm (the part outside of the nucleus). Vitamin D is vital for our immune systems to work correctly. Low vitamin D levels in animal research cause abnormal immune system activity. Some abnormalities are like those we see in lupus. See chapters 3 and 38 for more information about vitamin D and the reasons we use it to treat lupus.

Generic available: Yes, for both over-the-counter vitamin D3 and prescription vitamin D2.

How vitamin D works: Vitamin D supplementation may improve immune system activity in people with low vitamin D levels. People with severe SLE tend to have lower vitamin D levels than patients with milder disease, and low vitamin D levels often occur during lupus flares.

A 2013 Johns Hopkins University study showed that SLE patients with vitamin D levels less than 40 ng/mL who were treated with a combination of vitamin D3 and vitamin D2 ended up with less lupus disease activity. A 2014 Spanish study gave vitamin D3 to patients with cutaneous (skin) lupus. After one year, they had less active skin inflammation than patients who did not take vitamin D3. A randomized controlled trial

Table 35.6 Potential Side Effects of Plasmapheresis

	Incidence	Side Effect Therapy
Nuisance side effects		
Mild infusion reactions	Common	Dealt with by infusion staff.
Removes some drugs from your system	Common	Some of your drugs are dosed again afterward.
Serious side effects		
Low blood pressure	Common	Dealt with by infusion staff.
Shortness of breath	Common	Dealt with by infusion staff.
Low calcium and potassium levels	Common	Dealt with by infusion staff.
Increased bleeding	Uncommon	Dealt with by infusion staff.
Increased infections	Uncommon	Treat infection.
Severe allergy (anaphylaxis)	Uncommon	Dealt with by infusion staff.

Note: Side effect incidence key (these are approximations as they can vary widely from study to study): rare <1% occurrence; uncommon 1%–5% occurrence; common >5% occurrence.

(the best type of research) in children with SLE showed that vitamin D supplements improved disease activity.

Vitamin D also increases your body's ability to absorb calcium and help keep bones healthy.

Do not take if you already have elevated vitamin D levels.

Dosage: Vitamin D3 doses of 400 IU (international units) to 10,000 IU daily are commonly used. A thin person with an excellent diet and a mildly low level may do well on 400 IU daily. In comparison, someone with a severely low level (below 10 ng/mL) and has had gastric bypass surgery (doesn't absorb the vitamin well) may need 10,000 IU daily. Vitamin D2 usually begins at 50,000 IU weekly.

If you miss a dose, take it as soon as you notice you forgot it, then resume your regularly scheduled dose. For example, if you take ergocalciferol every Saturday and realize on a Friday that you forgot the previous Saturday's dose, go ahead and take a capsule that Friday, and then resume your regularly scheduled weekly dose the next day. You can even make up for missed doses. Let's say you go on a long vacation and because you forget to bring your vitamin D with you, you miss three weekly doses. When you return, you can take one capsule per day three days in a row, then resume your regularly scheduled weekly dose after that. Using this method, it is easy to keep vitamin D levels in the needed range. Ask your doctor.

Alcohol/food interactions: No known interactions with alcohol. Taking it with a fatty meal can increase absorption.

What to monitor while taking vitamin D:

• calcium and phosphorus levels (high phosphorus blood levels with vitamin D supplementation can lead to increased calcium deposits in the body).

• 25-OH vitamin D level three months after starting it and three months after each dose change. The physician can then adjust the dose every few months (using blood levels as a guide) until the target level is reached. Although we aim to have a level of around 40 ng/mL as recommended in the Johns Hopkins 2013 study, we do not truly know the best blood level. More research is needed.

Potential side effects of vitamin D: Dose-related side effects are rare; they should not occur with 25-OH vitamin D levels (chapter 4) of less than 88 ng/mL. However, if you routinely take too much vitamin D (more than the amount recommended by your doctor), your vitamin D levels could become too high and cause nausea, stomach upset, kidney injury, high blood pressure, nausea, constipation, low red blood cells, and calcium build-up in organs such as the heart, blood vessels, kidneys, and lungs.

Pregnancy and breast-feeding: Take during pregnancy and breast-feeding only if your blood levels are being checked by your doctor.

Geriatric use: It is commonly used in older people, who have a higher chance of being vitamin D–deficient, and as part of the treatment of osteoporosis (see chapter 24).

Vitamin D and surgery: Can be taken up to the day before surgery.

KEY POINTS TO REMEMBER

1. Thalidomide has a very high success rate in helping severe cutaneous lupus, but it also has lots of potential side effects.

2. Thalidomide causes severe birth defects. Two simultaneous birth control methods must be used if you have not undergone menopause.

3. The prescribing of thalidomide is very tightly controlled through THALOMID REMS. See thalomidrems.com.

4. Dapsone, which is a drug used to treat leprosy, can be very helpful for bullous lupus (chapter 8).

5. Dapsone can help prevent pneumocystis pneumonia in patients receiving mycophenolate or cyclophosphamide when they are taken with high-dose steroids.

6. Dapsone can potentially cause hemolytic anemia (mainly in G6PD deficient patients). A complete blood cell count should be checked regularly while taking it.

7. Danazol is a male-type hormone (androgen) that can help with some lupus problems, especially low platelet counts.

8. DHEA therapy can potentially help with mild lupus problems and increase bone density. It can help decrease the need for prednisone.

9. The quality of over-the-counter DHEA is unreliable. It is best to get it from a compounding pharmacist using a prescription.

10. IVIG may be used for infections in patients deficient in IgG immunoglobulins (hypogammaglobulinemia) and those with severe lupus who are not responding to the usual treatments.

11. Plasmapheresis is a treatment in which dangerous SLE autoantibodies are removed from the body.

12. Plasmapheresis is reserved for hospitalized, critically ill SLE patients, especially those with cryoglobulinemia, thrombotic thrombocytopenic purpura, or pulmonary hemorrhage.

13. Vitamin D supplements may help reduce lupus disease activity.

Prescription Pain Medicines

Angelique N. Collamer, MD, FACP, *Contributing Editor*

Most SLE patients have pain. The most common types are joint pain, muscle pain, nerve pain, and pleurisy (chapter 10) pain. Chapter 7 provides many recommendations for decreasing aches and pains. Reread that chapter if pain is a significant problem.

Because we feel pain because of the body's pain nerves sending messages to the brain, many pain drugs work by decreasing nerve activity. Examples include drugs for depression and seizures (chapter 27). In this chapter, we discuss nonsteroidal anti-inflammatory drugs (NSAIDs) and opioids. See chapters 7 and 27 for other options.

Non-Steroidal Anti-Inflammatory Drugs (NSAIDs)

NSAIDs (pronounced IN-saydz or IN-sehdz; the IN can also be pronounced EN) are the largest group of pain drugs used in SLE. They are also used for serositis (such as pleurisy and pericarditis) and other types of pain, such as headaches. There are many different NSAIDs (table 36.1).

Generic available: Yes.

How NSAIDs work: NSAIDs are weak anti-inflammatory drugs. They decrease the production of inflammation-producing prostaglandins.

Low-dose over-the-counter (OTC) NSAIDs have minimal anti-inflammatory effects. NSAIDs have analgesic (pain-relieving) properties with the amount of analgesia depending on the dose. High doses tend to decrease pain the most. It is best to take the lowest amount needed for pain to reduce the risk of side effects.

For inflammation, they need to be taken at high doses regularly. It may take one to three weeks (when regularly taken at a high amount) to reduce inflammation. For lupus inflammation (such as pleurisy or inflammatory arthritis), your doctor will probably ask you to take your NSAID at the full dose "around the clock."

One NSAID may work well in one person and not in another. Your doctor may need to try various NSAIDs to determine which is best for you. Also, NSAIDs need to be used regularly for a few weeks before knowing if they work.

Dr. Collamer contributed to this article in her personal capacity. The views expressed are her own and do not necessarily represent the views of the Walter Reed National Military Medical Center, the Uniformed Services University, or the United States government.

How a lupus patient can have pain when in remission

Active SLE most commonly causes pain due to inflammation of the joints (arthritis) or the linings of the heart, lungs, or abdomen (serositis). These are treated with antimalarials (chapter 30), immunosuppressants (table 22.1), and NSAIDs. These pains go away when SLE is in remission. Inflammation-induced pain is also called a type 1 symptom (chapter 5).

Type 2 symptom pains are due to overactivity of the body's pain nerves, often causing "all over" body pain, as in fibromyalgia (chapter 27). These do not respond to immunosuppressants and can occur when SLE is in remission.

A third type of pain is from permanent damage. Examples include foot nerve damage (lupus peripheral neuropathy) and avascular necrosis hip pain (chapter 25).

Finally, people can have pain unrelated to lupus. For example, osteoarthritis joint pains are common in patients 35 years old and older.

Do not take if you have kidney disease, uncontrolled high blood pressure, active stomach ulcers, a history of strokes or heart attacks, severe liver disease, or congestive heart failure.

Use caution if you have high blood pressure, diabetes, previous stomach ulcers, previous congestive heart failure, heart attack, or stroke, or if you are on blood thinners (such as Plavix, Eliquis, Coumadin, or heparin).

Dosage: NSAIDs come in pill, capsule, liquid, and topical forms. They all come in different doses and have different dosing schedules.

If you take aspirin to prevent heart attacks and strokes, check with your doctor. The combination of aspirin and an NSAID increases ulcer risks.

Also, take aspirin first thing in the morning and wait at least two hours before taking naproxen or ibuprofen. Taking the NSAID earlier reduces the aspirin's blood-thinning properties (needed to prevent heart attacks and strokes). Doctors have studied this only with naproxen and ibuprofen. Even so, it is probably good to take all NSAIDs at least two hours after aspirin.

If you miss a dose, you should generally skip that dose and take the next regularly scheduled dose. However, since NSAIDs come in so many different dose forms, this may not apply to all. Ask your doctor.

Alcohol/food/herbal interactions: Avoid alcohol, which increases the risk of stomach ulcers. NSAIDs are best taken with food to decrease stomach upset.

What to monitor while taking NSAIDs: blood pressure, liver and kidney function, and blood counts.

Potential side effects of NSAIDs (table 36.2): In addition to increasing inflammation, prostaglandins help keep the body healthy by protecting the stomach, stabilizing blood pressure, regulating kidney function, supporting blood platelets, and more. While reducing pain and inflammation by decreasing prostaglandins, NSAIDs can also

Table 36.1 NSAIDs

Type	Name	Pros/Cons
Non-acetylated salicylates	diflunisal, choline	*Pros*: Fewer stomach ulcers. Do not increase bleeding. *Cons*: Weaker pain relief and anti-inflammatory properties.
COX-2 inhibitors	celecoxib (Celebrex) and meloxicam (Mobic)	*Pros*: Fewer stomach ulcers and bleeding problems. Celecoxib can be taken with warfarin. Both can be taken once daily. *Cons*: 50% of people allergic to sulfa (sulfonamide) antibiotics may get a rash from celecoxib.
Nonspecific (COX-1 and COX-2) NSAIDs	diclofenac (Cambia; Lofena, Zipsor; Zorvolex), etodolac (Lodine), fenoprofen (Nalfon), ibuprofen, indomethacin (Indocin), flurbiprofen, ketoprofen, ketorolac, meclofenamate, nabumetone, mefe-namic acid, naproxen (Anaprox; Naprelan; Naprosyn), oxaprozin (Daypro), piroxicam (Feldene), sulindac, tolmetin	*Pros*: Diclofenac, ketoprofen, nabumetone, piroxicam, etodolac, and naproxen have convenient once-daily forms. Ibuprofen and naproxen are available over the counter. Nabumetone causes the least bleeding in this group and possibly fewer ulcers. Many consider naproxen the NSAID of choice in SLE (less likely to cause heart attacks and strokes). *Cons*: Diclofenac has an increased risk of liver inflammation. Indomethacin is more likely to cause headaches and trouble thinking.
NSAID + anti-ulcer drug combinations	diclofenac/misoprostol (Arthrotec), ibupro-fen/famotidine (Duexis), naproxen/esomeprazole (Vimovo)	*Pros*: Fewer stomach ulcers. More convenient than taking the drugs separately. *Cons*: More expensive than the individual drugs bought separately.

cause side effects (stomach ulcers, high blood pressure, kidney failure, bleeding, and many others).

Many patients are at high risk of NSAID side effects and should probably avoid them (even OTC naproxen and ibuprofen).

People at increased risk for stomach ulcers should take steps to avoid ulcers from NSAIDs (table 28.5). Ask your doctor.

While taking NSAIDs,

- contact your physician or seek emergency care at once if you throw up blood, develop abdominal pain, have bloody stools, or develop black tarry stools (melena). These could be warning signs of a bleeding ulcer. NSAIDs can decrease ulcer pain, so many people have no preceding stomach upset or pain from a bleeding ulcer from NSAIDs.

- tell your doctor if you develop heartburn, diarrhea, constipation, rash, elevated blood pressure, shortness of breath, yellowish-colored whites of eyes (jaundice), or swelling of the ankles.

- let doctors know you are on an NSAID before they prescribe anything to ensure any new drug does not contain NSAIDs and there are no drug interactions.

- do not take two or more different NSAIDs (except low-dose aspirin; see above).

Pregnancy and breast-feeding: Avoid celecoxib. Other NSAIDs can be taken up to the third trimester. Low-dose aspirin should be taken by all SLE patients throughout pregnancy (chapter 41). If you have difficulty having a baby (conceiving), do not take NSAIDs (except low-dose aspirin). Occasionally, NSAIDs can cause trouble getting pregnant.

NSAIDs can be taken during breast-feeding.

Geriatric use: Older people have a higher chance of side effects.

NSAIDs and surgery: Ask your rheumatologist and surgeon. Most people should stop NSAIDs 1–10 days before surgery, depending on the drug.

Non-acetylated salicylates and the COX-2 inhibitors (see table 36.1) can be continued up to surgery; they do not increase bleeding. However, they can raise blood pressure and decrease kidney function, so many surgeons would rather have them stopped. One exception is if they supply profound pain relief and if there is a chance of your having severe pain if stopped.

LUPUS IN FOCUS

Aspirin use in SLE

Aspirin is an NSAID. At high doses, it reduces inflammation by decreasing prostaglandins, and it is FDA-approved for this purpose in SLE. However, we do not use aspirin in this way anymore; high-dose aspirin has too many side effects.

When used in low doses, aspirin decreases production of a substance called thromboxane. Lower amounts of thromboxane (due to low-dose aspirin) "thin" the blood, help prevent blood clots, and reduce some pregnancy complications (such as preeclampsia, chapter 41). Therefore, we use low-dose aspirin in SLE to reduce heart attacks and strokes (chapter 21), improve pregnancy outcomes (chapter 41), and decrease blood clots in patients with antiphospholipid antibodies (chapter 9).

Table 36.2 Potential Side Effects of NSAIDs

	Incidence	Side Effect Therapy
Nuisance side effects		
Heartburn, nausea, and stomach pain	Common	Take with food, reduce the dose or stop the drug, or take a drug that reduces stomach acidity.
Cramping or diarrhea	Common	Take with food, reduce the dose or stop the drug, or treat the symptoms.
Increased bleeding and bruising	Common	Usually, no treatment needed for bruises; stop NSAID for bleeding.
Fluid retention, ankle swelling (edema), weight gain	Common	Decrease salt, take a fluid pill (diuretic), wear compression stockings, or stop the NSAID. Ask your doctor.
Headache, drowsiness, dizziness, difficulty concentrating	Common	Reduce the dose or stop the drug. These are most common with indomethacin.
Elevated liver enzyme blood tests	Common	Usually not problematic. If very high, reduce dose or stop the drug.
Ringing in the ears or decreased hearing	Uncommon	Reduce dose or stop the drug.
Rash	Uncommon	Stop NSAID. Use cortisone cream.
Decreased blood cell counts	Rare	No intervention if mild. If severely low, stop NSAID.
Serious side effects		
Elevated blood pressure	Common	Reduce NSAID dose or stop the drug.
Gastritis, esophagitis, stomach ulcers	Common	Stop NSAID and take medicine to decrease stomach acidity.
Bleeding ulcers (vomit blood or have bloody stools or black tarry stools)	Common	Seek medical attention immediately. Stop NSAID.
Decreased kidney function	Common	Discontinue NSAID.
Aseptic meningitis (brain inflammation)	Rare	Stop NSAID.
Severe allergic reaction (anaphylaxis)	Rare	Seek medical attention immediately.
Hepatitis (liver inflammation, damage)	Rare	Stop NSAID.
Worsening of aspirin-sensitive asthma	Rare	Treat asthma. Stop NSAID.

Note: Side effect incidence key (these are approximations as they can vary widely from study to study): rare <1% occurrence; uncommon 1%–5% occurrence; common >5% occurrence.

Aspirin is more complicated. If you take aspirin to prevent strokes, heart attacks, and blocked arteries, and you are at very high risk for these during surgery, it may be better to continue taking it. Discuss this with your cardiologist, neurologist, or vascular doctor.

Some surgeries (such as brain, spine, inner ear, and retina surgery) have such a high risk for bleeding that aspirin should always be stopped.

Aspirin usually does not have to be stopped for cataracts or dental procedures.

If you are told to stop aspirin, you should stop it 5–10 days before surgery to reduce bleeding (ask your doctor).

More information: rheumatology.org/patients/nsaids-nonsteroidal-anti-inflammatory -drugs.

KEY POINTS TO REMEMBER

1. NSAIDs can help lupus arthritis and serositis.

2. You should get blood work (blood counts, kidney function, and liver function) and check your blood pressure regularly while taking NSAIDs. Check home blood pressures.

3. Lower doses can help with mild discomfort.

4. For severe pain and inflammation, NSAIDs work best when taken regularly on a set schedule, at higher doses; it can take one to three weeks for pain relief.

5. One NSAID will often work better in a particular person than another. Trying different ones (trial and error) until the best one is found is often needed.

6. Potential side effects include stomach ulcers, high blood pressure, kidney problems, heart attacks, and strokes.

7. You should generally avoid NSAIDs if your kidneys do not work correctly or if you have had congestive heart failure, have an active stomach ulcer, have uncontrolled high blood pressure, or have severe liver damage (cirrhosis).

8. If you are at increased risk of stomach ulcers, see table 28.5.

Opioids

Morphine is probably the most well-known opioid. It is made from the poppy plant, is a strong pain killer, and is highly addictive. Opioids (also called narcotics) are drugs with morphine-like activity. Opioids are controlled substances (or scheduled drugs) in the United States since they can cause addiction and dependency (discussed later). At the same time, they can be safer than other pain relievers (such as NSAIDs, gabapentin, pregabalin, and duloxetine) in some people. Some commonly prescribed opioids include tramadol, codeine, hydrocodone, oxycodone, methadone, morphine, and fentanyl.

Generic available: Yes.

How opioids work: Opioids attach to opioid receptors on pain nerves and in the brain, decreasing how the brain senses pain. They can also decrease cough (codeine and hydrocodone) and reduce severe shivering due to surgery or drugs.

Pills can start to work as fast as 10 minutes (oxycodone), while others may take as long as an hour.

Do not take if

- you are at high risk of addiction (discussed below).

- you cannot stop drinking alcohol.

- you have been diagnosed with increased intracranial pressure (such as pseudo-tumor cerebri) or have had a brain injury.

Use caution

- when driving, using machinery, or working in high places. Do not do these when starting an opioid. Wait until your body becomes used to the drug.

- if you have a history of seizures (they increase the risk of seizures).

Dosage: Opioids come in pill, oral liquid, oral dissolving, injectable, and topical patch forms. They are available in both immediate-release and extended-release forms. Never crush or chew the slow-release forms; otherwise, you could develop severe, life-threatening side effects because a larger amount of the medicine would be absorbed at once. Usually, lower doses are taken by people with decreased kidney or liver function.

If you miss a dose, The immediate-release forms can be taken as needed if you are not physically addicted to the drug. If you use an extended-release form, you must take it regularly on schedule and never miss doses. If you miss a dose, you are at risk of developing withdrawal side effects. Ask your doctor.

Alcohol/food interactions: Alcohol increases drowsiness, accidents, respiratory depression (where you stop breathing), and even death. If you take an opioid with acetaminophen (Tylenol), do not drink more than two servings of alcohol in 24 hours to decrease the risk of liver damage (see chapter 38 for alcohol serving sizes).

Fatty meals increase absorption. Take opioids on a regular, consistent pattern with or without food to prevent changes in effects.

What to monitor while taking opioids:

- any side effects (see below)

- signs of psychological addiction (see below)

- urine or blood drug toxicity tests to ensure you are not taking other addictive drugs and that you are taking your opioid.

Potential side effects of opioids (table 36.3): Physical dependence occurs when the body becomes used to a drug. It is an expected side effect when opioids are taken regularly. Taking them occasionally usually does not cause physical dependency. If the drug is stopped abruptly in someone with physical dependence, withdrawal symptoms occur. Although withdrawal symptoms are very uncomfortable, they are usually not dangerous for most people as long as they are not doing activities such as driving, using machinery, caring for others, and the like. People with heart conditions are at increased risk for heart complications from opioid withdrawal and should be monitored by a cardiologist and pain management specialist.

Table 36.3 Potential Side Effects of Opioids

	Incidence	Side Effect Therapy
Nuisance side effects		
Constipation, bloating, stomach upset	Common	May need daily anti-constipation medicine. Exercise regularly, eat extra fiber (fruits and vegetables), and drink plenty of water.
Nausea, vomiting	Common	Reduce dose or stop the drug; or take an anti-nausea drug.
Itching	Common	Decrease the dose or take an antihistamine (Claritin, Alavert, Benadryl) regularly.
Muscle spasms	Uncommon	Reduce the dose or take muscle relaxants.
Serious side effects		
Drowsiness and difficulty thinking	Common	Reduce dose or stop the drug.
Withdrawal symptoms (discussed in the main text)	Common	Do not be late taking your medicine. Take your medicine as soon as you notice the symptoms.
Decreased production of sex hormones causing infertility, decreased libido, fatigue	Uncommon	Reduce dose or stop the drug.
Difficulty breathing (respiratory depression)	Uncommon	Mainly a concern in the elderly or in those with severe lung disease (such as COPD). Use lower doses in these patients.

Note: Side effect incidence key (these are approximations as they can vary widely from study to study): rare <1% occurrence; uncommon 1%–5% occurrence; common >5% occurrence.

Physical dependency withdrawal symptoms include moodiness, depression, restlessness, difficulty sleeping, runny nose, teary eyes, chills, flu-like symptoms, body pain, stomach upset, nausea, vomiting, diarrhea, yawning, and goosebumps. If you are trying to stop opioids, it is vital to work with your doctor and slowly decrease the drug. Withdrawal symptoms can be reduced by drugs such as clonidine, diazepam, promethazine, or loperamide.

Most people who fear taking opioids do so because of their fear of psychological dependence, or addiction, which is the term we use in the rest of the text. Addiction (which doctors do not want to occur) is very different from physical dependency (which is expected to happen). Someone who is addicted continues to take the opioid despite the presence of opioid-induced problems and/or in order to experience euphoria (a feeling of excitement and happiness). Euphoria can cause the person to have the desire to keep taking the drug as an "escape" from real-world problems.

Unlike someone who is physically dependent, someone who is addicted has lost control over their use of the drug. They may take extra doses, crave them, or continue to use them even though they are causing side effects. Some signs of addiction include hoarding pills while continuing to get the prescription filled (to use later) and getting into arguments with others about their opioids. Addicted people may neglect home, work, and school responsibilities and stop enjoyable activities or hobbies. They may become preoccupied with taking the drug or use it up faster than prescribed. They may convince themselves they need it for their health and pain while really using it because of addiction. Addiction often leads to problems in relationships with others, including with their treating physicians who are trying to get them off the opioid. Many do not realize they are addicted until they are off the drug. Only then do they recognize their addiction in hindsight.

Most prescribing doctors will have you read and sign a pain contract, listing side effects, withdrawal symptoms, and the rules you must follow to get your prescriptions. It should also spell out what steps to take if addiction occurs. Keep a copy at home. The pain contract helps protect you and your prescribing doctor from potential problems.

If you develop signs of addiction, discuss it with your doctor immediately. Addiction can be treated with drugs to help you get off the medicine. Psychological treatment can help with other addictive issues (such as dealing with stress and past traumatic events).

Many opioid preparations include acetaminophen (Tylenol). APAP on opioid labels stands for N-acetyl-para-aminophenol, acetaminophen's chemical name. An example is hydrocodone/APAP. Brand names such as Vicodin, Lorcet, Lortab, and Percocet are not as easy to figure out since they do not specifically state "Tylenol" or "APAP" on the label. Knowing whether an opioid has acetaminophen is essential to ensure you do not take too much OTC acetaminophen for pain along with your opioid.

You can tell how much acetaminophen is contained in each tablet as follows: if it says hydrocodone/APAP or oxycodone/APAP, and the dose is 5/325 mg, the first number is the mg of the hydrocodone or oxycodone (5 mg); the second number is the amount of APAP (acetaminophen) in each tablet (325 mg).

Do not take more than 2,000–4,000 mg daily of acetaminophen. Ask your doctor for your maximum recommended dose.

While taking opioids, tell your doctor if you develop side effects or signs of addiction.

Pregnancy and breast-feeding: Try to avoid opioids during pregnancy because they can cause physical dependency in newborns. Signs can be crying, diarrhea, fever, irritability, tremors, vomiting, stroke, and breathing problems in the newborn baby.

Some are safe to take during breast-feeding; others should be avoided. Ask your doctor.

Geriatric use: Lower doses are usually used due to increased side effects.

Opioids and surgery: Ask your doctor, surgeon, and anesthesiologist for instructions. Stopping an opioid can cause withdrawal symptoms. Your surgical team may need to give you an alternative around the time of surgery.

KEY POINTS TO REMEMBER

1. Opioids are narcotics; they work like morphine.

2. They can potentially become habit-forming.

3. When taken regularly, opioids are expected to cause physical dependence. If the drug is stopped abruptly or not taken on time, the person goes through withdrawal.

4. Withdrawal symptoms include moodiness, depression, restlessness, difficulty sleeping, runny nose, teary eyes, chills, flu-like symptoms, joint and muscle pain, stomach upset, nausea, vomiting, diarrhea, repetitive yawning, and having goosebumps.

5. Check if your opioid has acetaminophen (APAP). If it does, make sure that you do not take too much OTC acetaminophen.

6. Ask your doctor for a pain contract before starting an opioid to know the rules for getting opioid prescriptions and what steps to take if addiction occurs.

7. If you develop signs of addiction, let your doctor know right away.

8. Do not crush or chew extended-release forms.

9. Long-acting opioids need to be taken regularly and on a set schedule. Otherwise, withdrawal symptoms may occur.

Future Treatments for Lupus

Sarfaraz Hasni, MD, MSc, *Contributing Editor*

We are entering an age of incredible advancements in treating lupus. The FDA approval of Benlysta in March of 2011 showed that it was possible to do successful lupus drug research. Benlysta then became the first drug approved to treat children with lupus (2019) and kidney inflammation (lupus nephritis, 2020). In 2021, we saw voclosporin (Lupkynis) approved for lupus nephritis, and then anifrolumab (Saphnelo) for SLE. Today, there are more ways for doctors to treat lupus than ever. This chapter includes treatments for lupus patients that may not be considered standard. It also mentions drugs that are currently in research.

Knowing how lupus occurs helps us recognize what therapies may treat, prevent, or even cure lupus in the future. A simplified version of lupus's causes and problems is shown in figure 37.1 (see also chapters 1, 3, and 4).

1. Lupus occurs in someone born with genes that can cause the immune system to become overactive.

2. Environmental triggers (such as ultraviolet light, hormones, smoking, or infections) then turn on these genes.

3. Then, immune system cells, such as monocytes (dendritic cells and macrophages), B-cells, and T-cells, communicate with each other to become more active than usual.

4. These overactive immune cells lose the ability to differentiate between the body's own proteins and foreign proteins.

5. The activated B-cells turn into plasma cells that make autoantibodies that attack the body's own tissues.

Scientists and doctors are doing research to understand these steps. Many of them can be potential treatment targets.

Figure 37.2 shows how many of the lupus treatments discussed so far in the book work on different parts of lupus and its causes. All lupus patients should practice UV light protection (tables 38.2, 38.3, and 38.4) and not smoke. They should ensure their

Dr. Hasni contributed to this article in his personal capacity. The views expressed are his own and do not necessarily represent the views of the National Institutes of Health, or the United States government.

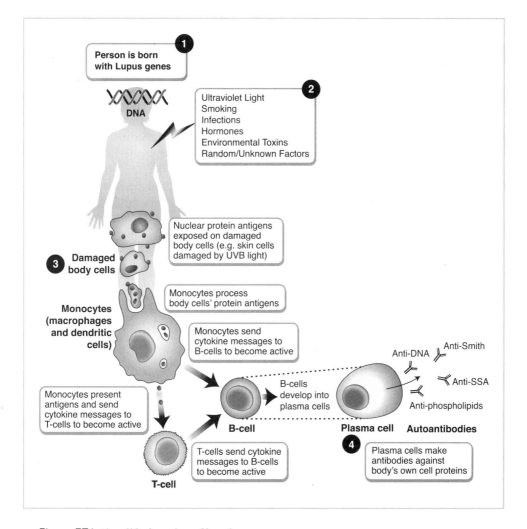

Figure 37.1 Simplified version of how lupus occurs

vitamin D levels are normal by taking supplements. All lupus patients should be taking an anti-malarial drug, such as hydroxychloroquine (chapter 30), unless they have problems with it. Steroids, stronger immunosuppressants, or biologics noted in figure 37.2 may be needed in people with moderate to severe lupus.

Research studies show us that drugs that are FDA-approved for other diseases and not commonly used for lupus could potentially help lupus patients. Some lupus experts are using some of these to treat SLE patients who have failed other drugs. These drugs will be discussed in this chapter, including abatacept and tocilizumab (FDA-approved for rheumatoid arthritis), and obinutuzumab (approved for leukemia). Many other drugs are not yet available (not FDA-approved for any disease) but are currently in lupus research studies.

How long it takes a drug to go from the test tube to the pharmacy

It typically takes 10 to 15 years for new drugs to come to market. The process begins when scientists discover the possible drug and use it in animal studies to see if it works and is safe. This typically takes three to six years.

Then the drug is studied in humans in research studies called clinical trials. The first three are labeled phase 1 through phase 3 clinical trials. All three human clinical trials typically take six to seven more years in total. If these studies are successful, the pharmaceutical company organizes all their research results and sends a New Drug Application (NDA) to the Federal Drug Administration (FDA), hoping for approval. The FDA can take up to two years before approval or denial. Most research drugs never make it through this strict process.

Since we will be referring to the different types of research studies (called clinical trials), we describe them here. Drugs seeking FDA approval go through multiple phases (stages):

- **Drug discovery phase:** Scientists discover a pathway involved in lupus and search for a drug aimed at that pathway.

- **Pre-clinical phase:** The drug is evaluated in animals.

- **Phase-1 clinical trials:** These look at the effects of the drug in humans.

- **Phase-2 clinical trials:** These look for the best drug dose and assess side effects.

- **Phase-3 clinical trials:** These much larger studies must show that the drug treats the disease without many side effects.

- **Phase-4 clinical trials:** These are done on FDA-approved drugs that are already marketed and prescribed. These are also called post-marketing surveillance trials and confirmatory trials. They can be performed for various reasons, such as determining whether side effects occur after long-term use, looking at other possible benefits, or answering additional questions posed by the FDA.

The therapies discussed below have shown some promise in helping lupus patients and are used by some lupus experts primarily when other therapies have failed. Most of these are add-ons to the standard lupus treatments.

Abatacept (Orencia)

Abatacept (pronounced AB-uh-TA-sept) is a biologic (chapter 33) that is FDA-approved for rheumatoid arthritis. In a 2012 report, a European group of lupus experts recommended using abatacept for difficult-to-treat arthritis and serositis in SLE. Several research studies evaluated abatacept for SLE patients, but none of them achieved its main goals (called the primary endpoints). However, abatacept appeared to help some lupus arthritis patients in these studies.

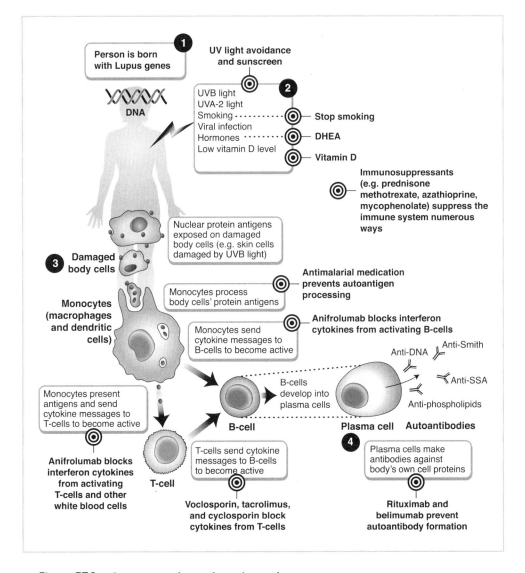

Figure 37.2 Where current lupus therapies work

Biosimilar available: No.

How abatacept works: Abatacept interferes with how the immune system's white blood cells, called antigen-presenting cells (APCs, see chapter 30), interact with T-cells. Macrophages and dendritic cells are examples of APCs (figure 37.1). Abatacept stops these APCs from telling the T-cells to become more active. This results in B-cells producing fewer autoantibodies that could attack the body.

If you have had TB in the past or have tested positive for TB, you need to let your doctor know before starting.

Do not take if you have chronic hepatitis B or other active infections.

673

Randomized controlled trials

There is a wide range in the quality of research studies. The highest quality type is the randomized, double-blind, placebo-controlled trial, or randomized controlled trial (RCT). Patients enter the study and are assigned to take either the study drug or a placebo (commonly called a "sugar pill"). The researchers randomly assign the patients to one or the other treatment group. Neither the researchers nor the study participants know who is taking the placebo and who is taking the drug. They are blind as to who gets what. Pharmacists keep track of which patients get which therapy but do not reveal this information until the end of the study, when the final results are calculated.

Dosage: Abatacept is given by IV (intravenous) and injections under the skin (subcutaneous, or SQ). One method is to receive an IV infusion of abatacept every two weeks three times in a row, followed by an IV infusion every four weeks after the first three infusions. Each infusion takes about 30 minutes.

Another method is to receive just one IV infusion followed by an SQ injection the following day and then an SQ injection weekly after that. The patient can do the SQ injections at home or have them done at the doctor's office.

If you miss a dose, reschedule your missed dose as soon as possible, then reset your infusion schedule starting from that date. For example, if you are scheduled to get your monthly (every four weeks) IV infusion on January 2 but have to reschedule it for January 10, your next injection should be four weeks after January 10. Ask your doctor.

Alcohol/food interactions: No known interactions.

What to monitor while taking abatacept: No extra labs required.

Potential side effects of abatacept: See table 37.1.

While taking abatacept, contact your primary care provider or go to an urgent care center immediately if you develop infection symptoms (table 22.3). Practice all measures to prevent infections (table 22.4).

Vaccines and abatacept: Do not get live vaccines. Instructions for other vaccines such as the flu shot, pneumonia shots, Shingrix, or the COVID-19 vaccine are as follows.

For intravenous (IV) abatacept, get your vaccine (including boosters) four weeks after your infusion, then wait one more week before the next abatacept infusion. In other words, have a total of five weeks between the two abatacept infusions instead of the usual four weeks. For the initial COVID vaccines (called the primary series) that require a shot three to four weeks after the first one, get your second abatacept infusion five weeks after the first vaccine and get the second vaccine during the five weeks between the two infusions.

For subcutaneous (SQ, SC) abatacept, do not take the abatacept dose before and after your vaccine. You do not need to skip any more doses of abatacept for the second shot of the COVID-19 vaccine. These recommendations may change, so ask your doctor.

For in-depth information, go to lupusencyclopedia.com/4th-covid-vaccines and lupusencyclopedia.com/2022-vaccine-recommendations.

Table 37.1 Potential Side Effects of Abatacept (Orencia)

	Incidence	Side Effect Therapy
Nuisance side effects		
Headache	Common	Take pain medicine.
Nausea	Uncommon	Take anti-nausea medicine.
Rash	Uncommon	Stop the drug. Can use cortisone cream or take an antihistamine.
Dizziness	Uncommon	Slow down infusion or stop the drug.
Serious side effects		
Infection	Common	Treat infection.
Elevated blood pressure	Uncommon	Slow down infusion. Treat with blood pressure medicine.
Infusion allergic reaction	Uncommon	Slow down infusion. The infusion nurse will treat it.
COPD exacerbation	Uncommon	See your doctor for treatment.
Bowel perforation	Rare	Seek immediate medical attention (emergency room).

Note: Side effect incidence key (these are approximations as they can vary widely from study to study): rare <1% occurrence; uncommon 1%–5% occurrence; common >5% occurrence.

Pregnancy and breast-feeding: Do not take during pregnancy. It is OK to use abatacept while getting pregnant but stop it once conception is confirmed.

There probably is not much in milk due to its large size, and the baby's stomach acid should destroy any swallowed molecules. However, it has not been studied.

Geriatric use: Older patients could be at increased risk of infections.

Abatacept and surgery: Check with your rheumatologist and surgeon. A standard recommendation is to schedule your surgery on the date of your usual abatacept dose. Then resume your abatacept on your usual schedule once the wound is healing well without infection (typically two weeks later). In patients with severe SLE who may flare if there is a delay in treatment, no changes in abatacept scheduling may be recommended.

Financial aid: Call 1-800-673-6242 or go to www.Orencia.com.

Drug helpline: 1-800-673-6242.

Website: Orencia.com and rheumatology.org/patients/abatacept-orencia.

Metformin (Glumetza, Riomet) and Pioglitazone (Actos)

After mice with lupus got better during treatment with metformin, it was tried in some SLE patients and showed promise. Although a 2020 study using metformin did not meet its major research goals, SLE patients who took metformin had less severe flares than placebo patients.

Why would a diabetes drug help lupus patients? We think it has to do with slowing down the metabolism of white blood cells (WBCs) and reducing insulin resistance. Areas of inflammation require more glucose (sugar) than normal, and the WBCs active in the inflammation show signs of insulin resistance. Metformin combats insulin resistance and reduces glucose availability. If these WBCs cannot get enough energy (glucose) due to metformin, they cannot function properly, and the result is less inflammation.

Pioglitazone, another diabetes drug, can reduce body inflammation. A 2022 NIH study showed that SLE patients who took pioglitazone have improvements in one part of their immune system (called NETosis, beyond the scope of this book). They also had improvements in cardiovascular function (chapter 21), such as less stiff artery walls, lower cholesterol levels, and less insulin resistance. This study did not prove that pioglitazone helps SLE, but the possible benefits deserve more study.

We do not use metformin or pioglitazone as main SLE treatments. But if we have a patient with prediabetes, metabolic syndrome, or diabetes (chapter 21) and their primary care doctor wants them to take metformin or pioglitazone, we encourage them to do so.

We do not go into detail here about how these drugs work, how they are taken, or what their side effects are. We will leave that up to the prescribing primary care providers.

Obinutuzumab (Gazyva)

As discussed in chapters 3, 33, and 34, B-cells (a type of white blood cell) are overactive in SLE and produce autoantibodies that attack the person's own body. Thus, drugs that lower B-cell activity, such as belimumab (Benlysta, chapter 34) and rituximab (Rituxan) help lupus patients.

A 2022 phase-2 clinical trial was published showing that the B-cell-depleting drug obinutuzumab worked well in lupus nephritis. All patients were treated with mycophenolate (chapter 32) and steroids plus either obinutuzumab or placebo (fake treatments). Two years after starting treatment, twice as many patients on obinutuzumab went into remission than those receiving placebo. There were also slightly fewer side effects in patients taking obinutuzumab than in the placebo group. Currently, a worldwide phase-3 clinical trial is being conducted. Another French phase-3 clinical trial is using obinutuzumab in lupus nephritis without using steroids.

This is an expensive drug approved by the FDA to treat certain lymphomas and leukemias (blood cancers).

Biosimilars available: No

How obinutuzumab works: It binds to the outer surface of B-cells on a particle (receptor) called CD20, which it causes the person's own immune system to attack the B-cell, which then dies. This results in fewer B-cells and autoantibodies that can attack the body, which means that there is less lupus inflammation and damage (as with rituximab; see figure 33.4B).

More specifically, the drug decreases kidney inflammation (reduces protein in the urine) and stabilizes or improves kidney function. Long-term goals are the prevention of kidney failure, dialysis, and kidney transplantation.

Do not take if you have chronic hepatitis B infection, tuberculosis (TB), or other active infections. It can be used if hepatitis B and TB have been treated appropriately.

Dosage: It is an intravenous (IV) infusion. A typical dosing schedule is to first get a dose of 1,000 mg, followed by a similar infusion two weeks later. This cycle is repeated six months later.

If you miss a dose, Ask your doctor.

Alcohol/food interactions: No known interactions.

What to monitor while taking obinutuzumab: blood cell counts, immunoglobulin levels (chapter 4), and chemistry panels.

Potential side effects of obinutuzumab: See table 37.2.

While taking obinutuzumab, contact your primary care provider or go to an urgent care center immediately if you develop infection symptoms (table 22.3). Practice all measures to prevent infections (table 22.4).

Vaccines and obinutuzumab: Your B-cells are necessary to respond well to vaccines. Since obinutuzumab gets rid of large numbers of B-cells, it is best to get vaccinations two to four weeks before each cycle's first obinutuzumab treatment. Do not get live vaccines.

For in-depth information, go to lupusencyclopedia.com/4th-covid-vaccines and lupusencyclopedia.com/2022-vaccine-recommendations. See the rituximab section.

Pregnancy and breast-feeding: Not recommended during pregnancy and breast-feeding. The manufacturer recommends not getting pregnant for six months after the last dose of obinutuzumab.

Geriatric use: Older people are at increased risk for infections.

Obinutuzumab and surgery: Ask your rheumatologist and surgeon. A standard recommendation is to schedule your surgery on the date of your usual dose. Then resume obinutuzumab, on your usual schedule, once the wound is healing well without infection (typically two weeks later). In SLE patients who may flare if there is a delay in treatment, no changes in scheduling may be recommended.

Financial aid: Go to gazyva.com/first-line-cll/financial-support/ways-to-save.html

Drug helpline: gazyva.com or call 888-835-2555

Website: gazyva.com

Sirolimus (Rapamune)

Sirolimus is FDA-approved to prevent organ transplant rejection. Several drugs commonly used to treat SLE were also designed initially as organ transplant rejection prevention drugs: azathioprine, cyclosporine, and mycophenolate mofetil.

There are currently (as of January 2023) phase-2 clinical trials using sirolimus in SLE being conducted. Some researchers have successfully used sirolimus in SLE, and we reviewed their results to write this section.

Generic available: Yes.

How sirolimus works: Sirolimus inhibits T-cell activation (figure 37.1). It also reduces type I interferons (chapter 34), which are important cytokines involved in SLE.

It decreases lupus disease activity and has been used successfully to treat lupus fatigue, arthritis, tendonitis, cutaneous lupus, and lupus nephritis.

Do not take if

- you have an active infection.

- an open sore or an open surgical wound.

FDA fast-tracked drug research

It usually takes 10 to 15 years for drugs to go from initial discovery to final FDA approval before use. This is too long for serious diseases that do not have adequate therapies. Therefore, the FDA grants some research drugs a "fast-track" designation, which allows the developer to meet with the FDA more often, prioritize meetings, and speed up approval. All the safety and effectiveness requirements must be met, as with other study drugs.

"Breakthrough therapy" is another designation that speeds up the review and approval process. "Priority review" applies to drugs that could be expensive to produce and may have difficulty recovering their research costs after availability, yet could greatly improve treating a disease that does not have many good treatments.

Since SLE is in such great need for better treatments, some lupus drugs in research receive FDA fast tracking. This occurred with Lupkynis, which received a priority review, and obinutuzumab, which was treated as a "breakthrough therapy."

- uncontrolled high blood pressure.
- severely low kidney function.

Dosage: Doses of 1 mg to 3 mg daily have usually been studied.

Alcohol/food/herbal interactions: No known interactions with alcohol.

Do not consume grapefruit; it increases sirolimus blood levels. High-fat meals change absorption. It is best to consistently take it with or without food (depending on which you tolerate best) to get a consistent result and minimize variability.

What to monitor while taking sirolimus:

- tests for blood counts, kidney function, and liver function
- blood pressure
- drug levels (sometimes).

Potential side effects of sirolimus: See table 37.3.

While taking sirolimus, contact your primary care provider or go to an urgent care center immediately if you develop infection symptoms (table 22.3). Practice all measures to prevent infections (table 22.4).

Vaccines and sirolimus: Do not get live vaccines. Inactivated vaccines can be given, although their effects may be blunted by sirolimus. Consider stopping sirolimus for one to two weeks after vaccines; ask your doctor.

For in-depth information, go to lupusencyclopedia.com/4th-covid-vaccines and lupusencyclopedia.com/2022-vaccine-recommendations.

Pregnancy and breast-feeding: Do not get pregnant while on this drug. Continue using effective birth control (chapter 41) for six months after stopping sirolimus.

Breast-feeding safety is unknown.

Table 37.2 Potential Side Effects of Obinutuzumab (Gazyva)

	Incidence	Side Effect Therapy
Nuisance side effects		
Rash, itchiness	Common	Usually mild; treat with cortisone cream or antihistamines; stop the drug if significant
Infusion reactions	Common	Benadryl, Tylenol, and steroids before and during infusions reduce the chances of this happening. Infusion staff will treat it if it occurs.
Elevated liver enzymes	Uncommon	Usually mild, requiring no treatment. Stop the drug if severe.
Stomach upset, nausea, diarrhea	Common	Usually mild and temporary; can take anti-nausea or anti-diarrhea drugs; stop infusion if severe.
Serious side effects		
Infections	Common	Treat infections; don't get infusion during infections.
Severe infusion reaction	Uncommon	Treated by the infusion center. Infusion most likely would not be repeated.
Low white blood cell counts and hypogammaglobulinemia	Common	Usually requires no treatment. Infusion may be delayed if it persists. If infections occur in people with hypogammaglobulinemia, IVIG helps (chapter 35).
Low red blood cells (anemia) and low platelet counts (thrombocytopenia)	Common	Usually, mild requiring no treatment. Infusion may be delayed if they persist.

Note: Side effect incidence key (approximations, as side effects can vary widely from study to study): rare <1% occurrence; uncommon 1%–5% occurrence; common >5% occurrence.

Geriatric use: Older people are at increased risk for infections and decreased kidney function.

Sirolimus and surgery: Ask your rheumatologist and surgeon. A standard recommendation is not to take sirolimus for one to three weeks before surgery, then resume it once the surgical wound has healed and there is no evidence of infection. However, in SLE patients at high risk of flaring, it may be continued throughout the surgery.

Financial aid: Call 866-706-2400 or go to lupusencyclopedia.com/patient-resources or pfizerrxpathways.com

Patient input in clinical trials

To decide if a drug works or not, we must have something to measure, give it a number, and compare the experimental drug and the placebo results. Measurements that doctors use in research assess inflammation, organ damage, prednisone amount that can be lowered, and many others. However, if these results look great but patients do not feel any better, what good is the drug?

This past decade has seen much work going into patient-reported outcome measures (PROM). PROM results regarding pain, energy, quality of life, and other issues come directly from patients. Several PROMs have been developed for lupus, including the Lupus Quality of Life Questionnaire (LupusQoL), the Lupus Patient Reported Outcomes, and the Lupus Impact Tracker (LIT). Research studies are showing their usefulness, and they are starting to be used to help figure out if treatments are worth it.

One example is the use of LupusQoL in patients on anifrolumab (Saphnelo, chapter 34). Not only did anifrolumab show significant improvements in lupus disease activity using the doctors' measurements, but it also improved quality of life results as measured by the LupusQoL by patients.

Drug helpline: none.
Website: pfizermedicalinformation.com/en-us/patient/rapamune

Stem Cell Transplant after High-Dose Cyclophosphamide

This aggressive treatment is performed only in highly specialized centers. One method is to remove cells (stem cells) from the person's bone marrow that can develop into mature immune cells and store them under refrigeration or freezing. Then the person receives high doses of chemotherapy (often cyclophosphamide, chapter 32) to completely kill all mature immune cells. The person's original stem cells are returned to the bone marrow to multiply and make a brand-new immune system. The doctors hope that the new immune system cells will not make the lupus autoantibodies that attack the body.

There are currently several stem cell transplant studies being done using various methods.

Generic available: Not applicable.

How stem cell transplantation works: Replaces the person's immune system with a new one that does not make autoantibodies.

What to monitor during stem cell transplantation: Patients stay in the hospital in special areas that use highly sophisticated anti-infection techniques. Hospital staff very closely watches the patients.

Potential side effects of stem cell transplantation (table 37.4): There is a very high risk for infections. Death (usually from infection) is also possible.

Table 37.3 Potential Side Effects of Sirolimus

	Incidence	Side Effect Therapy
Nuisance side effects		
Edema	Common	Take a fluid pill (diuretic), use compression stockings, lower the drug dose, or stop the drug.
Acne, rash	Common	Treat rash or stop the drug.
Headache	Common	Treat the headache. Lower the dose of the drug or stop the drug.
Insomnia	Common	Take in the morning. Treat insomnia. Lower the dose of the drug or stop the drug.
Muscle and bone pain	Common	Treat the pain. Lower dose of the drug or stop the drug.
High cholesterol	Common	Treat the high cholesterol.
Stomach upset, constipation, diarrhea, nausea	Common	Treat the symptoms. Lower dose of the drug or stop the drug.
Elevated liver enzymes	Uncommon	No intervention if mild; otherwise, lower the dose of the drug or stop the drug.
Serious side effects		
High blood pressure	Common	Treat the blood pressure. Lower dose of the drug or stop the drug.
Infections	Common	Treat infection. Don't take sirolimus during infections.
Anemia, low platelet counts, low white blood cell counts	Common	No intervention if mild; otherwise, lower the dose of the drug or stop the drug.
Decreased kidney function	Common	Lower the dose of the drug or stop the drug.
Cancer (primarily skin)	Uncommon	Consider yearly exams by dermatologist. Treat the cancer and stop the drug.

Note: Side effect incidence key (approximations, as side effects can vary widely from study to study): rare <1% occurrence; uncommon 1%–5% occurrence; common >5% occurrence.

Tocilizumab (Actemra)

Tocilizumab (pronounced toe-sĭ-LĬZ-ooh-MAB) is a biologic approved by the FDA for rheumatoid arthritis and a vasculitis called giant cell arteritis. It works by interfering with the cytokine (a chemical message immune system cells use to talk to each other)

Table 37.4 Potential Side Effects of Stem Cell Transplantation

	Incidence	Side Effect Therapy
Serious side effects		
Infection	Common	Treat infection
Death	Common	Not applicable

Note: Side effect incidence key (approximations, as side effects can vary widely from study to study): rare <1% occurrence; uncommon 1%–5% occurrence; common >5% occurrence.

called interleukin-6 (IL-6). IL-6 is produced by macrophages and T-cells and causes inflammation and increased immune system activity. SLE patients have higher levels of IL-6 than usual.

A phase-1 clinical trial was performed in 16 SLE patients. Tocilizumab showed decreases in anti-dsDNA levels (chapter 4) and lupus disease activity. All seven patients with lupus arthritis improved. Since then, there have been several reports of successfully using tocilizumab in rheumatoid arthritis overlap with lupus (rhupus) and in severe SLE. There are no current active studies. We may consider tocilizumab as a potential possibility in rhupus patients.

Generic available: No.

How tocilizumab works: Tocilizumab prevents IL-6 from stimulating immune system cells.

Caution: You need to be tested for TB before starting tocilizumab. If you have had TB in the past or you test positive for TB, you need to let your doctor know.

Dosage: In the SLE phase-1 trial, it was given intravenously (IV) every two weeks. For rheumatoid arthritis, it is given every four weeks.

If you miss a dose, reschedule your missed dose as soon as possible, then reset your infusion schedule starting from that date. For example, if you cancel your January 2 infusion, and you reschedule it for January 10, your next infusion should be two to four weeks after January 10. Ask your doctor.

Alcohol/food interactions: No known interactions.

What to monitor while taking tocilizumab: Blood counts, liver enzyme blood tests, and cholesterol.

Potential side effects of tocilizumab (table 37.5): The most common side effects are low white blood cell counts, elevated cholesterol, and elevated liver enzymes (ALT and AST).

While taking tocilizumab, contact your primary care provider or go to an urgent care center immediately if you develop infection symptoms (table 22.3). Practice all measures to prevent infections (table 22.4).

Pregnancy and breast-feeding: Not recommended during pregnancy. It may be used during breast-feeding.

Table 37.5 Potential Side Effects of Tocilizumab (Actemra)

	Incidence	Side Effect Therapy
Nuisance side effects		
Elevated cholesterol	Common	Treat with cholesterol-lowering drugs.
Elevated liver enzymes	Common	Monitor if mildly high.
Serious side effects		
Low white blood cell count or very high liver enzymes	Common	Decrease the dose or stop the drug if severe.
Infections	Common	Treat infection. Don't take tocilizumab during infections.
Infusion allergic reaction	Common	Treat the reaction. Slow down the rate of infusion. May need to stop the drug if severe.
Low platelet counts	Uncommon	Decrease dose or stop the drug if severe.
Intestinal perforation	Rare	Seek emergency medical attention for severe abdominal pain.

Note: Side effect incidence key (approximations, as side effects can vary widely from study to study): rare <1% occurrence; uncommon 1%–5% occurrence; common >5% occurrence.

Geriatric use: Older patients have a higher chance of infections.

Tocilizumab and surgery: Ask your rheumatologist and surgeon. A standard recommendation is to schedule your surgery on the date of your usual dose. Then resume your tocilizumab, on your usual schedule, once the wound is healing well without infection (typically two weeks later). In SLE patients who may flare if there is a delay in treatment, no changes in scheduling may be recommended.

Financial aid: Call 866-681-3261 or go to actemra.com.

Drug helpline: Call 800-228-3672.

Website: actemra.com. See also rheumatology.org/patients/tocilizumab-actemra.

Experimental (Research) Lupus Drugs

Numerous drugs are undergoing research for treating lupus. These lists constantly change as new research drugs are added. If you are interested in reviewing drugs being studied for lupus, go to clinicaltrials.gov.

We desperately need more minority patients for lupus research

Lupus occurs much more commonly in people with African ancestry than in White people. While we have more Black patients than white patients in our clinics, fewer than 20% of the patients in lupus research studies are Black. This means that we have inadequate research for one of our most important patient groups. Belimumab (Benlysta) clinical trials are case in point. Benlysta is the first drug designed and approved for SLE. Recruiting volunteers from Black patients was difficult, and there were so few Black patients in the studies that it was unclear whether Benlysta worked in them. Consequently, the FDA placed a warning on the package insert, saying that Benlysta may not work in Black patients. This resulted in many Black patients not receiving this safe and effective SLE drug.

Since the first clinical trials, several research studies showed that Benlysta helps Black patients. We have many Black patients on Benlysta who are in remission or have low (mild) disease activity, requiring few if any steroids. Realizing the benefits in Black patients, the FDA removed this warning (the possibility of not working in Black patients) from the product label (or package insert).

We do understand why many patients do not want to take part in research. One reason may be the mistrust of the medical community related to earlier problems with improper (and dangerous) experiments performed on Black people. And even today, some patients still meet prejudice and bias from some health care providers.

Still, the vast majority of physicians want only the best for all patients. In addition, laws governing clinical trials have changed dramatically such that research patients are treated with the utmost respect and are completely informed about all parts of any research they take part in. They can also withdraw from studies if they wish.

SLE clinical trials have additional safeguards. Since lupus can damage the body, it is unethical to have lupus patients only on a placebo (sugar pill). Today, all SLE patients in research studies must be on their usual lupus drugs. Usually, the research drug is added to these standard-therapy drugs. The research results in patients who have this added drug and those who take only the standard therapy lupus drugs are compared to see if it provides added benefits.

We hope that anyone reading this will strongly consider taking part in research. We need to better understand the cause of lupus so that someday we can find a cure. But we must have patients in the studies to do this.

Clinical trials need different participants to further understand lupus in diverse populations. You should feel empowered to ask your doctor to find clinical trials and research studies that may be right for you. Other resources that may help find out what clinical trials are being conducted and how you can participate are:

- CenterWatch at centerwatch.com/clinical-trials
- the National Institutes Lupus Clinical Trials Unit at niams.nih.gov/labs/hasni-lab
- the Lupus Foundation of America at lupus.org/advancing-research/get-involved-in-research
- the Lupus Research Alliance at lupusresearch.org/research/get-involved-in-research

KEY POINTS TO REMEMBER

1. We are entering an exciting period in treating lupus, with many potential therapies being studied.

2. Some treatments being studied as potential lupus therapies are currently available to treat other diseases. These include abatacept, obinutuzumab, sirolimus, metformin, and stem cell transplantation.

3. There are many drugs in the research pipeline for lupus treatment (go to clinicaltrials.gov).

4. Please consider participating in lupus clinical trials. This is the only way we will be able to find better, safer treatments, and hopefully a cure for lupus. Go to the websites listed above.

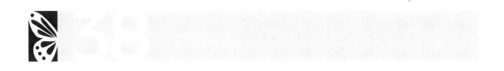

Non-Drug Therapies for Lupus

Vasileios C. Kyttaris, MD, and Sarah L. Patterson, MD, *Contributing Editors*

One thing that sets lupus apart from so many other disorders is that many things under someone's control can make it worse, while others can make it better. Controllable factors that worsen lupus (and that you should avoid) include ultraviolet (UV) light exposure, smoking, poor dental health, inflammation-causing foods, supplements that worsen lupus (such as Echinacea), stress, and lack of high-quality sleep. In addition to avoiding these, there are steps you can take to reduce inflammation, including eating anti-inflammatory foods, good dental care, taking vitamin D (if your level is low, chapter 35), exercising regularly, maintaining normal body weight, taking turmeric (chapter 39), and practicing daily mindfulness (chapter 39).

There is no doubt that it takes a lot of extra effort to incorporate healthy habits into your lifestyle. But if you make the effort, we promise that you will do better with your lupus.

IMPORTANT NOTE: None of the recommendations in this chapter and the next should take the place of your lupus medicines. It is important to take your SLE drugs regularly. By doing this, plus practicing healthy habits, you can help get your lupus under better control and reduce the need for toxic drugs such as steroids.

Ultraviolet Light

People with lupus must protect themselves from UV light (specifically UVA-2 and UVB light, figure 38.1). Unless you live in a dark hole or cave, UV light bombards your skin almost constantly. Light is made up of electromagnetic waves, as are X-rays, microwaves, and radio waves (figure 38.1). We see visible light in terms of color. Similar to the rainbow, visible light wave frequencies go from lower to higher: Red to Orange to Yellow to Green to Blue to Indigo to Violet (easy to remember with the name ROY G BIV). Light "beyond" violet is called ultraviolet (*ultra-* is Latin for "beyond) and is not naturally visible to the human eye.

Scientists divide UV light into UV-A, UV-B, UV-C light. The sun emits all three, but the atmosphere filters out UV-C light. Only UV-A and UV-B light reach Earth. UV-A light is further divided into UVA-1 and UVA-2 light, based on their biological effects. UVA-1 is not harmful and may even be protective. In contrast, UVA-2 and UV-B light worsen lupus. Even small amounts of UVA-2 and UV-B light contact the skin and damage cells lying just beneath the surface, leading to chemical reactions with the cell's proteins and

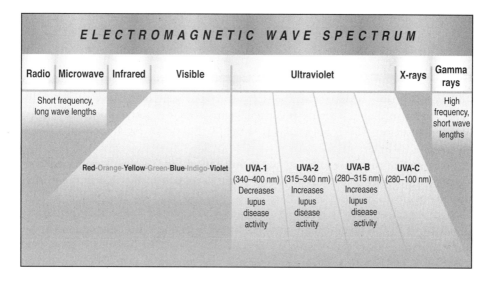

Figure 38.1 Electromagnetic wave spectrum

DNA. Proteins deep within the cells migrate from the damaged nuclei up to the cell surface and attach themselves outside. The lupus immune system recognizes them by way of its antinuclear antibodies, which cause the immune system to become more active, leading to inflammation and damage throughout the body. This increased lupus activity sometimes manifests as a rash on the skin, but only in about 30% of SLE patients. In those who do not get a rash, this UV-induced cell damage can cause SLE inflammation throughout the body.

The amount of UV-light induced inflammation is proportionate to the amount of light exposure, so the more exposure, the more damage.

Since the sun is the major source of UV light, being out in the sun, especially in the middle of the day, causes the most damage to skin cells and a greater chance for worse lupus disease activity. While some lupus patients develop cutaneous lupus (chapter 8) from sun exposure, others may not feel well, develop fever, or feel a burning discomfort instead.

You are also exposed to UV light indoors. There are three major types of light bulbs. The one invented by Edison is the incandescent light bulb, which gives off a small amount of harmful UV light. These were the most common bulbs used up through the 1990s with their familiar round shaped glass connected to a glass neck and then metal screw threads.

Fluorescent bulbs are commonly long, cylindrical, and coated in white and are often used in large office buildings. They light up due to electrical reactions with the gas inside the tube, which interacts with the white tube coating. Fluorescent bulbs give off more UV light than incandescent bulbs. Although they are better for the environment than incandescent bulbs, they are not as good for lupus patients.

Halogen light bulbs emit the largest amounts of UV light and should be avoided. These are not used as often in homes but are commonly used in other settings, such as garages, factories, and stages. Therefore, people in these occupational situations (such as stage entertainers, factory workers, and mechanics) need to pay special mind to this hazard (table 38.1 and table 38.2). If using them, cover halogen and fluorescent bulbs with UV-blocking covers.

The total amount of UV light exposure depends on both the light's strength and the total exposure time. Although incandescent and fluorescent bulbs emit much less UV light than the sun, lupus patients should apply sunscreen to exposed skin surfaces when in lit indoor spaces. This is not a concern with LED (light-emitting diode) bulbs, which do not emit UV light.

I have an SLE patient who is a dental technician whose SLE clearly worsened from UV exposure at work. Her lupus was much easier to control during vacations and after retirement.

Wear sunscreen in the winter and on cloudy days. Up to 80% of UV light penetrates clouds and is still present during winter, albeit in smaller doses. In addition, sand, snow, water, and concrete reflect UV light, so if you are at the beach, surrounded by snow, near water, or in an urban area, you are exposed to higher amounts of UV light than the sun itself emits. Sitting underneath an umbrella on the beach or sitting in the shade on a boat is not safe for lupus patients unless it is early morning or early evening. Also, snow reflects about 85% of sunlight, nearly doubling your UV exposure. Concrete reflects 15%, making exposure on a city sidewalk higher than walking in a grassy park.

Learning to protect your skin from even small amounts of UV light is just as important as avoiding the sun at noon in the summertime (table 38.3). Sunscreen lotions need to be a part of your daily routine. Regular sunscreen usage has been shown to improve

Table 38.1 Occupations with Increased UV Light Exposure

Food and drink irradiators

Hairdressers

Nail technicians (use UV drying lamps)

Laboratory workers

Lighting technicians

Lithographers and printers

Police

Outdoor workers (construction workers, farmers, and so on)

Paint and resin curers

Physiotherapists

Plasma torch operators

Welders and metal factory workers

Stage entertainers

Office workers with halogen-light desk lamps

Anyone working around water, snow, glass, and concrete reflecting sunlight

Anyone who regularly uses photocopier machines with the lid open

Table 38.2 UV Light–Emitting Devices to Avoid

Bactericidal lamps

Blacklight lamps

Halogen lamps

Spotlights

Stage lights

Movie projector lights

Carbon, xenon, and other arcs

Dental polymerizing equipment

Fingernail-drying lamps

Fluorescence equipment

Hydrogen and deuterium lamps

Metal halide lamps

Mercury lamps

Plasma torches

Phototherapy lamps

Printing ink polymerizing equipment

Welding equipment

systemic problems in SLE and reduce cutaneous lupus reactions. I consider it a medicine for lupus and include it on patients' medication lists.

It is best to use sunscreen with the highest tolerable sun protection factor (SPF). Dermatologists specializing in lupus recommend an SPF of at least 70; 100 is even better. These higher SPF sunscreens tend to be thicker, and some people have trouble tolerating them. In those cases, a lower SPF is better than wearing no sunscreen. It may take some experimentation with different brands and SPFs until you find a good fit. Some people prefer the spray-on types, while others prefer lotions. However, spray-on brands may not give as much protection as lotions. Many popular moisturizers also have sunscreen.

Make sure to apply sunscreen as early in the morning as possible. Reapply it 30 minutes before going outside to allow it to penetrate the skin and exert its effects.

There are two major categories of sunscreen, physical (also called mineral) and chemical. The advice above regarding the amount of sunscreen to use applies to chemical sunscreens. Look for the following active ingredients in chemical sunscreens: octinoxate, oxybenzone, avobenzone, octisalate, octocrylene, and homosalate. However, people with sensitive skin and those who worry about chemical sunscreens being absorbed into the body may want to consider physical sunscreens instead. Look for the active ingredients zinc oxide and titanium dioxide.

If you have difficulty tolerating off-the-shelf sunscreen and skincare products due to allergies, see a dermatologist to help find something that will work for you.

Wear UV-protectant clothing and sunglasses outside. A typical cotton shirt has an SPF of only 5 or 6. While some companies make special UV-protectant clothing, you can

Table 38.3 UV Light Protection Measures

- Wear sunscreen on all exposed skin areas every day, even if you stay indoors.
- Use the highest SPF tolerable (SPF 70 or higher is preferable).
- Use "broad-spectrum" sunscreen (blocks UVA and UVB).
- Use water-resistant sunscreen labeled "80 minutes" or higher.
- Apply sunscreen 30 minutes before going outside.
- Apply enough sunscreen (see main text).
- Do not forget your lips, ears, nose, neck, upper chest, hands, and feet. Consider sunblock sticks for the lips, ears, and around the eyes.
- Sunscreen gel may be best for oily skin; lotions may be best for dry skin.
- When outside, reapply every 2 hours; inside, reapply every 4 to 6 hours.
- Avoid the sun between 10:00 A.M. and 3:00 P.M. (standard time). A good rule of thumb is avoiding outdoor activities if your shadow is shorter than your height.
- Always wear a wide-brimmed hat outside.
- Consider wearing tightly woven loose-fitting pants and long-sleeve shirts.
- Wear tightly woven, dark, dry fabrics (which keep out UV rays most effectively).
- Wear sun-protective clothing with a UPF of 30 or higher (50 is better).
- Consider using Rit SunGuard when you wash your clothes to increase their SPF.
- Do not use UV drying lamps when you get your nails done.
- *Never* sunbathe! If you become tan, you did not protect yourself adequately from UV light.
- Instead of a natural tan, use artificial tanning sprays, lotions, and gels.
- Wear UV-protective glasses.
- Always drive with the windows up.
- Consider UV tinting for car, work, and home windows.
- Change all indoor bulbs to LED bulbs.
- If you have fluorescent or halogen bulbs, cover with fluorescent light filter covers that block UV light.
- Ask employers if they can tint windows with UV protection and use UV-blocking fluorescent light filter covers over fluorescent and halogen lights. See lupusencyclopedia.com/can-you-work-with-lupus-lupus-patients-and-the-ada.

make the clothing you have more protective by adding a product such as Rit SunGuard powder when you wash them. It increases the SPF of clothes as high as 30, lasting for up to 20 washings, so using it in the wash several times a year would be enough for most people. Also, ensure you wear clothing with a tight weave. Hold the fabric up to the light. If you see light coming through it, find a tighter-weaved substitute (table 38.4).

Instead of SPF, clothing is rated on a scale called the UV protection factor (UPF). Clothes with a UPF of around 30 block out at least 96% of UV light. Wear fabrics with a UPF of 30 or higher (50 is even better) for the best protection.

You are probably not using enough sunscreen

Most people do not use enough sunscreen. The average person only applies about one-third of the correct amount. An often-quoted rule of thumb is to use a shot-glass amount of sunscreen for the entire body, including the legs.

However, it is hard to envision a shot glass full, and much of the time, you don't need it on your legs (when you wear pants). A more practical method is to measure with your fingers. Squirt a line of sunscreen on the palm side of your index and middle fingers from where the finger begins (at the palmar crease) to the fingertip. These two strips of sunscreen should be used on one body part. There are 11 body parts: head and neck, each arm, upper back, lower back, chest, abdomen, each upper leg and thigh, and each lower leg and foot. Some dermatologists recommend applying one strip of sunscreen to each body area first, then applying the second strip 30 minutes later.

Table 38.4 Clothing and UV Protection

Fabrics with more UV protection

Bamboo (tightly woven Lycra or cotton blends)

Cotton (unbleached, viscose, and bamboo blends)

Denim (black and dark blue)

Lycra

Polyacrylonitrile

Polyester (100%, as well as shiny blends)

Rit SunGuard–treated clothing

Satin silk

Tightly woven (hold up to the light as in the main text)

UV protective clothing

Wool

Fabrics with less UV protection

Cotton (bleached)

Jeans (white, undyed)

Knits

Polyester crepe

Viscose

Worn, old fabric

Nail-drying lamps for manicures emit significant UV light. I have had patients flare after having gel nails dried by them. Do not get manicures or pedicures that require UV nail-drying lamps or enter an establishment using them to ensure you are not exposed accidentally.

Car windshields and windows prevent most UV light from entering, so you should drive with the windows up. Consider professionally installed UV-protectant window tinting for your vehicle. It doesn't need to be dark in color. Some areas do not allow car window tinting. However, a doctor's note saying that tinting is medically necessary usually satisfies government requirements. Windows at home can be tinted, as can windows at your place of employment, if your employer is willing to have this done (go to lupusencyclopedia.com/can-you-work-with-lupus-lupus-patients-and-the-ada).

Smoking

Do not smoke! Not only does smoking cause cancer and permanent lung damage, but it has other far-reaching effects (table 38.5). For example, smokers develop autoimmune diseases more often and more severely than nonsmokers. This has been demonstrated in disorders such as SLE and rheumatoid arthritis. SLE patients who smoke do not respond as well to treatment as nonsmokers. Why this occurs, we do not know. Nor do we know why smoking reduces the effects of antimalarial drugs, such as hydroxychloroquine, but it does. This is especially troublesome because hydroxychloroquine has numerous benefits (table 30.1) and is one of our safest drugs. If a person is unable to stop smoking while taking hydroxychloroquine, we may need to add a stronger immunosuppressant and/or steroid to their treatment. These drugs have many more potential side effects than hydroxychloroquine.

The number one cause of death in US lupus patients is cardiovascular disease, which causes strokes, heart attacks, and blood clots. Smokers are at a much higher risk of getting these complications than nonsmokers. Smoke chemicals cause the body's blood vessels to become thickened, hard, and clogged with plaque. Nicotine causes the arter-

---

Table 38.5 Cigarette Smoking Effects in Lupus

- Reduces hydroxychloroquine (Plaquenil) effectiveness
- Worsens Raynaud's (chapter 11)
- Lowers sleep quantity and quality
- Increases gum disease, altering the microbiome, which can worsen lupus (chapter 3)
- Worsens Sjögren's dryness (chapter 14)
- Increases cardiovascular complications (chapters 11 and 21)
- Increases LDL (bad) cholesterol; lowers HDL (good) cholesterol
- Increases blood clots, especially if antiphospholipid antibody positive
- Increases cancer risks, especially lung cancer (chapter 23)
- Increases lung infections (chapter 22)
- Decreases lifespan

---

ies to constrict (get smaller), resulting in less blood flow to vital organs such as the brain and heart.

Lupus patients who smoke endanger their health from many directions. Some people are fortunate and can readily quit when they learn of the dangers they are putting themselves in. But because nicotine is highly addictive and because smoking is usually an ingrained habit, most smokers have great difficulty quitting. Most primary care providers can recommend smoking cessation classes and even prescribe drugs to decrease the urge to smoke. Also, the US government supplies services free of charge to help. You can go to smokefree.gov or call 800-784-8669 or 877-448-7848 to get help.

Dental Hygiene

Should good dental hygiene be considered a treatment for lupus? We believe so.

There is much evidence for bad dental health (periodontal disease) increasing the risk for rheumatoid arthritis. However, there has been less research for SLE. A 2020 study evaluated 10 research papers and showed that SLE patients have a higher rate of periodontal disease (chapter 3). A 2014 Brazilian study compared patients with lupus nephritis (kidney inflammation) who received periodontal treatment with their immunosuppressant therapy to patients who did not receive periodontal treatment. Patients receiving periodontal treatment ended up with less lupus disease activity.

There are some theoretical reasons why good dental health may help SLE. First, the bacteria on diseased teeth (biofilm) and inflamed gums alter their normal microbiome (chapter 3). Some bacteria in periodontitis cause the production of anti-SSA autoantibodies (chapter 4). Anti-SSA is especially common in lupus and Sjögren's disease (chapter 14).

In SLE, immune system molecules called toll-like receptors (TLRs, chapter 30) become more numerous, increasing inflammation. Periodontitis can increase TLR levels, theoretically worsening lupus disease activity. Periodontal treatment reduces their amount, which could potentially help SLE.

Brush your teeth and use antibacterial rinses twice daily; floss daily, improve dry mouth (chapter 14), don't smoke, avoid sweets, and have regular dental cleanings for good dental health. See lupusencyclopedia.com/prevent-early-tooth-loss-when-you -have-dry-mouth-from-lupus-or-sjogrens-syndrome.

Diet

Some dietary habits may lower inflammation, decrease flares, and help you feel better. Eating a balanced, healthy diet is one of the most important. The Standard American Diet is very unhealthy—and the abbreviation for it, SAD, is telling. It is loaded with high amounts of bad fat, simple sugars, high-fructose corn syrup, and salt, while being deficient in vitamin-rich, healthy foods such as whole grains and fruits, vegetables, and nuts.

Researchers think that the high-sugar, high-fat Western diet may cause unhealthy changes to our DNA (epigenetics, chapter 3). These DNA changes can persist, at least for a while, even after changing the diet. A 2018 research study switched mice from a healthy diet to a typical Western diet. They developed increased body inflammation on this SAD diet. After returning to a healthy diet, the inflammation improved, but very slowly. Don't eat a SAD diet!

We have an obesity epidemic in the United States. Many experts link it to the abundance of fast food and foods rich in high-fructose corn syrup. Fructose sugar is associated with increased fat production (and therefore obesity), increased heart disease rates, and other medical conditions such as gout (an arthritis due to uric acid). It is essential to read ingredient labels and avoid those products that have fructose corn syrup listed in the first few ingredients. Some common examples include breads, crackers, packaged sweets, cola, fast food, fruit drinks (such as Hawaiian Punch and Minute Maid), frozen sweets, breakfast foods, fruit preserves, and condiments. Also, many foods labeled "low-fat" are less healthy than their high-fat counterparts because fructose corn syrup takes the place of the fat.

Most of what we know about diet and lupus is new, and more research is occurring rapidly. We present recommendations based on the best medical evidence at this time (January 2023). We are confident that if you follow the advice in this section, you will experience significant improvements in your health (table 38.6).

Table 38.6 Recommended Diet in Lupus

- Cover at least half your plate at each meal with a variety of non-starchy vegetables and fruits.
- Choose low glycemic index (GI) carbohydrates rather than high glycemic. Check out the GI of common foods at health.harvard.edu/diseases-and-conditions/glycemic -index-and-glycemic-load-for-100-foods.
- Eat whole grains rather than refined grains (which are high-glycemic).
- Choose non-meat proteins (such as beans, legumes, nuts, whole soy foods, and nonfat Greek yogurt) and limit red meat.
- Eat healthier fats such as monounsaturated or omega-3 polyunsaturated fatty acids (flaxseed, chia seed, cold-water fatty fish, walnuts, avocados, olive oil).
- Increase fiber (vegetables, fruit, whole grains, psyllium) to cause satiety (feeling full) and improve the gut microbiome.
- Adjust calories based on your energy expenditure (how much you exercise) and whether you need to gain, lose, or maintain weight. Most people should eat fewer calories that get turned into fat.
- Season food with anti-inflammatory spices such as turmeric, ginger, and cinnamon.
- Avoid foods with hydrogenated oil, partially hydrogenated oil, or high-fructose corn syrup as ingredients.
- Limit saturated fat (from meat and whole-fat dairy products), processed flour, added sugar, simple carbohydrates, and high-fructose juices.
- Use alcohol in moderation (follow serving sizes mentioned later in the main text).
- Model your diet after the Mediterranean diet, which consists of vegetables, fruits, whole grains, beans, legumes, low-fat or fat-free dairy products, fish, poultry, non-tropical vegetable oils, and nuts (discussed later in the chapter in more detail).
- If you are highly motivated and want to adopt a more specific diet, consider the ITIS diet (see table 38.7).

What level of vitamin D should SLE patients aim for?

The Johns Hopkins Lupus Center (Baltimore, Maryland) treated SLE patients with low vitamin D levels with over-the-counter vitamin D3 and prescription-strength vitamin D2 (ergocalciferol). In 2013, they published their results. They achieved lower disease activity and less protein in the urine in those whose levels rose by at least 20 ng/mL to a level of at least 40 ng/mL or higher. Therefore, we aim for a level of around 40 ng/mL or higher. Vitamin D is an important lupus medicine.

Consume foods rich in vitamin D. Vitamin D is essential for the immune system's proper function. Most SLE patients have low vitamin D levels (chapter 3), and those with the worse disease and most flares have the lowest levels. Low vitamin D is also common in antiphospholipid syndrome, which causes recurrent blood clots (chapter 9). Most SLE patients require vitamin D supplements; however, you may also want to consider vitamin D-rich foods (table 24.7).

We successfully use prescription vitamin D-2 (ergocalciferol) and over-the-counter vitamin D-3 (cholecalciferol) to normalize vitamin D levels. Note, though that the quality of over-the-counter (OTC) vitamin D varies widely. A 2013 study assessing OTC brands found that the pills contained anywhere between 52% and 135% of the label-stated dose. If you use OTC vitamin D-3, choose a brand that has passed third-party quality testing, such as USP dietary supplement verification (it would state this on the label). Also, stick with the same brand and regularly check your vitamin D blood level, so you and your doctor know if you are taking the correct dose.

Eat foods rich in omega-3 and omega-6 fatty acids. Certain fats appear to be more beneficial than others. Studies show that a diet rich in omega-3 fatty acids decreases several inflammation measures in the body, including lower inflammation-causing cytokines (chapter 33). Good omega-3 fatty acid foods include cold-water fatty fish (such as salmon, sardines, herring, black cod, and mackerel), flax seeds (one of the highest concentrations), chia seeds, hemp seeds, walnuts, and whole soy foods.

Like omega-3 fatty acids, omega-6 fatty acids are polyunsaturated fats (healthier fats, unlike saturated fats discussed below). While omega-6 fatty acids had bad press in the past, we now know that they are essential for good health, especially when used in place of unhealthy saturated fats. They lower bad cholesterol (LDL, chapter 21), increase HDL (good cholesterol), and help normalize sugar (glucose) by improving the body's response to insulin. The American Heart Association states that omega-6 fatty acids are healthy for the heart and circulation, and they may reduce body inflammation.

Many foods are rich in omega-6 fatty acids, but not all are equally healthy. Those that are not included animal fats and lard. Vegetable oils (such as safflower oil and canola oil) are better omega-6-rich alternatives. Healthier sources include sunflower seeds, tofu, eggs, peanut butter, almonds, and walnuts.

Walnuts have the advantage of being rich in both omega-3 and omega-6 fatty acids. I buy raw walnuts in bulk (less expensive that way) and eat a small handful daily. An advantage of raw walnuts is they tend to be less tasty than other nuts, so I am less likely to binge on them. Three to four walnuts (six to eight halves) supply the National Institutes of Health's recommended daily amount of omega-3 fatty acids.

There is some evidence that omega-3 fatty acid foods may help SLE. We can study lupus in the laboratory by using mice genetically destined to develop lupus. Lupus mice fed omega-3 fatty acid-rich diets developed less immune system activity, fewer autoantibodies (such as anti-DNA and antiphospholipid antibodies), and less lupus nephritis activity (reduced urinary protein and kidney damage).

Two separate Irish randomized controlled trials (chapter 37) showed that SLE patients eating 3 grams a day of omega-3 fatty acids over 6 months ended up with lower lupus disease activity

We recommend that SLE patients eat foods rich in omega-3 and omega-6 fatty acids. This may help reduce cardiovascular events (such as heart attacks and strokes) and improve lupus disease activity.

Limit saturated fats. An unhealthy fat called saturated fat is found primarily in meat and dairy products. Saturated fats are solids (rather than liquids) at room temperature. While this quality prolongs shelf life and makes premade foods convenient, these fats can increase inflammation and disease. Examples of foods high in saturated fat—which we recommend that people with SLE limit—include meat products (beef, pork, poultry, all processed meats), fried foods, whole milk, cheese, butter, biscuits, pastries, ice cream, coconut oil, and palm oil. Artificial versions of saturated fats (hydrogenated or trans fats) are the unhealthiest and should be avoided. Examples of foods that have hydrogenated and trans fats include shortening, margarine, and many processed foods such as premade or packaged pastries, frozen pizzas, and canned frosting.

Saturated fats may also worsen memory (a common SLE problem). A 2012 study showed a correlation between fats eaten in the diet and memory decline. Women who ate a diet high in saturated fat had worse memory problems over four years than those who ate a diet with low amounts of saturated fats.

Eat non-meat protein and fat. There are plenty of healthy foods that supply protein and good fats and can be eaten in place of saturated fatty foods. Healthy alternatives include legumes (lentils, beans, peanuts), peas, fish, nuts, seeds, peanut butter, avocado, cultured Greek yogurt, and monosaturated oils (olive, canola, safflower, sesame, corn, soybean).

Non-meat proteins are much healthier than meat proteins. Eating processed meats and red meats (burgers and steaks) is associated with worse health outcomes, including a higher risk of heart disease, diabetes, and cancer. On the other hand, people who eat less meat live longer. People with rheumatoid arthritis who eat a vegetarian diet have less inflammation and pain.

Therefore, we recommend replacing red meat with other protein sources such as legumes, nuts, Greek yogurt, and whole grains. If you must eat meat, choose the leanest cuts and trim off visible fat. Better yet, stick to fish and lean, skinless poultry.

Other foods affecting inflammation. Sugar, high-fructose corn syrup, and simple/refined carbohydrates (sugar-related substances) may increase inflammation. These are found in white bread, pastries, soda, sugar-sweetened beverages, and most pasta and desserts. A 2012 study showed that SLE patients who ate high-carbohydrate diets had higher disease activity and higher cholesterol than SLE patients who ate fewer carbohydrates.

How much water should you drink per day?

The United States National Academies of Sciences, Engineering, and Medicine has figured out that an adequate daily fluid intake is 15.5 cups daily for men and 11.5 cups for women. Since we get approximately 20% of our fluids from food sources, this translates into men needing to drink 12.5 cups of liquids daily, and women to drink 9 cups.

Foods shown to lower inflammation include vegetables, fruits, whole grains, beans, legumes, nuts, and some spices (such as black pepper, ginger, and turmeric; see chapter 39). Targeting vegetables and fruits with various colors (carrots, spinach, red bell peppers, cherries, raspberries, and blueberries) is an excellent anti-inflammatory strategy. A rule of thumb is to cover at least half your plate with varying colors of vegetables and fruits. Healthy whole grains may also reduce inflammation and include oatmeal, brown rice, quinoa, barley, and whole wheat. Read about resistant starches below.

Probiotics and prebiotics. Before discussing prebiotics and probiotics, it is important to understand the living organisms in our gut and their relationships with lupus. We encourage you to read the section on the microbiome and resistant starches in chapter 3 before proceeding.

An important question is whether altering the microbiome could make lupus better or worse. While we know that dietary changes (for example, switching from a SAD to a vegetarian diet) alter the microbiome, we are still learning how those changes affect systemic autoimmune diseases.

Research shows that abnormal gut microbiomes occur in people with a wide variety of autoimmune diseases, including rheumatoid arthritis, dermatomyositis, polymyositis, ankylosing spondylitis, inflammatory bowel disease, scleroderma, and SLE. They also show that the gut microbiome in patients with well-controlled disease differs from those with more active disease.

A 2019 Yale University (New Haven, Connecticut) lupus microbiome study showed some interesting results. Anti-SSA (anti-Ro, chapter 4) is one of the earliest autoantibodies found in people predisposed to developing lupus and it appears many years before the disease. The researchers took germ-free mice (mice born and raised in a sterile environment) and placed a type of bacteria that naturally has Ro protein (antigen) into the mice's intestines. The immune system of these mice ended up producing anti-SSA antibodies, just as we see in lupus and Sjögren's patients. This study provides evidence for a mechanism by which bacteria living in an animal's gut can cause that animal to make autoantibodies.

Another study placed *Enterococcus gallinarum* (a bacterium) into the guts of germ-free mice. The bacteria went through the intestinal wall and increased immune system activity, leading to anti-dsDNA and anti-RNP (both commonly seen in SLE). These unwanted immune system problems from *E. gallinarum* were prevented when the mice were given antibiotics and vaccines that target the bacteria. Other studies have also shown that *E. gallinarum* can promote autoimmunity in research animals.

SLE patient studies have found DNA from this same bacteria, *E. gallinarum*, in their blood and liver, and they have increased antibodies directed toward *E. gallinarum*. This knowledge combined with what was seen in the lupus mice raises questions as to whether *E. gallinarum* in the gut may play a role in SLE and if ridding it from the gut could potentially help SLE.

Understanding the microbiome and its effects on the immune system will help us understand probiotics and prebiotics.

Prebiotics are foods that are consumed by gut bacteria and that promote increases in beneficial organisms. Fiber is one type of prebiotic. It is found in vegetables, fruits, whole grains, and psyllium (a high-fiber plant and the main ingredient in Metamucil). Fiber is poorly absorbed into our body but can be consumed and fermented by gut bacteria, producing short-chain fatty acids (SCFAs). These SCFAs can help reduce inflammation.

Resistant starch (discussed in chapter 3) is a type of prebiotic. In the resistant starch experiment described in chapter 3, the mice fed the resistant starches developed milder SLE and at older ages than the mice that did not eat resistant starches. They had lower levels of inflammation molecules (such as type I interferon, chapter 34), milder anemia (chapter 9), less major organ involvement (the liver, spleen, and kidneys), and lived significantly longer.

In addition to improving gut bacteria, resistant starch appears to have other health benefits, including better glycemic (blood sugar) control, preventing constipation, lowering cholesterol, and reducing the risk of colon cancer. Butyrate is a short-chain fatty acid that increases in the gut when people eat resistant starches. It is thought to have anti-cancer properties and improves bowel wall integrity.

Considering the above, lupus patients should consider including resistant starches (a prebiotic) in their daily diet.

Examples of resistant starches include plantains, green bananas (ripe bananas have less healthy starch), potatoes, potato starch, peas, whole grains (such as quinoa, oats, barley, and brown rice), and legumes (like beans and lentils).

Heating and cooling change the chemical structure of resistant starches. For example, cooked potatoes contain three times more resistant starch if you refrigerate them overnight and eat them the next day. Brown rice has the highest amount when cooked, then cooled, then reheated without water. Oats have the highest amount if not cooked (let uncooked oats soak overnight in milk or yogurt before eating). Also, if you refrigerate oatmeal after cooking it, then eat it cold—it has more resistant starch than when it is still warm.

One potential side effect of resistance starches is that their fermentation in the large intestine leads to hydrogen production, which causes gas (flatulence) and bloating. This can be avoided by eating a small amount first, then slowly increasing your intake over time.

Probiotics are foods containing health-beneficial live organisms. While prebiotics feed beneficial gut bacteria, probiotics are meant to replenish beneficial gut bacteria.

The studies mentioned previously suggest that alterations in gut bacteria are associated with changes in lupus disease activity. The next step is to wonder whether the introduction of beneficial bacteria through probiotics may help lupus. Studies have shown that probiotic bacteria alter the lupus immune system in lupus mice.

Examples of probiotic foods

Probiotic foods may increase good gut bacteria: live culture yogurt, kefir, fermented cabbage (sauerkraut and kimchi), tempeh, and kombucha. Aged cheeses (Swiss, Provolone, Gouda, cheddar, Edam, Gruyère, feta, Emmental, and Parmesan) have some probiotics.

Think of prebiotics as nutrients for the beneficial gut bacteria provided by probiotic foods. Consider including prebiotics and resistant starches in your daily diet along with probiotic foods.

When lupus mice are given some probiotic bacteria, lupus disease activity (including lupus nephritis, liver inflammation, and heart inflammation) is less than in mice that did not receive the probiotics. In some studies, the mice fed these probiotics also lived significantly longer. Probiotic bacteria species that improved lupus in mice include *Bifidobacterium bifidum*, *Ruminococcus obeum*, *Blautia coccoides*, and numerous species of *Lactobacillus*.

But while some studies showed that *Lactobacillus reuteri* (*L. reuteri*) reduced inflammation and lupus disease activity in lupus mice, others found *L. reuteri* to be associated with worse lupus disease activity. Many probiotic supplements contain *L. reuteri*. We do not know whether these would be harmful or helpful for SLE patients.

As mentioned earlier, other bacteria, such as *E. gallinarum*, can also worsen lupus in mice. Though this exact strain is not typically used as a probiotic, some probiotic supplements include other *Enterococcus* species.

There are a lot of immune system similarities between lupus mice and lupus humans, and we learn a lot about SLE through animal research. However, they are not exactly the same. We do not know if the research results in the mice would be the same in human SLE patients.

Because of these unknowns, we do not recommend probiotic supplements for lupus patients. We need good research to show which may be helpful and which are harmful.

In summary, more research is needed to know how prebiotics and probiotics affect immune function in lupus patients. Meanwhile, there is enough information to know that some prebiotics (such as resistant starches) are important for overall health. It would be an added benefit if they could also help lupus, but this is not known. Because of the reasons above, we suggest people get probiotics from food sources (if they wish to consume probiotics) but avoid prepackaged probiotic supplements.

Gluten. People with gluten hypersensitivity and gluten-sensitive enteropathy (celiac disease) need to eat a gluten-free diet (chapter 15). Some of our lupus patients who do not have these problems also report feeling better when eating less gluten. While some health professionals believe that eating large amounts of gluten can increase gut inflammation, no studies to date have shown a direct link between eating gluten and developing lupus or having more severe lupus. Feeling better on a gluten-free diet may be due to other effects, such as replacing simple carbohydrates and processed food containing gluten (such as, bread, pasta, chips) with more whole grains, vegetables, and fruit. Unless you have a diagnosed gluten sensitivity, SLE patients do not need to completely avoid gluten, but if you follow the recommendations in this chapter—such as limiting low glycemic carbohydrates, filling half your plate with vegetables, and avoiding processed foods—you will find yourself on a low-gluten diet.

Anti-inflammatory diets. Some food components and ingredients can increase or decrease inflammation by affecting blood sugar, antioxidant levels, fatty acid signaling molecules, and the bacteria that live in our gut. There is a lot of interest among patients, health care providers, and nutrition researchers in finding a specific diet that optimally reduces inflammation.

One example is the ITIS diet (table 38.7), designed by the University of California, San Diego, to be used as a complementary therapy in addition to drugs treating rheumatoid arthritis (RA), another autoimmune disease with similarities to lupus. Half of the patients who ate the ITIS diet had improvements in joint pain and fatigue. While the ITIS diet was designed for RA, not SLE, it includes foods that lower inflammation and could help other systemic inflammatory conditions.

Another diet with potential anti-inflammatory properties is the Mediterranean diet, discussed in more detail below. On the other end of the spectrum, the standard American diet (or SAD diet), which contains large amounts of high-calorie processed foods, saturated fat, and added sugar, is pro-inflammatory and associated with increased cardiovascular disease and death.

The Mediterranean Diet. This diet reduces the risk of cardiovascular disease (such as heart attack and stroke), improves brain health, and may decrease inflammation. The Mediterranean diet is a pattern of eating based on the typical diets of countries near the Mediterranean Sea, such as Greece, Italy, and Spain. Interest in this diet began when experts noted longer life expectancies and lower rates of heart attacks in some countries. The Mediterranean diet has lots of vegetables, fruits, olive oil, whole grains, beans, and moderate amounts of fish, chicken, low-fat dairy, nuts, and small amounts of wine. It limits red meat, sugary drinks (including fruit juices), salt, processed foods, and processed meats. Note that a Mediterranean diet does not mean eating lots of pizza and pasta.

Two randomized controlled trials (chapter 37) evaluated the Mediterranean diet in RA patients. The first study found that the patients who ate a Mediterranean diet had significantly decreased RA disease activity (reduced joint inflammation) after 12 weeks. The second study found that RA patients who ate a Mediterranean diet had less pain and morning stiffness.

A 2021 Spanish study showed that SLE patients who ate a Mediterranean diet had less disease activity than when they were not on the diet. They were also less likely to develop obesity, diabetes, or high blood pressure.

This study was conducted at just one point in time, so we will need another study with multiple time points to know if eating a Mediterranean diet reduces disease activity in SLE patients. That being said, since there is plenty of data showing that the Mediterranean diet is good for overall health, we encourage our lupus patients to follow such a diet.

Learn more about the Mediterranean diet from a reliable resource such as the American Heart Association: heart.org/en/healthy-living/healthy-eating/eat-smart/nutrition-basics/mediterranean-diet.

Table 38.7 The ITIS Anti-Inflammatory Diet

Recommendations (What to Eat)	Diet Strategies (How to Implement)
Daily omega-3 fatty acid foods	Fatty and white fish 4 days a week
Reduce saturated fats	Daily flaxseed, avocado, sesame, or tahini. Avoid red meats, butter, fried food, precooked foods
Daily green leafy vegetables and fruits	Broccoli, cabbage, zucchini, Brussels sprouts, etc.
	Daily homemade green juice (green vegetables plus fruits)
Daily prebiotics and probiotics	Vegetables and fruits as above, plus miso or no-sugar added yogurt daily
Daily enzymatic fruits	Pineapple, mango, papaya as snacks
Eat anti-inflammatory condiments	Turmeric, black pepper
	Eliminate sauces such as ketchup
Reduce nightshade vegetables *(note: these have not been shown to be harmful in SLE)*	Reduce eggplant, tomatoes, potatoes. *We don't agree with this part of the diet.*
Increase anti-inflammatory vegetables	Eat garlic, onion, pumpkin, etc.
Replace red meat proteins	Eat turkey or chicken twice weekly
	Eat legumes twice weekly (lentils, beans, etc.)
	Eat more whole grains (quinoa, barley, etc.)
Reduce gluten *(note: this has not been shown to help SLE, but it is a healthy dietary habit)*	Reduce wheat foods (bread, pasta, etc.)
	Substitute with corn tortillas, rye bread, etc.
Reduce dairy (except live culture yogurts)	Instead, drink almond, rice, oat, or coconut milk
Eat chia seeds (pain-reducing tryptophan)	Put on salads and in juices

Source: Reproduced with permission from Monica Guma, MD from: Bustamante MF, et al. Design of an anti-inflammatory diet (ITIS diet) for patients with rheumatoid arthritis. Contemp Clin Trials Commun. 2020 Jan 21;17:100524.

Fasting and weight loss. Intermittent fasting has become a popular lifestyle change for healthy eating and weight control. I have been practicing intermittent fasting for over three years. I eat only from 3 P.M. to 10 P.M. daily. From waking up to when I start eating at 3:00 P.M., I drink only water (usually noncaloric, fruit-flavored, without artificial sweeteners) and black coffee. I lost over 40 pounds, have easily kept it off, and feel more energetic. My cholesterol, glucose sugar levels, and kidney function have improved

LUPUS IN FOCUS

Should you avoid nightshade vegetables?

Nightshade vegetables include tomatoes, potatoes, eggplants, tomatillos, pimentos, and peppers. A common, unfounded belief that they may have inflammatory properties is not based on good research, so we do not recommend avoiding these foods. Many have substances with good health benefits, such as lycopene (an antioxidant) in tomatoes and capsaicin (pain-reducing) in peppers. Nightshade vegetables were included in the ITIS diet mentioned earlier.

LUPUS IN FOCUS

Garlic and lupus

Some doctors recommend staying away from garlic because it contains substances (allicin, ajoene, and thiosulfinates) that could theoretically increase immune activity. Yet, no medical studies show that garlic causes lupus flares.

The ITIS diet mentioned above includes garlic. It was based on medical evidence about certain foods and inflammation, including a 2018 study in which garlic was used because of its phytochemical contents. Phytochemicals are substances that help plants resist infections. Many experts thus suggest that garlic has health benefits.

While we do not know whether garlic helps the immune system in SLE patients, we do not think it is harmful.

a lot. This lifestyle change has been much easier than any restrictive diet I've been on in the past.

So, how about people with autoimmune disorders like lupus? Several separate studies show that lupus mice on a calorie-restricted diet live longer and have less inflammation in their skin, kidneys, salivary glands (as in Sjögren's), and blood.

Before considering fasting in your lifestyle, make sure to ask your doctor. It could be dangerous for diabetics treated with insulin.

Overweight SLE patients tend to have higher lupus disease activity. Having extra fat increases systemic inflammation, which increases the need for steroids, which causes even more weight gain. It is easy to see how this becomes a vicious cycle. Being overweight also increases the chances of cardiovascular complications (such as strokes, heart attacks, and blood clots), which are some of the most common causes of death in SLE. Therefore, changing the diet to lose weight should be a priority for overweight SLE patients.

Other dietary considerations. Establishing the best diet is more complicated for people with multiple medical problems. We recommend that you consult an experienced dietician. Many insurance companies will help cover the cost of seeing a dietician to improve your current health and prevent health problems down the road.

Vitamins

Except for vitamin D supplements in those who are deficient, most other vitamins do not appear to be medically necessary.

Minerals could potentially make a difference. A 2014 Iranian study showed that lower copper levels were seen in SLE patients with higher disease activity. Also, SLE patients had lower zinc and selenium levels than healthy people. These results still need to be confirmed. Rather than taking extra mineral supplements, it may be better to ensure an adequate food intake of these minerals. This would include legumes, low-fat dairy, eggs, nuts, seeds, leafy green vegetables, dark (not milk) chocolate, tofu, and whole grains. Note that most of these are important parts of an anti-inflammatory diet.

As mentioned in chapter 4, biotin is a common supplement taken by many of our patients. Be aware that it can cause artificial abnormal lab results, including thyroid, iron, and anti-dsDNA results. If you take biotin, make sure to stop it three days before lab work.

Alcohol

Alcohol may reduce inflammation and protect against lupus. A 2020 Harvard University (Cambridge, Massachusetts) research study of over 200,000 women measured immune system substance levels seen in lupus. Those who drank alcohol had lower stem cell factors, an abnormality seen in SLE. Chapter 3 addressed the lower rates of lupus onset in women who drink moderate amounts of alcohol. Whether it can also decrease lupus disease activity or not has not yet been proven.

Moderate alcohol intake may decrease the risks of cardiovascular disease problems (heart attacks, strokes, blood clots) and increase HDL good cholesterol levels.

However, heavy alcohol drinking (especially binge drinking) increases the risk of death from heart disease (sudden cardiac death). It may also increase the risk of breast, esophagus, mouth, throat, colon, pancreas, liver, and lung cancers.

Heavy alcohol use also increases the risk of depression, gout (arthritis due to uric acid), pancreatitis (inflammation of the pancreas), low blood cell counts, nerve damage, brain damage, dementia, liver damage (cirrhosis), and heart muscle damage. Any amount of alcohol can impede reflexes and increase the risk of a motor vehicle accident while driving, putting others' lives at risk.

Before drinking alcohol, first double-check with your doctor to ensure it is not forbidden with your medicines. Prednisone, non-steroidal anti-inflammatory drugs (NSAIDs), acetaminophen, antidepressants, opioids, and methotrexate can potentially have more side effects if taken with alcohol.

If you drink alcohol, drink a moderate amount or less. Women (and men older than 65 years) should not drink more than 1 serving within any 24-hour period. In contrast, men younger than 65 should not drink more than 2 servings. One serving is approximately 12 ounces of beer, 8 ounces of malt liquor, 5 ounces of wine, 3 to 4 ounces of fortified wine (such as sherry and port), 2.5 ounces of 24% alcohol liqueur, or 1.5 ounces of 80-proof liquor. There is evidence that red wine may have more health benefits than other alcohol forms, but this has not yet been proven.

If you do not drink alcohol, we do not recommend that you begin. If you drink more than the recommended amounts above, you should reduce your intake. If you are a woman, consider taking a daily folic acid supplement. There is some suggestion that alcohol may increase the risk of breast cancer in some women. Taking daily folic acid may reduce this risk.

If you are at increased risk of harm from alcohol (such as having a history of drug or alcohol abuse, liver disease, or a family history of breast cancer), consider abstaining.

Exercise

Regular exercise is essential for SLE patients (table 38.8). As mentioned many times in this book, one of the most common causes of death in lupus is cardiovascular disease (heart attacks, strokes, and blood clots). Regular exercise (chapter 7), especially aerobic exercise, decreases the chances of developing these complications by improving cardiovascular health, lowering bad cholesterol (LDL), increasing good cholesterol (HDL), reducing bad inflammatory HDL (oxidized HDL, chapter 21), reducing blood pressure, improving diabetes control, and decreasing fat weight.

Most SLE patients are overweight or obese (chapter 21) for many reasons, including the need for steroids and decreased activity levels as a natural response to pain and fatigue. Obesity increases the chances of dying prematurely from cardiovascular complications. Obesity also increases immune system activity and inflammation, resulting in the need to use more steroids, which can cause more fat gain. Aerobic exercise (such as bicycling, brisk walking, jogging, swimming, or using a treadmill or elliptical machine) helps to burn up calories, while toning exercises (weight and strength training) can increase the amount of calorie-burning muscle mass.

SLE patients are at increased risk for brittle bones (osteoporosis, chapter 24). The bones must "learn" to become strong by feeling stress through weight-bearing activities such as weight training, walking, and low-impact aerobics. Performing 30 minutes of weight-bearing exercise 5 days a week is recommended.

Table 38.8 Exercise Benefits for SLE

- Decreases heart attacks, strokes, and blood clots
- Decreases bad cholesterol (LDL); increases good cholesterol (HDL)
- Decreases pro-inflammatory HDL cholesterol levels
- Improves high blood pressure, diabetes, and weight control
- Increases muscle mass
- Increases bone density to fight osteoporosis
- Improves sleep quality
- Increases energy levels
- Decreases depression and anxiety
- Improves memory
- Improves quality of life, self-esteem, and sense of well-being

People with lupus often have sleep problems. This can occur from pain, medications that cause trouble sleeping, depression, fibromyalgia, and stress. Regular exercise improves sleep quality (chapter 6). Exercise should be done at least a couple of hours before bed; otherwise, the mind may be too active, making it more difficult to sleep.

Fatigue is one of the most common SLE problems and one of the most difficult to manage. Numerous studies show that regular exercise improves energy in SLE. There is a lot of interesting science behind why this happens. For example, a 2022 NIH study showed that SLE patients (non-exercisers) with bad fatigue who were placed on a supervised exercise regimen, ended up with significantly less fatigue and a better quality of life. From a scientific standpoint, the SLE patients started off with abnormal mitochondria. Mitochondria are microscopic parts (called organelles) inside of cells that produce energy. They are the "powerhouse of the cell." Regular exercise repaired and improved the SLE patients' mitochondria while also increasing their energy levels.

Exercise can, at first, be difficult for someone who feels too tired to exercise. It is best to start an exercise program gradually, increasing the amount slowly over time. Start with just a few minutes at a time, five days a week. Every week or so, increase the number of minutes until you get to 30 minutes or more of exercise a day.

Regular exercise also improves the quality of life beyond improving sleep and energy levels. It helps decrease depression and anxiety, improve memory, lead to better self-esteem, and increase one's sense of well-being.

How much should you exercise? In its 2018 Physical Activity Guidelines for Americans, the US Department of Health and Human Resources recommends getting at least 150 minutes of moderate aerobic exercise per week and two days a week of moderate muscle strengthening for all major muscle groups.

Some SLE patients have physical difficulties that could place them at increased risk of injury if they exercise incorrectly. It is best to get some professional help in learning to exercise properly in these situations. Get a physical therapist referral from your doctor or get help from a licensed personal trainer at a fitness center. Also, there are community exercise classes for arthritis patients. Water exercise classes are a good choice for many people, as are exercise classes for seniors. The Arthritis Foundation and YouTube are other sources of information on exercise programs.

Stress

SLE can flare during times of stress. This has been shown to occur with major stressful events, such as divorce or the death of a loved one, as well as with intermittent everyday stress, such as the hassles of commuting. One study showed that increased stress was associated with worse memory problems in SLE. This association was independent of issues of depression and anxiety (both of which cause memory problems and are worse with stress).

The immune system becomes more active during stressful periods. This may be connected to why lupus may occur more often and flare more often in people suffering from stress. A 2006 study found that certain genes can make it more difficult to produce important chemicals in the brain, such as serotonin, which is essential for mood stabilization and pain relief. This report showed that SLE patients with this gene abnormality had increased lupus nephritis flares when exposed to stress.

Experiencing stress while having a chronic disease, such as lupus, can become a vicious cycle. SLE patients who are prone to stress can develop increased lupus flares, which are of course, stressful themselves. Thus, stress reduction techniques should be an important part of treatment for SLE patients. A 2010 study found that a group of lupus patients who learned proper coping methods ended up with decreased depression, anxiety, daily stress, and pain symptoms. They also had an overall better quality of life than the lupus patients who did not learn how to deal with stress.

The 2022 California Lupus Epidemiology Study showed that after periods of increased stress, SLE patients developed worse disease activity. SLE patients with less stress or stable levels of stress did not. The authors recommended that teaching our patients about stress reduction techniques should be part of their treatment. Therefore, it is crucial to learn to manage stress appropriately.

Some strategies for decreasing stress are listed in table 38.9. However, if you cannot learn these techniques by yourself, consider seeing a professional who can help you learn to deal with stress (a counselor, psychologist, or sociologist).

An often-overlooked aspect of dealing with stress is how we deal with others. How we interact with family, friends, and co-workers plays a significant role in coping with medical illnesses and stress. Do not feel and act as if you are in this alone. People with a good, thoughtful support structure are better equipped to deal with their medical problems and stressors than isolated people. It is essential not to isolate yourself. Instead, work on making interpersonal connections with other people; you never know when you may need their help. Getting involved in groups that do hobbies you are interested in or volunteering are social activities that can help.

If you have a partner, it is important that they understand your condition. It can be especially supportive if your spouse or significant other goes with you to doctor visits if your schedules allow it. That way, they can learn more about your disorders and better understand what you are going through. If your schedules don't allow your partner to go to the doctor with you, you can consider other activities such as attending educational lupus seminars together, or you can at least provide them with educational material to read. Unfortunately, if your relationship was already difficult, inserting a chronic medical condition, such as SLE, can worsen things. In that case, professional help such as counseling may be needed to learn proper communication skills for reconnecting in a loving, giving, two-way relationship.

Sleep

Most people do not get enough sleep. Inadequate sleep is linked to many medical conditions, including obesity, body pain, fibromyalgia, depression, diabetes, and migraines. Research suggests that insufficient sleep is also associated with abnormal immune system activity. A 2018 study showed that SLE patients' relatives who got less than seven hours of sleep a night had a higher risk of developing SLE. Inadequate sleep in SLE is associated with increased depression, difficulties with memory, fatigue, obesity, and fibromyalgia. In addition, increased disease activity disrupts normal sleep, so it needs to be taken seriously. All SLE patients need to learn to purposefully schedule at least eight hours of sleep a night and practice good sleep hygiene (table 6.2). Taking a supplement called melatonin can help people sleep. While some lupus experts previ-

Table 38.9 Stress-Reduction Techniques

- Identify stressors in your life; work on decreasing their ill effects.
- Practice daily mindfulness (such as breathing exercises, chapter 39).
- Set realistic expectations (rather than unrealistic goals) and plan ahead.
- Say "no" to increased amounts of work and duties.
- If you have children, say "no" to nonessential activities; stick to those that are important for family and health.
- Ask for help in doing activities.
- Proactively lighten your load.
- Prioritize the important things in your life; cut out less important activities.
- Do yoga and/or tai chi.
- Get biofeedback training to learn to decrease anxiety and stress.
- Prepare well ahead of time for major activities.
- Learn to practice good time management.
- Plan for periods of rest and relaxation in your routine *every day.*
- Learn to say positive things to yourself; compliment yourself for doing something well.
- Do not think negative things about yourself.
- When running errands or going to appointments, get ready early, and give yourself more time than you think you need.
- Arrive early for all occasions.
- Schedule appointments and errands during less busy times, such as early Saturday mornings. This can greatly decrease stress from traffic and waiting in long lines.
- Learn to not argue. Accept that everyone has differing opinions or ways of doing things and that many conflicts are not important. Take deep breaths (as you learn to do from mindfulness), relax, leave before an argument begins or before you say something you may regret.
- Live at or below your means. Too many people try to "keep up with the Joneses" or other family members and friends. Staying out of debt can greatly decrease stress. Always ask yourself, "Is this something I truly need, or just something I want?" before you buy it.
- When you feel stressed, put the stressor into perspective; compare it to the important things in life (health, family, religion). "Don't sweat the small stuff."
- Exercise regularly.
- Schedule at least eight hours of planned sleep a night. Practice good sleep hygiene (table 6.2).
- Do not skip healthy, planned meals.
- Avoid unhealthy foods (sweets, carbohydrates, fatty foods, and fast food).
- Get counseling to learn better communication skills if you have difficulties with relationships.
- At work, request job accommodations needed for your medical condition. See lupusencyclopedia.com/can-you-work-with-lupus-lupus-patients-and-the-ada
- If it is possible, work from home; not commuting reduces stress.
- Take the depression and anxiety tests (tables 13.3 and 13.5). If you score high, take the results to your doctor to see if you need treatment.

ously recommended against melatonin, recent research suggests that melatonin is not harmful in lupus.

Brief Summary

The importance of non-drug therapies in lupus cannot be overemphasized. A 2011 study by the Centers for Disease Control and Prevention showed that four health risk behaviors were responsible for most premature deaths. These were poor nutrition, not exercising, drinking excessive alcohol, and smoking. Not smoking cigarettes provided the best protection from all causes of death. By comparison, there was a 63% overall reduction in deaths in people who ate a proper diet, exercised, drank alcohol in moderation (defined earlier), and do not smoke cigarettes. There was also a 66% reduction in cancer deaths and a 65% reduction in cardiovascular deaths (heart attacks and strokes). Moderate alcohol consumption showed the largest benefit for lowering cardiovascular deaths.

Patients may tire of their doctors telling them to "eat right, exercise regularly, don't drink too much, and don't smoke!" This study showed that what doctors tell their patients is right. The people in this study who did all four of these healthy habits added more than a decade (11 years on average) to their lifespan. We strongly recommend that SLE patients implement the lifestyle changes in this chapter. It takes a lot of work, but it is worth it in the end.

Make sure to read and follow all of "The Lupus Secrets" recommendations in chapter 44. It includes a summary of these essential lifestyle practices.

KEY POINTS TO REMEMBER

1. The treatment of lupus should include healthy habits as well as taking medicines.

2. All people with lupus (whether they get lupus rashes or not) need strict UV light protection (table 38.3), including wearing sunscreen religiously every day.

3. There are many reasons why lupus patients should not smoke.

4. If you cannot stop smoking on your own, go to www.smokefree.gov or call 800-QUIT-NOW.

5. Increase foods rich in omega-3 and omega-6 fatty acids in your daily diet.

6. Eat a diet rich in vegetables, fruits, whole grains, nuts, and low-fat dairy.

7. Limit the amounts of non-fish meat proteins, sugar, salt, and animal fat.

8. Avoid processed foods and foods that have fructose corn syrup in their ingredients.

9. Engage in at least 30 minutes of physical activity every day.

10. Practice stress-reduction techniques and mindfulness regularly (table 38.9 and chapter 39).

11. Schedule at least eight hours of sleep daily; use good sleep hygiene (table 6.2).

Integrative (Complementary) Medicine

Neda F. Gould, PhD, Dana DiRenzo, MD, MHS,
and Neha S. Shah, MD, *Contributing Editors*

Therapies that do not fall under conventional Western (allopathic) medicine are often based on cultural and historical traditions instead of scientific proof. "Alternative medicine" is the term used when these therapies are used by themselves. "Integrative medicine" (also called complementary medicine) is used when they are practiced along with conventional, Western medicine.

The National Center for Complementary and Integrative Health (NCCIH), a section of the US National Institutes of Health, promotes and funds complementary medicine research. A list of active research studies can be viewed at clinicaltrials.gov/ct2/results ?recr=Open&no_unk=Y&spons=NCCIH.

A lot of research is being conducted on most of the therapies discussed in this chapter. However, as of January 2023, the NCCIH did not list any lupus-specific integrative medicine research studies. The NCCIH is also a great resource for finding out more about these therapies: www.nccih.nih.gov/health/atoz.

SLE patients can safely combine integrative therapies with the medical regimens prescribed by their physician, and this chapter supplies some guidance. Some of these therapies can be greatly helpful, especially diet, exercise, and other lifestyle habits. These are also integrative medicine interventions and were discussed in chapter 38. Since the publication of the first edition of this book, some of the therapies in chapters 38 and 39 have had much more research supporting their use. We go over some of these findings.

We are honored to have three experts in their fields contributing to this important chapter.

Choosing among the many different integrative therapies can be daunting. If we had to select those in this chapter with the most beneficial evidence, we would recommend mindfulness, yoga, tai chi, and turmeric. When considering integrative therapies, weigh the potential pros and cons. For those not proven to work, ask yourself if it is truly worth your time and money to pursue them. Always ask your doctor whether it is safe, given your medical condition. If you see an integrative medicine provider, ask them to send notes with diagnoses and therapy recommendations to your conventional medical doctor (and vice versa) so that open communication exists, giving you the best overall, coordinated medical care. This chapter is divided into categories used by the NCCIH. Some therapies overlap between these major categories, and some treatments use a combination of types.

Mind-Body Medicine

These techniques are based on the realization that mental and emotional factors influence physical health and well-being. They use behavioral, social, psychological, and spiritual methods. Many of these (such as yoga, tai chi, biofeedback, hypnosis, mindfulness, and relaxation techniques) are now accepted in mainstream medicine. These therapies are most commonly used for pain, anxiety, sleeping problems, headaches, and depression.

Mindfulness

If you read only one section and choose just one type of integrative medicine, mindfulness would be the best choice. Mindfulness is defined as bringing attention to the present moment—to what is happening inside and outside our bodies. Its opposite is mindlessness or being on autopilot. Practicing mindfulness can be as simple as doing five minutes of daily breathing exercises.

Mindfulness research shows it helps with stress, anxiety, pain, and depression. A 2022 Johns Hopkins University (Baltimore, Maryland) study showed that practicing mindfulness for just 10 minutes daily using a smartphone app led to improvements in sleep, fatigue, pain, anxiety, mood problems, and managing stress. Fatigue improved most of all. This is important since fatigue is one of the hardest SLE problems to treat. Also, imagine having less pain and feeling better by practicing mindfulness instead of taking pain drugs and antidepressants.

You are more likely to practice mindfulness if you understand how it works. Let's look at the so-called fight-or-flight response. When placed in a dangerous situation, our brain and nervous system react to protect us by turning on our sympathetic nervous system (SNS, chapters 11 and 13). The SNS causes the immediate release of stress hormones, such as adrenaline and cortisol, which in turn activate many body reactions. Your body needs to be on full alert to save you from the perceived danger. The pupils dilate so you can see better, your heart pumps faster and harder, you breathe harder to get more oxygen to the muscles and brain, your reflexes become quicker, your muscles tense up, and you sweat so that your body can cool down from the heat buildup. You are super alert, and your brain and muscles are primed to get you out of danger. This reaction is necessary to keep us alive. After the threat has passed, the SNS calms down, and you relax.

In some people, though, the fight-or-flight response is turned on too often or too quickly when dangerous situations are not present. These false alarms do not help us

---

LUPUS IN FOCUS

Mindfulness improves the quality of life in SLE

A 2017 Iranian research study evaluated 23 SLE patients who learned to do breathing exercises, yoga, the concept of "acceptance," and how to deal with depressive episodes. After seven weeks, they reported greater improvements in psychological symptoms and quality of life compared to patients who did not practice mindfulness.

in a healthy way. They are forms of anxiety. While stress hormones and increased SNS activity are helpful for short periods during danger, they can harm your body and brain when occurring inappropriately, especially when this happens repeatedly or on an almost continuous basis.

These stress hormones (such as cortisol) can create unhealthy changes in the brain, causing us to react inappropriately to our environment (anxiety, depression, addiction), to develop sleep problems, and to gain weight (from excessive eating). Headaches, trouble thinking, and painful muscle spasms can occur. In addition, blood pressure can rise, and arteries can become hardened, increasing the risk of heart attacks and strokes (chapter 21).

Chronic activation of the stress response can lead to increased inflammation (just what you do not want with lupus). The nervous system directly cross-talks with immune system cells and causes them to secrete molecules that increase inflammation.

The good news is that everyone can learn to retrain their brain and body to not overreact. With mindfulness, you train your mind to relax, concentrate on the present, learn not to judge your actions negatively, and not worry about what happened yesterday or what will occur tomorrow. Practicing mindfulness causes positive brain changes with long-lasting health benefits.

In the future, whenever you are in stressful situations (traffic incidents, long slow grocery store lines, or unpleasant confrontations with people), before reacting on impulse, take a few deep breaths and tap into what you have learned from practicing mindfulness. Your body, mind, and loved ones will thank you.

Biofeedback

Biofeedback is a type of therapy in which you can teach your brain to control biological processes that are generally not under conscious control. The biofeedback therapist checks various biologic functions such as blood pressure, brain waves, heart rate, muscle tension, and temperature and guides the patient to change these conditions using their mind. It can help Raynaud's phenomenon, pain, stress, and sleep problems.

LUPUS IN FOCUS

How to start practicing mindfulness

Mindfulness should become as important a lifestyle habit as exercising, eating well, maintaining proper body weight, and getting eight hours of good quality sleep each night.

Check out YouTube videos such as "5-Minute Mindfulness Meditation," and "5-Minute Meditation You Can Do Anywhere." Smartphone apps such as "Breath Ball: Breathing Exercise," "10% Happier," "Calm," "Smiling Mind," "Headspace," "Insight Timer," and "iBreathe" can also be helpful.

Choose a regular time of day to practice mindfulness. Bedtime is good for those with insomnia. Begin with 5 minutes and see if you can build to 20–30 minutes. Finding a quiet room free of other people, pets, and noises is best. Sit on a comfortable chair, on a yoga mat, or lie down on a comfortable surface.

Prayer

Prayer has not been formally studied in lupus, but it has been studied in other conditions. A 2016 review evaluated the top 12 prayer studies. Seven of them showed positive health benefits, including anxiety and physical function.

Hypnotherapy

Hypnotherapy (hypnosis) is a relaxation therapy. The hypnotherapist guides the subject into heightened relaxation and increased focus. It has been used for anxiety, smoking cessation, weight control, and pain.

Aromatherapy

Aromatherapy uses the inhalation of essential oils, such as chamomile, lavender, geranium, cedar, and lemon. Proponents suggest they can help with mood, sleep, stress, pain, and nausea. Some research suggests that lavender and chamomile may help with sleep. No studies have proven their use in lupus.

Art Therapy

Art therapy is a type of psychotherapy in which the patient uses art to communicate. Patients need no art experience. It can help one deal with the emotional stresses of illness. You can find a practitioner by contacting the American Association of Art Therapists at https://arttherapy.org.

Whole Medical Systems

Whole medical systems are systems of diagnosis and practice that are based on a particular philosophy, such as the power of nature or the presence of energy. Traditional Chinese and Ayurvedic practices are two of the oldest examples. The main focus of whole medical systems is often on prevention and balance.

Traditional Chinese Medicine

Traditional Chinese medicine (TCM) is based on the theory that disease and illness result from improper energy flows. A proper balance of the opposing forces of yin and yang is necessary. TCM uses a combination of diet, Chinese herbs, massage, meditation, and acupuncture.

Chinese Herbal Therapy

At least eight studies show that TCM may help lupus. Most were published in Chinese medical journals without review by worldwide lupus experts.

One example is a 2018 Chinese SLE randomized, controlled trial (RCT, chapter 37) that evaluated a Chinese herbal formula called Zi Shen Qing (Zishenqing). Half of the participants took the herbal therapy; the other half took 200 mg daily of hydroxychloroquine (HCQ, Plaquenil). The results showed that Zi Shen Qing worked better at reducing lupus disease activity after three months than HCQ. It helped reduce the need for steroids without significant side effects.

However, they used a much lower dose of HCQ than we normally use. Also, HCQ usually takes six months to one year for its full effects, and this study was only 3 months. It would be best to repeat the study with a larger number of patients, using standard doses of HCQ, for at least a year.

TCM also uses *Tripterygium wilfordii hook F* (TwHF, Thunder god vine) for joint pains, fever, chills, swelling, and inflammation. TwHF decreases inflammation-producing cytokines (chapter 33). It is an approved treatment in China for rheumatoid arthritis (RA), an autoimmune disease related to lupus. It is not FDA-approved.

TwHF has been shown in small studies to be as effective as methotrexate for RA. A 2015 study showed that using TwHF with methotrexate was superior to using methotrexate or TwHF alone.

There have been no well-designed studies evaluating TwHF in lupus. Five low-quality studies assessed 249 lupus patients and suggested improvements in fatigue, joint pain, fever, rash, lupus nephritis, and low platelet counts.

However, side effects included intestinal problems (diarrhea, nausea, vomiting), hair loss, dry mouth, headaches, rash, mouth sores, weight changes, irregular menstrual cycles, infertility, heart disease, and high blood pressure. It is not safe to take during pregnancy.

Chinese herbal safety cannot even be assured in China itself. One study evaluated 430 Chinese herb samples from local hospitals, medical centers, and herbalist shops in Taiwan. One-third of the herbal products were contaminated with Western medicines, including phenylbutazone, which can cause severe side effects.

Some Chinese herbal supplements can cause kidney disease and are routinely discouraged by kidney specialists (nephrologists).

LUPUS IN FOCUS

Learn about any herbs before taking them

"Natural" does not mean "safer."

Echinacea can cause lupus flares. *Ginkgo biloba* can cause increased bleeding. Feverfew can cause pregnancy complications. St. John's wort (used by some people for depression) can cause dangerously high blood pressure when consumed with aged cheeses or red wine.

Some of the most powerful and potentially toxic medicines (when not dosed and monitored correctly) come from plants. These include colchicine (from the Autumn crocus) for gout (an arthritis due to uric acid), digoxin for heart disease (originating from the digitalis plant), quinidine for heart disease, quinine for malaria (both from cinchona tree bark), paclitaxel for cancer (from the Pacific yew tree), and *Tripterygium wilfordii hook F* for RA.

Before taking any herb, learn about it on the NCCIH's website at nccih.nih.gov/health/herbsataglance.

Acupuncture and Acupressure

Acupuncture involves inserting very tiny needles into the skin on specific body areas (called acupoints). This affects energy flow (called qi, pronounced CHEE) in different body parts and restores a balance of yin and yang. Acupressure uses pressure or pushing on acupoints instead of inserting needles.

A 2018 review of 13 research studies involving over 20,000 people suggested that acupuncture may help chronic pain and headaches. Acupuncture is covered by some American insurance plans.

Complications are rare but have included nerve damage, infections, and punctured organs. Acupuncture needles should not be placed in areas of infection or cancer. Let your acupuncturist know if you are pregnant, have a pacemaker, have low white blood cell or platelet counts, or take blood thinners.

There are no large acupuncture lupus studies. One small 2008 study showed no help with lupus pain or fatigue. Another Chinese study suggested that earlobe acupuncture improved discoid lupus rashes and well-being in 15 patients. However, there was no placebo group for comparison. Acupuncture has no proven benefit for the immune system, so beware of false claims.

Earlobe acupressure (auriculotherapy) is recommended for insomnia treatment in the 2020 Chronic Insomnia Clinical Guidelines. Auriculotherapy ear seeds are tiny and have an adhesive to apply to your outer ears and are available for purchase on the internet.

Acupressure has also been used to treat pain, nausea, and motion sickness. However, these uses are not proven by well-done research studies.

Tai Chi (Taiji, Tai Chi Chuan)

Tai chi is a Chinese mind-body exercise incorporating dance-like movements, meditation, and martial arts. Numerous studies have shown tai chi to help fibromyalgia, anxiety, pain, depression, and quality of life. Classes are easy to find at exercise centers, hospitals, martial arts clinics, and seniors' centers, as well as online. Tai chi is best performed in a group setting.

A 2017 Ohio State University study looked at tai chi in SLE. After 10 weeks, lupus patients practicing tai chi had less inflammation (specifically, less IL-6, IL-8, interferon-gamma, and TNF-alpha, chapter 33).

Ayurvedic Medicine (Ayurveda)

Ayurvedic medicine originated with Indian Hindu healers over 3,000 years ago. It believes that disease comes from an imbalance of the body's life force and focuses on disease prevention. It includes diet, herbs, massage, meditation, breathing exercises, yoga, fasting, and internal cleansing. Although there are no extensive studies of using Ayurveda in SLE, some successful cases have been reported in the medical literature. Ayurvedic practices that can improve health include a healthy diet, massage, mindfulness (breathing exercises and meditation), yoga, fasting (chapter 38), and the use of ginger and turmeric (curcumin). If looking for a certified Ayurvedic practitioner, go to the National Ayurvedic Medical Association at www.ayurvedanama.org.

Yoga is a body-mind practice using meditation, regulated breathing, and holding specified poses or stretches. Yoga has been studied in over 300 randomized controlled trials, demonstrating improvements in anxiety, strength, flexibility, balance, mood, memory, pain, and quality of life.

At least 18 studies have demonstrated anti-inflammatory effects. A 2018 Washington, DC, study showed improved balance and body awareness in SLE patients.

Challenging yoga poses may be modified to meet the needs and level of any patient under the guidance of a certified yoga instructor. Avoid poses that cause pain.

SLE patients should avoid forms of hot yoga, such as Bikram yoga.

Homeopathy

Homeo- comes from the Greek word for "like;" *-opathy* comes from the Greek word for "disease." Homeopathy is based on the principle that "like cures like." The idea is that if something causes illness in large doses, tiny amounts may be the cure.

Homeopathy treatments are aimed at the symptoms of disease and a person's personality and lifestyle. No homeopathic therapies have been proven helpful for lupus or any rheumatic condition. A 2012 review of homeopathic treatments reported 1,159 side effects, including four deaths. Allergic reactions and intoxications were the most common.

Naturopathy

Naturopathy emphasizes preventing and treating disease through a healthy lifestyle and addressing the "whole person." Therapy focuses on finding and addressing the root cause of disease instead of treating symptoms alone. Naturopathic doctors may use herbs, homeopathy, exercise, mind-body treatments, sleep improvement, diet, stress reduction, hydrotherapy, and other interventions.

Before beginning naturopathic treatments, you should check with your medical doctor to ensure they are not bad for your lupus or have dangerous interactions with your medications. Especially make sure that your naturopathic doctor sends all notes to your other doctors (and vice versa).

Biologically Based Practices

Integrative medicine that uses treatments found in nature is labeled "biologically based." Examples include foods (such as prebiotics, chapter 38), vitamin and mineral supplements, spices, herbs, hormones, and even cannabis (medical marijuana). This section will discuss some that may or may not help SLE. Others, such as omega-3 fatty acids, probiotics, prebiotics, DHEA, and vitamin D, are discussed in chapters 35 and 38.

Supplements

The 1994 Dietary Supplement Health and Education Act (DSHEA) defines a dietary supplement as a product having one or more of the following: "a vitamin, mineral, amino acid, herb, other botanical, concentrate, metabolite, constituent, or extract."

A downside of US dietary supplements is that manufacturers do not have to provide proof of effectiveness, safety, or quality. Even if the company finds out about potential side effects after a supplement goes to market, it does not have to report this to the FDA. Instead, it is the FDA that bears the burden of proof proving whether any supplement is unsafe or ineffective. Only then can it exert its power to remove dangerous supplements and protect the public.

Over-the-counter (OTC) supplements often state inaccurate quantities of ingredients. For example, many OTC vitamin D3 and DHEA (chapter 35) products have much smaller or greater amounts than are on the label.

One way around this problem is to obtain supplements from compounding pharmacists, who are specially trained in preparing high-quality products such as DHEA. Chapter 35 discusses how to deal with the problem with vitamin D3.

Ginger

A 2021 University of Michigan research study showed that one of the active ingredients of ginger, 6-gingerol, reduced inflammation, reduced anti-dsDNA and antiphospholipid antibodies (chapter 4), and decreased blood clots in mice with lupus and antiphospholipid syndrome (chapter 9). However, no human studies have been done.

If you decide to take a ginger supplement, be careful of the brand. ConsumerLab .com independently evaluated 15 brands and could not recommend 7 of them due to poor quality.

Potential side effects of ginger include stomach upset, heartburn, diarrhea, and mouth soreness. It can interfere with platelet function, so be careful with blood thinners, including aspirin. Stop taking ginger one week before surgery to prevent bleeding. It may also lower blood sugar levels, so be cautious with diabetic drugs.

Curcumin (Turmeric)

Curcumin is the active ingredient in the spice turmeric (a member of the ginger family). In the laboratory, curcumin decreases inflammation-producing cytokines (chapter 33) and reduces animal autoimmunity. An Oklahoma study showed that curcumin-treated lupus mice had less cutaneous (skin) lupus, kidney inflammation (lupus nephritis), and organ damage, as well as fewer autoantibodies than placebo-treated mice. In the same study, the mice prone to getting Sjögren's (chapter 14) developed less salivary gland inflammation and fewer swollen lymph nodes. A subsequent 2020 study showed that curcumin-treated lupus mice ended up with less kidney damage and better kidney function.

An Iranian study showed that lupus nephritis patients who took one capsule of turmeric three times a day with food had lower kidney inflammation (reduced urine protein and blood) and better blood pressure than placebo-treated patients.

Although curcumin is poorly absorbed, some of its effects may occur through the gut microbiome (chapters 3 and 38) and not depend on absorption. Curcumin (turmeric) dissolves better in oil than water, so take most brands with a fatty meal. Make sure the fats are healthy (chapter 38). When you use turmeric in food, adding black pepper helps absorption.

Turmeric's potential side effects include allergic reactions, diarrhea, nausea, headaches, and elevated liver blood tests. Rare cases of hepatitis (liver inflammation) have been seen. If you are prone to oxalate kidney stones, avoid large amounts of turmeric. Many pure curcumin products contain little to no oxalate, making them a better choice (read the labels). Turmeric and curcumin decrease platelet function (chapter 9), so be careful with blood thinners (including aspirin). You should stop taking it for at least one week before surgery. Curcumin also lowers blood sugar, so be careful with diabetic drugs.

In large amounts, curcumin can lower calcineurin inhibitor (CNI: cyclosporin, tacrolimus, and voclosporin) blood levels. CNIs are used for lupus nephritis. At recom-

Avoid herbal supplements if you take voclosporin (Lupkynis)

Voclosporin is used for lupus nephritis (kidney inflammation). St. John's wort can reduce voclosporin blood levels. Cat's claw, Echinacea, black licorice, chamomile, and red clover increase levels.

It is safest to avoid all herbal supplements while taking voclosporin.

mended doses, curcumin does not enter the liver in high enough concentrations to cause problems. Do not consume large quantities if you take voclosporin (Lupkynis) or other CNIs.

Curcumin binds to iron and can cause or worsen iron deficiency anemia. Do not take curcumin within a few hours of iron supplements.

Melatonin

Melatonin is a hormone released by the brain's pineal gland. It signals the brain to prepare for sleep when it senses decreased light. Therefore, melatonin can help sleep.

In 2013 and 2019, scientific review articles argued that melatonin may help autoimmune disorders. In the lab, melatonin increases valuable T cells called Tregs (regulatory T cells), which can calm down an overactive immune system. SLE patients tend to have fewer Tregs, resulting in increased inflammation and autoimmunity. From a theoretical perspective, if melatonin increases Tregs in lupus patients, it could lower disease activity. However, this has not been studied.

Some doctors recommend that lupus patients not take melatonin, even though there is no research to support this. The only human melatonin study for systemic autoimmune disease is in RA patients. It did not worsen their condition. There are no human lupus studies.

Phytotherapy

Phytotherapy uses supplements or drugs that come from plants or herbs. Chinese herbal therapies were discussed above in the TCM section.

Pycnogenol (French maritime pine bark) can decrease inflammation by interfering with TNF-alpha (a cytokine, chapter 33). Since TNF-alpha occurs in high levels in SLE, it could theoretically help SLE. One small *Pycnogenol* SLE study with 11 patients suggested that it may help SLE, but this study is much too small to accept the results. *Pycnogenol* can increase bleeding, so be careful if you are on any blood thinners, including aspirin.

Echinacea can boost the immune system and worsen autoimmune diseases. The Lupus Clinic at Johns Hopkins has had patients develop SLE flares from Echinacea. Two even needed cyclophosphamide (chapter 32) for lupus nephritis flares. SLE patients should not take Echinacea or other supplements touted as "boosting" the immune system. In SLE, we need to calm down the overactive immune system.

When you consume an herbal supplement, you rarely know the amount of the active ingredients. Concentrations of active ingredients can vary greatly, depending on many

LUPUS IN FOCUS

Green tea and lupus

A 2017 randomized, controlled trial evaluated green tea extract capsules (2,000 mg per day) in SLE patients. They had reduced disease activity and better quality of health after three months. This study needs repeating.

factors such as how much rain and sun the plants received, the nutrients in the soil, plant maturity at harvest, and how it was processed. This makes it almost impossible to accurately label what is in the product without extracting the actual active ingredients.

As with other dietary supplements, the FDA does not regulate phytotherapy products. So, you really do not know what you are getting. Phytotherapy products should be considered unregulated drugs. They have significant effects, both positive and negative. Researchers need to figure out the active ingredients, standardize the amounts, and do adequate studies to prove effectiveness and safety. We should hold these products up to similar standards as prescription drugs.

Medical Marijuana (Cannabis, Cannabinoids, THC, CBD)

For more detailed information go to lupusencyclopedia.com/cbd-for-lupus.

Cannabinoids are the active compounds of the cannabis plant. There are 140 different cannabis-derived cannabinoids, each of which acts differently. The two most studied and well-known are cannabidiol (CBD) and tetrahydrocannabinol (THC). THC is the cannabinoid responsible for the "high" intoxicating effects. CBD does not make people high. Since CBD does not cause a "high" in users, US federal law allows CBD-containing hemp (industrial hemp) to be grown if it contains less than 0.3% THC. CBD from industrial hemp is available in all 50 states.

CBD is not FDA-regulated, so it has quality problems. A 2017 study of 84 online CBD products found that 70% of them were mislabeled, having significantly more or less CBD than stated on the label. A 2020 study showed that only one out of five CBD products purchased in Mississippi contained the stated amount of CBD. Dangerous amounts of lead, mercury, and other contaminants have also been seen. Consider checking lab reports on CBD purity on websites such as ConsumerLab.com.

Recreational and medical cannabis from regulated dispensaries are found in the states that legalized it. Products have varying amounts of THC and CBD. If you decide to use medical cannabis, make sure you get it from a reputable dispensary. Potential dangers of homemade products include unknown THC and CBD quantities, mold, pesticides, and contamination with other drugs.

How cannabinoids work: Many cells have cannabinoid receptors (attachments) on their surfaces to which cannabinoids can attach; they are called cannabinoid 1 (CB1) and 2 (CB2) receptors. When CBD, THC, and other cannabinoids bind to these receptors, they cause cellular chemical changes. CB2 receptors are on most immune system cells, including T cells and B cells (chapter 33). When cannabinoids bind to CB2, they can lower the activity of these cells, resulting in less inflammation.

When CBD, THC, and other cannabinoids interact with nerve and brain cells, the result can be less nausea, reduced pain, less seizure activity, and fewer muscle spasms. THC (but not CBD) produces intoxication and euphoria through these interactions.

Note, however, that while you could get improvements in pain (especially neuropathy or nerve damage pain, chapter 13), nausea, or sleep, these effects are not proven. Also, effects may vary greatly depending on quality, method of administration (such as edibles versus creams), and the amounts of CBD and THC.

A 2017 National Academies of Sciences, Engineering, and Medicine review of 35 RCTs (chapter 37) concluded that cannabinoids may help chronic pain. Another 2017 study from Portland, Oregon, found evidence that cannabinoids may help nerve pain, but not other pain types.

Subsequently, a 2018 Canadian Evidence Review Group evaluated RCTs on medical cannabis. There was insufficient evidence of benefit in chronic pain, including nerve pain. Although they recommended avoiding medical marijuana for acute pain, headaches, and rheumatologic conditions, they noted that if all standard, proven therapies fail someone, it could be considered for nerve pain or to help decrease pain and suffering in dying patients.

Better high-quality research is greatly needed.

Do not use cannabinoids if

- you have liver cirrhosis.

- you have had cannabinoid allergic reactions.

- you are diagnosed with "cannabis use disorder," or if you have a history of alcohol or drug abuse.

How cannabinoids are taken: Cannabinoids can be used in many different forms—smoked, vaped, ingested (in edibles, capsules, concentrates, and tincture drops), topicals (ointments, creams), and as an aerosol sprayed on the insides of the cheek.

Do not smoke or vape cannabis if you are a lupus patient. Smoking tobacco is very dangerous in lupus (chapter 38). Cannabis smoke has many of the same hazardous chemicals and carcinogens (cancer-causing substances) as tobacco. Smoking cannabis increases the chances of having heart attacks and strokes, which are among the most common causes of death in SLE (chapter 21). Smoking cannabis can also lead to chronic bronchitis and permanent lung damage. This increases infection risks, which is another leading cause of death in SLE. In addition, smoking cannabis worsens dry mouth, can cause thrush (chapter 22), and increases periodontal disease (chapter 38), all of which are dangerous problems in SLE.

What to monitor on cannabinoids: Liver function, weight, blood counts, and kidney function.

Potential side effects of cannabinoids (tables 39.1 and 39.2): OTC CBD products, which can contain trace amounts of THC of less than 0.3%, can cause positive THC drug screens. If insurance physicals, security clearances, or your job demands no THC use and uses urine toxicity screens, avoid OTC CBD.

There are many potential drug interactions. Ask your doctor.

While taking cannabinoids,

- do not drive, climb, or use machinery 24 hours after using THC.

- taper it off slowly if you use a cannabis product regularly to prevent withdrawal problems, such as seizures.

- store cannabis products (especially tempting edibles) in a secure place, away from children and pets.

Pregnancy and breastfeeding: Do not use while breastfeeding or while pregnant. THC increases the risk of permanent fetal brain damage, which can lead to autism, hyperactivity, lower IQ, memory problems, and psychiatric illness.

Cannabis smoking decreases sperm counts by around 30% and should be avoided in men trying to have a baby.

Geriatric use: Older individuals have a higher chance of side effects, so lower doses are usually needed. Cannabinoids can cause dangerous falls.

Cannabinoids and surgery: Cannabinoids should be avoided before surgery to prevent dangerous interactions with anesthetics.

More information: lupusencyclopedia.com/cbd-for-lupus

Folk Medicine

Folk medicine uses herbs and other biological substances believed to have medicinal value. Although some of these might be safe and effective, research is lacking. Some folk remedies, such as snake or bee venom, may be dangerous and potentially fatal. Some have been found to have detectable amounts of prescription medicines, heavy metals, and other toxic substances. Folk medicine therapies cannot be recommended.

LUPUS IN FOCUS

Side effects versus benefits of medical cannabis

What if we prescribed a drug causing side effects in 1 out of 6 people, and only 1 of every 19 had pain relief? Our patients would think we were crazy. Guess what? These are results from the best cannabinoid research pain studies (such as arthritis and fibromyalgia).

While CBD is popular, studies fail to prove pain-relieving effects. Research studies suggest that THC/CBD combination products may be beneficial, but this is not proven.

Medical marijuana and edibles from medical and recreational dispensaries average 20% THC and 2% CBD, although actual amounts range from 0 to 45% THC and 0 to 40% CBD. The THC amount in most products was two to three times higher than needed for pain relief. This places people at higher risk for dangerous psychotic side effects without added pain relief.

Since the potential for side effects of using medical marijuana is much greater than its proven benefits, we cannot recommend its use for pain until more rigorous studies are done.

Table 39.1 Potential Side Effects of Pure CBD (Epidiolex)

	Incidence	Side Effect Therapy
Nuisance side effects		
Stomach upset, nausea, diarrhea, weight change, loss of appetite	Very common	Take with food, decrease the dose, or contact your doctor.
Rash	Common	Contact doctor. Stop the drug.
Elevated liver enzymes	Common	No action needed if mild. May need to lower the dose or stop the drug if moderate to severe.
Anemia	Common	No action needed if mild. May need to lower the dose or stop the drug if moderate to severe.
Serious side effects		
Drowsiness, fatigue, insomnia, difficulty thinking, moodiness, aggression/anger, suicidal thoughts	Very Common	Lower the dose or stop the drug.
Infection and fevers	Common	Stop the drug and seek medical attention immediately.
Rash, hives, angioedema	Uncommon	Stop the drug and seek medical attention immediately.

Note: Side effect incidence key (these are approximations as they can vary widely from study to study): rare <1% occurrence; uncommon 1%–5% occurrence; common >5% occurrence.

Manipulative and Body-Based Practices

These therapies treat medical conditions through various forms of manipulation of body parts.

Chiropractic Therapy

Chiropractors believe that a misaligned spinal column can be a significant source of some medical problems. They use spinal manipulation, massage, acupressure, electrical stimulation, heat, cold, exercise, and other techniques to realign the spine.

Chiropractic is not helpful for autoimmune problems such as SLE. Spinal manipulation could potentially be dangerous if you have osteoporosis (brittle bones), a history of stroke, hardening of the arteries, or a history of spinal surgery.

Table 39.2 Potential Side Effects of Pure THC (Dronabinol)

	Incidence	Side Effect Therapy
Nuisance side effects		
Euphoria, "high"	Very common	Reduce the dose or stop the drug.
Abdominal pain, nausea, vomiting, weight changes, diarrhea	Common	Lower the dose or stop the drug. Contact your doctor.
Facial flushing, heart palpitations, fast heart rate	Common	No action needed if mild. May need to lower the dose or stop if moderate to severe.
Muscle weakness or pain	Uncommon	Lower the dose or stop the drug.
Increased sweating	Uncommon	No action needed.
Elevated liver enzymes	Uncommon	No action needed if mild. May need to lower the dose or stop if moderate to severe.
Serious side effects		
Thinking abnormalities, altered judgment, sexual indiscretion activity, drowsiness, memory loss, anxiety/depression, incoordination, confusion, flu-like symptoms, headaches, nightmares, speaking problems, ringing in the ears, psychiatric symptoms (hallucinations, paranoia)	Very Common	Lower the dose or stop the drug.
Low blood pressure, lightheadedness, passing out (syncope)	Common	Stop the drug and seek medical attention if at risk of falling.
Rash, hives, angioedema, mouth sores	Uncommon	Stop the drug and seek medical attention immediately.
Seizures	Rare	Stop the drug and seek medical attention immediately.

Note: Side effect incidence key (these are approximations as they can vary widely from study to study): rare <1% occurrence; uncommon 1%–5% occurrence; common >5% occurrence.

Massage

Massage involves physically manipulating body tissues to decrease pain, anxiety, stress, and improve circulation. Although massage therapy has not been studied formally in SLE, it may be beneficial for depression and anxiety and help decrease pain. The American Massage Therapy Association recommends avoiding vigorous massage, deep tissue massage, and heat treatments in inflamed areas of SLE patients.

Colonic Irrigation and Cleansing

Proponents of colonic irrigation and cleansing believe that unhealthy toxins in the colon contribute to disease. Therefore, they use liquid to cleanse the colon. No studies prove it helpful for any condition. It can cause dehydration, electrolyte abnormalities, bowel perforation, and infection risks. Avoid it if you have heart disease, kidney or liver problems, or take certain medications. Steroids can thin out the bowel wall, increasing the risk of bowel perforation. SLE patients should avoid these treatments.

Energy Medicine

This group of therapies tries to manipulate body energy fields to improve health. They are generally safe.

Qi Gong (Qigong, Chi Kung, Chi Gung)

Qi gong is a Chinese exercise using slow movements and breathing exercises. Qi gong may help decrease pain, such as neck and back pain. We are unaware of any studies proving benefit in SLE, but since pain is common in SLE, it could theoretically help some people.

Reiki

Reiki is a Japanese healing art based on the idea that healing energy can be intuitively transmitted from the healer to the patient by placing the hands on parts of the patient's body. It can also be practiced from a distance without touching. A 2011 study on cancer patients suggested improvements in pain, sleep, relaxation, anxiety, and well-being. There are no studies proving benefit in SLE.

Therapeutic Touch

Therapeutic touch is also called "the laying on of hands," similar to Reiki, but it usually does not involve touching. The hands are held a few inches away from the patient and swept down from the head to the lower part of the body. Practitioners say they can sense and manipulate the person's energy field (aura), attempting to return the mind and energy to a peaceful state. Some studies suggest its use in fibromyalgia, osteoarthritis, pain, and anxiety disorders. No studies prove its use in lupus.

Magnetic Therapy

No well-done studies prove that magnets reduce pain or benefit disease. There are studies showing them not to help back pain, carpal tunnel syndrome, and degenerative arthritis. A 1995 Russian study suggested that pulsed magnetic fields could help lupus, but it was poorly done without a placebo control group.

1. Practice mindfulness daily.

2. Mindfulness, yoga, tai chi, and turmeric (curcumin) have some of the strongest evidence to support their use.

3. The US National Center for Complementary and Integrative Health is 100% committed to studying integrative therapies.

4. Having an integrative medicine doctor as part of your medical team could be beneficial.

5. Avoid herbal products and colon cleansings; they are not proven safe and effective for lupus.

6. Do not take supplements that stimulate ("boost") the immune system, such as Echinacea. They can worsen SLE.

7. Most lupus patients should take vitamin D (chapters 35 and 38).

8. DHEA and omega-3 fatty acid supplements can potentially help SLE (see chapters 35 and 38).

9. Therapies that may help pain and anxiety include biofeedback, mindfulness, tai chi, yoga, acupuncture, relaxation techniques, art therapy, massage therapy, Qi gong, Reiki, and therapeutic touch.

10. If you use any of these for your SLE, use them to complement conventional Western medicine and not replace it.

PART V

Other Practical Matters

Understanding Your Symptoms

Sarthak Gupta, MD, *Contributing Editor*

A symptom is what you feel or notice as part of a medical condition. Knowing the possibilities and how urgent they are can help you understand how to respond to them.

There are many potential causes for each symptom. For example, chest pain could be due to lung inflammation (such as pleurisy), a heart attack, acid reflux, a lung blood clot, overstimulation of nerves, or rib pain. This chapter looks at the causes and helps you figure out whether the problem is an emergency or whether you can wait to see your doctor. Situations that need immediate medical attention at an urgent care center (UCC) or an emergency room (ER) are noted in table 40.1.

For situations that are typical of a lupus flare, contact your doctor right away. Also, be prepared with a "Flare Plan" (table 5.2) ahead of time.

Fever

The basic approach to fever in SLE patients is that it is an infection until proven otherwise. This is because infection is one of the most common causes of death in SLE. Rapid diagnosis and treatment are important. Check your temperature if you feel hot, feverish, sweating, or having chills. If you have a fever, as defined in chapter 6, contact your doctor. **Sweats, chills, and shivering with a fever can potentially mean a bacterial infection, and urgent medical attention may be needed.**

Some examples of infection symptoms include cough (pneumonia or bronchitis), pain while urinating or increased frequency of urination (urinary tract infection), red and painful skin (cellulitis, skin infection), headache and congestion (sinusitis), runny nose with sneezing (upper respiratory tract infection), and diarrhea (intestinal infection).

Some drugs, such as prednisone, NSAIDs (table 36.1), and acetaminophen (Tylenol), can mask a fever. Still contact your doctor if you develop infection symptoms on these drugs and do not have a fever.

SLE can cause fever (chapter 6), requiring NSAIDs, acetaminophen or even immunosuppressants (table 22.1) in severe cases. Do not assume that SLE is the cause without

---

Dr. Gupta contributed to this article in his personal capacity. The views expressed are his own and do not necessarily represent the views of the National Institutes of Health, or the United States government.

Table 40.1 When to Seek Immediate Medical Attention

NOTE: Seek medical attention (UCC, ER, or doctor) if any of the following conditions occur along with the symptoms noted. Use Table 5.2 for possible lupus flares.

Condition	Symptoms
Fever (defined in chapter 6)	• Any type of fever, occurring by itself or in conjunction with any of the conditions in this table
Fatigue	• Shortness of breath, chest pain, stomach pain, headache -Difficulty thinking -Weight loss
Joint and muscle pain	• If it feels like a lupus flare
Rash	• New or worsening lupus rash
	• If it occurs soon after starting a new medicine (call the doctor who prescribed it)
	• Burning, painful area of skin, especially if it has blisters (possible shingles)
	• Red, hot, painful skin (possible cellulitis)
	• New spot or mole, especially if it is enlarging or if it is a sore that is not healing
Raynaud's phenomenon	• Fingers or toes develop open sores or become dark purple, black, and painful without returning to normal after warming up
Chest pain	• First episode or any new type of chest pain
Trouble breathing	• Any new episode of shortness of breath
Difficulty urinating	• Urinary frequency, urgency, or discomfort when you urinate (UTI symptoms)
	• Inability to urinate, with a burning sensation or pressure in the lower abdomen
	• Weakness or loss of sensation in your legs
	• Back pain
Numbness	• Weight loss
	• Leg bruising
	• Sudden loss of sensation in an arm, leg, or face
Muscle weakness	• Face muscle weakness (droopy face)
	• Double vision
	• Difficulty talking, slurred speech
	• Weakness in an arm or leg
	• Difficulty raising the arms to brush your hair or difficulty standing from a chair without using your arms to push yourself up

Table 40.I (*continued*)

Headache	• Sinus congestion or thick nasal secretions
	• New type of headache, especially if "the worst headache I've ever had in my life"
	• Nausea and vomiting (unless it is a classic, recurrent migraine that has been evaluated and diagnosed before)
	• Worsens in different body positions
	• Arm or leg muscle weakness, numbness
	• Abrupt visual changes (unless it is a migraine that has been previously diagnosed)
Stomach upset	• Nausea, vomiting
	• Black/tarry stool, blood in the stool
	• Severe pain
Blurred vision	• Red and/or painful eyes
	• Headache
	• Double vision

considering infection first. If you have had a fever before with lupus flares, then it is usually accompanied by other lupus problems such as joint pains, hair loss, chest pain when you take in a deep breath (pleurisy), cutaneous (skin) lupus, or mouth sores.

Fever can also occur with other dangerous problems such as lung blood clots, which can also cause chest pain and shortness of breath.

Sometimes, it can be difficult to tell whether a fever is from SLE or infection. In this case, it may be best to treat both possibilities.

We recommend that our patients call and see their doctor if they get a fever. If it develops in the evening or weekend, they should go to an ER or UCC.

Fatigue

Around 20% of the population, most of whom do not have an illness, admit to significant fatigue. This is usually due to being overworked or not getting enough sleep. The percentage is much higher in SLE (chapter 6).

Fatigue means having a lack of energy (mental or physical) to do activities that should be effortless, such as doing the dishes or sweeping the floor. Fatigue can also develop from a nonstrenuous activity, such as bathing and getting dressed. It is normal, and expected, to have occasional fatigue, especially when we're overworked or get less than eight hours of sleep. But when it is persistent or occurs most of the time, and interferes with quality of life, it is a problem.

Blood pressure medicines, antidepressants, antihistamines, immunosuppressants, pain drugs, muscle relaxants, and even steroids can cause fatigue. If it develops soon after you start a new drug, call your doctor. They would commonly reduce the dose or

What to do if you develop a drug side effect

The wrong thing to do is put up with it. Too many patients do this thinking they are supposed to have side effects in exchange for the drug working for them. However, we do not want patients to have side effects. Most side effects are not harmful (what we call nuisance side effects), but some can be dangerous. For example, a little stomach upset on naproxen could be an ulcer, requiring an anti-acid. If you develop a side effect, look up the drug in the index and review the drug's table of side effects; it also gives advice on what to do. However, also contact your doctor.

For example, hydroxychloroquine (HCQ) is an important SLE drug (table 30.1), so if a patient were to get stomach upset on HCQ, we would not tell them to stop taking it. Instead, we would recommend that they take it with dinner, split up the dose, or take bismuth subsalicylate (Pepto Bismol) with it. If those measures did not work, then we'd recommend that they cut the pills into quarter or half portions with a pill splitter (the portion sizes do not need to be exact with HCQ) and start with one tiny portion a day with food. In a week, increase to one of those tiny pieces twice daily, and so on. We tell them their job is to figure out the maximum dose they can tolerate without stomach upset.

try something different. Fatigue can also be a symptom while coming down or off a medicine. For example, decreasing steroids too quickly may cause fatigue from adrenal insufficiency (chapter 26).

Sometimes fatigue can point to a more urgent medical problem. **New-onset fatigue accompanied by shortness of breath, chest pain, stomach pain, trouble thinking, numbness or weakness in an arm or leg, difficulty talking, fever, headache, or weight loss calls for urgent medical attention.**

Some disorders, such as muscle weakness, can be mistaken for fatigue. For example, if you have difficulty raising your arms to brush your hair or have trouble standing up from a chair without using your arms to push you up, these could be caused by lupus myositis or thyroid disease, among other possibilities. If you have actual muscle weakness, see your doctor.

If you get less than seven to eight hours of high-quality sleep a day, have trouble falling asleep, wake up throughout the night, or feel exhausted when you wake up (as if you did not get a good night's sleep), you may have a sleep disorder. Poor lifestyle habits (not scheduling enough sleep, not exercising, smoking cigarettes, drinking alcohol too close to bedtime, and so on) can affect sleep. So can a disorder that interrupts sleep, such as depression, anxiety, fibromyalgia, or sleep apnea. To look for possible causes of sleep problems (and therefore find possible ways to help that problem), go to tables 6.4, 13.3, and 13.5, and read how fibromyalgia is diagnosed in chapter 27. If you have a high score on these tests, you may have one of these problems, and you should show the results to your doctor. You should also see your doctor if you adhere strictly to the sleep hygiene and fatigue management suggestions (tables 6.1, 6.2, and 6.3), but still have trouble with sleep and fatigue. A sleep study may be helpful.

Joint and Muscle Pain

Ninety percent of SLE patients get joint and muscle pain. See chapter 7 for a complete discussion.

If you develop a new pain that is tolerable, it is better to contact your doctor than go to a UCC or ER for several reasons. One is that UCC or ER personnel will probably assume lupus to be the cause and give patients dangerous amounts of unnecessary steroids. Your doctor can provide better and safer treatments, such as joint cortisone injections, that are not done in the ER. Also, ER personnel do not have the expertise to perform an adequate joint exam, which is to accurately diagnose the cause of joint pain. Too often, they rely on x-rays, which can identify bone and cartilage damage but not inflammation or soft tissue problems. For example, if you go to the ER with hip pain, an x-ray might show osteoarthritis, but if the real cause is bursitis, the x-ray would not pick it up. Bursitis treatment is different from osteoarthritis treatment. The best treatment cannot be given unless the cause of the pain is accurately identified.

Gout (arthritis due to uric acid) can also cause red, painful foot swelling, especially around the big toe. Rheumatologists are the specialists who treat gout.

There are, however, situations when you should go to a UCC or an ER. One is if you have severe, intolerable joint pain.

Rashes and Other Skin Problems

Rashes are among the most common problems in lupus (chapter 8). If you have been doing well for a while, but then your lupus rash recurs or gets worse, see your rheumatologist or review your "Flare Plan" (table 5.2).

People with lupus can develop rashes from non-lupus problems. Drugs are a common cause. An allergic reaction to a drug typically shows up as a rash 7 to 10 days after starting the medication. If you develop hives or a red rash soon after starting a new drug, contact the prescribing doctor at once. Note, though, that some drugs cause subacute cutaneous lupus to appear or worsen weeks to years after starting them (chapter 8).

People with lupus are at increased risk of skin cancer. This can occur from a viral infection called human papillomavirus (chapter 22) and possibly from some immunosuppressants (chapter 23). Show your doctor any new, growing, or nonhealing areas of skin.

An area of red, hot, tender skin (especially on the lower legs) could be a skin infection called cellulitis. If this happens, you should see a doctor right away for antibiotics.

Shingles can result in a painful, blistering rash (chapter 22). **It is crucial to seek medical attention for shingles at once.** Rapid treatment can prevent permanent nerve damage and chronic pain.

Anti-malarials, such as hydroxychloroquine (HCQ), can cause skin discoloration. This often develops slowly on the front of the legs, forehead, or neck, typically after months to years of use and is not a dangerous condition. It may get better when the doses of these drugs are decreased. They should not be discontinued since their health benefits outweigh any cosmetic side effects.

Skin discoloration can also occur in areas previously affected by cutaneous lupus inflammation, such as on the cheeks or the ears (chapter 8). This is part of the healing process.

Many people with SLE have Raynaud's phenomenon (chapter 11). **Severe pain and change of color of a toe or finger to dark purple, or even black, that does not improve after rewarming suggests a complete loss of blood flow and warrants urgent medical attention.**

Chest Pain

Chest pain can be caused by something as simple as indigestion, gastroesophageal reflux, or a muscle spasm. However, some causes (heart attack, pulmonary embolism, or aneurysm) are potentially deadly and require prompt medical evaluation. One of the most common causes of death in lupus is cardiovascular disease (heart attacks, strokes, and blood clots). **If you ever get chest pain for the first time, seek immediate medical attention.** Do not wait to see if it will go away or schedule an appointment to see your doctor later.

Some people get recurrent chest pain from a previously diagnosed cause that does not require immediate medical attention. In this case, ask your doctor what you should do when it occurs.

Chest pain examples are discussed below.

Heart Attacks (Myocardial Infarctions)

A heart attack (myocardial infarction, chapter 21) occurs when a blockage in a coronary (heart) artery causes a part of the heart muscle to die. The typical symptoms are severe, crushing pressure-like chest pain under the breastbone that may radiate to the jaw, neck, or left arm. It usually worsens with exertion and improves with rest. Similar (but milder) pain that comes and goes could be due to intermittent decreases in heart muscle blood flow. This is called angina. **Any new chest pain should be treated as a medical emergency.** Rapid treatment can minimize heart muscle damage and prevent death.

LUPUS IN FOCUS

Should you go to the ER or an urgent care center (UCC)?

Some tests can only be done in a hospital. Blood clots in the lungs or legs (pulmonary embolisms and deep venous thrombosis), heart attacks, and strokes can be diagnosed and treated in an ER connected to a hospital. UCCs are usually not adequate. *If you have shortness of breath, chest pain, stroke symptoms (chapter 13), or a painful, red, swollen calf, go to the ER.*

Most infections (unless severe) and many matters not listed above (such as cuts that need sutures or a sprained ankle) can be evaluated and treated at a UCC. Also, wait times are typically shorter in UCCs than in ERs.

Lung Blood Clots (Pulmonary Embolism)

A pulmonary embolism (PE) occurs when a blood clot blocks a lung blood vessel (chapters 9, 10, 11, and 21). This can be life-threatening. Sometimes it is preceded by symptoms of a clot in the leg called deep vein thrombosis, which may cause pain and swelling in one of the calf muscles, sometimes accompanied by red-colored, warm skin. PE may occur after sitting or lying for a long time in one spot, such as after surgery, being sick in bed, or after a long car or plane trip. PE can cause rapid-onset stabbing chest pain with shortness of breath. The chest pain may worsen with deep breathing, as in pleurisy. Sometimes the person may cough up blood. Other symptoms such as light-headedness, dizziness, fever, and a feeling of dread or anxiety, may also occur. **Seek immediate medical attention if you have any of these.**

Thoracic Aortic Aneurysm

A thoracic aortic aneurysm (chapter 11) occurs when a part of the largest artery, the aorta, swells like a balloon and is in danger of rupturing. It can cause deep, throbbing chest pain or back pain, shortness of breath, cough, or hoarseness. **An aortic aneurysm is a medical emergency requiring lifesaving surgery.**

Gastroesophageal Reflux Disease

Gastroesophageal reflux disease (GERD, chapter 28) is due to acidic stomach contents traveling up into the esophagus (located in the chest cavity under the breastbone). Although many people will feel heartburn, sometimes chest pain or dry, nagging cough may be the only symptoms. Often the chest pain worsens with lying down or improves after taking an antacid such as Tums or Maalox. Other problems, such as esophageal muscle spasms, can also cause chest pain. **Never assume that new-onset chest pain is due to GERD; go to your closest ER.**

Musculoskeletal Chest Wall Pain

Musculoskeletal (MSK) chest wall pain occurs when ligaments, tendons, muscles, ribs, or cartilage are the pain source. Costochondritis is one example of MSK chest wall pain. Its symptoms include tenderness over the area where the ribs connect to the breastbone at cartilage connections, often at the left lower side of the breastbone, but potentially anywhere on the chest. Fibromyalgia is another common cause of MSK. Other causes that could be life-threatening need to be excluded, though, so **if you develop MSK chest wall pain, go to the ER.**

Trouble Breathing

Any new episode of breathing difficulty is a medical emergency that requires immediate attention at an ER. It is essential to ensure no heart or lung problems (chapters 10, 11, 21). A low red blood cell count (anemia) can also cause shortness of breath. Other possibilities, such as weight gain or lack of exercise, are common causes of gradually increasing shortness of breath with activity. However, they are usually considered after other dangerous causes are excluded.

Difficulty Urinating

Urinary tract infections (UTIs) are among the most common reasons for urination problems in SLE. A bacterial infection usually causes bladder wall irritation and uncontrollable bladder contractions, which cause a sense of urgency to urinate and increased urinary frequency. A burning discomfort or pain may accompany urination. A UTI may or may not cause fever. Let your doctor know if you develop UTI symptoms. If you wait too long, the infection could travel up to the kidneys or even enter the blood, causing a severe and potentially life-threatening condition called sepsis.

Some pain drugs, such as tramadol and antidepressants, can interfere with how the bladder muscles squeeze out urine. Signs include having trouble urinating and feeling pressure in the lower abdominal area where the bladder is. If you have recently started a new drug, call your doctor at once.

As men get older, most develop a problem called benign prostatic hypertrophy (BPH). The prostate is an organ encircling the urethra at the lower part of the urinary bladder. It helps to keep the bladder closed until it is time to urinate. As men get older, the prostate enlarges. The enlarged prostate squeezes on the urethra, causing difficulty urinating (imagine squeezing a garden hose). They may develop smaller urinary streams and have trouble starting urination. It may take them longer to urinate, and they may not be able to empty their bladders. This can cause them to urinate more often (including getting up throughout the night to urinate). This is rarely a medical emergency unless it occurs abruptly.

A rare lupus problem occurs when the nerves going to the urinary bladder are compromised, causing the bladder not to squeeze out urine correctly. One potential cause is lupus myelitis (chapter 13), in which lupus attacks the spinal cord, causing paralysis, loss of sensation in the legs, and difficulties with urination and defecating. Sometimes, the opposite can occur, with no control over urination and urinating when you do not want to (incontinence). Incontinence can also be caused by other spine problems such as herniated disks, spinal cord tumors, infections, or broken bones in the back. **You need immediate medical attention if you cannot urinate and feel pressure building up in the lower abdominal area** (where the bladder is).

Another rare cause of urination problems is lupus cystitis (chapter 12). This is seen exclusively in women of Asian ancestry. Immunosuppressants are needed; a correct and prompt diagnosis is essential.

Along with UTIs, the most common cause of urination problems in women is incontinence, especially stress incontinence. This occurs in some women when they age due to the pelvic muscles not working normally. Women can also develop an overactive bladder, causing frequent urination or bladder incontinence that worsens with time. See your primary care provider, gynecologist, or urologist (bladder specialist) for these problems.

Numbness

Decreased skin sensation, or numbness, is most commonly a nerve problem. Some nerve problems are medical emergencies, the best known of which are strokes (chapters 13 and 21). Strokes occur from brain damage and are referred to as "heart attacks of the brain." **Seek urgent medical care if you have abrupt weakness or loss of feeling of an arm, leg, or one side of the face.** If doctors diagnose a stroke within the first couple of hours, they can use blood thinners to reverse the stroke and prevent permanent brain damage.

Numbness can also occur from nerve problems such as lupus myelitis (chapter 13).

Lupus vasculitis can cause numbness from mononeuritis multiplex (chapter 13). A common clue to this is difficulty flexing the foot upward (foot drop). Most people with mononeuritis multiplex from vasculitis are usually very sick and often have other symptoms such as fever, weight loss, and bruising on the legs (called petechiae or palpable purpura, chapter 8). **If you develop foot drop, urgent medical attention is needed.**

Peripheral neuropathy (chapter 13) is the most common cause of numbness from SLE. It is due to small-nerve damage in the arms and legs. It most commonly causes a gradual onset of decreased sensation in the feet, sometimes followed by similar problems in the hands, often in a "stocking and glove" distribution. This is usually not an emergency, but it does require your doctor's attention.

Muscle Weakness

Muscle weakness refers to when muscles are truly weak. This is different from generalized fatigue. **Abrupt onset of arm or leg weakness can potentially mean a stroke. An abrupt onset of weakness in both legs could mean spinal cord damage from lupus (myelitis) or other emergencies, such as Guillain-Barré syndrome. These problems require immediate medical attention.**

Strokes and cranial neuropathies (chapter 13) can sometimes affect facial muscles, causing one side of the face to look very different, as well as problems with double vision, talking, smiling, or opening and closing the eyes. **Any of these symptoms should prompt seeking immediate medical attention.**

Difficulty raising your arms to brush your hair or difficulty standing up from a chair without using your hands can sometimes be due to muscle inflammation (lupus myositis, chapter 7). This condition should be assessed and treated quickly to prevent severe muscle weakness problems. **Any new onset of any form of muscle weakness is a medical emergency requiring immediate medical attention.**

Headache

Any type of new headache, especially severe, needs to be taken seriously. See chapter 13 for complete details and descriptions.

Sinusitis is an infection of the sinuses of the bones of the face. Sinuses are air-filled cavities that lighten the weight of the skull and transmit sound waves. Fluid can build up if the sinus passages are blocked by mucous or inflammation (allergies, infection, or Sjögren's, chapter 14). This typically causes face pain associated with a sense of fullness or congestion. The headache may feel worse when the head is lowered or if pressure is applied to the bones of the face. Fever and thick nasal secretions are other symptoms. Infections such as sinusitis can potentially be dangerous in SLE patients and need to be identified and treated quickly.

Ruptured brain aneurysms typically cause an abrupt onset of severe headache often described as "the worst headache I've ever had in my life." **A ruptured aneurysm is a life-threatening situation usually requiring emergency surgery.**

Brain tumors can cause headaches 50% of the time. Brain tumor headaches may cause nausea and vomiting (just as a migraine can) and worsen with body positions (similar to sinusitis headache).

A medication overuse headache is one that develops in someone who uses pain relievers such as opioids, acetaminophen (Tylenol), or NSAIDs for recurrent migraine or tension headaches. Over time, these pain relievers may cause the headaches to worsen. Proper treatment is to stop all pain medicines.

The evaluation and treatment of chronic headaches can be complex. A headache expert, most commonly a neurologist, best manages these situations.

Stomach Upset

The most common reason for stomach upset in SLE patients is medications. Even multiple vitamins and calcium supplements can cause stomach upset. If you develop stomach upset soon after starting a new drug, contact your doctor. They will often stop the drug or lower its dose. Sometimes drugs that calm the stomach's acidity may help. GERD and ulcers also cause stomach upset (chapter 28).

Mesenteric vasculitis is one of the most devastating SLE complications (chapter 15). Fortunately, it is rare. It occurs when SLE causes inflammation in the intestinal arteries, causing decreased blood flow and death to part of the intestines. Usually, people are very sick and have other symptoms such as fever and weight loss. **Abdominal pain, nausea, and vomiting can be severe enough to require emergency medical care.**

Inflammation of the abdominal cavity lining (the peritoneal cavity) is called peritonitis (chapter 15). This may cause abdominal pain, fever, and tenderness of the abdomen.

Pancreas inflammation (pancreatitis) can be life-threatening. **Symptoms include nausea and vomiting with upper abdominal pain, sometimes spreading to the back, and require emergency medical care.** The most common causes of pancreatitis are gall bladder stones, drugs, and alcoholism. However, lupus can rarely cause it (chapter 15).

Blurred Vision

You need to see an eye doctor for blurred vision. Many quickly blame their hydroxychloroquine (HCQ) and want to stop taking it. Please do not do this because HCQ is the safest lupus drug with many benefits (table 30.1). Most of the time, blurred vision in lupus patients is due to other problems, such as cataracts (clouding of the lens), dry eyes (chapter 14), or a change in glasses prescriptions. Vision problems from HCQ retina problems are rare as long as you get your proper annual eye tests (chapter 30). Always let your eye doctor figure out the causes. **Blurred vision associated with eye pain, red eye, headache, or double vision can signify something more dangerous, such as an eye infection, glaucoma, vasculitis, uveitis, nerve damage, or stroke. If these symptoms occur, seek immediate medical attention.**

Is the Problem Lupus or Not?

Since SLE can affect nearly every body part, it is common to blame lupus for many problems, even when lupus is not the cause. If you have been told that any of your symptoms are "due to" lupus, it is best to discuss with your rheumatologist to confirm.

On the flip side, some lupus symptoms may be confused for other things. If you have lupus and are admitted to the hospital for anything (other than a planned surgery or procedure), always ask the admitting physician to have the hospital's rheumatologist look at you, even if the admission problem is not lupus-related. For example, lupus pneumonitis (chapter 10) can look just like bacterial pneumonia, but the treatment would be to use immunosuppressants instead of antibiotics (or use both). A stroke or heart attack from SLE may need special therapy, such as warfarin, in addition to the standard treatments. It may be necessary for some of your lupus drugs to be changed during admission. Having a rheumatologist guide these decisions will be beneficial. Also, additional stress (from infection or hospital admission, among other things) could make your SLE worse in the weeks afterward, so try to schedule an appointment with your rheumatologist at discharge.

KEY POINTS TO REMEMBER

1. Some problems and symptoms occurring in lupus patients require immediate medical attention (such as an ER). Use the recommendations in table 40.1 and all bold font sections above to help guide you.

2. Some problems are common in SLE, such as headache and fatigue. This chapter discusses many of these.

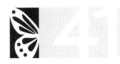

Prepare for Pregnancy, Breast-Feeding, Contraception, Menopause

Jill P. Buyon, MD, *Contributing Editor*

With proper preparation for and monitoring during pregnancy, most women with SLE will have a good outcome and a healthy baby. This is a huge change compared to previous decades. As recently as the 1980s, most women with SLE were told not to get pregnant.

However, the risks of complications, such as a miscarriage, preeclampsia (high blood pressure with protein in the urine), early delivery, and lupus flares are still real. If you have SLE and follow the advice in this chapter, your chances of having a successful pregnancy will significantly increase. If you desire to breast-feed, this chapter advises on what drugs are safe. You can also look up all your drugs in the index, locate them in the book, and see what to do with them before pregnancy, during pregnancy, and while breast-feeding.

We encourage women with SLE interested in becoming pregnant to read chapter 18 first, then return to this chapter.

But note that it is also crucial to know how to prevent unintended pregnancy. Some drugs require strict birth control. This chapter gives you the practical tools to prevent pregnancy when your doctor advises you to avoid it and have a successful pregnancy when desired.

Menopause advice is provided at the end of the chapter.

How to Have a Successful Pregnancy

The first step is to assess your risk for having a difficult pregnancy. Review risk factors in table 41.1. Put a check mark next to each item that applies to you. You can ask your rheumatologist for assistance if need be. You can also ask your rheumatologist to do any of the labs listed if they have not been done. Some of these, such as anti-SSA (also called anti-Ro) and antiphospholipid antibodies (aPLAs: lupus anticoagulant, cardiolipin antibodies, and beta-2-glycoprotein I antibodies), are essential. It helps to check them even if they were checked in the past. Previously positive anti-SSA and aPLAs can become negative over time with treatment. They are not problematic if they become negative.

Add up your checkmarks to estimate your risk of having a complicated pregnancy. The higher your score, the higher your chances of having complications. If you score 0 and follow everything in this chapter, your chance of having a healthy baby is excellent.

You have no control over some factors in table 41.1 (such as being Hispanic or African American or being positive for lupus anticoagulant). You do, however, have control

Table 41.1 Pregnancy Complication Risk Factors

Risk Factors You Can Potentially Control	What You Can Do
Have had active SLE (such as lupus nephritis, fluid around lungs, or bad anemia) within the previous 6 months	Avoid pregnancy until SLE is under control for 6 months.
Elevated blood pressure	Work with your doctor to keep blood pressure less than 130/80.
Not taking an antimalarial such as hydroxychloroquine	Take an antimalarial if tolerated.
BMI > 25 kg/m²	Work on weight loss before pregnancy.
High cholesterol	Work on lowering bad cholesterol (LDL) and increasing good cholesterol (HDL).
Uncontrolled thyroid disease (not including subclinical hypothyroidism, chapter 17)	Work with your doctor to normalize your TSH.

Risk Factors Not under Your Control

C3 or C4 level currently or recently lower than your usual

Platelet count is currently or recently lower than your usual

Anti-ds DNA is currently or recently higher than your usual

Positive for anti-thyroid antibodies or have Hashimoto's or Graves' disease, chapter 17

SSA antibody positive

Antiphospholipid antibody positive: anticardiolipin antibodies, beta-2-glycoprotein-I antibodies, **and especially lupus anticoagulant**

African, Hispanic, or Asian **descent**

Take a blood pressure pill (even if your blood pressure is perfect)

Poor socioeconomic factors (see main text)

Note: Items in **bold** are the most important. Read full details in the main text.

of others, and you should deal with them to maximize your chances of having a successful pregnancy.

As of January 2023, the most extensive pregnancy research study is the PROMISSE study, published in 2017. It showed that the most important risk factors that increase the chances for bad pregnancy outcomes are being positive for lupus anticoagulant, being of African or Hispanic ethnicity, and taking a blood pressure drug (even if blood pressure was under good control). Lower socioeconomic status, in terms of education and income on the personal and community levels, was also a factor. Participants were instructed not to get pregnant until after six months of stable lupus disease and to take hydroxychloroquine (HCQ) during pregnancy. Therefore, these two risk factors (having active disease at the time of pregnancy and not taking HCQ) could not be evaluated.

Some problems cause such a high risk of poor pregnancy outcomes that experts strongly recommend not getting pregnant (table 41.2). Having pulmonary hypertension (high blood pressure in the lung's arteries) is one. Severe interstitial lung disease (ILD) is another. However, it is safe to get pregnant if ILD is mild. If you have ILD and pulmonary hypertension and want to know about pregnancy, ask your lung and heart specialists.

Here are practical steps you can take to maximize your chances of having a successful pregnancy.

1. ***Ensure that SLE is under control for at least six months before pregnancy.*** This is the most crucial initial step. Avoid an unplanned pregnancy by using birth control measures (discussed below). If you decide you would like to have a baby, talk to your rheumatologist and find out how you should prepare. If your SLE has not been under reasonable control, your first goal is to get it under control before trying to get pregnant. After six months of reasonable lupus control, it is safer to attempt pregnancy.

A study of 275 pregnancies showed that if a woman with SLE had active disease within three months of getting pregnant, she was four times more likely to lose her baby. When the disease was under control for six months before pregnancy, the chances of a good outcome approached that of a healthy woman.

Some of the risk factors in table 41.1 are signs of active SLE. These include elevated urine protein, abnormal kidney function, low complement levels, elevated anti-ds DNA, and a low platelet count. While it is best to get all these tests within normal ranges in pregnancy preparation, this is not possible for everyone. Reasonable control of SLE varies from patient to patient. Some may have chronic high anti-dsDNA or low complements, which are not likely to become normal, but their SLE may be doing well.

Another example is kidney involvement. Some patients may have residual protein in the urine but otherwise have normal kidney function and no active inflammation

Table 41.2 Reasons Not to Get Pregnant

- Have pulmonary hypertension (felt to be an absolute contraindication by some)
- Had stroke or heart attack
- Have chronic kidney disease stage 4 or 5 (eGFR < 30 mL/min)
- Have severe interstitial lung disease with poor oxygenation (ask lung specialist)

(lupus nephritis). While these women may be at higher risk for lupus nephritis flares during pregnancy than those who have never had kidney disease, they may still do well. What is important is to refrain from pregnancy when there is a lot of protein in the urine, decreased kidney function, or active lupus nephritis.

Regarding the platelet count, doctors generally do not use stronger medicines than HCQ if the platelet count remains above 20,000 platelets/microL (also notated as 20,000/ μL, or 20,000 platelets per microliter). Normal platelet count levels are higher than 140,000/microL in many labs. However, in SLE, they are not dangerous unless they are much lower. It is unusual to have a bleeding problem if the platelets remain above 20,000/microL.

Although bleeding occurs during all vaginal and cesarean deliveries, if the platelet count stays above 20,000/microL, the baby's delivery is usually safe without additional treatments. However, if an epidural is needed at the time of vaginal delivery, the anesthesiologist may want the platelets to be above 80,000 and may recommend steroids.

Ask your rheumatologist if additional treatment for your lupus is warranted if you have any abnormal tests (elevated urine protein, low complement levels, high anti-ds DNA, and low platelets). Consider egg freezing if pregnancy is delayed (see below).

2. *Ensure that blood pressure is under good control.* Many experts recommend keeping the top number (systolic blood pressure) less than 140 mmHg and the bottom number (diastolic blood pressure) below 90 mmHg during pregnancy. You may need to frequently see your primary care provider (or cardiologist or nephrologist) for medication adjustments.

Working on diet, weight loss, and exercise helps. So does staying away from high-sodium (salty) foods. Use a home blood pressure machine. If your blood pressure is consistently higher than the recommended levels, see your doctor for drug adjustments. Also, make sure your device is accurate. Take it with you to a doctor's visit and compare its results with your doctor's.

Many blood pressure drugs cannot be used during pregnancy. For example, angiotensin-converting-enzyme inhibitors and angiotensin receptor blockers (ACEi and ARBs, table 12.4), commonly used in lupus nephritis, should not be used during the second and third trimesters. Someone who needs an ACEi or ARB may continue it in the first trimester but would need to change to a pregnancy-safe drug by the second trimester.

Most doctors advise changing ACEi and ARBs during the several months leading up to conception. Hydrochlorothiazide (HCTZ), methyldopa, hydralazine, calcium channel blockers, and labetalol are safe pregnancy alternatives.

3. *Ensure that you take your anti-malarial regularly.* Whatever you do, ***do not stop taking your hydroxychloroquine (HCQ, Plaquenil).*** One of the worst things to occur during pregnancy is a lupus flare. HCQ helps prevent them.

HCQ also decreases miscarriage risks, reduces antiphospholipid antibody levels, and lowers the chances of having a baby with neonatal lupus if you are anti-SSA positive (chapter 18).

HCQ does not cause any problems with the baby. Instead, HCQ increases your baby's survival chances.

4. ***If you are taking a drug that is unsafe in pregnancy, ask that it be changed to a pregnancy-safe drug before attempting pregnancy.*** Table 41.3 lists drugs used in lupus

Table 41.3 Lupus Drugs and Pregnancy

Drug	Management during Pregnancy
abatacept (Orencia)	Stop before pregnancy. Don't take during pregnancy (not studied).
adalimumab (Humira)	Safe
anifrolumab (Saphnelo)	Stop before pregnancy (not studied).
aspirin (81 mg–162 mg)	Use throughout pregnancy if no bleeding risks.
azathioprine (Imuran)	Safe
baricitinib (Olumiant)	Stop when trying to get pregnant.
belimumab (Benlysta)	Stop before pregnancy. (This may change, so ask your doctor.)
bisphosphonates (table 24.9)	Avoid pregnancy for 6 months after stopping.
certolizumab pegol (Cimzia)	Safe
chloroquine	Safe
colchicine	Safe
cyclophosphamide	Stop 3 months before trying to get pregnant. Used for life-threatening SLE in 2nd and 3rd trimesters.
cyclosporine	Safe
etanercept (Enbrel)	Safe
golimumab (Simponi)	Safe
heparin	Safe
hydroxychloroquine (Plaquenil)	**Safe!** Absolutely take the drug if there are no reasons not to.
infliximab (Remicade)	Safe
IVIG	Safe
leflunomide (Arava)	Use the cholestyramine elimination protocol (chapter 32). Need 2 negative drug level results before pregnancy. These recommendations may change; ask your doctor.
methotrexate	Stop 1 month before trying to get pregnant.
methylprednisolone (Medrol)	Use lowest needed dose.
mycophenolate (CellCept, Myfortic)	Stop 6 weeks before trying to get pregnant.
NSAIDs (table 36.1)	Stop before 3rd trimester; avoid celecoxib (Celebrex).
prednisone	Use lowest needed dose.
quinacrine	Do not use (safety unknown).

Table 41.3 (*continued*)

rituximab (Rituxan)	Stop before pregnancy. Can be used during pregnancy if needed.
statins for cholesterol	May be continued in some patients; ask your doctor.
sulfasalazine (Azulfidine)	Safe
tacrolimus	Safe
thalidomide	Stop for 1 month before trying to get pregnant.
tocilizumab (Actemra)	Stop before pregnancy. Don't take during pregnancy (not studied).
tofacitinib (Xeljanz)	Stop before pregnancy.
upadacitinib (Rinvoq)	Stop before pregnancy.
ustekinumab (Stelara)	Stop before pregnancy. Don't take during pregnancy (not studied).
voclosporin (Lupkynis)	Stop before pregnancy.
warfarin (Coumadin)	Stop before pregnancy; switch to heparin if needed.

and their pregnancy safety. Some drugs must be stopped for some time before getting pregnant. While waiting, use effective, safe birth control (discussed later). Drugs that should be stopped followed by a waiting period before getting pregnant include mycophenolate (six weeks), cyclophosphamide (three months), methotrexate (one month), thalidomide (one month), and bisphosphonates (six months). Janus kinase inhibitors (tofacitinib, upadacitinib, baricitinib) and belimumab safety are unknown and should be stopped before pregnancy. However, belimumab appears to be safe among women in some research, as of April 2023, so this recommendation could change (ask your doctor).

If you get pregnant while taking unsafe drugs listed in table 41.3, stop the drug immediately and contact your doctors.

Your doctor usually needs to replace an immunosuppressant that is stopped with a safe alternative. Azathioprine is the most common substitution. Since it can take up to three months for azathioprine to work, it is best to make this drug substitution at least three months before pregnancy to ensure it keeps your SLE under control.

Some of the drugs considered to be contraindicated during pregnancy may be needed if your SLE becomes active. In the case of a severe lupus flare, high-dose steroids, intravenous gammaglobulins (IVIG), plasmapheresis (chapter 35), cyclophosphamide, or rituximab (Rituxan) can be used. If cyclophosphamide is necessary, it is safer to give it during the second and third trimesters (preferably the third). Rituximab may be used, if needed, at any time.

These drug planning recommendations can be quite complex. Ensure your rheumatologist writes down all recommendations. Later in this chapter, we will look at an example of a lupus patient planning her pregnancy.

Statins (table 21.5), which are cholesterol-lowering drugs that can reduce heart attacks and strokes, most likely do not pose risks to the fetus. In 2021, the FDA asked statin producers to remove the pregnancy contraindication from their statins, stating that they could be used in patients at high risk for cardiovascular events during pregnancy. Of interest, a 2016 Greek and United Kingdom collaboration study showed that women with antiphospholipid syndrome who took pravastatin and blood thinners had a higher rate of successful pregnancies than women treated with blood thinners alone. Using pravastatin in this manner needs more study.

5. *Observe special considerations with NSAIDs.* It is common to use an NSAID (table 36.1) for lupus arthritis or pleurisy during pregnancy. Acetaminophen is preferred. NSAIDs should be stopped after about 30 weeks. If they are not stopped, there is the potential that a blood vessel (the ductus arteriosus) could close prematurely, resulting in problems with the baby's lung circulation.

NSAIDs may decrease some women's chances of getting pregnant (conceiving). If you are trying to conceive and are unsuccessful, consider stopping NSAIDs if you are taking one.

In October 2020, the FDA recognized that NSAIDs could cause kidney problems in the fetus or oligohydramnios (too little fluid in the womb) at around 20 weeks of pregnancy. If NSAIDs are required at 20 weeks and later, it is recommended to use the lowest dose possible for the shortest amount of time.

6. *Take low-dose aspirin throughout pregnancy.* Taking low-dose aspirin (81 mg to 162 mg daily) lowers the risk of preeclampsia (chapter 18). You should begin aspirin while attempting pregnancy if you are not at high risk for bleeding (ask your doctor) and continue up to delivery. An exception is when a Cesarean section is planned, in which case aspirin may need to be stopped 5–14 days before surgery (ask all your doctors).

7. *Protect your baby with vaccines.* Get your recommended vaccines: COVID-19, pneumococcal, the flu shot yearly in the fall, and all recommended vaccines, including a tetanus vaccine (chapter 22). These can protect you and your baby.

8. *Do not take any drugs during pregnancy unless approved by your rheumatologist and obstetrician.* Your rheumatologist can usually address your SLE drugs, but you need to check with your obstetrician about other medicines. Do this before pregnancy.

9. *Do not smoke.* There are many reasons why lupus patients should not smoke (chapter 38). It is more critical during pregnancy because it increases the risk of preeclamp-

LUPUS IN FOCUS

Register in a pregnancy drug registry if you are on the drug while pregnant

Drug clinical trials (research studies) do not include pregnant women. We can learn about pregnancy drug safety only by monitoring what happens when women on certain drugs accidentally become pregnant. Many drugs have pregnancy registries that collect information from women who become pregnant and track how they do. If you get pregnant while on a medication, enroll in that drug's pregnancy registry (if there is one). Also, contact the MotherToBaby study at 866-626-6847 or mothertobaby.org.

sia, death of the baby, congenital malformations, preterm delivery, and a baby born smaller than normal. The unhealthy effects of smoking during pregnancy continue after delivery. Babies born to mothers who smoke are at increased risk for sudden infant death syndrome, lung and ear infections, asthma, colic, shorter height, obesity, and hyperactivity. They also have short attention spans and tend not to perform well in school, particularly in reading and spelling. Even secondhand smoke has been associated with an increased risk of stillbirth (death of the baby), congenital malformations, and having a baby born smaller than normal.

10. *Do not drink alcohol.* Drinking alcohol during pregnancy increases the chances of stillbirth and congenital malformations related to fetal alcohol syndrome. There is no safe alcohol amount during pregnancy.

11. *Exercise regularly during pregnancy unless told otherwise.* Regular exercise is important during pregnancy because it decreases the chances of complications, including diabetes and preeclampsia. However, physical activity restrictions may be needed for pregnant women with some medical conditions. Ask your obstetrician.

12. *Eat a healthy diet.* Remember that you are eating for two during pregnancy but don't overeat. Consider seeing a dietician to learn what foods (and amounts of food) are best. Extra precautions need to be taken to decrease the risk of foodborne illnesses (such as hepatitis A, listeria, toxoplasmosis, or brucellosis). If you eat a healthy diet full of whole grains, vegetables, fruit, and an adequate amount of protein and dairy products, you may not need vitamin supplements, except for folic acid, as discussed next.

13. *Take supplements as directed by your obstetrician.* Unfortunately, most Americans do not eat a healthy diet, and most women need to take extra vitamins and minerals during pregnancy. Discuss this with your obstetrician, dietician, and rheumatologist.

If you are at increased risk of osteoporosis (chapter 24), you may need calcium and vitamin D supplements. The calcium recommendation is 1,000 mg a day during pregnancy to allow for the developing baby's skeleton's increased calcium needs.

Most SLE women are vitamin D deficient and should take vitamin D (chapters 35 and 38). Speak with your obstetrician or rheumatologist about the amount you need.

All pregnant women should take a daily supplement that contains at least 0.4 mg of folic acid one month before conception and continue it for several months after pregnancy. This helps prevent spina bifida (a spinal cord problem).

14. *See a high-risk obstetrician.* All SLE pregnancies are potentially high risk. We recommend that all patients see a high-risk obstetrician (maternal-fetal medicine specialist) before pregnancy. This applies especially to anyone who checked off any of the items in table 41.1. Try to see someone experienced in SLE.

15. *If you have any major organ involvement from SLE, see a specialist for that organ system during pregnancy.* This is especially true for heart, lung, kidney, or central nervous system involvement. Suppose you have had lupus nephritis before, but it is in remission when you get pregnant. In that case, you do not have to see a kidney doctor (nephrologist) if your urinary protein and blood eGFR are normal. Be sure, though, that your rheumatologist feels comfortable monitoring your kidneys.

If confirmed by cardiac catheterization, pulmonary hypertension (chapter 10) is such a high risk for poor pregnancy outcomes that many experts recommend that all women who have it should not get pregnant. Even so, a successful pregnancy is possible in some situations.

16. *Follow up with your rheumatologist regularly during pregnancy.* If SLE is under good control at conception, and you are not at high risk for complications (table 41.1), see your rheumatologist at least once each trimester. During these visits, labs checking for SLE disease activity, anti-dsDNA, and complements are done. You may need to be seen more often if you develop any active SLE problems such as rash, joint pain, pleurisy, difficulty breathing, extreme fatigue, ankle or eye swelling, or fever. If there is a history of lupus nephritis, more frequent monitoring may be needed. In general, your urine is checked every time you see the obstetrician. Any increases in urine protein should be immediately communicated to your rheumatologist. Early intervention for lupus flares can significantly increase the chances of a successful outcome.

17. *If you are positive for anti-SSA, have your baby's heart monitored.* SSA antibodies can cause congenital heart block (CHB), in which the baby's heart beats too slowly (chapter 18).

The 2020 American College of Rheumatology (ACR) guidelines recommend that anti-SSA-positive women have their baby's heart monitored using pulsed Doppler fetal echocardiography (fetal heart monitoring, usually by a pediatric cardiologist), which safely uses sound waves to assess the heart. This should begin around the 16th to 18th week and be continued through the 26th week. If you have had a baby in the past with CHB, you should have fetal heart testing weekly. If you have not, less often may be OK.

You can now monitor your own baby's heart with a handheld Doppler monitor at home. A study showed that mothers can identify abnormal rates and rhythms, and more studies are underway to further evaluate their use.

18. *If you are aPLA-positive, ask your rheumatologist if you should take blood thinners.* APLAs (especially lupus anticoagulant) increase the risk of blood clots in the placenta (the connection between the mom and baby). This increases the risk of miscarriage, stillbirth, preeclampsia, and other complications. Unless at high risk for bleeding, all women with SLE should take low-dose aspirin, 81 to 162 mg daily, throughout pregnancy. This may lower the risk of preeclampsia. HCQ also reduces these complications.

However, if you have had several early miscarriages in the past (three or more), have had a late pregnancy loss or stillbirth, or have ever had a blood clot of any kind, then you may have antiphospholipid syndrome (APS). Women with APS should probably also be taking a stronger blood thinner, such as low molecular weight heparin (LMWH, like

LUPUS IN FOCUS

Should all anti-SSA-positive women undergo fetal heart monitoring?

In women who have never had a baby with congenital heart block (CHB), 500 fetal heart monitoring ultrasounds are needed to identify one case of CHB. Because undergoing fetal ultrasounds requires a lot of time, is expensive (but usually covered by insurance), and can cause anxiety, some doctors question its use. But then CHB is potentially treatable if caught early, and if severe CHB occurs, it is permanent.

In our opinion, prevention is best.

enoxaparin or Lovenox) during pregnancy. If you do, take calcium and vitamin D, and perform regular weight-bearing exercises to prevent broken bones from heparin-induced osteoporosis.

There is an increased risk of blood clots during the first 6 to 12 weeks after delivery, especially in women with APS. To prevent these, the ACR guidelines for reproductive health management recommends that all women with APS (including those who have never had a blood clot) continue blood thinners (such as heparin or warfarin) 6 to 12 weeks after delivery. Women with APS who have had blood clots before should continue the blood thinner after that.

Warfarin (Coumadin) can cause congenital birth defects during the first trimester. It must be switched to LMWH, ideally before attempting pregnancy. If you become pregnant while on warfarin, contact your doctors immediately.

19. *If you are on thyroid drugs, make sure your TSH is normal before and during pregnancy.* Approximately 1 out of every 20 women with SLE has autoimmune thyroid disease, which increases the risk of preterm delivery. Normalizing the TSH with medicine lowers this risk. Ensure your thyroid status is monitored and treated closely during pregnancy.

Thyroid function test interpretation during pregnancy can be complicated. It is best for an endocrinologist (thyroid specialist) to monitor these tests during pregnancy. Also, remember to stop biotin supplements three days before all blood tests to ensure it doesn't interfere with results (chapter 4).

Treating those with subclinical hypothyroidism (chapter 17) or those with positive thyroid autoantibodies (such as anti-TPO, chapter 4) without significant thyroid level abnormalities does not reduce pregnancy complications. Thyroid supplements should not be taken in these situations.

20. *If you have been on steroids during pregnancy and need a C-section, alert your obstetrician because you may need stress doses.* Cesarean delivery (also called C-section or Cesarean section) is a stressful event. Naturally, the adrenal glands secrete a large amount of steroids during the event to help the body manage the stress. However, people who have taken steroids in high enough doses or for a long time are at increased risk of the adrenal glands not working correctly and not providing these increased amounts. This is called adrenal insufficiency (chapter 26). Women with adrenal insufficiency may need additional doses of steroids at C-section surgery to compensate for this. Alert your OB/GYN and high-risk obstetrician to ensure that the appropriate increase

---

LUPUS IN FOCUS

Taking steroids after delivery to prevent flares

Previous studies suggested that lupus flares were more frequent after delivery, and so it was commonplace to give steroids after delivery to prevent them. The PROMISSE study showed that modern methods of pregnancy care, such as using hydroxychloroquine in all patients, resulted in severe flares occurring less than 2% of the time after delivery. Therefore, using prophylactic steroids after surgery is no longer recommended.

in steroids is given at delivery. Note that stress doses of steroids are not needed for vaginal delivery.

Wear a medical alert bracelet stating that you may have adrenal insufficiency or have been on chronic steroids. If you were to go into labor prematurely in an area where the doctors do not know you, they need to recognize that you need the steroids.

Pregnancy Case Example

BG (not her real initials) developed SLE right before marriage. She had severe disease with arthritis and lupus nephritis. She is positive for anti-SSA and lupus anticoagulant (fortunately has never had a blood clot). Her SLE has been under excellent control with mycophenolate mofetil, HCQ, and low-dose aspirin for about a year.

She has risks on three levels: maternal (risk of lupus flare in her kidneys and joints), placental (blood clots, miscarriage, preeclampsia, and other poor pregnancy outcomes because of the lupus anticoagulant), and fetal (congenital heart block from anti-SSA).

She and her husband had been looking forward to having a baby. After discussing this with her rheumatologist, she was taken off mycophenolate (which should be stopped at least three months before trying to conceive) and put on azathioprine (safe to take during pregnancy and can work well for lupus nephritis and arthritis). She was advised to wait at least three months before attempting pregnancy. This was done because azathioprine can take three months to be fully effective and to ensure it does not cause side effects. Meanwhile, she used an IUD, the contraceptive of choice in SLE (discussed later).

Three months later, her labs looked fantastic with no SLE activity. She continued taking HCQ, aspirin, and azathioprine throughout pregnancy. As instructed, she saw her rheumatologist every month to ensure that her lupus (especially the lupus nephritis) did not flare. She was also seeing a high-risk obstetrician. All doctors communicated with each other with notes and lab results throughout her pregnancy.

Since she was positive for anti-SSA, there was a minimal but real increased risk of fetal heart block (see chapter 18). Therefore, during her 16th week of pregnancy, she began having fetal heart monitoring done by a pediatric cardiologist. The fetus never developed heart block.

She never developed preeclampsia and delivered vaginally at term. Her well-planned pregnancy was successful.

Assisted Reproduction and In-Vitro Fertilization

There are lower fertility rates in SLE for many reasons (chapter 18). Young women with SLE may need to delay becoming pregnant while their SLE is active. Then, when they are medically ready to proceed, their older age can mean that they are less fertile. Make sure to read about oocyte cryopreservation at the end of this section. Endometriosis (chapter 18) can occur in SLE and cause difficulties getting pregnant. In addition, women who have taken cyclophosphamide can develop infertility. In these situations, assisted reproduction techniques such as in-vitro fertilization (IVF) and other options such as donating sperm and eggs to a surrogate mother may be worth considering. In some cases, adoption may be the only practical solution.

LUPUS IN FOCUS

Assisted reproduction and IVF results are improving for SLE patients

In a 2017 study, 37 women with SLE underwent 97 rounds of IVF (around 3 rounds for each). Of these, 26 women (70%) ended up with healthy babies, while 28% of the 97 IVF procedures resulted in a live, healthy baby. This is a rate similar to women without SLE.

Only four women had a lupus flare, but two were not regularly taking their medications (like HCQ). Similarly, four women with aPL antibodies developed blood clots, but two occurred in women with antiphospholipid syndrome who were not taking their blood thinners. In other words, 50% of the complications may have been avoided if the women had been adherent to therapy.

One of the methods used to help fertility problems is ovarian stimulation in which women receive hormones that increase egg production. The eggs are then fertilized with the father's sperm (IVF), and the embryos are placed in the woman's uterus. The specifics of IVF and other assisted reproductive techniques are beyond the scope of this book, but we will mention some important practical points.

It is essential to test for antiphospholipid antibodies (aPLAs, chapter 9) beforehand. APLAs increase the risk of blood clots. IVF is safest for women who are aPLA-negative. In women who are aPLA-positive and at high risk for clotting, blood thinners (aspirin or LMWH) may be needed before and after (but not during) egg retrieval.

Follow all the advice in the "How to Have a Successful Pregnancy" section above for the best results with assisted reproduction.

One of the most important advances in assisted reproduction is the ability to successfully freeze eggs (called oocyte cryopreservation, OC). If you are told not to get pregnant and can afford OC, you should do it. Another reason to consider OC is if you are young (but at a reproductive age) and want to delay pregnancy.

There are some essential facts about OC. First, you can do OC while taking drugs forbidden during pregnancy (such as methotrexate and mycophenolate). Second, eggs harvested and frozen at a young age (such as at 25) are much more likely to result in a successful pregnancy than those harvested at an older age (such as at 34). Plus eggs harvested at a young age (say, 25) and used to get pregnant when older (say, 42) are much more likely to result in a successful pregnancy than natural techniques with the 42-year-old eggs. Although research is ongoing, fertility experts believe that frozen eggs survive and can be successfully used throughout your reproductive life.

Frozen eggs can be useful in several SLE scenarios. While treatments have significantly advanced and most of our patients do very well, some develop severe SLE with issues such as pulmonary hypertension, heart muscle damage (cardiomyopathy, chapter 11), or severe kidney function loss and should not get pregnant because of these problems. Other SLE patients may have other reasons they cannot get pregnant, such as waiting too late in life. In these cases, the frozen eggs could be implanted into

Pregnancy recommendations for different antiphospholipid antibodies (aPLAs) and the antiphospholipid syndrome (APS)

SLE patients who are positive for aPLAs but do not have APS are usually treated differently than those with the syndrome (those who have APS, chapter 9). However, for pregnancy, both groups should follow some of the same recommendations. For example, for contraception, we recommend that both groups avoid oral contraceptive pills (OCP, birth control) containing estrogen. Estrogen-containing OCPs increase the risk of blood clots in aPLA-positive patients.

APLAs are also not all created equal. People who are lupus anticoagulant (LAC) positive or who have very high levels of beta-2 glycoprotein I (B2GP1) antibodies or anticardiolipin (ACLA) antibody (as opposed to mild elevations), or who have "triple positivity" (positive for LAC and B2GP1 and ACLA) are at higher risk for blood clots. Some experts will use stronger blood thinners (such as heparin) during IVF and pregnancy in these patients.

a surrogate mother after fertilization with the father's sperm (IVF). Your baby can have your genetics but be carried through pregnancy by someone else.

Men with Lupus and Pregnancy

If you are a man with SLE and wish to get your partner pregnant, your choices are more straightforward. The primary concern is that if a dangerous medication is present in the seminal fluid (the ejaculate), it could potentially affect the egg. Fortunately, this is a concern with only two drugs. If you are on cyclophosphamide, you need to wait three months before attempting conception. If you are on thalidomide, you need to wait one month. You can continue all other drugs.

Although sulfasalazine can occasionally cause fertility issues, it is rarely used in SLE.

Once pregnancy is established, there are no risks. A man with SLE can take all his drugs (including cyclophosphamide and thalidomide) and have sexual intercourse without causing danger to the unborn baby. However, get approval from your obstetrician; there are some situations where sexual intercourse is not recommended during pregnancy.

Elective Abortions

The decision to have an abortion can be a part of the family-planning process. It may also be necessary when the mother's health is in jeopardy or if the fetus has a birth defect. The decision-making process and the procedures are beyond the scope of this book. However, elective abortions seem to be safe overall in SLE. A 2020 US report of 562 SLE patients (93 of whom had aPLAs) who underwent elective abortions did well without flares of their SLE or the need for hospitalization.

As of January 2023, there are no formal guidelines regarding abortion in SLE. Also, in 2022, the US Supreme Court ruled that each state oversees abortion rights in that state. If you are thinking of having an abortion, discuss this with your doctor, obstetrician, or a local family planning center to know your local options.

Breast-Feeding

Breast-feeding your newborn can provide health benefits to your baby and you. Many SLE patients can safely breast-feed and should consider doing so. But keep in mind that if you cannot breast-feed for medical reasons or prefer not to, your baby can do fine on baby formula.

Some drugs enter breast milk (table 41.4) and potentially cause problems in the baby. The primary medications that need to be avoided are methotrexate, mycophenolate mofetil (CellCept, Myfortic), cyclophosphamide, leflunomide (Arava), thalidomide, tofacitinib, upadacitinib, baricitinib, and statins. Pregnancy-safe drugs, such as azathioprine and hydroxychloroquine, are also safe during breast-feeding. Therefore, most pregnant SLE patients can continue their pregnancy drugs while breast-feeding. However, if SLE flares during or right after pregnancy, medications considered unsafe for breast-feeding may be needed to control the patient's SLE.

Azathioprine is probably safe to continue during breast-feeding. However, for extra cautious women who are concerned about the theoretical risks, an alternative is to have the baby's white blood cell count checked 10 to 15 days into breast-feeding to ensure that there are no effects on the baby's immune system. Another alternative is to pump and discard breastmilk for the first four hours after taking azathioprine, then breast-feed after that.

Contraception (Birth Control)

It is essential to ensure that SLE has been under good control for at least six months before attempting pregnancy. It is also essential to prevent pregnancy while taking drugs such as mycophenolate, methotrexate, leflunomide, cyclophosphamide, and thalidomide. In the case of some of these medications, such as thalidomide, contraception is so crucial that using at least two forms of birth control is recommended.

Birth control techniques vary in safety and effectiveness. Permanent forms, such as tubal ligation ("getting your tubes tied") or vasectomy (male sterilization), are 100% effective. We discuss only reversible procedures, ranging from the most effective first (IUDs and progestin implants) to the least effective (spermicides and coitus interruptus, or "withdrawal method"). **Due to their high success rates, IUDs and progestin implants are the best choices for most patients.** Hormonal contraceptives, where appropriate for some patients, are the next most effective.

Most rheumatologists are not well-trained in the subtleties of contraception; discussion with your gynecologist is essential.

Intrauterine Devices (IUDs). An IUD is a device inserted into the uterus by a gynecologist. There are two major types. The copper IUD interferes with sperm movement to the uterus (womb), preventing fertilization. The levonorgestrel-containing (LNg) IUD releases the female hormone progestin to prevent pregnancy. Since the copper IUD can

Table 41.4 Lupus Drugs and Breast-Feeding

Drug	Safety Concerns
abatacept (Orencia)	Probably safe (but not studied)
adalimumab (Humira)	Safe
anifrolumab (Saphnelo)	Do not use (not studied); theoretically could be safe; ask doctor.
aspirin (low dose)	Safe
azathioprine (Imuran)	See main text
baricitinib (Olumiant)	Do not use
belimumab (Benlysta)	Probably safe
bisphosphonates (table 24.9)	Do not take (not studied)
certolizumab pegol (Cimzia)	Safe
chloroquine	Safe
colchicine	Safe
cyclophosphamide	Do not use
cyclosporine (Sandimmune, Neoral)	Safe
etanercept (Enbrel)	Safe
golimumab (Simponi)	Safe
heparin	Safe
hydroxychloroquine (Plaquenil)	Safe
infliximab (Remicade)	Safe
intravenous immunoglobulin (IVIG)	Safe
leflunomide (Arava)	Do not use
methotrexate	Do not use
methylprednisolone (Medrol)	Breast feed anytime if ≤16 mg; if taking more than 16 mg, wait at least 4 hours after last dose to breast feed.
mycophenolic acid (CellCept, Myfortic)	Do not use
non-steroidal anti-inflammatory drugs (including celecoxib)	Safe
prednisone	Breast feed anytime if ≤20 mg; if more than 20 mg, wait at least 4 hours after last dose to breast feed.
quinacrine	Do not use (not studied)
rituximab (Rituxan)	Safe
statins for cholesterol	Do not use (not studied)
sulfasalazine (Azulfidine)	Safe
tacrolimus	Safe
thalidomide	Do not use
tocilizumab (Actemra)	Probably safe (but not studied)
tofacitinib (Xeljanz)	Do not use
upadacitinib (Rinvoq)	Do not use
ustekinumab (Stelara)	Probably safe (but not studied)
voclosporin (Lupkynis)	Do not use (not studied)
warfarin (Coumadin)	Safe

LUPUS IN FOCUS

Contraception when taking mycophenolate (CellCept, Myfortic)

Mycophenolate can lower estrogen and progesterone hormone levels, which in turn reduces hormone-based contraception effectiveness (including over-the-counter levonorgestrel, Plan B One-Step). IUDs are the recommended contraception for women on MMF. Combining a progestin-based method (implants and pills) with a barrier-type (condom, spermicide) is another option.

The FDA has enrolled these drugs in a Risk Evaluation and Mitigation Strategy (REMS) program, the purpose of which is to decrease side effects. If you can potentially become pregnant, you should read the REMS information about mycophenolate before starting it and discuss contraception with your doctor. Then sign the REMS form stating that you understand everything (mycophenolaterems.com).

increase menstrual bleeding and cramping and the LNg IUD can decrease them, the latter is preferable for many women.

IUDs are the most suitable form of contraception in SLE. Out of 125 couples using copper IUD for one year, only one gets pregnant. The chances are even lower (1 out of 500) with the LNg IUD. Copper IUDs can last 12 years or longer; LNg IUDs can last 7 years.

Progestin Implants. A progestin implant is a tiny, plastic rod containing the female hormone progestin. It is inserted under the skin of the inner upper arm. It continuously releases progestin into the bloodstream, preventing pregnancy for around three years. Although these implants can cause unpredictable vaginal bleeding that can be bothersome, menstrual bleeding tends to be lighter, which is desirable in many. Fewer than 1% of couples who practice this method for one year get pregnant.

Depo-Provera Shots. Depomedroxyprogesterone acetate (Depo-Provera) is injected under the skin or into muscle and lasts for three or four months. It can be used in women who cannot take estrogen-containing oral contraceptive pills. Potential side effects include blood clots, osteoporosis, weight gain, and vaginal bleeding. **Avoid Depo-Provera if at risk for osteoporosis or if positive for aPLAs (which means most SLE patients,** chapter 24). About 4% of couples using this for one year will get pregnant.

Oral Contraceptive Pills (OCPs). The most effective oral contraceptive pills (birth control pills) contain estrogen and progestin. In addition to preventing pregnancy, they can lower the risks of certain cancers, such as uterine, endometrial, and ovarian cancers. However, they can potentially cause blood clots, worsen migraines, worsen liver disease, or increase breast cancer risk. OCPs with low-dose estrogen (30 mcg or less of ethinyl estradiol) are generally safe in most women who have well-controlled lupus and do not increase flare risks. They are probably safe in women with mild, stable active lupus, such as arthritis or active rash. They have not been studied in women with moderately active and severely active SLE (such as active lupus nephritis).

Because OCPs can cause blood clots, they should be avoided by women at higher risk of blood clots, especially those who are positive for aPLAs (table 41.5). About 8% of couples using this for one year will get pregnant.

Table 41.5 Who Should Avoid Estrogen-Progestin Combination OCPs and Consider an IUD

- Have moderately to severely active SLE (or consider progestin-only types)
- Antiphospholipid antibody–positive (or consider progestin-only types)
- Have poorly controlled blood pressure, very high cholesterol, pulmonary hypertension, atrial fibrillation, coronary artery disease, or have had a heart attack or stroke
- Have migraine headaches
- Smokers
- Have nephrotic syndrome (chapter 12)
- Had breast cancer in the past
- Have liver cirrhosis, liver cancer, or hepatic adenoma (a benign liver lesion)
- If you have decreased kidney function, avoid OCPs containing drospirenone

Progestin-Only Pills. These may be an alternative for women who cannot take estrogen-containing OCPs. They can be used by aPLA-positive patients and SLE patients with active disease. However, they are less effective, can cause irregular menstrual bleeding, and must be taken at the same time every day to prevent pregnancy. About 7% of couples using this for one year will get pregnant.

Transdermal Patches. Transdermal patches, which stick to the skin, contain a combination of estrogen and progestin, which are absorbed through the skin. They are typically changed weekly. They cause higher estrogen blood levels than hormonal pills and vaginal rings. These could result in higher rates of lupus flares and blood clots, so **they should be avoided in women with SLE or aPLAs.**

Vaginal Rings. Vaginal rings release estrogen and progesterone but have not been studied in SLE. They release approximately the same amount of estrogen into the bloodstream as OCPs. **They are probably safe in women with inactive SLE and negative for aPLAs.** About 8% of couples who use this for one year will get pregnant.

Levonorgestrel (Plan B One-Step). Levonorgestrel is classified as emergency contraception and is available over the counter. It needs to be taken within 72 hours of unprotected intercourse as a one-tablet or two-tablet regimen. It is most effective if taken within 24 hours. It is 97% effective in preventing pregnancy when taken as recommended. It is safe for SLE patients, although it may be less effective in women taking mycophenolate.

Diaphragms. A diaphragm is a soft, dome-shaped device inserted into the vagina and over the cervix (entrance to the womb) to function as a physical barrier against sperm. It should be used along with spermicidal preparations (described below) for the best results. It does not prevent sexually transmitted diseases (STD), which female condoms (below) can do. Diaphragms can cause irritation, and some women are allergic to them. Around 12% of couples using this for one year will get pregnant (it is just 6% with perfect use). It is only helpful if you remember to use it.

Condoms. Condoms are physical barriers to help prevent sperm from reaching the vagina and reduce STD transmission. Male condoms fit over the penis; female condoms are fitted from outside the vagina and extend down to the cervix. With perfect use, pregnancy occurs around 3% of the time using male condoms and 4% with female condoms. Around 1 out of 5 couples using this for one year will get pregnant. Condom use is safe in SLE.

Cervical Caps. A cervical cap (such as FemCap in the United States) is shaped like a sailor's cap and inserted into the vagina, like a diaphragm. It is available only by prescription and is best fitted by a doctor. It should be used with spermicidal preparations. It is more effective in women who have never had a baby. In that case, around one out of six who use this method (with spermicide) get pregnant within one year. For those who have had a baby, the number is closer to one out of three.

Coitus Interruptus. This is commonly called pulling out, the withdrawal method, or the "pull and pray" method and involves the man removing his penis from the vagina before ejaculation. Although it is safe in SLE, it is not very effective, not only because it requires self-control on the man's part, but also because pre-ejaculation fluid often contains enough sperm to cause pregnancy.

Fertility Awareness–Based Contraception. Also called natural family planning or the rhythm method, this involves avoiding sexual intercourse when the woman is physiologically able to get pregnant. The methods used to estimate the fertile period are complicated. They involve tracking menstrual cycle length, evaluating cervical secretions, and monitoring body temperature. Even with perfect knowledge and use, around one out of four couples doing this for one year get pregnant. This is not a reliable form of contraception.

Spermicides. Spermicides contain a chemical that immobilizes sperm and requires placement at the cervix (entrance to the womb or uterus) before intercourse. Over-the-counter preparations contain nonoxynol-9, and the prescription form is an acidic preparation (brand name of Phexxi). It must be used one hour before intercourse; it is ineffective if used afterward. It is best used with a barrier technique, such as a condom or diaphragm. It should not be used as primary contraception due to low effectiveness. Close to 30% of couples using this for one year get pregnant.

LUPUS IN FOCUS

What do I do if I accidentally get pregnant?

If you get pregnant on pregnancy-safe drugs (azathioprine, hydroxychloroquine, tacrolimus, cyclosporine, NSAIDs, prednisone), and your SLE has been under excellent control, then you should be just fine. You should take daily low-dose aspirin (if you are not at high risk for bleeding) and follow all the advice in this chapter. Make sure and contact your rheumatologist and OB/GYN doctor right away.

If you are on any pregnancy-unsafe drugs or your lupus is active, your situation is more complicated. Discontinue pregnancy-unsafe medications and immediately contact your rheumatologist and OB-GYN. You should also see a high-risk obstetrician (maternal-fetal medicine specialist) or a pregnancy medication specialist.

If you wish to terminate the pregnancy, see your OB-GYN to discuss your options.

Menopause Treatments

The effects of SLE on menopause and how SLE does after menopause are discussed in chapters 18 and 19. This section will discuss treatment for the symptoms of menopause in SLE patients.

Menopause begins when the ovaries (egg-producing organs) produce less estrogen, a female hormone that supports pregnancy and reproduction. Estrogen usually begins to decrease several years before menstrual cycles stop. This is known as the perimenopausal (*peri-* means "around the time of") period. The decrease in estrogen can produce unwanted symptoms, especially hot flashes, in around 80% of women. Around one-fourth of women will have symptoms that affect their quality of life. Hot flashes typically occur abruptly in the upper chest and face. They can be accompanied by heavy sweating, heart palpitations (fluttering), chills, shivering, and a feeling of anxiety. When they occur at night, they can interrupt sleep. This can worsen fatigue in SLE patients who may already have energy problems.

Menopausal hormone therapy (MHT) using estrogen is highly effective against hot flashes. (MHT is called hormone replacement therapy by some doctors.) MHT can also help with other menopausal problems, such as insomnia, joint pain, depression, and moodiness.

MHT can cause mild to moderate (but not severe) lupus flares. This is important to keep in mind.

Another possible side effect is blood clots, so women positive for aPLAs should avoid MHT. If used at all, it should be used for the shortest time needed and generally stopped by age 60. Also, abide by the same recommendations as for estrogen-progestin OCPs (table 41.5).

The anti-depressants paroxetine (Paxil) and citalopram (CeleXA) are recommended as the drugs of choice for hot flashes in women who cannot take MHT. However, they are less effective. Paroxetine should be avoided by women on tamoxifen (a breast cancer drug). Alternatives for women on tamoxifen are escitalopram and venlafaxine. Gabapentin (chapter 27) can be tried for sleep problems.

KEY POINTS TO REMEMBER

1. Before getting pregnant, ensure your SLE has been under excellent control for at least six months. Discuss getting pregnant with your doctors.

2. If you are anti-SSA-positive, your baby's heart should be monitored regularly, starting at weeks 16 to 18.

3. Take low-dose aspirin throughout pregnancy if you are not at high risk for bleeding.

4. Review the safe medicines to take during pregnancy (table 41.3) and breast-feeding (table 41.4).

5. Continue hydroxychloroquine throughout pregnancy (if tolerated).

6. See your rheumatologist at least once each trimester during pregnancy (or monthly if at higher risk, ask your doctor).

7. See a high-risk obstetrician if you get pregnant; ask about their experience treating SLE patients.

8. If at risk of adrenal insufficiency (chapter 26), wear a medical alert bracelet, and ask your OB/GYN and rheumatologist if you need extra steroids if you get a C-section.

9. Do not take OCPs if you have any problems listed in table 41.5.

10. If positive for aPLAs or your SLE is active, your best birth control choice is an IUD.

11. If your SLE is in low disease activity (or remission) and you are negative for aPLAs, an IUD is your best option for contraception, followed by progestin-implants, OCPs, progestin-only pills, and vaginal rings.

12. If you take mycophenolate, an IUD is your best choice. A progestin-based contraceptive combined with a barrier protection (such as condoms) is the second-best choice.

13. Mycophenolate can reduce the effectiveness of Plan B.

14. Estrogen can be used for menopausal hot flashes in SLE patients who are negative for aPLAs and are in remission or have stable, low disease activity. Abide by the recommendations in table 41.5.

15. If told not get pregnant or you choose to delay pregnancy for other reasons, consider freezing your eggs (oocyte cryopreservation), if it is affordable. The younger you are, the better the results. It has numerous advantages.

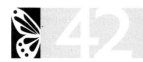

Preparing for Surgery and Travel

Deborah Lyu Kim, DO, FACR, *Contributing Editor*

How to Have a Successful Surgery

Preparing for and having a successful surgery present unique challenges for lupus patients, who are at higher risk for infections and other complications. This section provides general information about preparing for surgery. However, it will not give all the information they need since all surgeries are different and have different preparation and recovery requirements. Always consult with all your doctors and the surgical team for specific advice. Note that surgeons are rarely familiar with many lupus drugs and situations (such as Sjögren's), so having a final word from a rheumatologist is essential if you have one.

Most surgical procedures are elective (routine) surgeries, not emergencies, which means that you will have adequate preparation time. But emergency surgeries are sometimes needed. You may not have time to do everything discussed in this section in those situations. Even so, much of this information can still be helpful. The steps for preparing for surgery are listed in table 42.1 and in this section.

Preparation for surgery begins with your first surgery appointment. Take all items in 42.2 with you. This will maximize your chances for a successful surgery.

Ask your surgeon if you need additional surgical recommendations from other doctors. Usually, you should get a surgical evaluation and medical advice from your primary care provider and rheumatologist. Some SLE patients have involvement of internal organs, such as the kidneys, lungs, heart, and liver. If you fall into this category, you may need recommendations from other specialists, such as your cardiologist (heart), pulmonologist (lungs), nephrologist (kidneys), or gastroenterologist (liver).

Medications

Ask all your doctors which drugs you should continue or stop taking before and after surgery. This section lists some common drugs used in lupus to help guide what you should do. We generally follow the 2022 American College of Rheumatology (ACR) surgical guidelines for hip and knee replacement surgeries. These recommendations may not apply to some surgeries, such as heart and vascular surgeries, and these exceptions will be pointed out. If you obtain any conflicting recommendations from your surgeon about these drugs, make sure to ask the prescribing physician to talk to your surgeon. Written or verbal communication between them is important.

Table 42.1 Surgical Preparation Checklist

- Gather the items in table 42.2.
- Have your doctors fill out drug stop and restart dates (table 42.3).
- See all major organ involvement doctors (such as lung and heart specialists).
- Prepare information about dealing with Raynaud's for your doctors and nurses.
- Prepare information about dealing with Sjögren's for your doctors and nurses.
- Bring all your drugs with you to the hospital in case the hospital does not carry them.

Table 42.2 What to Bring to the Surgeon and Anesthesiologist

- Your medical records
- The following lists:
    - all prescription drugs with doses, how often taken, and what they are for
    - all over-the-counter drugs (including vitamin and herbal supplements)
    - all your medical problems (including what your lupus problems are)
    - all past surgical procedures
    - all drug allergies and intolerances (include sulfonamide antibiotics, chapter 5)
- Names and phone numbers of your doctors
- Names and phone numbers of your emergency contacts
- Surgical preparation instructions from your rheumatologist, primary care provider, and specialists
- Advanced directives and power-of-attorney papers (if you have them)

LUPUS IN FOCUS

Total hip replacement surgery and SLE

SLE patients may be at higher risk for total hip replacement (THR) complications than people without lupus. A 2019 Chinese study showed that SLE patients who were older than 45 and had an overlap syndrome (chapter 2), fever, high anti-dsDNA (chapter 4), or were not in remission or low disease activity were at higher risk for complications. Therefore, if possible, SLE patients should try to postpone total hip replacement until a period when their SLE is under excellent control.

A 2014 United Kingdom study also showed that steroids, alcohol consumption, or having antiphospholipid syndrome also increased THR risks.

If you take many drugs, it can be challenging to remember when to stop and start each drug. We recommend using a chart like the one shown in table 42.3 to keep track. Ask the doctor who prescribed each drug when that medicine should be stopped before surgery and resumed afterward. Then write these stop and start dates on a calendar that includes your surgical date to simplify and organize this information. Some dates

Table 42.3 Drug Stop and Restart Dates for Surgery

Date of Surgery: _____

Medication Name	Prescribing Doctor	Stop Date	Restart Date

may have to be changed. For example, if your surgical wound does not heal well after surgery or an infection occurs, you may have to delay restarting immunosuppressants (table 22.1).

Hospitals do not carry all drugs. Therefore, it is best to bring your own medicines to the hospital. **Ask your surgeon to write an order saying that you can take your own medication for any not carried by the hospital.**

This section discusses several drugs commonly used for lupus: steroids, NSAIDs (table 36.1), blood thinners, immunosuppressants, pain drugs, Raynaud's and Sjögren's medicines, and supplements and herbal products.

Steroids. You usually should not stop steroids for surgery. As in chapter 26, the adrenal glands produce more steroids during stressful events such as surgery. This surge of steroids ensures that bodily functions react appropriately to the surgery. Unfortunately, the adrenal glands stop working correctly if you take steroids for an extended period or at high doses (see table 26.3). You may need extra steroids for surgery (chapter 26). Doctors often refer to this as providing a "stress dose." You should ask your rheumatologist if you need stress doses of steroids. Then let your surgeon and anesthesiologist know. If taking steroids briefly, you may be able to stop them for surgery.

Another steroid problem is that they can interfere with wound healing. Higher doses are associated with poor surgical site healing, which increases infection risks. Therefore, your doctors will want you to be on the lowest possible doses of steroids before and after surgery (except for any required stress doses).

Aspirin-Like Drugs. Most NSAIDs (including aspirin) prevent blood platelets (chapter 9) from clotting properly. If you take them before surgery, you could bleed excessively. Once bleeding dangers have decreased enough, you can often restart them as soon as 24 hours after surgery. It is important to find out when to stop them before surgery and when you can restart them after surgery. If you take them for pain, it is best to restart them as soon as you are allowed after surgery to prevent the recurrence of nonsurgical pains.

Some surgeries have such a low bleeding risk that NSAIDs (such as aspirin) do not need to be stopped. For example, cataracts, minor dental, and skin surgeries generally have low bleeding risks.

Other surgeries have such a high bleeding risk that NSAIDs are always stopped before surgery. These include operations on the brain, around the spinal cord, inside the middle ear, and in the back of the eye (retina).

The effects of NSAIDs on clotting differ depending on the drug. For example, aspirin's effects on clotting last longer than other NSAIDs. This means that aspirin needs to be stopped sooner than others. Although in general, you should stop aspirin 7 to 10 days before most major surgeries, this recommendation does not apply to everyone or all surgeries. Patients taking aspirin to prevent cardiovascular (CV) events such as heart attacks and strokes may be at such high risk for them that they should not stop aspirin. The risk of a CV event may be higher than the chances of a bleeding problem from aspirin. This may include people with stents (tubes that keep blood vessels open) inside the arteries of their heart, arms, or legs. Stopping aspirin may cause a stent to become blocked with a blood clot, causing complications such as a heart attack. If you have significant heart, blood vessel, or brain problems, ask your cardiologist (heart doctor), vascular surgeon, or neurologist (brain doctor) if you should stop aspirin.

Non-acetylated salicylates and COX-2 inhibitors (salsalate, diflunisal, celecoxib, and meloxicam) do not thin the blood. So, they do not need to be stopped for bleeding purposes, but they may need to be stopped to prevent blood pressure and blood flow problems, as mentioned below. If stopped for these reasons, meloxicam should be stopped at least five days before surgery. Three days is usually sufficient for the others.

All other NSAIDs can cause bleeding problems and should be stopped before major surgery. Many doctors recommend stopping them at least three to four days beforehand. Aspirin is usually stopped 7 to 10 days before. The effects of ibuprofen and ketoprofen (immediate-release pills) do not last very long. They can usually be stopped 24 hours before surgery. Other NSAIDs' effects last much longer, so those should be stopped well in advance. For example, piroxicam should be stopped 11 days before surgery.

All NSAIDs (other than low-dose aspirin) can increase blood pressure or decrease kidney blood flow. Therefore, they may need to be stopped before surgery. Ask all your doctors, especially your cardiologist (if you have one) and your surgeon.

Other Blood Thinners. Some SLE patients need to take blood thinners, such as warfarin (Coumadin), clopidogrel (Plavix), enoxaparin (Lovenox), fondaparinux (Arixtra), dabigatran (Pradaxa), rivaroxaban (Xarelto), apixaban (Eliquis), or dalteparin (Fragmin). When and whether to stop these is complex and depends on why they are being used. Ask all your doctors, especially your hematologist, and cardiologist, if you have one.

Immunosuppressants. Many lupus patients need to take drugs that suppress the immune system. While taking these drugs can increase infection risks, they are important for controlling SLE inflammation; stopping them could cause a flare.

The consequences of an SLE flare are often worse than the potential risks of taking an immunosuppressant. For example, SLE flares increase infection risks due to immune system abnormalities from the flare. An SLE flare can also significantly interfere with rehabilitation. And if steroids are needed for the flare, this increases infection risks more than other immunosuppressants and can interfere with surgical wound healing.

The decision to continue or stop these drugs needs to be carefully considered based on your SLE severity, your risk for flaring, and the type of drugs you take. For example, it would be reasonable to stop immunosuppressants in someone with mild lupus and a low risk of flaring while continuing them in someone with severe SLE.

Although methotrexate is an immunosuppressant, it does not appear to increase surgical infections. Therefore, you may not need to stop it. There are exceptions, though.

LUPUS IN FOCUS

Steroids are more dangerous for surgery than other immunosuppressants

A 2019 research study evaluated over 10,000 major surgeries (joint, heart, and abdominal) in US Medicare patients. Prednisone as low as 5 mg daily increased the risk of death and readmission to the hospital within one month of surgery. By contrast, biologics and other immunosuppressant drugs (such as azathioprine, mycophenolate, and leflunomide) did not increase the risk of death or readmission rates. Steroids are the primary immunosuppressant responsible for side effects, such as infections (chapter 22), more so than biologics and non-steroid immunosuppressants.

The researchers concluded that surgeries should not be postponed in rheumatologic patients if they had recently received a biologic or a non-steroidal immunosuppressant if that surgery is needed quickly.

For non-urgent surgeries (elective surgeries), the American College of Rheumatology published recommendations on how to deal with immunosuppressant drugs around the time of surgery. These recommendations are under each drug description in this book (such as what to do with methotrexate in chapter 32 and belimumab in chapter 34).

One is if you have chronic kidney disease. In that case, you may need to stop methotrexate since dangerous levels of methotrexate could occur if your kidney function were to decrease during and after surgery. The ACR also lists leflunomide as a drug that does not have to be stopped for surgery. Do not stop hydroxychloroquine; it is not an immunosuppressant.

Every drug commonly used for lupus includes a section on what to do during surgery. Look up your drugs in the index and find their surgical recommendations in the main section about each drug. However, always double-check with your prescribing doctor.

Pain Drugs. If you take pain drugs daily for pain control, you may need to continue them throughout surgery or have them switched to a surgery-safe alternative. Stopping some of them, especially opioids, can cause withdrawal symptoms and severe pain. Ask your prescribing doctor.

Sjögren's Drugs. Lupus patients with Sjögren's may take cevimeline (Evoxac) or pilocarpine (Salagen), which help make more saliva and tears. But because these two medications can cause airway passages to constrict, lower blood pressure and heart rate, and cause urination problems, some experts recommend they not be taken around surgery in people at high risk for these conditions. Both are out of the system quickly after stopping them, so it is sufficient to not take them the day before your surgery.

Female Hormone Drugs. Drugs with estrogens and related hormones increase the risk for blood clots, so it is best to stop them before surgery. Ask your prescribing doctor and surgeon.

For transgender women (male to female reassignment) who take higher doses of estrogen, some experts recommend lowering the doses a few weeks before surgery, stopping them before surgery, then waiting a week after surgery before restarting low doses. After a couple of weeks, a patient may resume full-dose estrogen.

Raloxifene (Evista) prevents and treats osteoporosis (chapter 24). It may be OK to continue raloxifene for surgeries at low risk for blood clots. However, it should be stopped at least 7 days before high-risk surgeries, then restarted once the risk for blood clots is gone.

Supplements and Herbal Products. Some products, such as turmeric, curcumin, fish oil, omega-3 fatty acids, vitamin E, garlic, ginkgo, and ginseng, can increase bleeding. Others, such as kava, valerian, and St. John's wort, can have dangerous interactions with anesthesia drugs. Ephedra (ma huang) can cause heart problems, while ginseng and turmeric (curcumin) can cause low glucose (sugar) levels. It can take a long time to get some of these supplements and herbal products out of your system, so it is best to stop taking all of them at least one week before surgery.

Raynaud's Phenomenon

If your fingers, toes, and ears become cold and turn colors with stress or cold temperatures, you may have Raynaud's (chapter 11). Hospitals, especially the operating room, tend to be colder than normal. This can cause reduced blood flow to the fingers and toes, causing them to become painful or develop open sores in Raynaud's patients.

Let the anesthesiologist and nurses know about your Raynaud's. They can increase the operating room temperature ahead of time. You should ask for more blankets, socks, a hat, and covers for the hands and feet to decrease the severity of Raynaud's attacks in the operating and recovery rooms.

Sjögren's Disease

Surgery can worsen Sjögren's dryness because operating room and hospital humidity tend to be very low. In addition, medications used for pain, anesthesia, and skin cleansing can be drying, while tubes inserted in the nose and throat can irritate dry areas.

Before your surgery, you will be told not to eat or drink anything. This usually does not include using artificial saliva, so if you need artificial saliva, it is generally acceptable to keep using it. Ask your surgeon and anesthesiologist about your brand.

Make sure to communicate with your surgeon, anesthesiologist, and nurses before and after surgery about your Sjögren's and about how important it is to make sure you maintain proper moisture. Even better, ask your rheumatologist to include instructions in their surgical recommendations. Ask your anesthesiologist to humidify your oxygen supply if oxygen is needed. Bring all eye, mouth, ear, nose, and skin moisturizers to the hospital with you. Use them immediately before your surgery (if allowed) and ask the nurses in the recovery room to use them right after surgery. Ask the anesthesiologist to use a moisturizing gel in your eyes when they are closed during surgery to prevent cornea (clear front part of the eye) damage. Remind the surgical team that tubes inserted into the nose or throat may need extra lubrication. Even if you do not typically use anything for your nose, bring a moisturizing nose spray or gel (such as Ayr brand). Also, bring a lip moisturizer, because you will need it.

During and after surgery, you may need antibiotics. This increases the risk of *Candida* (yeast, chapters 22 and 14) infections. Sjögren's patients are at higher risk for these. Symptoms include soreness and redness of the tongue and corners of the mouth, a sore throat, a white coating inside the mouth, or a vaginal discharge. Consuming probiotic-rich foods, such as live-culture yogurt (chapter 38), before and after surgery may help. Also, ask your doctors for anti-fungal drugs.

1. Be prepared when you see your surgeon and anesthesiologist by going over the checklist in table 42.2 before your appointment.

2. List all drugs—prescription, over-the-counter, and supplements (table 42.3). Ask each prescribing doctor when to stop and restart each of these.

3. Take all of your drugs with you to the hospital just in case some of them are not available from the pharmacy.

4. If you have Raynaud's or Sjögren's, let your surgeon, anesthesiologist, and surgery nurses know and read the sections above.

5. Request that extra measures be taken to keep you warm during and after surgery if you have Raynaud's.

6. Take all moisturizing products with you if you have Sjögren's and use all of them before and after surgery. Use lip and nose moisturizers even if you do not usually use them.

Travel Tips

Traveling with SLE can present its own challenges. Making sure that you stay as healthy and safe as possible is essential.

Preventing Infection

One of the most important things to find out when traveling to another country is whether you need to take any special infection-prevention measures. Patients on immunosuppressants (table 22.1) are at higher risk of bad outcomes if they get infections. Sometimes vaccines are recommended and even required. Some vaccines, such as for MMR and yellow fever, have live virus and should be avoided by patients on strong immunosuppressants (chapter 22). Some countries have an increased risk of malaria and taking additional antimalarials may be necessary. Hydroxychloroquine may prevent malaria in areas without chloroquine resistance but does not help in most areas.

Some places have a high risk for infections from contaminated water and food. Traveler's diarrhea can occur, for example. Having a supply of antibiotics from your doctor while you travel is helpful. Insect-borne (mosquitos, flies, ticks) illnesses are common. Wear repellants on skin and clothing, wear protective clothing, and avoid being outside during the insect's prime feeding period.

Use strict protection such as condoms if you engage in sexual contact. Hopefully, you have already had your vaccine against human papillomavirus (chapter 22).

Infections can easily occur from swimming in freshwater. Wear footwear even on beaches to avoid contact with animal (and even human) feces and infections such as hookworm.

Traveling increases the risk of respiratory illnesses (influenza, colds, COVID-19). Be extra diligent with hand-washing and ensure you are vaccinated. If the COVID-19 pandemic is still ongoing in the area where you are traveling, abide by strict social distancing (chapter 22) and mask-wearing.

It is best to see a travel medicine specialist for advice before traveling. Find a clinic close to you at istm.org/AF_CstmClinicDirectory.asp. You can also check with the Centers for Disease Control at cdc.gov/travel. Select the country you are traveling to, and the site will provide sound advice. Plan your travel strategy a minimum of one month before.

Other Traveler Health Safety

Always protect yourself from ultraviolet (UV) light (tables 38.3, and 38.4), and make sure you take an adequate supply of sunscreen and UV-protective clothing.

All SLE patients, especially those positive for antiphospholipid antibodies (chapter 9), are at increased risk for leg and lung blood clots. Prolonged sitting and lying down (in a car, train, or plane) further increase these risks. Travel times of more than four hours have double the risk compared to shorter trips. Do not wear anything that has a tight waistband or that squeezes the tops of your legs. Compression stockings below the knees can help. Drink lots of water to stay well hydrated. If you do not take low-dose aspirin, ask your doctor if you should. Aspirin thins the blood and could potentially reduce clotting. Make sure to get up and walk around regularly. While sitting, move and squeeze your feet and leg muscles repeatedly. Use a timer on your smartphone to remind you to do this every half hour or so.

If you have severe lung and heart issues, such as pulmonary fibrosis or pulmonary hypertension, see your lung or heart specialist beforehand. Some people need to take oxygen on the plane since jet planes can have lower oxygen levels at high altitudes.

Dryness of the airway passages in the head (sinuses and Eustachian tube) from Sjögren's can result in excruciating pain from air pressure changes during takeoff and landing. Using saline sprays and gels in the nose can be helpful to prevent this. Consider using decongestants (such as phenylephrine, Sudafed) in pill form and nasal spray (such as oxymetazoline, Afrin) 30 minutes to 1 hour before take-off and landing. If Sjögren's causes you to have sinus and nasal congestion, consider taking guaifenesin (Mucinex) and fluticasone (Flonase) daily before and during your trip. Also, check tables 14.2, 14.5, and 14.6 for more advice.

If traveling between time zones, jet lag can cause sleepiness, weakness, and mental fog. Napping at your destination at least 8 hours before bedtime there and for no more than 30 minutes can be beneficial. If you use a non-UV-producing light to normalize your biological clock (table 6.2), bring it with you. Use your light in mid to late mornings as soon as you arrive at your destination, or go outside, using your UV protection at those times. Another choice is taking 1 mg to 10 mg (3 mg usually suffices) of melatonin (chapter 39) on the night of arrival and for the next five nights. There are also smartphone apps (such as Timeshifter) that give personalized recommendations on the basis of your flight times and time zones.

It is usually safe to fly during an uncomplicated pregnancy. Most airlines allow pregnant women to fly up to their 37th week (32 weeks for twins). To help prevent complications, take precautions such as staying well hydrated and wearing below-the-knee venous compression stockings.

Medications and Travel

Bring an adequate supply of your drugs with you. If you need to fill your prescriptions early, ask your doctor to write an explanation for your pharmacist explaining your need for an early refill.

During lupus flares (see table 5.2), some patients need extra steroids, such as a methylprednisolone (Medrol) dose pack. If you have adrenal insufficiency, you need extra steroids for stressful situations such as injury or infection (see table 26.1). Bring these with you in case you need them.

Some drugs, such as belimumab (Benlysta), need to stay cool. Pack them in insulated packaging along with cold packs. When booking your hotel, ask for a room with a refrigerator ahead of time.

KEY POINTS TO REMEMBER

1. If traveling to a foreign country, you should see a travel medicine specialist. Go to istm.org/AF_CstmClinicDirectory.asp and cdc.gov/travel at least one month before your trip.

2. On plane flights, take measures to prevent blood clots and inner ear and sinus problems.

3. If you have severe lung or heart problems, see your specialists for advice before flying.

4. Using a non-UV light therapy lamp and melatonin can help reduce jet lag severity. Consider using apps such as Timeshifter.

5. Make sure you properly prepare your drugs and have enough for your trip. Include extra steroids, if needed, for possible lupus flares and adrenal insufficiency.

6. This section includes a long list of practical information. Highlight all areas that apply to you and organize them into a checklist to simplify their use.

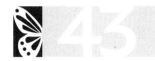

Communicating with Your Health Care Provider

Sarthak Gupta, MD, *Contributing Editor*

Behind the Scenes of Your Office Visit

New patient visits take about 25 to 45 minutes, on average. Follow-up visits may allow only 10 to 20 minutes, on average.

However, there can be many variations. For someone who is very ill and who requires an extensive evaluation, a visit can easily take an hour or more. For someone whose lupus is doing well, the visit could take just five minutes. It is hard to know beforehand.

Wait times also vary. If the doctor sees several sick patients in a row, then all of the patients scheduled afterward may end up with long wait times. The most common reason for patients having unexpected long wait times is an unusually large number of complicated patient visits earlier in the day. However, in a well-run office, this should not happen frequently. If you do have long waits every time you are at the doctor's office, this may be due to the office scheduling too many patients in too short a time. This is one measurement you can use to decide what doctor you want to stay with.

In addition to seeing patients in the exam room, the doctor also needs to review the patient's chart, labs, x-rays, and other tests; call the lab or radiology center for any missing test results; review the drug list for appropriateness, accuracy, and potential drug interactions; and read other doctors' notes. I usually do this right before seeing the patient so that everything is fresh in my mind and I am fully prepared for the visit. This can take anywhere from 5 to 20 minutes depending on the complexity of the case and can add to the patient's wait time in the reception area. During that time, the patient may be wondering why the doctor is not seeing them yet, while they are actually working diligently on the patient's health care.

After the patient leaves the room, the visit is not over. The doctor needs to write down or type the visit details. These days, this documentation is usually done through electronic medical records (EMR; or electronic health records [EHR]). The doctor must accurately record the history, physical exam, test findings, diagnoses, treatment, and what other tests are needed. The doctor may also include additional information that helps other health care providers understand the decisions and cite recent research studies. This note should accurately state exactly what was going on with the patient and the

Dr. Gupta contributed to this article in his personal capacity. The views expressed are his own and do not necessarily represent the views of the National Institutes of Health, or the United States government.

doctor's thoughts regarding the patient's current status. It should also be thorough enough so that any health care provider reading it could understand the patient's medical condition and any plans for testing and treatment.

In short, much work goes on at the patient's office visit before the doctor enters the examination room and does not end until after the office visit is documented in the records while at the same time making sure to give the patient the best quality of care possible.

In the process, unexpected issues can arise. Your doctor may need to answer phone calls from other doctors and hospitals about sick patients and tend to emergency situations. Or problems such as the computer system crashing can occur.

Every physician's office has different appointment times and days that are less likely to be busy. Often these tend to be the first appointments in the morning or afternoon. Most of the time, if the first patient of the morning or afternoon arrives early, we will see that patient quickly to stay ahead of schedule. If your appointment is toward the end of the morning or afternoon, you run the risk of earlier patients having complicated problems, and their visits taking longer than expected.

Getting the Most from Doctor Visits

There are many things you can do to maximize your visit. Table 20.5 outlines some of these. We elaborate here.

Before your appointment, make a short list of goals and questions. Maybe you have a new problem, or you want to know if you can cut back on your steroids, or you need to prepare for an upcoming surgery. Often, the doctor's visit goals differ from yours, yet both are important. Hand the doctor your questions and concerns at the beginning of the visit. Then your doctor can plan on answering them in an unrushed, organized way. Do not hand your doctor a list of ten questions at the end of the visit. Your doctor most likely thought the visit was over and may have more patients waiting in exam rooms. The answers to your questions will most likely be rushed and be less than satisfactory.

Keep a personal copy of your medical records and bring it to each visit. You can keep your medical information on your computer, make changes as they occur, and print out important lists, test results, or other doctors' notes before each visit. An abbreviated medical record can be just one to two pages listing your doctors' names and contact numbers, your medical problems and surgeries, your updated medication list (table 29.6), and your drug intolerances (make sure to include sulfonamide antibiotics, chapter 5). Also, keep track of drugs that did not help you in the past. This prevents a drug from being prescribed that you may have forgotten you tried in the past. Note medicine changes by other doctors or if you have any new medical problems.

If you have a long list of problems, do not write them all down. We cringe when a patient hands us 5 pages of incredibly detailed notes that can take 15 minutes to read. To be fair, patients are trying to convey what has happened as accurately as possible. Keep in mind that the doctor is only human, can only read so much at a visit, and cannot solve every problem.

We recommend choosing your top three concerns and being brief. If you do this, your doctor will be most appreciative, and you will get the best results. Thoroughly addressing those three most important problems is much better than addressing a large number of problems inadequately.

On the day of your visit, plan to arrive early. Schedule enough time to be at your doctor's office at least 15 minutes before your appointment time. This means leaving plenty of time to allow for the possibility of heavy traffic or other delays. If you arrive early, you will be calm, your blood pressure will be reliable, you can fill out the necessary paperwork, and do the essential things required by your insurance carrier.

Plan to wear appropriate clothing. As arthritis doctors, we often need to examine body parts covered with clothing, such as the hips, knees, and shoulders. If you have a problem with a particular body part, avoid layers that take a long time to remove (suspenders, long underwear, stockings that go up to the hips, several different shirts/sweaters, and so on). For example, we have many patients with bad knee arthritis who get knee injections. Most of them get into the habit of wearing loose-fitting shorts or sweatpants with no stockings, making evaluating and treating their condition easier.

Be courteous to all office staff. Most patients are wonderful and charming to everyone. But some are not. Your medical care does not begin and end with the doctor. It starts when you pick up the phone to call the office. From there, your path to and from the doctor is paved with essential members of our health care team. If you do not treat them with respect, you will find it more challenging to get the best health care possible.

For their part, doctors want to surround themselves with the best possible staff. If a staff member repeatedly gives you subpar service, let someone know. It is usually more effective to go directly to the office manager. Reserve the time with your doctor for your medical problems. You do not want your office visit with the doctor to be taken up by discussing a staff or office issue for 10 minutes.

During your visit, try to discuss relevant issues with the specific doctor you are seeing. Specialists should manage the problems in which they are trained. Briefly tell each doctor if any new medical problems have occurred. We want to know about new medical issues, surgeries, and such. When seeing you lupus doctor, you do not have to go into great detail if the issues are not lupus-related. But because lupus can affect every body part, you should at least mention any new problems, so that your lupus doctor can sort out what may or may not be lupus-related. The same holds true for visits with other specialists, such as those who treat lungs, heart, skin, and kidneys.

LUPUS IN FOCUS

Your concerns may be very different from your doctor's

Most of you reading this are troubled by fatigue, pain, "lupus fog," and feeling worn out. A 2018 Australian study showed that these concerns were evaluated in less than half of doctor's visits.

Most rheumatologists concentrate on SLE's immune system effects, such as lupus rashes, inflammatory arthritis, and kidney inflammation. This is because active SLE causes ongoing permanent organ damage and increases heart attack and stroke risks. Identifying active problems and treating them are important for our patients to live longer and better.

Still, fatigue, "lupus fog," and diffuse (all-over) pain can lower your current quality of life. These are called type II symptoms (chapter 5), as opposed to the immune system inflammatory symptoms (noted in the previous paragraph). Type II symptoms are rarely due to inflammation. They are usually due to the complicating problems of fibromyalgia, depression, anxiety, insomnia, and so on. Many doctors feel powerless to address these issues and leave them out of the conversation.

How can you get help? First, if any of these is your primary concern, write it down as one of the three questions you hand over to your doctor at the start of the visit. Second, you need to understand how difficult these are to treat medically and that lifestyle changes (like exercise, diet, and sleep hygiene) are the most effective ways to address many of them. Refer to chapter 44, "The Lupus Secrets," and see lupusencyclopedia.com/lupus-secrets.

All doctors treating SLE patients should regularly communicate with each other by at least sending copies of office visit notes and test results to each other. If your doctors do not do this, consider getting different health care providers (if this is possible). You deserve the best medical care possible, and communication between doctors is essential for this to occur. The only doctor who usually is not expected to send out notes is the primary care provider, who should instead be getting notes from all the specialists you see.

Answer all staff and doctors' questions truthfully. Even what seems like very personal questions may be important for your medical condition. For example, questions about sex, alcohol, and drugs may make many patients uncomfortable. They may even consider it no one's business. If you feel that way, just be honest and respectfully decline to answer, but do not give false answers.

Let the doctor know if you are not taking your drugs exactly as prescribed. We have often wondered why patients were not doing well, only to find out that although they always answered "yes" to taking an important drug, they were not taking it regularly or not at all. For example, if you have been prescribed a drug to be taken three times a day, but you usually remember to take it only twice a day, let your doctor know. In this case, they can try to find an alternative drug taken once or twice daily.

If you cannot afford your medicine, let your doctor know. Sometimes doctors can come up with alternate, less expensive drugs or have samples available. You can also find out what similar medicines may be more affordable from your prescription plan and let your doctor know.

Talking to Your Doctor

When evaluating patients, the first thing doctors do is ask them to describe their problems. This part of the evaluation is called taking the patient's history. Sometimes, symptoms alone can lead to an accurate diagnosis. The physical exam and tests help narrow down the causes, though, if there are many possibilities. Proper communication with your doctor helps obtain a correct diagnosis and ensure that necessary tests are done.

The history is usually followed by the physical examination. After that the doctor tells you what they think is going on and what the plan is as far as testing or treatment changes. Understanding this order can help you know what to expect (history—then physical—then summary).

Your doctor may start the history portion of the visit with, "How have you been doing?" or "How can I help you today?" or "What brings you here today?"

Immediately give your doctor your short list of questions and goals for the visit.

Then briefly express what has been happening. It is usually best to do this starting from the beginning. "Doctor, I was doing well until about two weeks ago when . . ." While describing what has been happening, focus on the main problems and avoid unrelated information. For example, if you have chest pain, describe the chest pain to your doctor, what you were doing when it happened, what it felt like, and what things made it worse or better (table 43.1).

Try to give the most important information in the shortest amount of time. Advice for remembering essential aspects of your situation, providing the most valuable information, and not getting sidetracked is in table 43.1.

Using the questions in table 43.1 as a guide, write a description of your problem ahead of time. Here is an example:

> Doctor, about 2 months ago, after I started taking naproxen, I got stomach upset. This came on slowly and infrequently but now occurs more often, about 5 times a day. It occurs at the top of my stomach, causing a mild achy, gnawing feeling that sometimes goes up into my chest. When I eat food or take some Tums, it helps. When I lie down, I often get heartburn, and the pain worsens. I occasionally feel nauseated and cough. I exercise without difficulty, and no one else I know has similar problems. I am concerned that I could have pancreatic cancer since my cousin had similar problems before being diagnosed with pancreatic cancer.

This account is very brief, but it is loaded with helpful information. This patient describes gastroesophageal reflux disease (GERD) brought on by taking naproxen, an NSAID (table 36.1), perfectly. However, a stomach ulcer is also possible. Chest pain from blocked arteries in the heart (angina from coronary artery disease, CAD) is unlikely, but possible. Although the symptoms described are not classic, women can have unusual symptoms with CAD, so CAD needs to be considered, too.

Table 43.1 Describing a Medical Problem to Your Doctor

- Start at the beginning, when the problem first started.
- Say what happened in the order it occurred.
  - What were you doing when you first noticed the problem?
  - Did it start gradually or suddenly?
  - Describe how it made you feel.
- In what part of your body is the problem?
- If there is pain, does it spread anywhere (radiate)?
- Is the problem constant (never a second without it), or does it come and go in a pattern?
- How often does it occur?
- What things make the problem worse (times of day, activities, body positions)?
- What makes the problem better?
- Over time, is it getting worse, better, or staying about the same?
- Is the problem mild, moderate, or severe?
- How severe on a scale of 1–10 (10 is the worst ever in your life; 1 would be hardly noticeable).
- Are there any associated problems or symptoms?
- How has the problem interfered with activities in your life?
- Has anyone else (family, friends, or co-workers) had similar symptoms?
- Have you ever had this problem before? If so, what happened?
- What is your biggest concern, or fear, about what may be going on?

Next, the doctor does a physical exam and orders a blood count to ensure no anemia from a bleeding ulcer. The patient may need to get an ECG (chapter 11) and heart stress test. For the moment, though, this is enough helpful information to stop the naproxen, give the patient advice on dietary changes for GERD, and prescribe anti-acid medication (table 28.3). At this point the doctor can also reassure the patient that they probably do not have pancreatic cancer. More tests can always be done if things do not get better quickly.

Describe your problem as specifically as you can. For example, if you say you are "tired," what do you mean? There are many different ways to feel fatigued (chapter 40), including being mentally exhausted, being overworked, being stressed, being sleepy, having shortness of breath, or having muscle weakness. Each of them can point to something different.

Describing how "tired" feels and explaining how it interferes with your life can help your doctor narrow down the cause. Think of writing it down in a book, like a story, for others to read and understand.

Dizziness is another condition that can have multiple different causes. If it feels as though the room is moving, it could point to vertigo, a problem with the inner ear, or the nerve that goes to the ear. If you get lightheaded when you stand, your blood pres-

The worldwide shortage of rheumatologists is getting worse!

In 2015, the American College of Rheumatology (ACR) counted 6,013 rheumatology care providers; 4,997 were full-time rheumatologists, and 598 part-time. The other 418 were nurse practitioners and physician assistants specializing in rheumatology. This was 13% fewer rheumatologists than needed. These numbers have been decreasing. Many rheumatologists are retiring, and fewer are entering the specialty. In 2020, 100 doctors who wanted to get into rheumatology training programs could not do so because there were not enough training slots.

By 2030, the number of rheumatology health care providers in the US is predicted to drop to 4,133 nationwide. That is 30% fewer than in 2015. There will also be a greater need for rheumatologists, because the number of older people with arthritis (the baby boomers) will be much higher. It is estimated that there will be only half the number of rheumatology health care providers needed to care for rheumatologic patients, like those with SLE.

Many areas of the United States have few to no rheumatologists. Many patients must travel hundreds of miles for rheumatologic care. In the United States, 21% of rheumatologists are located in the Northeast; only 4% are in the Southwest.

In 2019, more than 60% of US patients had to wait more than a month to get a new patient appointment with a rheumatologist. More than a quarter of patients had to wait more than two months.

It's much worse for pediatric SLE patients. Only one out of four children with arthritis can see a pediatric rheumatologist. In 2023, one-third of the available pediatric rheumatology training positions were unfilled. Children fortunate to have a pediatric rheumatologist have an average of an hour's drive. Nine states have no pediatric rheumatologists, and six states have only one (as of 2021).

This is not just a US problem. A 2019 United Kingdom study showed that patients waited an average of over six months after the onset of rheumatologic symptoms before being able to see a rheumatologist.

sure may be too low, or you could be dehydrated or anemic (low red blood count), or you could have a nerve or heart problem causing blood pressure problems. The causes of vertigo and lightheadedness are different, yet both cause "dizziness." It is easier to figure out when you describe it in detail using simple everyday language.

Understanding What Your Doctor Says

When your doctor tells you about drug changes, your diagnosis, what possible issues could be causing a symptom, or what tests are needed, ask that this information be written down in easy-to-understand language. It can be overwhelming to be told many different things at a doctor's visit. To a doctor, what may seem straightforward may be complicated to a nonmedical person. Never be afraid to say, "I don't understand . . . can you explain that or write it down in simpler terms?" Make sure you leave the visit understanding what is going on. It is usually not necessary to know everything (such as what every lab result means), but it is crucial to understand the big picture.

Don't wait until the doctor is ending the visit to ask for an explanation. Let them know early on in the visit that you do not understand something.

Doctors spend much of their time talking to other health care providers, so the complex language of medicine is second nature. Although they want patients to understand what is going on, they can forget how to say things in understandable, everyday language and sometimes need to be reminded.

Most medical problems can have a number of possible causes. These are the problem's "differential diagnosis." In most differential diagnosis lists, one or two items are usually the most likely causes. Doctors call those items the "top of the differential diagnosis."

Let's make a nonmedical comparison. You lie in bed during a windy night and hear a creaking sound. The possible causes include a ghost, a robber, the house foundation settling, or the wind causing a part of the house to creak. Of these, the most likely cause is the wind, so it is at the top of the differential diagnosis. However, any of them is possible (if you believe in ghosts), so you get up and walk through the house. You don't see a ghost, the doors are locked, there's no robber, and then you notice the wind causing a shutter to creak. You've confirmed it is the wind.

Medical situations are similar. Consider, for example, anemia, when the red blood cell count is low (chapter 9). There are many possible reasons for anemia. Finding the exact cause is important for treating it properly. Many think that they must be low in iron and need an iron supplement, but iron deficiency is only one possibility. Taking iron supplements does not help other causes, which need additional tests to determine.

Before ordering any tests, the doctor comes up with a list of possibilities (the differential diagnosis). These include iron deficiency, gastrointestinal bleeding (such as from colon cancer or an ulcer), vitamin B-12 deficiency, folic acid deficiency, anemia of chronic disease (from lupus inflammation), hemolytic anemia from SLE (chapter 9), or due to a drug like methotrexate.

In a menstruating 49-year-old woman taking methotrexate, the most common causes of anemia may be anemia of chronic disease, iron deficiency, and methotrexate-induced anemia. These would be at the top of the differential diagnosis. They would also be at the top of the list for diagnostic testing, but the doctor would still have to consider other possibilities and arrange tests to ensure that the less likely, but possibly more dangerous problems do not exist.

For example, this patient with anemia may be sent for a colonoscopy to ensure that there is no evidence of colon cancer, which can cause anemia due to slow intestinal bleeding. In reality, colon cancer may not be very likely, but it would be very dangerous if not diagnosed.

Telehealth

Since the COVID-19 pandemic started in March 2020, telehealth visits have become commonplace. This format has proved adequate for patients who are doing well, especially those in remission. We can see some things on video, like rashes, hair loss, and

Table 43.2 Making the Most of Telehealth Visits

- Do everything in tables 40.1 and 40.2.
- Have your wifi connection strength optimized to ensure adequate, uninterrupted connections. Even better, have your computer "hard-wired" to the internet via Ethernet cable.
- Ask all household members to stay off their smartphones, internet, and other wifi devices during visits.
- Close all other programs on your computer, internet browser tabs (including email), and smartphone before a visit
- Practice connecting via the internet on your computer, laptop, tablet, or smartphone (such as via FaceTime on iPhones) with friends or family.
- Have the camera at eye level; have your face fill the video screen.
- Have lighting (such as windows) in front of you, not behind you.
- Wear earbuds or headphones to maximize your hearing ability.
- Be in a quiet location; place pets in another room.
- Turn all unused devices off during the visit, such as cellphones and voice assistants (Amazon's Alexa, Google Assistant), or place on vibrate or "airplane mode."
- Check your blood pressure, heart rate, and temperature before each visit.
- If you think you need an in-person physical examination, let your doctor know.
- If the telehealth platform has a chatbox, ask your doctor to type out any terms, instructions, or websites so you understand them.

mouth sores during flares. If we need a physical exam, we schedule our patients to come into the office, often by the next day.

Ways to get the most out of your telehealth visits are described in table 43.2.

KEY POINTS TO REMEMBER

1. Strive to make your doctor visits as productive as possible (see table 20.5).

2. Describe problems to your doctor in a way that will increase your chances of getting an accurate diagnosis and treatment (table 43.1).

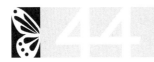

The Lupus Secrets Checklist

A Note for Patients

Some recommendations should be followed by all lupus patients in order to maximize their health. The "Lupus Secrets" checklist below summarizes these do's and don'ts. I call them "secrets" not because I want them to be a secret, but because most people do not know about these steps to better health with lupus, and so they seem like secrets.

Download a copy of the "Lupus Secrets" from lupusencyclopedia.com/lupus-secrets .html.

Most physicians and nurses do not have time to go over the items on this list with their patients, even though they are important. I recommend that you go through the list and highlight each item that you did not know you should do or that you are not doing. Work on including each item in your life and health practices. Working on one change at a time may be the best way to ensure these become lifelong habits. Double-check any of these recommendations with your doctor, as your situation may need to be addressed differently.

A Note for Health Care Providers

Wouldn't you love to have the time at each visit to teach each lupus patient how to manage their disease completely? Usually, that's not possible. The "Lupus Secrets" is a list of do's and don'ts that are based on the best medical evidence as of January 2023. Read through it and share it with all your lupus patients. It can help them lower their lupus disease activity and minimize its complications. You may not agree with some because they are not based on randomized, controlled trials. Just cross those out and ask your patients to do the rest.

I credit Doctors Daniel Wallace and Bevra Hahn for starting me on this journey. They included a short version of patient self-care recommendations in *Dubois' Lupus Erythematosus* when I was a rheumatology fellow in the early 1990s. When I read it, I immediately realized the importance of empowering lupus patients to manage their disease with much more than just taking medications. Their patient self-care recommendations helped me form my initial list of "Lupus Secrets," and I have regularly added to this list as our knowledge has improved. Today, I care for over 200 lupus patients, most of whom are in remission or have low disease activity. My patients' use of "The Lupus Secrets" has been important in achieving this goal.

Download a copy from lupusencyclopedia.com/lupus-secrets.html. There you will also find free downloadable handouts on topics such as fatigue management, sleep hygiene, UV light protection, memory improvement, and stress reduction.

I'd like to share some words from a patient who has followed "The Lupus Secrets" for over 20 years. In 2020, she flared after being in remission for many years. Her hydroxychloroquine (HCQ) whole blood level was subtherapeutic, which led to a conversation in which she admitted missing doses. It turned out that her pharmacist had told her to always take HCQ with food, and since she frequently skipped meals, she also skipped doses. After I explained that she does not have to take HCQ with food—doing so just helps those with a sensitive stomach—she resumed her drug regimen and quickly went back into remission. Here is a portion of her thank-you card:

> Dr. Thomas . . . this has really been a wake-up call for me. . . . I want to live a long time. No one in my family lived past the age of 60.

This patient was 73 years old when she wrote this. She has lived longer than any of her family members, many of whom had died from SLE. She has SLE, and she lives by the Lupus Secrets.

The Lupus Secrets

• Take an up-to-date medication list (or a bag of all your pill bottles) that includes your drug intolerance list to every doctor's visit. Carry this list with you at all times (table 29.8)

• Avoid sulfonamide ("sulfa") antibiotics (like Bactrim); include them in a drug intolerance list that you carry at all times (chapters 1 and 5).

• Keep a personal record of labs, biopsy results, x-rays, and doctors' notes (especially those that established your SLE diagnosis) (chapter 1).

• When you see specialists, ask them to send your rheumatologist a note and all test results, even if you don't think it is important. Lupus can affect every part of the body.

• Take 81 mg of aspirin a day (if you are not at high risk of bleeding) to decrease your risk for heart attacks, strokes, and blood clots (ask your doctor first) (chapters 11 and 21).

• If you are fatigued, do everything in tables 6.1, 6.2, 6.3, and 6.4.

• Get eight hours of quality sleep per night (tables 6.2, 6.3, 6.4, and chapter 38).

• If you have trouble sleeping, follow the recommendations in tables 6.2, 6.3, and 6.4.

• For lupus pains, do everything in table 7.1.

• See a rheumatologist or other lupus specialist regularly—usually every three months—even if you feel great. Kidney inflammation occurs in around 45% of SLE patients. Urine samples help us identify the problem early when it is easier to treat (chapter 12).

• If you have memory issues, use table 13.4 as a guide.

- Tell your doctor if you feel depressed or down in the dumps, especially if you have thoughts about hurting yourself. Take the questionnaires in tables 13.3 and 13.5. If you score high, show your doctor the results.

- If you have dryness problems, follow the guidelines in tables 14.2–14.8.

- If you have heartburn, use table 15.2 as a guide.

- All SLE patients should have a home blood pressure monitor. Check it before each doctor visit and give the results to your doctor. Many experts recommend a BP goal of < 126/80 when measured at home and < 131/80 when measured by your doctor (ask your doctor, your situation may differ) (chapter 21).

- Maintain normal LDL and total cholesterol levels; ask for a statin if they are high (chapter 21).

- High HDL is not necessarily good in SLE (chapter 21).

  - We cannot measure pro-inflammatory and oxidized HDL in the clinic; that is possible only in research studies.

  - Pro-inflammatory HDL occurs in 45% of SLE patients, increasing heart attacks and strokes.

  - Regular exercise is the best way to decrease bad HDL.

- If you get a fever, call/see your primary care provider or go to an urgent care center ASAP (chapters 22 and 40).

- Get a flu shot every fall. September and October are the best months to do so in the Northern Hemisphere, or March and April in the Southern (chapter 22).

- Get pneumococcal pneumonia vaccines (chapter 22).

- Keep up to date on all vaccines (chapter 22).

- Ask your doctor if you should time immunosuppressants (table 22.1) with your vaccines (table 22.6).

- Keep up-to-date on cancer screening tests (for example, breast, cervical, colon).

- Get the human papillomavirus (HPV) vaccine (Gardasil) series to prevent HPV-associated cancers for anyone 9 years or older, and up to 45 years old if you are not in a permanent, monogamous relationship (chapters 22 and 23).

- Consume adequate calcium (chapter 24).

- If your vitamin D level is less than 40 ng/mL, ask your doctor for a vitamin D supplement; recheck your level every 3 months to ensure it stays around 40 or higher (chapters 35 and 38).

- If you take steroids (such as prednisone), ask if you need a drug to prevent osteoporosis. Get enough calcium from food or additional supplements (chapter 24).

- If you take steroids regularly, wear a medical alert bracelet (chapters 26 and 31).

- If you take steroids, practice everything in table 31.4 to minimize side effects.

• Take your drugs regularly. Learn how to not miss doses (table 29.5).

• Take hydroxychloroquine (HCQ, Plaquenil), chloroquine, or quinacrine unless you cannot tolerate them (chapters 29 and 30).

• Ask your lupus doctor to regularly measure your HCQ whole blood level to ensure it is not too high or too low.

• Prevent eye side effects from HCQ and chloroquine (chapter 30):

  - Get a Visual Field 10-2 plus an SD-OCT yearly.

  - FAF or mfERG can be substituted if the previous two are unavailable.

  - If you are Asian, you also need a VF 24-2 or VF 30-2 (three tests per year).

  - Use an Amsler grid monthly when taking HCQ or chloroquine (figure 30.5).

• Ask your lupus doctor about DHEA (chapter 35 and table 35.4).

• Do not get pregnant until cleared to do so by your lupus doctor (chapters 18 and 41). Follow all the advice in chapter 41.

• If you get pregnant, see your lupus doctor more often and consider seeing a high-risk obstetrician (chapters 18 and 41).

• If you are anti-SSA positive and get pregnant, alert your OB/GYN: you need weekly fetal heart monitoring beginning at 16 weeks of pregnancy (chapters 18 and 41).

• If you run into financial problems, go to lupusencyclopedia.com/patient-resources

• Ensure your work environment is conducive for your SLE. Go to lupusencyclopedia.com/can-you-work-with-lupus-lupus-patients-and-the-ada

• If your SLE is severe and you can no longer do your job, go to lupusencyclopedia.com/can-you-work-with-lupus-lupus-patients-and-the-ada

• Continue to educate yourself about lupus; join a lupus educational organization. More information is available at lupusencyclopedia.com/patient-resources

The following are healthy lifestyle practices that may help reduce lupus inflammation.

• Do not smoke. Smoking causes lupus to be more active, keeps HCQ from working, increases strokes and heart attacks (among the most common causes of death in SLE), increases lung cancer (occurs more commonly in SLE), and causes broken bones from osteoporosis (chapters 3, 21, 23, 24, and 38). For help quitting, go to smokefree.gov or call 1-800-QUIT-NOW.

• Ask your doctor if you can drink alcohol (especially red wine) in small amounts (chapter 38).

• Exercise regularly (chapters 7, 21, and table 38.8).

• Maintain normal weight (chapters 21 and 38).

• Use daily sunscreen and avoid UV light (chapter 3 and tables 38.2, 38.3, and 38.4).

• Eat an anti-inflammatory diet (chapter 38 and tables 38.6 and 38.7)

- Avoid foods that may flare lupus (such as alfalfa and mung bean sprouts) (chapter 3)

- Eat omega-3 fatty acid-rich foods such as cold-water fatty fish, walnuts, flaxseed, and chia seed daily.

- Consider foods that may improve your gut microbiome, including prebiotics such as resistant starches (overnight oatmeal, green plantain, lentils, whole grains) and probiotic foods such as like live-culture yogurt.

- Consider turmeric (curcumin) in food or as a supplement, but only under a doctor's direction. Curcumin can interact with blood thinners and other drugs and cause lab abnormalities.

• Maintain good dental health: brush twice daily, floss daily, don't smoke. It improves your mouth microbiome. Have gingivitis and periodontitis treated if they occur, and have your teeth cleaned regularly by your dentist (chapters 3 and 38).

• Learn to reduce stress (table 38.9).

• Spend at least five minutes a day practicing mindfulness (chapter 39).

• Do not take Echinacea (an herbal supplement promoted to treat colds) or any supplement promoted to "boost" the immune system (chapters 3 and 39).

• Every day, tell yourself, *"Today will be a good day; there are many things within my power that I can do to feel better and live a long, healthier life."*

Remember: Knowledge is power!

I wish you all the best in life and health!

Donald Thomas, MD

Page numbers in **bold** refer to pages containing definitions or main sources of terms.

For material available online at lupusencyclopedia.com, entries include the word *online* followed by a letter designation, for example, *online-A*. The letters refer to the following online locations:
A. lupusencyclopedia.com/health-insurance-for-lupus-patients-affordable-health-care
B. lupusencyclopedia.com/can-you-work-with-lupus-lupus-patients-and-the-ada
C. lupusencyclopedia.com/patient-resources

196; causes of, **410**, **412**; cholesterol and, 563; cutaneous lupus and risk of, 144; HCQ and, 563; sudden cardiac death and, **415**; symptoms of, 732

heart failure with preserved ejection fraction (HFpEF), 216

heart rate: aerobic exercise and, 136–37; arrhythmias and, **413–14**; bradycardia and, 230; POTS and, 231; SLE and fast heart rate (tachycardia), 229

heart valve infections, **453**

heat therapy (thermotherapy), **140**

Helicobacter pylori, 533

HELLP syndrome, 359–60

hematocrit (HCT), **67**

hematuria, 60, 539

hemoglobin (HGB), 57, 58, **67**, 203

hemoglobin A1c, **70**, 417

hemolysate folate, **70**

hemolytic anemia, 66, 649

hemophagocytic lymphohistiocytosis (HLH), **181–82**

hemoptysis, 213

Henoch-Schönlein purpura, 31

HEp-2 cells, 75

heparin, 198, 214, 363, 742, 752

hepatic vasculitis, 332

hepatitis, 332–33

hepatitis A and B vaccines, **447**

hepatitis B, **456**

hepatitis C, **456**

hepatomegaly, **331**

hepatosplenomegaly, **331**

herpes simplex virus (HSV), 43, 158, **442**

herpes zoster (shingles), **173**, 396, **441–42**, **448–49**, **458**, 731

HFpEF (heart failure with preserved ejection fraction), 216

HGB (hemoglobin), 57, 58, **67**, 203

hiatal hernia, GERD and, 525, 528

high blood pressure. *See* blood pressure

high-density lipoprotein (HDL) cholesterol, 421–22, 429, 778

high-resolution computed tomography (HRCT), 206–7, 217

high-risk obstetricians, 745

hip fractures, osteoporosis and, 468, 481

hip joint, AVN and, 494–95

Hispanic ethnicity, 376, 380–82

histamine type 2 (H2) blockers, 529

histone antibodies, 9, **85**

HIV (human immunodeficiency virus), 6, 433, **442–43**

hives (urticaria), **162**, 446

Holter monitor, 414

homeopathy, 715

honeycombing, on CT scans, 212

Horner's syndrome, ptosis and, **344**

HPV (human papillomavirus), 43, **446**, 462–63, 778

HRCT (high-resolution computed tomography), 206–7, 217

HSV (herpes simplex virus), 43, 158, **442**

human immunodeficiency virus (HIV), 6, 433, **442–43**

human papillomavirus (HPV), 43, **446**, 462–63, 778

human T-cell lymphotropic virus, 43

Humira (adalimumab), 9, 10, 129, 449, 464, **625–29**, 742, 752

hyaline casts, 61

hydralazine, 10, 48

hydrazine, 48

hydrocortisone, 505

hydrotherapy, for FM, 514

hydroxychloroquine (HCQ, Plaquenil), 117–18, 198, 200, 206, 224, 278, **560–75**; adherence to, 548; Afib and, 573; alcohol and, 572; antigen processing and, 560; AVN risk reduced with, 495; benefits of, 541, **560–63**; blood clot risk decreased with, 562–63; blood levels, **85**; breastfeeding and, 573, 752; bull's eye maculopathy and, 564; cancer and, 465; COVID-19 pandemic and, 413; cutaneous lupus treatment with, 154; for CVD, 425–26; desensitization and, 575; dosing, **565–67**, 571–72; elderly people and, 573; eye exams and, 466, **567–70**, 779; functioning of, 570; heart attacks and, 563; with immunosuppressants, 562; life expectancies with SLE and, 563; lupus nephritis treatment with, 253; maculopathy and, 342; measuring levels of, 542; myasthenia gravis and, 294; for neonatal lupus prevention, 365; pregnancy and, 360, 573, 741, 742; QT-interval prolongation and, 572; race and, 382; rashes and, 172–73, 575; safety of, 431; side effects of, 573, 574, 730; skin discoloration form, 731–32; strength of, 562; surgery and, 573; timing and effectiveness of, 541; for UCTD, 27, 561; vaccines and, 573; warnings with, 570–71